Backyard Chicken Care for Veterinary Technicians and Nurses

Dedicated to the memory of the feathered lives entrusted to our care, whose lessons continue to shape how we learn, teach, and practice as credentialed veterinary technicians.

Backyard Chicken Care for Veterinary Technicians and Nurses

Sarah Meyer, CVT, FVTE
Assistant Professor, Fellow of Veterinary Technician Educators
Pensacola State College
Pensacola, FL, USA

Stephanie Freeman, CVT
Companion Animal Clinic
Cantonment, FL, USA

WILEY

Published by John Wiley & Sons, Inc., Hoboken, New Jersey.

Library of Congress Cataloging-in-Publication Data applied for:

Paperback ISBN: 9781394349449

Cover Design: Wiley
Cover Images: Stephanie Freeman, CVT, Sarah Meyer, CVT, FVTE

Set in 9.5/12.5pt STIXTwoText by Straive, Pondicherry, India

Printed and bound by CPI Group (UK) Ltd, Croydon, CR0 4YY

C97813943449_280726

Contents

Acknowledgment

This text is the result of colleagues and fellow guardians who believe that the advancement of backyard chicken care is grounded in excellent veterinary care, lifelong learning, and the goal of improving each chicken's quality of life. We are grateful to Darcy Dickinson Smith (Funky Chicken Rescue), Unusual Pet Vets, and Cindy Justice Liles (Baking and Eggs), for the contribution of invaluable images to enhance reader engagement. A generous thanks goes to all those who encouraged us in this venture and continue to support our enamoration with chickens.

1

Acquiring Chickens and Common Breeds

When contemplating the addition of chickens to one's "homesteading" lifestyle, the consideration of the expense and responsibility of caring for them must occur. As with all animal guardianship, animals are not a necessity but rather a "luxury" for those with disposable income. There is no doubt about the intrinsic value and joy that animals bring to our lives, but their proper care requires an honest reflection of a guardian's financial budget and available time. The cost of everyday preventive care, veterinary care for ill birds, nutritional needs, equipment (upkeep and replacement), appropriate predator-proof housing, cleaning supplies, enrichment, and upgrades to living arrangements must be included in a guardian's planning. All too often, people forget that animal guardianship is a privilege, not a right. Chickens are living, intelligent, and sentient beings deserving the Five Rights of Animal Welfare and respect from their caregivers.

Five rights (or freedoms) of animal welfare
Right to live in a clean environment
Freedom from pain, injury, and disease
Right to express normal behavior
Freedom from hunger and thirst
Right to live without fear and distress

Table by Sarah Meyer.

Once the downy cuteness of a chick wears off, the fact that a chicken's life span can reach or exceed 10 years can be an unwelcome reality to new chicken caregivers. The animal's daily physical and psychological needs lose priority and novelty, and chickens are neglected. Many towns have ordinances in place prohibiting roosters, and caregivers are faced with finding a suitable home. Oftentimes, cruel ignorance leads to dumping roosters in the countryside or public parks to fend for themselves. There are fates worse than death, and roosters are severely misunderstood and mistreated for exhibiting normal behaviors.

The intention of bringing chickens into a family, regardless of sex, should be thoroughly researched, and contingencies for future adverse events must be considered. Being a responsible chicken guardian requires dedicated mindfulness, rationality, and forethought. The purpose of this text is multifaceted—provide a credible resource for veterinary staff in clinical practice and empower caregivers with information to provide excellent care to their feathered family members.

1.1 "What Breed Is Best?"

The first step in selecting the right breed is figuring out the reason chickens are desired. Eggs? Meat? Enjoyment? Many breeds have dual purposes, meaning they are used for meat and egg production. In this chapter, each bird's original intended use is listed: egg production, meat production, dual purpose, or ornamental. Commonly, the ornamental breeds are "just for fun," competition, and companionship. The selection of specific breeds should consider that intentional trait-focused breeding can increase susceptibility to breed-associated hereditary disorders. Prolific egg-laying breeds are predisposed to reproductive malignancies early in life, and their nursing care should be considered. Meat-breed birds can develop orthopedic and cardiovascular disorders due to obesity.

Novice chicken guardians discover a breed's nuances and develop preferences of certain breeds over time. Experienced guardians keep their favorite breeds depending on personal preferences and the use of the birds. Many backyard flocks comprise mixed-breed chickens with hybrid vigor, and these birds tend to have longer lifespans.

1.2 Step Two: Size Matters

The second step is determining what breed fits the planned living space. Of course, the larger the bird and the number of birds, the more space is necessary to prevent overcrowding, which can result in psychological and physical ailments. Some breeds are not compatible with confinement, certain types of housing, and space available. Chapter 3, Husbandry, Housing, and Biosecurity, details spacing recommendations.

Chickens vary from bantam-sized to extra-large, heavy-bodied breeds. The bantam breed is very small, so they will not be ideal for meat birds or egg production. In general, bantams are the miniature version of a standard chicken breed; they are not an actual breed of chicken. The eggs laid will not be regular-sized eggs, but rather extra small and proportional to their body size. Medium-sized chickens will comprise most of the egg layers and a larger carcass is desirable for consumption. It is recommended that at least 4 sq. ft. per medium chicken be provided. Large-breed chickens are typically dual-purpose. Most large-bodied chickens are heritage breeds, as they were originally bred within small communities for both eggs and meat. It is recommended to provide at least 6 sq. ft. per large bird. Extra-large birds can be some of the friendliest chickens; however, ample space must be provided for these big friends. They require at least 8 sq. ft. per extra-large bird.

1.3 Step Three: Location, Location, Location

The third consideration in selecting the right breed is the geographical location. Some chickens do not thrive in colder climates; some will suffer in hotter or humid climates. Depending on their origin, a purebred chicken was adapted not only for purpose or use but also for different climates. Cold-hardy breeds will be the plumper breeds with smaller combs. Heat-hardy breeds will be the leaner-bodied breeds with larger combs for effective heat convection. All-season breeds can flourish in multiple climates. Hatcheries often provide this key information in their catalogs for keepers to consider when selecting breeds for their location.

1.4 More Than a Pretty Face

All too often, a breed is selected based on its physical characteristics, not its hardiness, which is unfortunate for the bird(s). When planning for chickens, keep in mind that chickens are a social species and prefer same-species companionship. Regardless of breed, chickens will be more psychologically stable with at least one fellow avian companion per enclosure.

1.5 Special Consideration When Ordering Chicks

While vaccines for chickens are not readily available outside of commercial hatcheries and production farms, vaccination is an option when purchasing chicks. Reputable hatcheries will vaccinate chicks at the time of purchase or when ordered (catalogs of breeds). Later in this book, preventable diseases are discussed; these diseases are either preventable through strict biosecurity measures or by vaccination. Commercial hatcheries are typically certified through an NPIP (National Poultry Improvement Plan), which was established to diminish Pullorum Disease (*Salmonella pullorum*) and now provides testing and monitoring of other poultry diseases. Small- and large-scale breeders and hatcheries can voluntarily earn NPIP certification, certifying that the facility is "clean." Purchase of NPIP-certified eggs (or chicks) or vaccinated chicks does not guarantee the health of the birds, but it is a responsible choice made by the new or experienced caregiver to "prevent the preventable."

The chicken breed list in this chapter is not exhaustive; rather, it includes commonly seen birds in clinical practice with a few author favorites. There is a plethora of sources for more extensive lists, including the American Poultry Association, state poultry associations, and state extension services. Each breed includes its origin, use, average body weight, egg production, primary feather color(s), egg color, temperament, life span, comb type, and breed-specific health concerns.

Ameraucana

Figure 1.1.

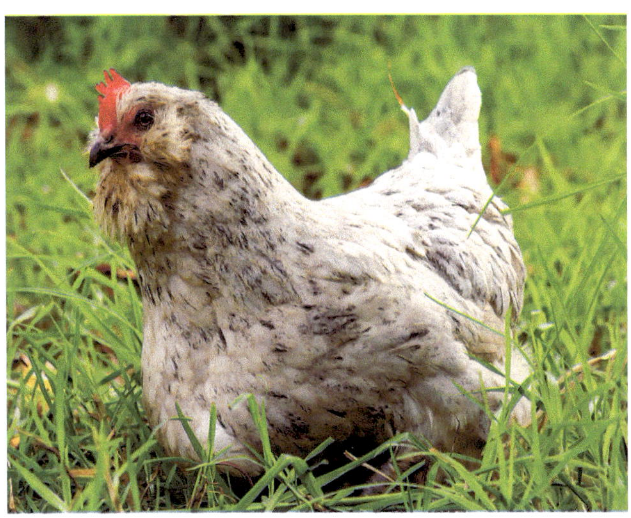

Figure 1.1 Ameraucana Hen. Megan Marie Weaver / Adobe Stock Photos.

Origin: United States
Use: Dual Purpose
Weight: Male–7 pounds, Female–4 pounds
Egg Production: Average of 250 eggs yearly
Color: Variety of colors
Egg Color: Blue
Temperament: Docile and sweet
Life Span: 7–8 years
Comb Type: Pea
Breed-Specific Health Concerns: Susceptible to cross beak

Andalusian
Figure 1.2.

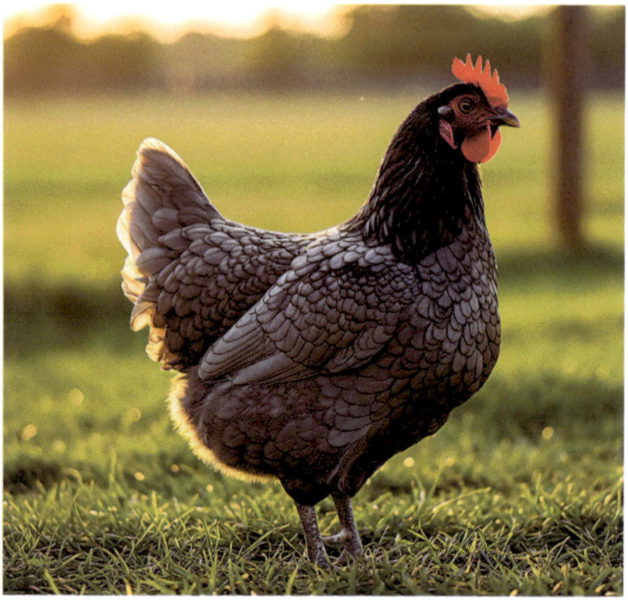

Figure 1.2 Andalusian Hen. Animal Lover / Adobe Stock Photos.

Origin: Province of Andalusia, Spain
Use: Egg Production
Weight: Male–7 pounds, Female–5.5 pounds
Egg Production: Around 150 eggs yearly
Color: Blue
Egg Color: White
Temperament: Friendly, curious, and flighty
Life Span: 5–8 years
Comb Type: Single
Breed-Specific Health Concerns: Prone to frostbite, feather eating, and faded plumage

Araucana
Figure 1.3.

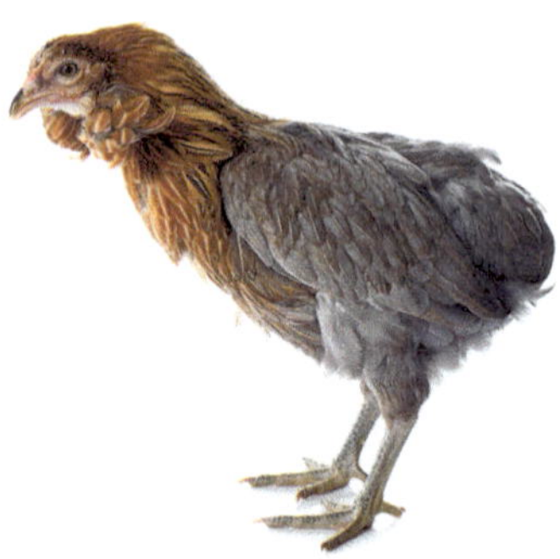

Figure 1.3 Araucana Hen. cynoclub / Adobe Stock Photos.

Origin: Chile
Use: Egg Production
Weight: Male–6.6 pounds, Female–5.5 pounds
Egg Production: Around 250 eggs yearly
Color: Variety
Egg Color: Blue
Temperament: Friendly and intelligent
Life Span: 7–10 years
Comb Type: Pea
Breed-Specific Health Concerns: Can be prone to ear infections if ear tufts are not kept clean, developmental abnormalities of the auditory canals, copulation issues, and defecation issues due to lack of a tail.

Austra White
Figure 1.4.

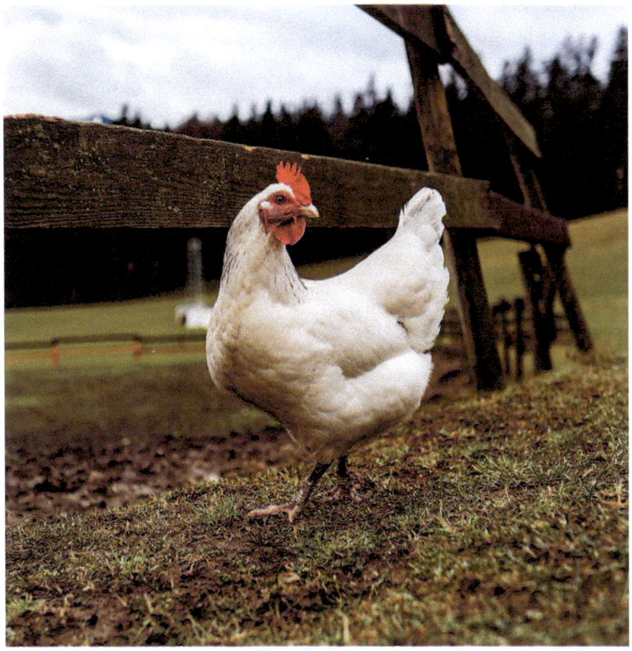

Figure 1.4 Austra White Hen. Funk Design / Adobe Stock Photos.

Origin: Oregon
Use: Dual Purpose
Weight: Male – 6.5 pounds, Female – 5 pounds
Egg Production: Around 220–280 eggs yearly
Color: White
Egg Color: Off-white and cream
Temperament: Active, quiet, and inquisitive
Life Span: 6–10 years
Comb Type: Single
Breed-Specific Health Concerns: Prone to frostbite

Australorp
Figure 1.5.

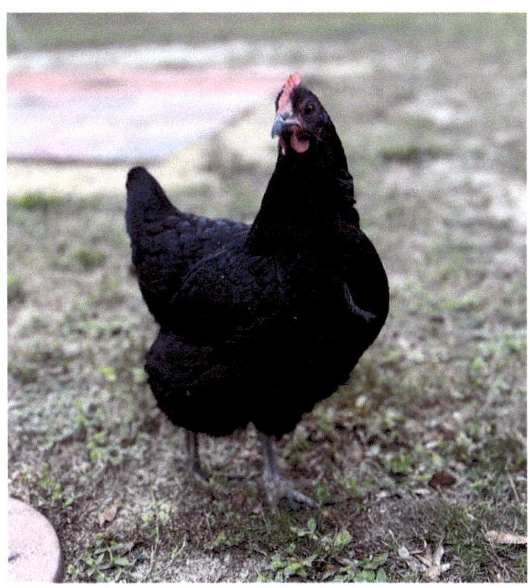

Figure 1.5 Australorp Hen. Stephanie Freeman.

Origin: Australia
Use: Dual Purpose
Weight: Male – 9 pounds, Female – 6.5 pounds
Egg Production: Around 250–300 eggs yearly
Color: Black
Egg Color: Brown
Temperament: Active and yet gentle
Life Span: 5–8 years
Comb Type: Single
Breed-Specific Health Concerns: None

Ayam Cemani
Figure 1.6.

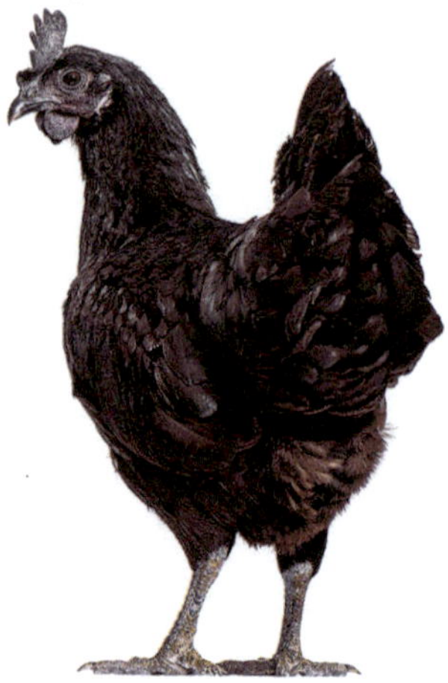

Figure 1.6 Ayam Cemani Hen. Eric Isselée / Adobe Stock Photos.

Origin: Indonesia
Use: Ornamental
Weight: Male–9.5–15 pounds, Female–7.5–9 pounds
Color: Black
Egg Production: 60–100 eggs yearly
Egg Color: Cream with a pinkish tinge
Temperament: Intelligent and friendly
Life Span: 6–8 years
Comb Type: Single
Breed-Specific Health Concerns: None

Barnevelder
Figure 1.7.

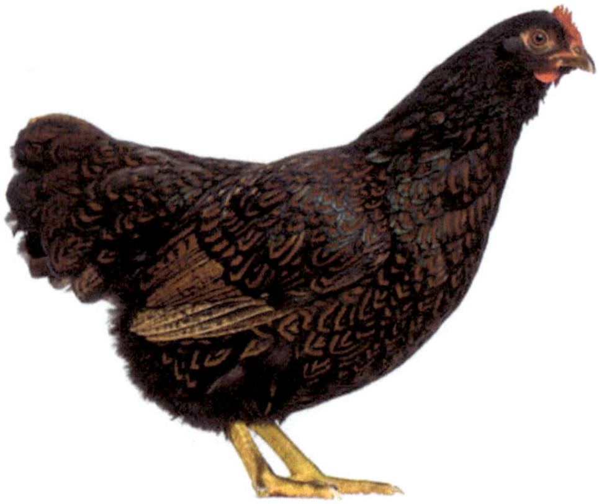

Figure 1.7 Barnevelder Hen. Eric Isselée / Adobe Stock Photos.

Origin: Netherlands
Use: Dual Purpose
Weight: Male–6–7 pounds, Female–5.5–6 pounds
Egg Production: Around 180–200 eggs yearly
Color: Black with red mottling
Egg Color: Dark brown
Temperament: Quiet, active, and docile
Life Span: 6–12 years
Comb Type: Single
Breed-Specific Health Concerns: None

Barred Rock

Figure 1.8.

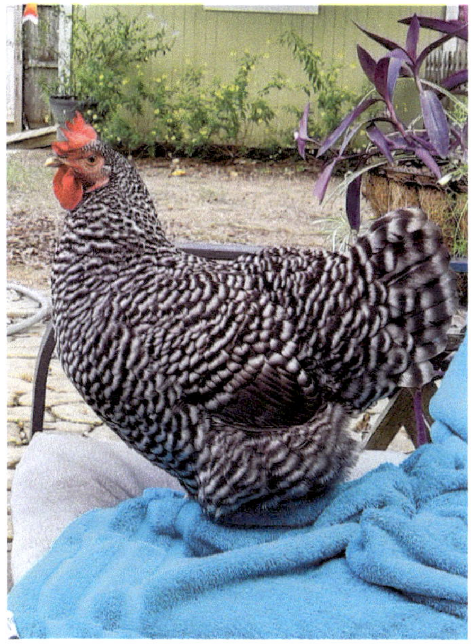

Figure 1.8 Barred Rock Hen. Sarah Meyer.

Origin: United States, Massachusetts
Use: Dual Purpose
Weight: Male–9–10 pounds, Female–7–7.5 pounds
Egg Production: Around 200 eggs yearly
Color: Dark gray and white striping
Egg Color: Light tan
Temperament: Inquisitive, friendly, and docile
Life Span: 6–12 years
Comb Type: Single
Breed-Specific Health Concerns: None

Black Copper Marans

Figure 1.9.

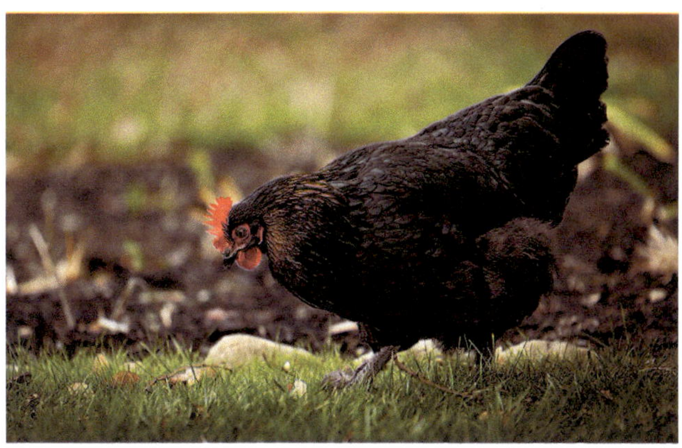

Figure 1.9 Black Copper Maran Hen. AGrandemange / Adobe Stock Photos.

Origin: France
Use: Dual Purpose
Weight: Male–8.5 pounds, Female–7 pounds
Egg Production: Around 200 eggs yearly
Color: Black with copper neck feathers
Egg Color: Dark brown
Temperament: Friendly and calm
Life Span: 8 years
Comb Type: Single
Breed-Specific Health Concerns: None

Brahma

Figure 1.10.

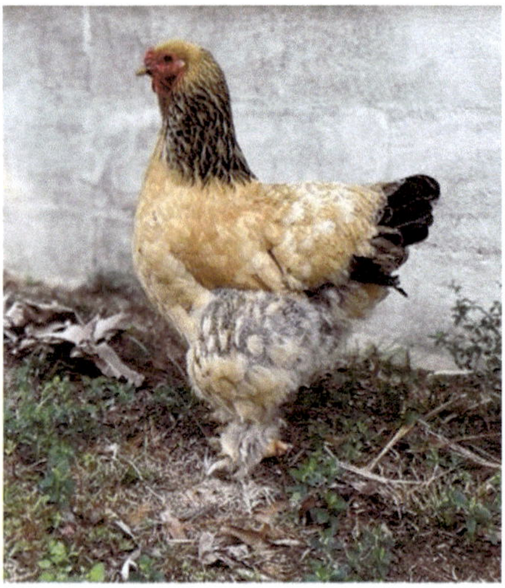

Figure 1.10 Brahma Hen. Stephanie Freeman.

Origin: United States
Use: Dual Purpose
Weight: Male–12 pounds, Female–9.5 pounds
Egg Production: Around 150–200 eggs yearly
Color: Light, dark, and buff
Egg Color: Brown
Temperament: Friendly and approachable
Life Span: 5–8 years
Comb Type: Pea
Breed-Specific Health Concerns: Prone to frostbite on toes from wet feathers

Bresse

Figure 1.11.

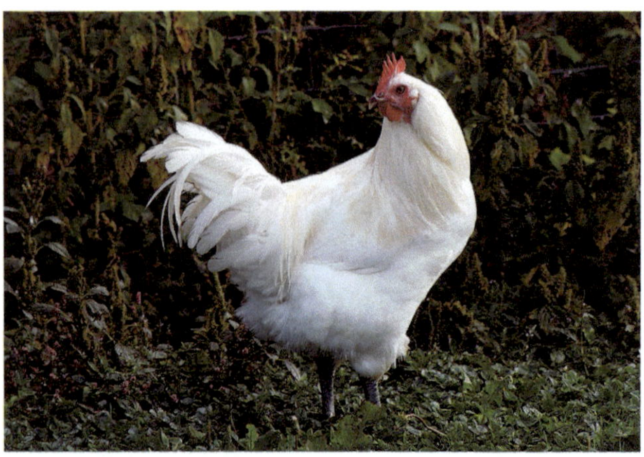

Figure 1.11 Bresse Rooster. Maurice Metzger / Adobe Stock Photos.

Origin: Bresse Province of France
Use: Dual Purpose
Weight: Male–6.5 pounds, Female–5.5 pounds
Egg Production: Around 250 eggs yearly
Color: White
Egg Color: White
Temperament: Skittish
Life Span: 6–7 years
Comb Type: Single
Breed-Specific Health Concerns: Disease resistant

Buckeye

Figure 1.12.

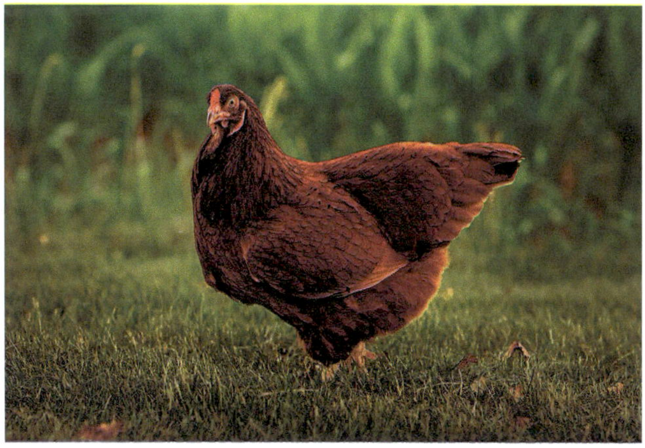

Figure 1.12 Buckeye Hen. Cavan / Adobe Stock Photos.

Origin: United States, Ohio
Use: Dual Purpose
Weight: Male–9 pounds, Female–6.5 pounds
Egg Production: Around 200 eggs yearly
Color: Dark red-brown
Egg Color: Brown
Temperament: Calm and Gentle
Life Span: 10+ years
Comb Type: Pea
Breed-Specific Health Concerns: None

Cinnamon Queen

Figure 1.13.

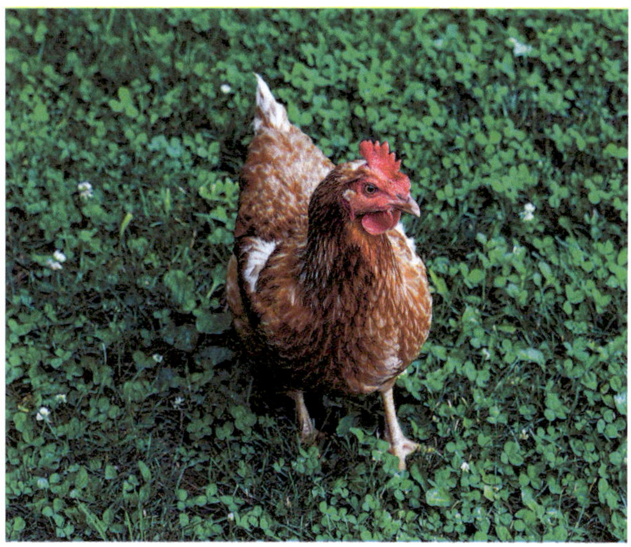

Figure 1.13 Cinnamon Queen Hen. Kathy / Adobe Stock Photos.

Origin: United States
Use: Dual Purpose
Weight: Male–8 pounds, Female–6 pounds
Egg Production: Around 300 eggs yearly
Color: Red with white splashes
Egg Color: Brown
Temperament: Friendly and curious
Life Span: 3–7 years
Comb Type: Single
Breed-Specific Health Concerns: Reproductive cancer, egg binding, and egg yolk peritonitis

Cochin
Figure 1.14.

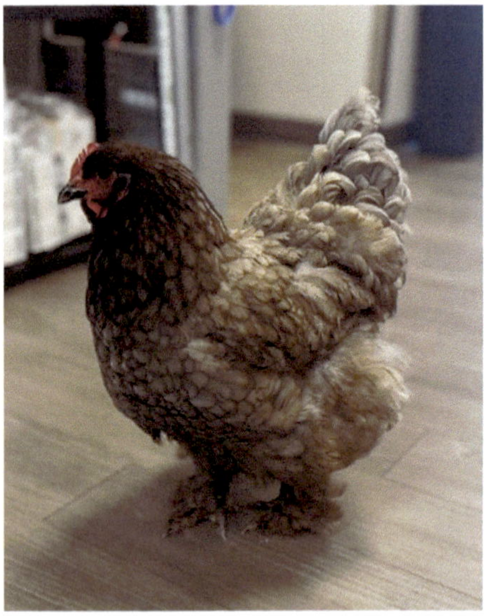

Figure 1.14 Cochin Hen. Stephanie Freeman.

Origin: China
Use: Ornamental
Weight: Male–12 pounds, Female–7–9 pounds
Egg Production: Around 150–180 eggs yearly
Color: Variety
Egg Color: Brown
Temperament: Friendly and gentle
Life Span: 8–10 years
Comb Type: Single
Breed-Specific Health Concerns: Prone to obesity

Cornish Cross
Figure 1.15.

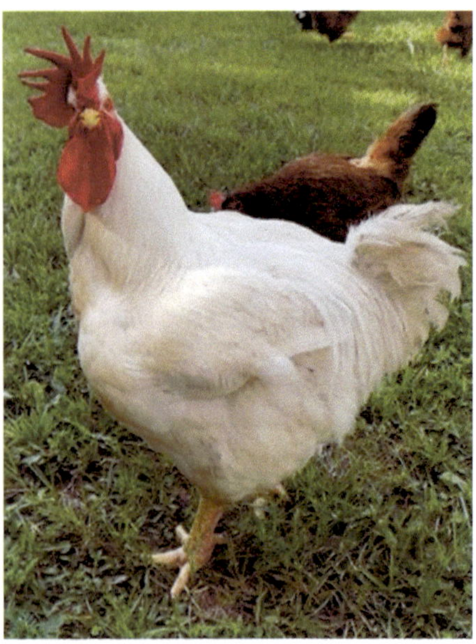

Figure 1.15 Cornish Cross Rooster. Stephanie Freeman.

Origin: United States
Use: Meat Production
Weight: Male–10 pounds, Female–6 pounds
Egg Production: N/A
Color: Variety
Egg Color: White
Temperament: Docile
Life Span: 10 weeks
Comb Type: Single
Breed-Specific Health Concerns: Congestive heart failure, joint issues, and obesity

Cream Legbar

Figure 1.16.

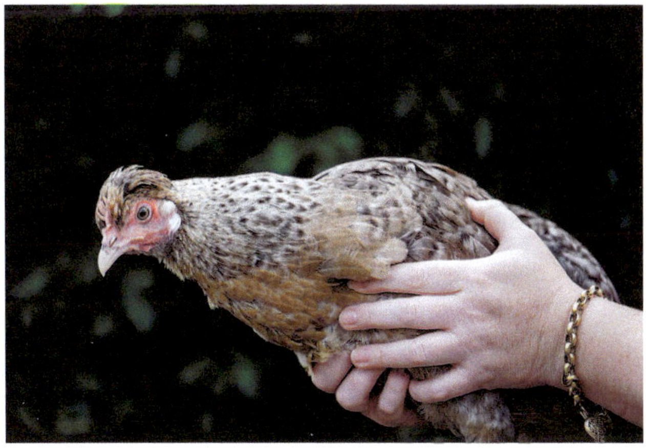

Figure 1.16 Cream Legbar Hen. Tabatha / Adobe Stock Photos.

Origin: United Kingdom
Use: Egg Production
Weight: Male–7.5 pounds, Female–5.5 pounds
Egg Production: Around 180 eggs yearly
Egg Color: Blue
Temperament: Easy-going and peaceful
Life Span: 5–10 years
Comb Type: Single
Breed-Specific Health Concerns: Prone to Marek's Disease and frostbite

Delaware

Figure 1.17.

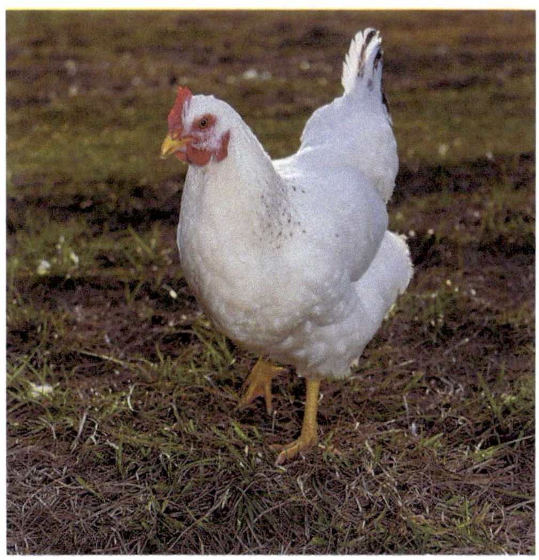

Figure 1.17 Delaware Hen. Guy Sagi / Adobe Stock Photos.

Origin: United States
Use: Dual Purpose
Weight: Male–8.5 pounds, Female–6.5 pounds
Egg Production: Around 100–150 eggs yearly
Color: White
Egg Color: Dark Brown
Temperament: Gentle
Life Span: 5–7 years
Comb Type: Single
Breed-Specific Health Concerns: None

Dominique
Figure 1.18.

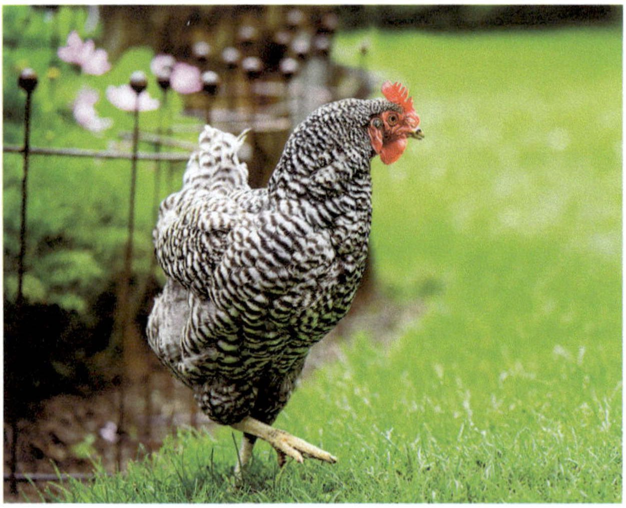

Figure 1.18 Dominique Hen. SHS Photography / Adobe Stock Photos.

Origin: New England
Use: Dual Purpose
Weight: Male–7 pounds, Female–5 pounds
Egg Production: Around 230 eggs yearly
Color: Gray and white striping
Egg Color: Brown
Temperament: Calm and hardy
Life Span: 6–8 years
Comb Type: Rose
Breed-Specific Health Concerns: None

Dorking
Figure 1.19.

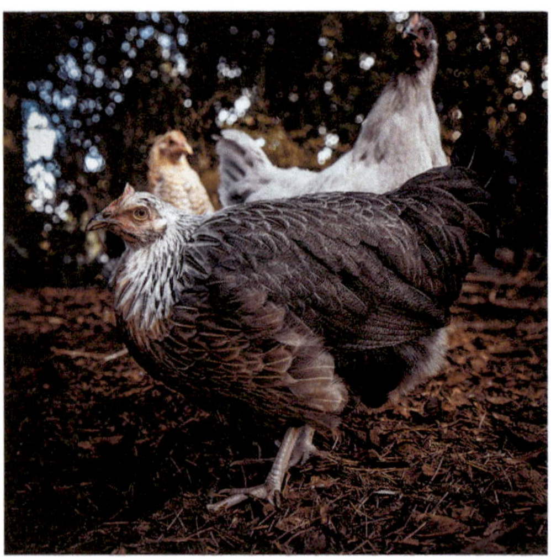

Figure 1.19 Dorking Hen. Adeline / Adobe Stock Photos.

Origin: United Kingdom
Use: Dual Purpose
Weight: Male–9 pounds, Female–7 pounds
Egg Production: Around 170–190 eggs yearly
Color: Variety
Egg Color: White or Cream
Temperament: Friendly
Life Span: 7 years
Comb Type: Single or Rose
Breed-Specific Health Concerns: Prone to obesity and more susceptible to respiratory infections

Belgian Bearded D'Uccle

Figure 1.20.

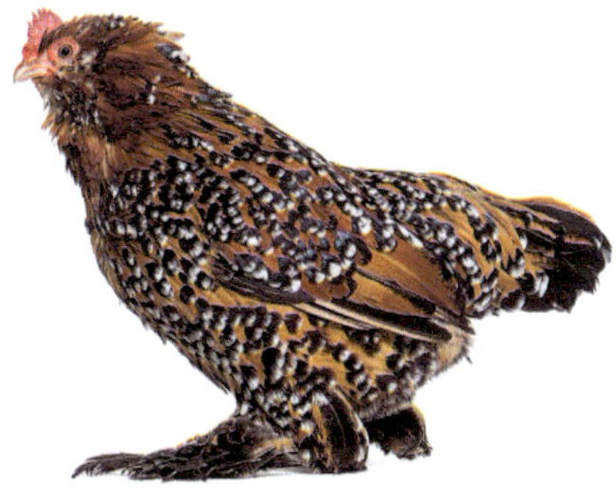

Figure 1.20 Belgian Bearded D'Uccle Hen. Eric Isselée / Adobe Stock Photos.

Origin: Belgium
Use: Ornamental
Weight: Male–26 ounces, Female–22 ounces
Egg Production: Around 100–150 eggs yearly
Egg Color: Cream
Temperament: Docile and friendly
Life Span: 7–8 years
Comb Type: Single
Breed-Specific Health Concerns: None

Easter Egger

Figure 1.21.

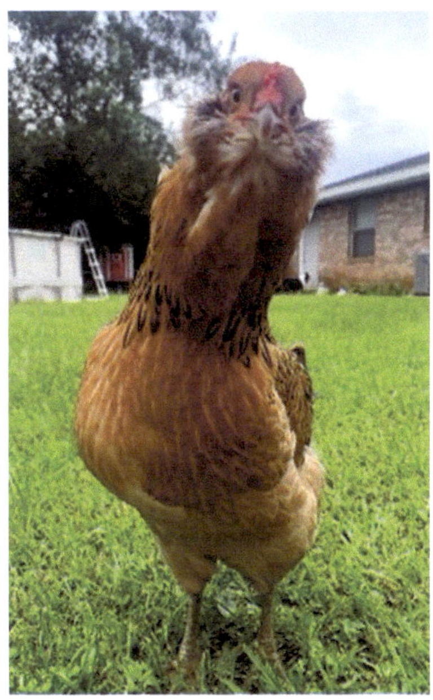

Figure 1.21 Easter Egger Hen. Stephanie Freeman.

Origin: Chile
Use: Dual Purpose
Weight: Male–5 pounds, Female–4 pounds
Egg Production: Around 260 eggs yearly
Color: Variety
Egg Color: Green, Blue, or Light Pink
Temperament: Friendly and docile
Life Span: 5–8 years
Comb Type: Pea
Breed-Specific Health Concerns: Prone to cross beak

Egyptian Fayoumi
Figure 1.22.

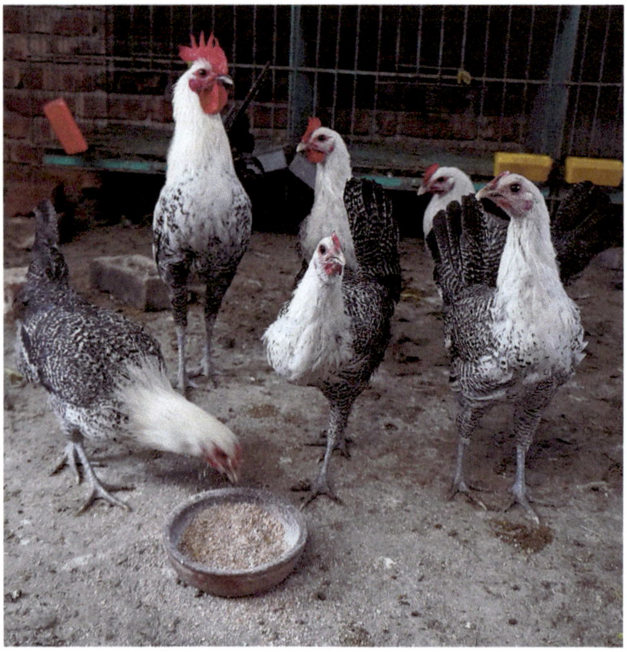

Figure 1.22 Egyptian Fayoumi Rooster with Hens. Almas / Adobe Stock Photos.

Origin: Egypt
Use: Ornamental
Weight: Male–4.5 pounds, Female–3.5 pounds
Egg Production: Around 150–200 eggs yearly
Color: Cream and gray mottled
Egg Color: Cream
Temperament: Independent, flighty
Life Span: 5–8 years
Comb Type: Single
Breed-Specific Health Concerns: None

Faverolles
Figure 1.23.

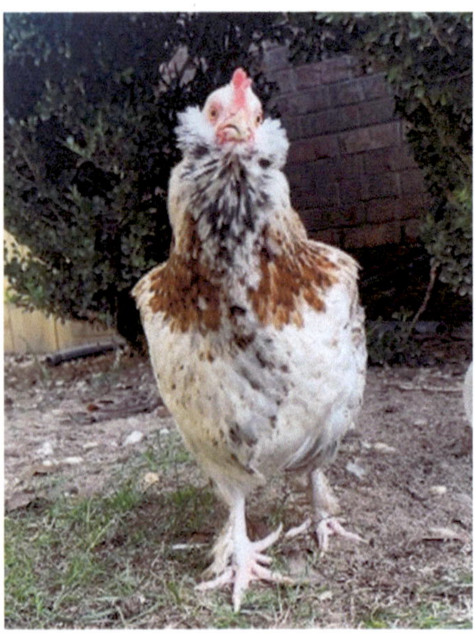

Figure 1.23 Salmon Faverolles. Stephanie Freeman.

Origin: France
Use: Dual Purpose
Weight: Male–8 pounds, Female–6.5 pounds
Egg Production: Around 150–200 eggs yearly
Color: Salmon or white
Egg Color: Cream
Temperament: Docile and gentle
Life Span: 5 years
Comb Type: Single
Breed-Specific Health Concerns: Prone to frostbite and external parasites

Indio Gigante

Figure 1.24.

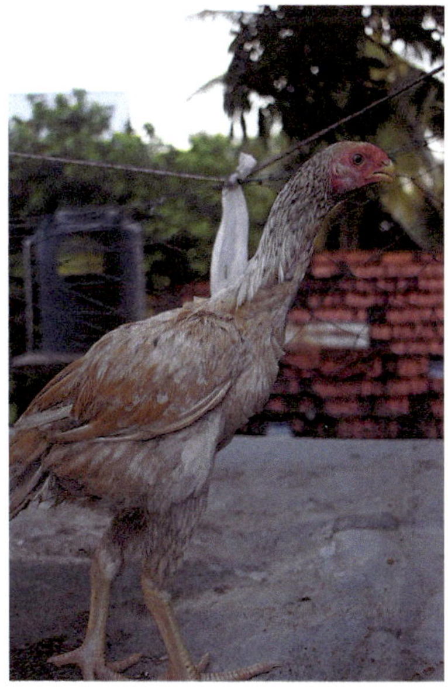

Figure 1.24 Indio Gigante Hen. Infinity Focus / Adobe Stock Photos.

Origin: Brazil
Use: Dual Purpose
Weight: Male–10–12 pounds, Female–8–10 pounds
Egg Production: Around 200 eggs yearly
Color: Variety
Egg Color: Tinted
Temperament: Calm and inquisitive
Life Span: 5–7 years
Comb Type: Single and small
Breed-Specific Health Concerns: Cold intolerant

Java

Figure 1.25.

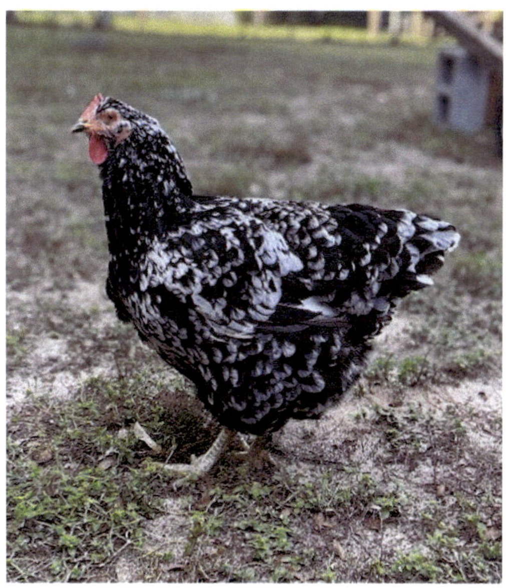

Figure 1.25 Mottled Java Hen. Stephanie Freeman.

Origin: United States
Use: Dual Purpose
Weight: Male–9.5 pounds, Female–7.5 pounds
Egg Production: Around 150–180 eggs yearly
Color: Mottled black, brown, and white
Egg Color: Brown
Temperament: Friendly and calm
Life Span: 5–8 years
Comb Type: Single
Breed-Specific Health Concerns: None

Jersey Giant
Figure 1.26.

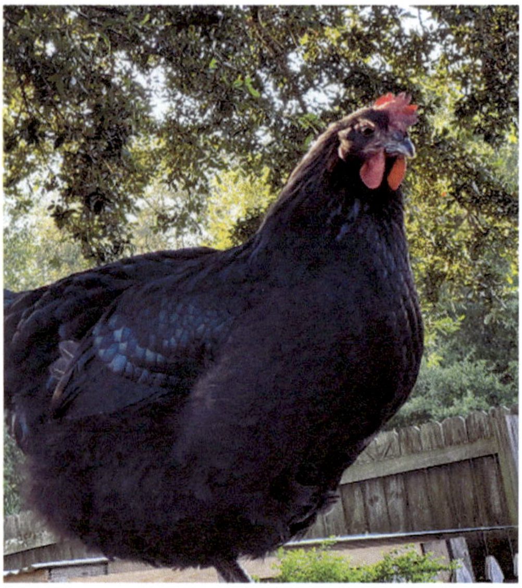

Figure 1.26 Jersey Giant Hen. Sarah Meyer.

Origin: United States
Use: Dual Purpose
Weight: Male – 13 pounds, Female – 10 pounds
Egg Production: Around 150–200 eggs yearly
Color: Black and white
Egg Color: Brown
Temperament: Calm and docile
Life Span: 8+ years
Comb Type: Single
Breed-Specific Health Concerns: More susceptible to heat stroke

Langshan
Figure 1.27.

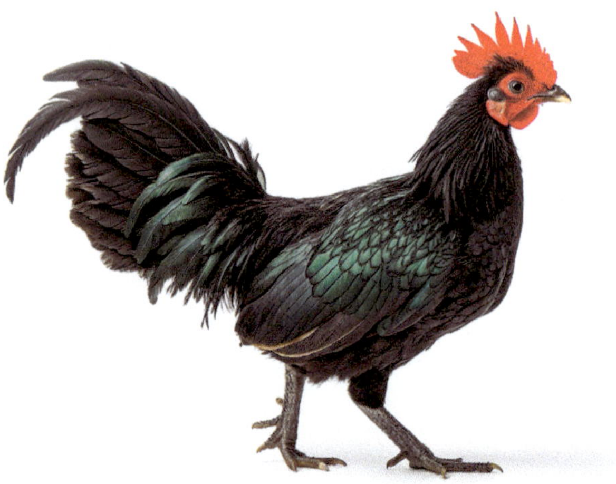

Figure 1.27 Langshan Rooster. Idea Lab / Adobe Stock Photos.

Origin: China
Use: Dual Purpose
Weight: Male – 9.5 pounds, Female – 7.5 pounds
Egg Production: Around 150 eggs yearly
Color: Black
Egg Color: Brown
Temperament: Docile and friendly
Life Span: 5–8 years
Comb Type: Single
Breed-Specific Health Concerns: None

Leghorn
Figure 1.28.

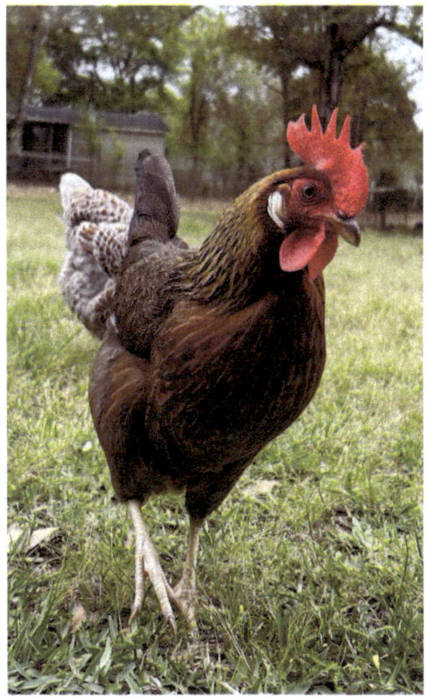

Figure 1.28 Leghorn Hen. Stephanie Freeman.

Origin: Italy
Use: Egg Production
Weight: Male–6 pounds, Female–4.5 pounds
Egg Production: Around 280–300 eggs yearly
Color: Variety, commonly solid white or brown
Egg Color: White
Life Span: 4–6 years
Comb Type: Single
Breed-Specific Health Concerns: Prone to frostbite

Minorca
Figure 1.29.

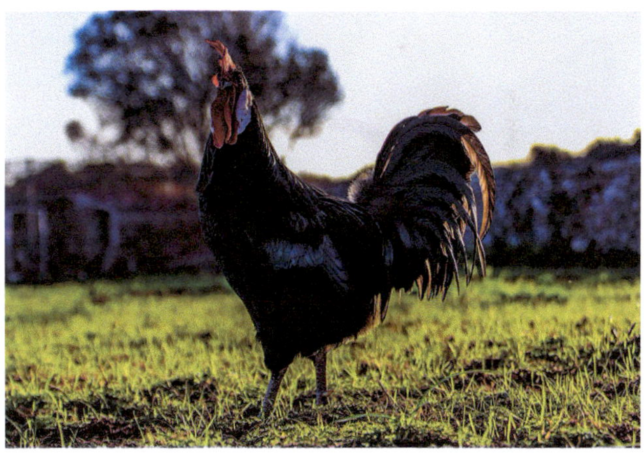

Figure 1.29 Minorca Rooster. Dani Olives / Wirestock / Adobe Stock Photos.

Origin: Spain
Use: Dual Purpose
Weight: Male–9 pounds, Female–7.5 pounds
Egg Production: Around 120 eggs yearly
Color: Black with white face; white
Egg Color: White
Temperament: Flighty
Life Span: 8–10 years
Comb Type: Single or Rose
Breed-Specific Health Concerns: Prone to frostbite

New Hampshire
Figure 1.30.

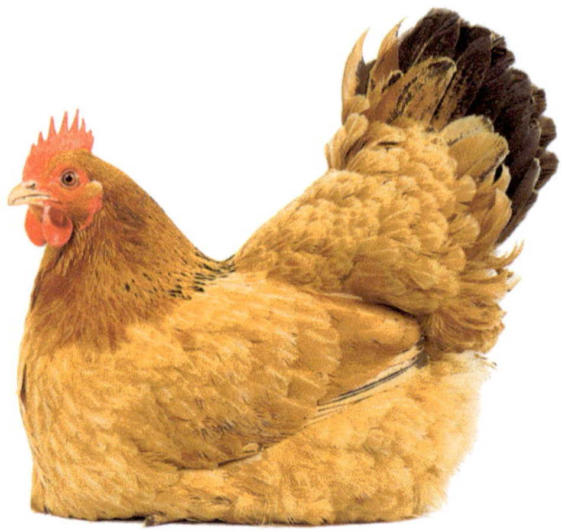

Figure 1.30 New Hampshire Hen. Leoniek / Adobe Stock Photos.

Origin: United States
Use: Dual Purpose
Weight: Male–8.5 pounds, Female–6.5 pounds
Egg Production: Around 220 eggs yearly
Color: Buff with black tail feathers
Egg Color: Brown
Temperament: Vary between docile and unfriendly
Life Span: 7–8 years
Comb Type: Single
Breed-Specific Health Concerns: Prone to frostbite

Old English Game
Figure 1.31.

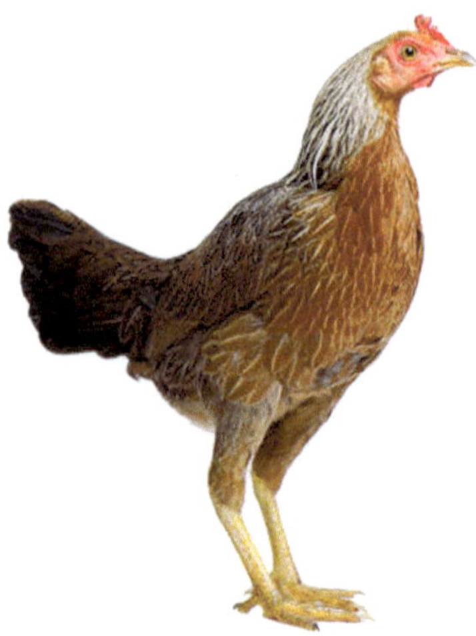

Figure 1.31 Old English Game Hen. ณัฐวุฒิ เงินสันเทียะ / Adobe Stock Photos.

Origin: United Kingdom
Use: Ornamental
Weight: Male–1.5 pounds, Female–1.5 pounds
Egg Production: Around 160–180 eggs yearly
Color: Variety
Egg Color: White
Temperament: Aggressive and noisy
Life Span: 10–15 years
Comb Type: Single
Breed-Specific Health Concerns: None

Olive Egger
Figure 1.32.

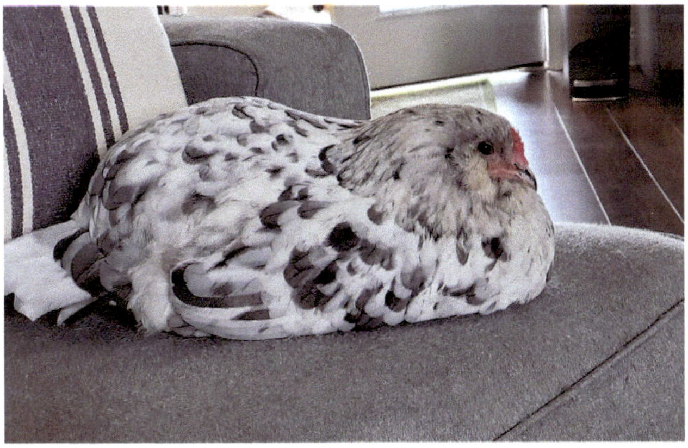

Figure 1.32 Olive Egger Hen. Sarah Meyer.

Origin: United States
Use: Dual Purpose
Weight: Male—7 pounds, Female—5 pounds
Egg Production: Around 260 eggs yearly
Color: Variety
Egg Color: Green
Temperament: Docile and friendly
Life Span: 5–8 years
Comb Type: Pea
Breed-Specific Health Concerns: None

Orpington
Figure 1.33.

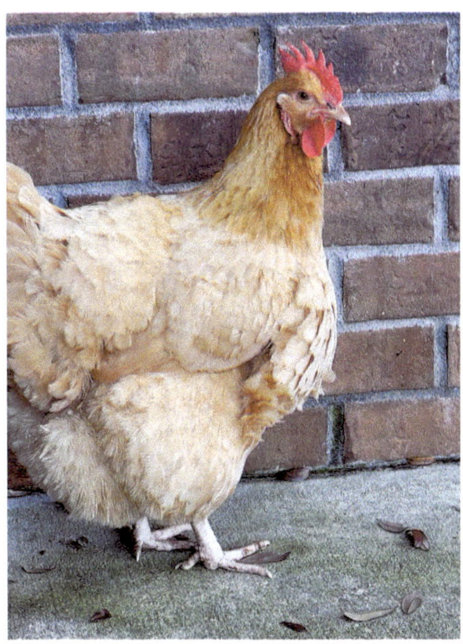

Figure 1.33 Orpington Hen. Sarah Meyer.

Origin: United Kingdom
Use: Dual Purpose
Weight: Male—8–10 pounds, Female—6–8 pounds
Egg Production: Around 170–200 eggs yearly
Color: Black, blue, buff, and white
Egg Color: Brown
Temperament: Docile and friendly
Life Span: 8 years
Comb Type: Single
Breed-Specific Health Concerns: Prone to heat stroke, obesity, crop disorders

Pekin Bantam
Figure 1.34.

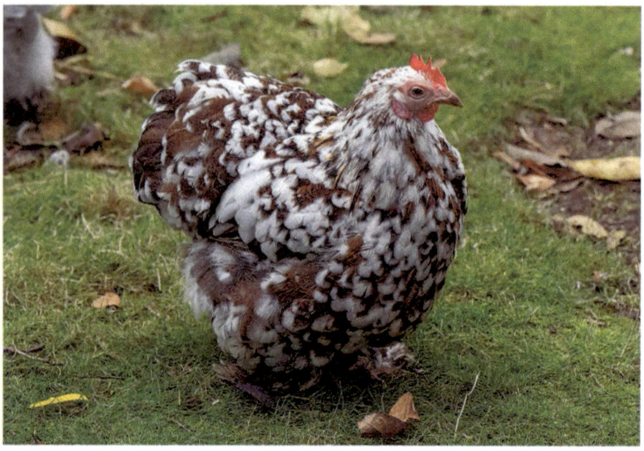

Figure 1.34 Pekin Bantam Hen. Alexandre Prevot / Adobe Stock Photos.

Origin: United Kingdom
Use: Ornamental
Weight: Male–2 pounds, Female–1.7 pounds
Egg Production: Around 120–140 eggs yearly
Color: White
Egg Color: Brown
Temperament: Docile
Life Span: 4–5 years
Comb Type: Single
Breed-Specific Health Concerns: Prone to obesity

Plymouth Rock
Figure 1.35.

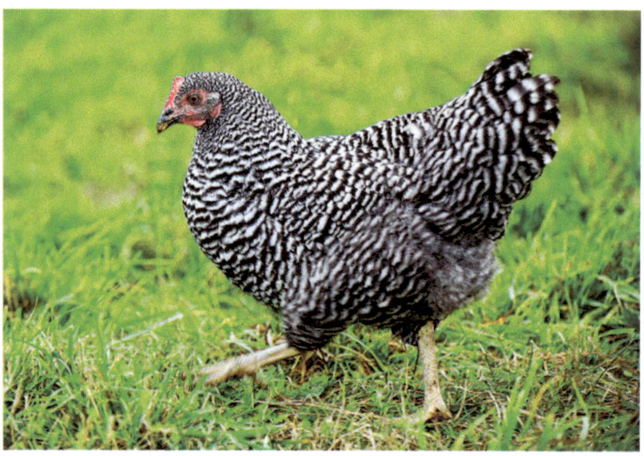

Figure 1.35 Plymouth Rock. Elenathewise / Adobe Stock Photos.

Origin: United States
Use: Dual Purpose
Weight: Male–9.5 pounds, Female–7.5 pounds
Egg Production: Around 200 eggs per year
Color: Gray and white striping
Egg Color: Brown
Temperament: Calm and docile
Life Span: 6–19 years
Comb Type: Single
Breed-Specific Health Concerns: None

Polish
Figure 1.36.

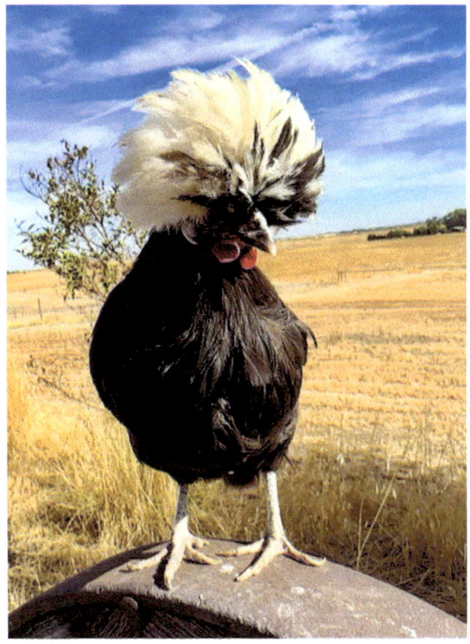

Figure 1.36 Polish Hen. Funky Chicken Rescue.

Origin: Spain
Use: Ornamental
Weight: Male–6 pounds, Female–4.5 pounds
Egg Production: Around 150–200 eggs yearly
Color: Variety
Egg Color: White
Temperament: Calm, gentle, and friendly
Life Span: 5–8 years
Comb Type: V
Breed-Specific Health Concerns: Prone to hydrocephalus

Red or Black Sex Link
Figure 1.37.

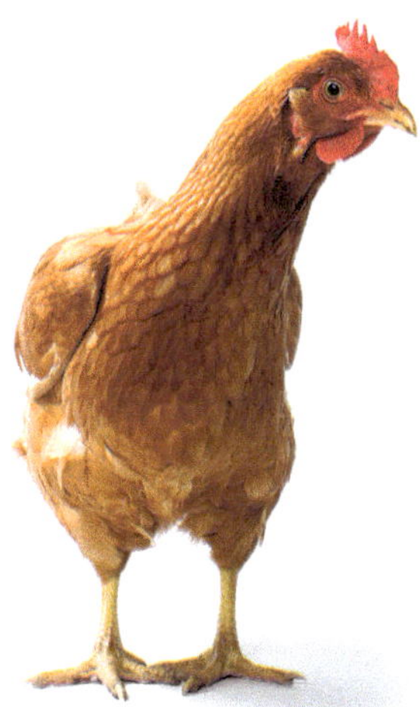

Figure 1.37 Red Sex Link Hen. Tony Campbell / Adobe Stock Photos.

Origin: United States
Use: Egg Production
Weight: Male–8 pounds, Female–6 pounds
Egg Production: Around 200–280 eggs yearly
Egg Color: Brown
Temperament: Docile and friendly
Life Span: 3–5 years
Comb Type: Single
Breed-Specific Health Concerns: Reproductive cancer, egg binding, and egg yolk peritonitis

Rhode Island Red
Figure 1.38.

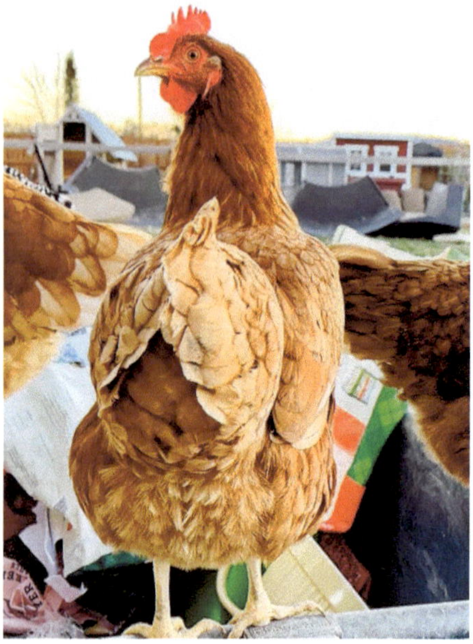

Figure 1.38 Rhode Island Red Hen. Funky Chicken Rescue.

Origin: United States
Use: Dual Purpose
Weight: Male–8.5 pounds, Female–6.5 pounds
Egg Production: Around 300 eggs yearly
Egg Color: Brown
Temperament: Docile and friendly
Life Span: 5–8 years
Comb Type: Single
Breed-Specific Health Concerns: None

Sebright
Figure 1.39.

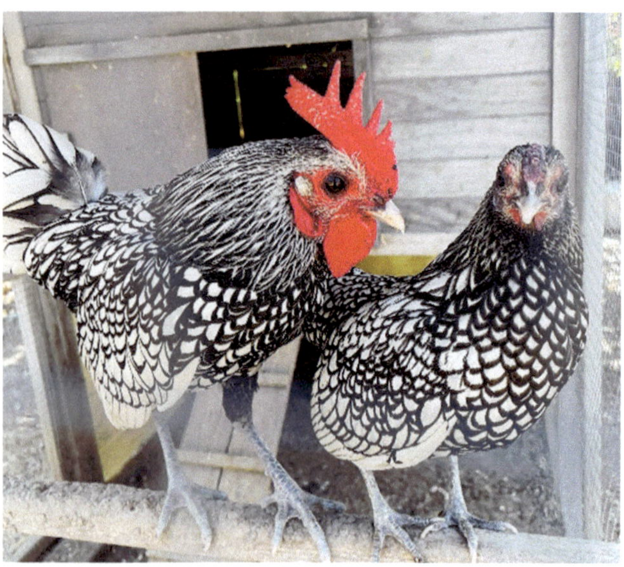

Figure 1.39 Sebright Rooster and Hen. Funky Chicken Rescue.

Origin: United Kingdom
Use: Ornamental
Weight: Male–22 ounces, Female–20 ounces
Egg Production: Around 60–80 eggs yearly
Color: Gold or silver spangled
Egg Color: Creamy White
Temperament: Sweet and Docile
Life Span: 8–12 years
Comb Type: Can vary, but the most common is single
Breed-Specific Health Concerns: Susceptibility to Marek's Disease

Serama

Figure 1.40.

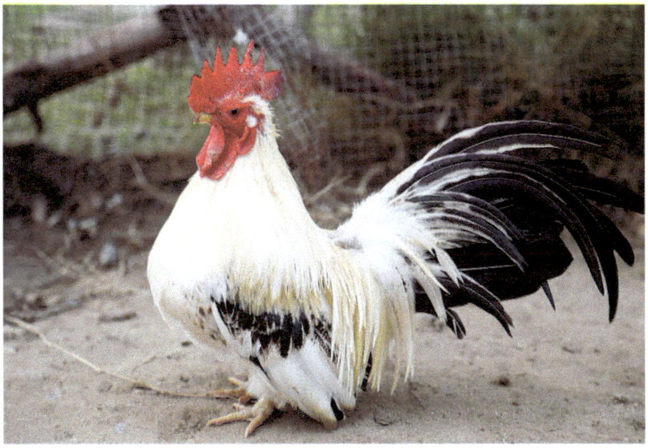

Figure 1.40 Serama Rooster. kimberrywood / Adobe Stock Photos.

Origin: Malaysia
Use: Ornamental
Weight: Male—0.8–1.2 pounds, Female—0.5–1.2 pounds
Egg Production: Around 150–200 eggs yearly
Egg Color: Cream
Temperament: Docile and friendly
Life Span: 7–10 years
Comb Type: Single
Breed-Specific Health Concerns: None

Sicilian Buttercup

Figure 1.41.

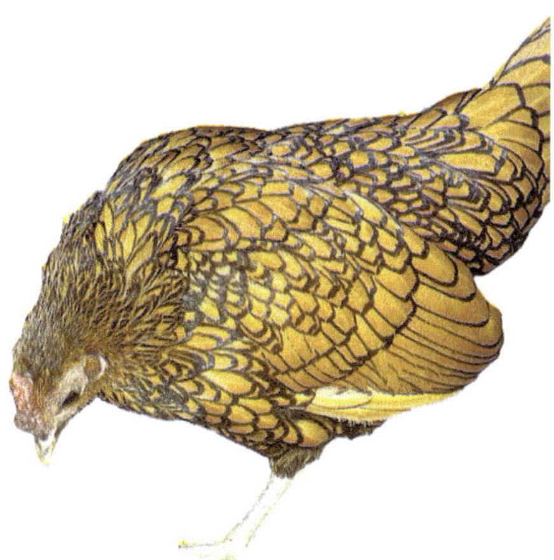

Figure 1.41 Sicilian Buttercup Hen. Herman Vlad / Adobe Stock Photos.

Origin: Island of Sicily
Use: Dual Purpose
Weight: Male—5–6 pounds, Female—4 pounds
Egg Production: Around 140–180 eggs yearly
Color: Gold spangled
Egg Color: White
Temperament: Can be flighty if not handled
Life Span: 5–8 years old
Comb Type: Two single combs that merge over the beak
Breed-Specific Health Concerns: Prone to frostbite

Silkie

Figure 1.42.

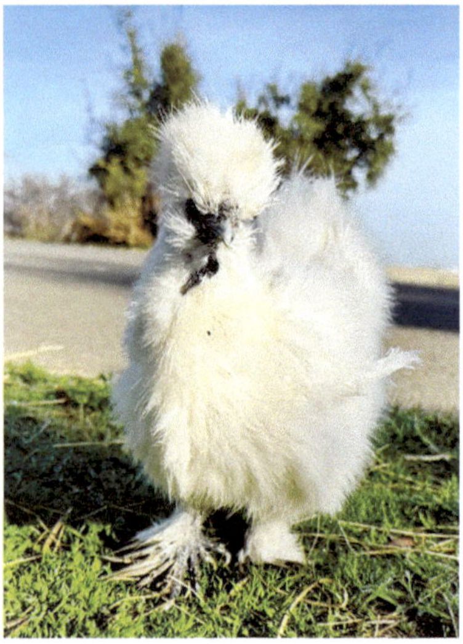

Figure 1.42 Silkie Hen. Funky Chicken Rescue.

Origin: China
Use: Ornamental
Weight: Male – 2–3 pounds, Female – 1.5–2 pounds
Egg Production: Around 120 eggs yearly
Color: Variety
Egg Color: Cream
Temperament: Docile and gentle
Life Span: 8–9 years
Comb Type: Walnut
Breed-Specific Health Concerns: Susceptible to Marek's Disease, wry neck, and head injuries

Sussex

Figure 1.43.

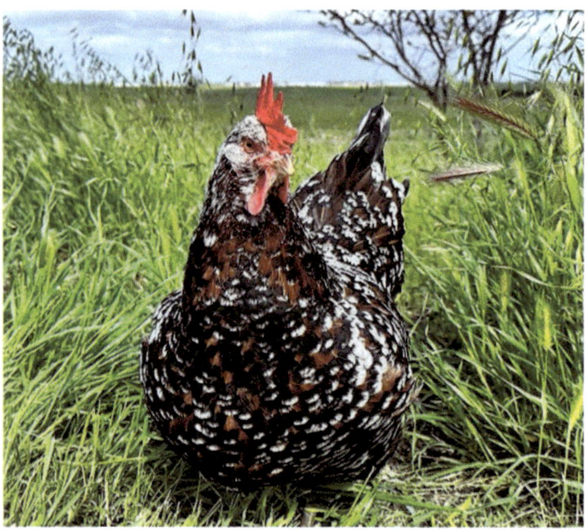

Figure 1.43 Sussex Hen. Funky Chicken Rescue.

Origin: United Kingdom
Use: Dual Purpose
Weight: Male – 9 pounds, Female – 7 pounds
Egg Production: Around 240–260 eggs yearly
Color: Red, black, white, and mottled
Egg Color: Cream
Temperament: Friendly and calm
Life Span: 5–8 years
Comb Type: Single
Breed-Specific Health Concerns: Prone to obesity

Transylvanian Naked Neck (Turken)

Figure 1.44.

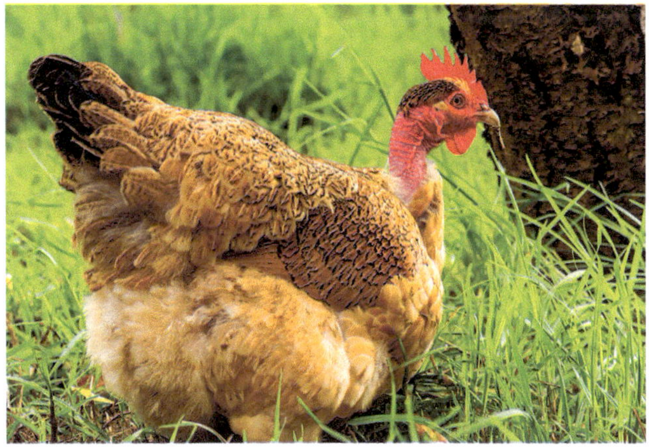

Figure 1.44 Transylvanian Naked Neck. Megan Marie Weaver / Adobe Stock Photos.

Origin: Europe
Use: Dual Purpose
Weight: Male—8.5 pounds, Female—6.5 pounds
Egg Production: Around 265 eggs yearly
Color: Black, buff, red, and white
Egg Color: Brown
Temperament: Docile and friendly
Life Span: 7–8 years
Comb Type: Single
Breed-Specific Health Concerns: Frost bite, hypothermia

Welsummer

Figure 1.45.

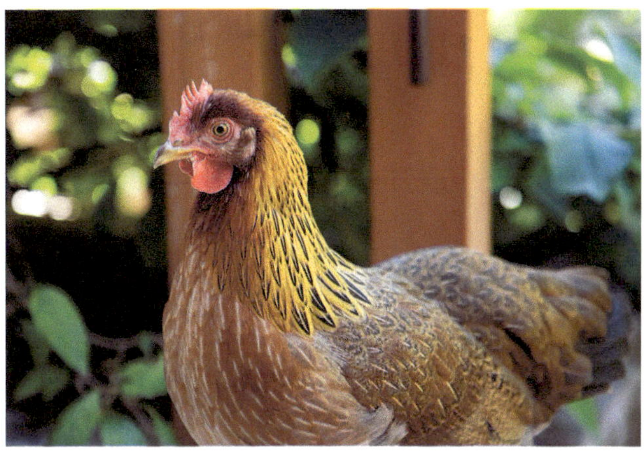

Figure 1.45 Welsummer Hen. Q2Studios / Adobe Stock Photos.

Origin: Welsum, Holland
Use: Dual Purpose
Weight: Male—8 pounds, Female—6 pounds
Egg Production: Around 150–200 eggs yearly
Color: Partridge; brown and gold
Egg Color: Dark Brown
Temperament: Friendly and docile
Life Span: 6–12 years
Comb Type: Single
Breed-Specific Health Concerns: None

White-Faced Black Spanish
Figure 1.46.

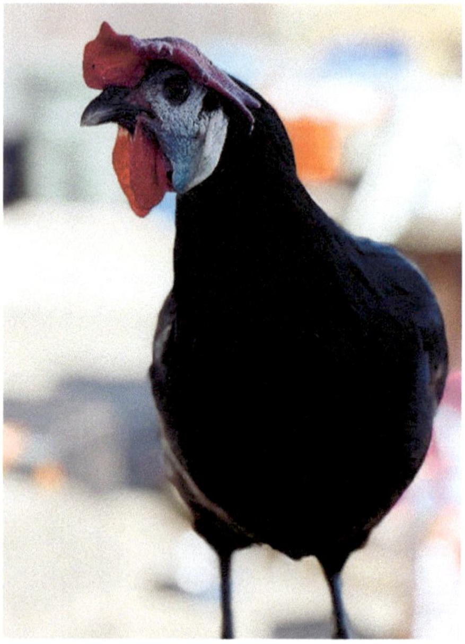

Figure 1.46 White-Faced Black Spanish Hen. Funky Chicken Rescue.

Origin: Caribbean Islands
Use: Ornamental
Weight: Male—8 pounds, Female—6.5 pounds
Egg Production: Around 180 eggs yearly
Color: Black with a white face
Egg Color: White
Temperament: Active and noisy
Life Span: 5–7 years
Comb Type: Single
Breed-Specific Health Concerns: Prone to frostbite

Wyandotte
Figure 1.47.

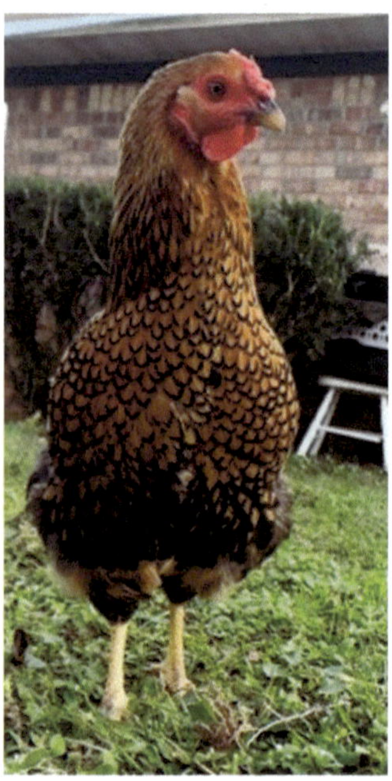

Figure 1.47 Golden Laced Wyandotte Hen. Stephanie Freeman.

Origin: New York
Use: Dual Purpose
Weight: Male—8 pounds, Female—6 pounds
Egg Production: Around 150–200 eggs yearly
Color: Variety
Egg Color: Brown
Temperament: Friendly and docile
Life Span: 6–12 years
Comb Type: Rose
Breed-Specific Health Concerns: Prone to obesity

Further Reading

Breeds of Chickens - Oklahoma State University [Internet]. 2021 [cited 2025 Dec 7]. Available from: https://breeds.okstate.edu/poultry/chickens/

Legal Protections for Chickens | Animal Legal & Historical Center [Internet]. www.animallaw.info. Available from: https://www.animallaw.info/intro/legal-protections-chickens

NPIP: Animal Health [Internet]. [cited 2025 Dec 7]. Available from: https://www.poultryimprovement.org/

Poultry Breeds - The American Poultry Association (APA) [Internet]. The American Poultry Association (APA). 2021 [cited 2025 Dec 10]. Available from: https://www.amerpoultryassn.com/poultry-breeds/

2

Life Stages and End of Life

2.1 Incubation

Research using credible sources, such as this text, must be conducted prior to attempting the incubation of eggs to gain healthy chicks. Incubating eggs, without a hen, can be quite challenging. Even with a hen, the eggs are not guaranteed to hatch, and the chicks are not guaranteed to thrive. The following information discusses utilizing a countertop incubator for hatching eggs. Most commercially available incubators have automatic turners, thermometers, and hygrometers. Even with automation, these incubators must be tested prior to placing fertilized eggs inside for incubation.

All variables must be exact, and some issues can still arise. Proper sanitation is key. If the egg environment is unsanitary, this will allow for bacteria and other contaminants to enter through the pores of the eggshell. After each successful (or unsuccessful) hatch, the incubator must be thoroughly disinfected. A soapy water scrubbing and rinse with clean water, followed by a wipe down with 70% rubbing alcohol or other evaporative disinfectant, will lessen the likelihood of "leftover" contamination from the previous hatch. Newborn chicks defecate in the incubator until they are placed in a brooder, and those stools can be a source of pathogenic microorganisms (Figure 2.1).

Always test the incubator with a thermometer and hygrometer to ensure that it is operating properly for at least 2–3 days before placing the fertile eggs inside. If either percentage is improper, do not use the incubator. After a fertilized egg is laid, it is viable for 6–7 days when kept at room temperature. Hatcheries include instructions for handling purchased fertilized eggs once received. If newborn chicks, versus fertilized eggs, are purchased, a brooder is necessary for growing babies, not an incubator. Once fertilized eggs are placed in an incubator, incubation takes 21 days until the chick is fully developed and ready to hatch on its own (Figure 2.2).

The incubator humidity should stay between 43% and 44%. The temperature should be 100–102°F; if the temperature exceeds 103°F, it will kill the embryos. Keeping the incubator out of direct sunlight and away from drafts will allow effective control of interior humidity and temperature. If the humidity becomes too low, the shell membrane will dry out, making it difficult for the chick to break through when hatching. If the humidity becomes too high, it could cause unviable chick developmental conditions (Figures 2.3 and 2.4).

During incubation, the eggs must be turned regularly three times daily to allow appropriate development of the embryo. If turned more frequently, ensure to always turn an odd number of times so the developing embryos are not in the same part of the shell overnight, every night. It is key not to turn the eggs after day 18 of incubation. This time is called lockdown, and the incubator should not be opened again until all chicks have hatched (Figures 2.5 and 2.6).

Figure 2.1 Fertile eggs before being placed in a prepared incubator. Courtesy of Sarah Meyer.

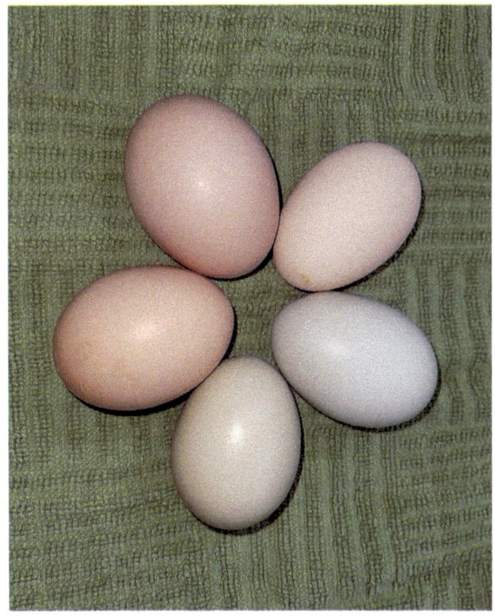

Figure 2.2 Internal egg anatomy. Oleksandr Pokusai / Adobe Stock Photos.

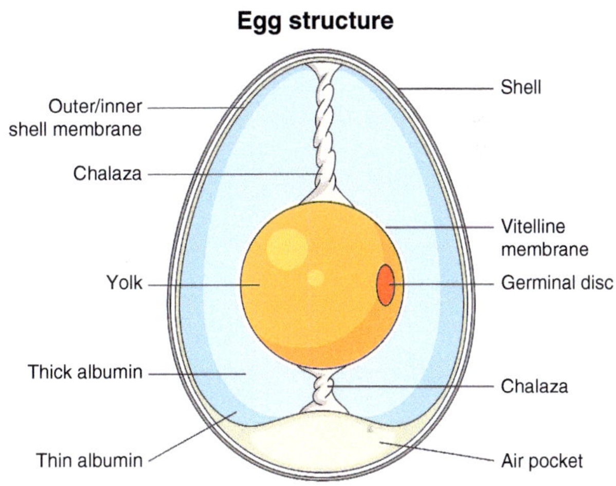

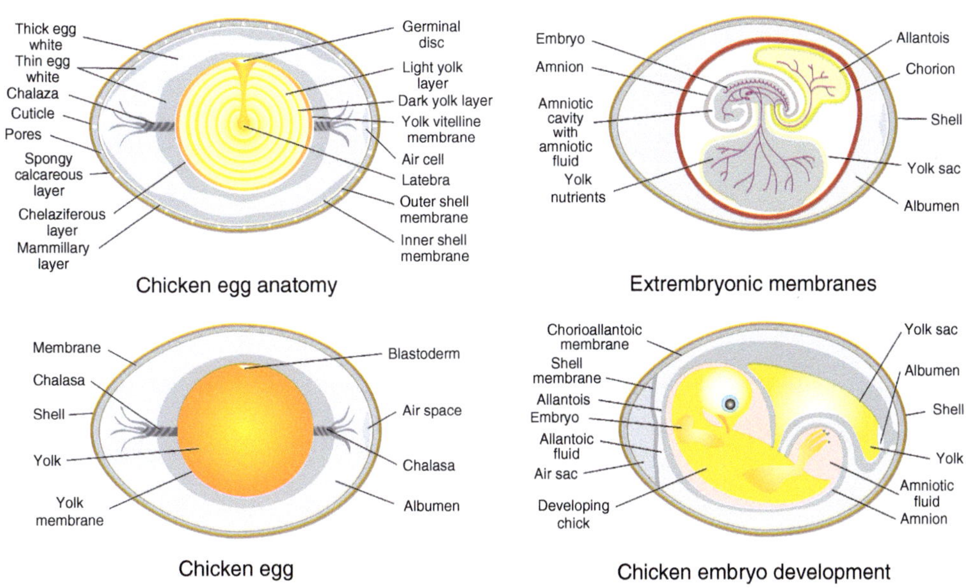

Figure 2.3 Embryonic development stages. vonuk / Adobe Stock Photos.

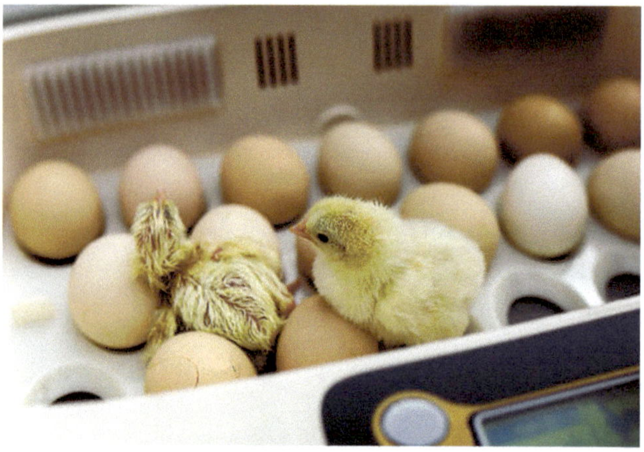

Figure 2.4 Home-use incubator. Ivan Kurmyshov / Adobe Stock Photos.

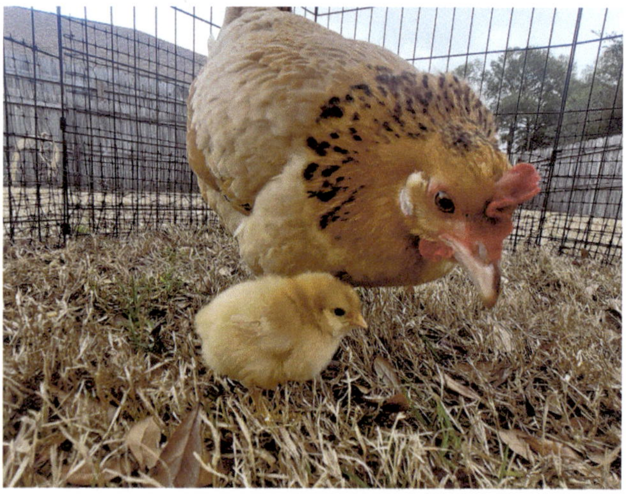

Figure 2.5 Hen and a 4-day-old chick. Courtesy of Sarah Meyer.

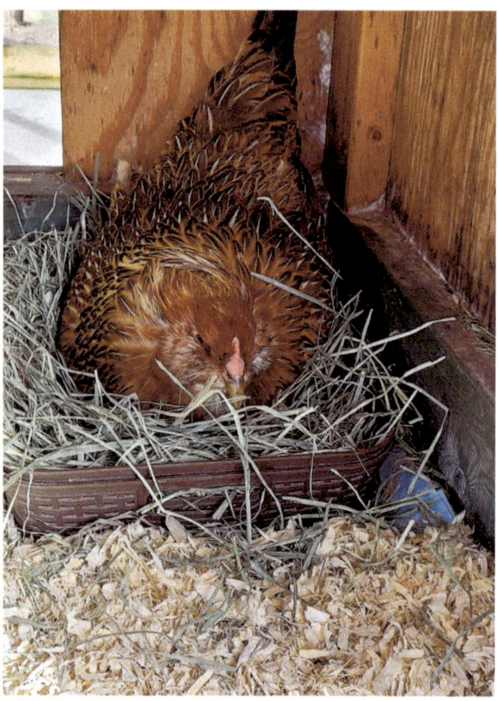

Figure 2.6 Hen on a clutch of eggs. Courtesy of Sarah Meyer.

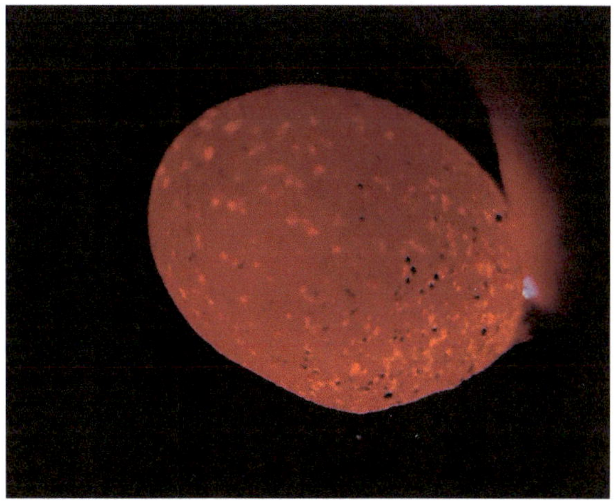

Figure 2.7 Egg candling. The presence of veins and a moving dark "spot" indicates a developing embryo. Courtesy of Sarah Meyer.

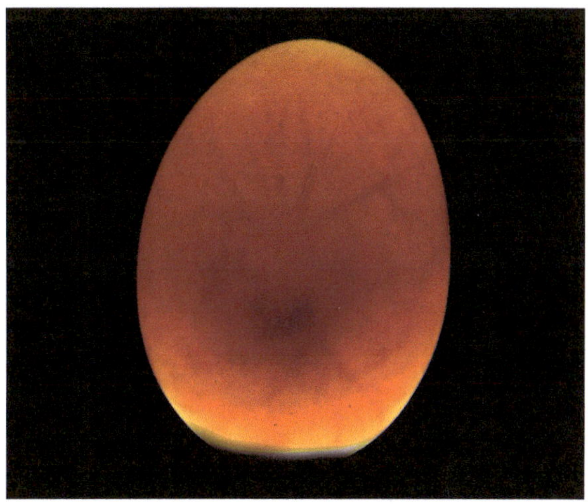

Figure 2.8 Visible veins, indicating embryo development. Олег Мальшаков / Adobe Stock Photos.

Candling the eggs with either a specific candling light or a bright flashlight should occur at least once during the incubation, prior to day 18. It is recommended to candle after 7–10 days of incubation. The presence of blood vessels and a larger dark "spot" is evidence of a developing embryo. The first 7–10 days of incubation are the first mortality peak. Unviable eggs should be removed as soon as possible, as they can rupture from decomposition gas buildup, which can then infect the other eggs with bacteria. Deceased embryos will normally have a blood ring around the embryo that is visible when candling (Figures 2.7 and 2.8).

2.2 Hatching

On day 20, the chick is preparing for hatch day, and the yolk is finishing being absorbed fully. This absorption allows the hatchlings to survive without food or water for up to 2–3 days. The "egg tooth" on the rostral tip of the beak will be used to start penetrating the membrane into the air cell. This will be evident as a hole in the shell when the chick starts to break (pip) through.

Day 21 is the hatching day. Normally, the hatching chick will begin unzipping the shell with their egg tooth, and they use their wings to help guide themselves in a circular motion. The chicks should remain in the incubator until completely dry and fluffed. Ensure that all eggs are hatched before opening the incubator to allow an ideal hatching environment by not interrupting the humidity or temperature levels. If the eggs have not hatched out by day 23, they are more than likely not viable. If curious, the eggs can be opened to investigate chick development. Otherwise, they must be disposed of respectfully (Figures 2.9–2.11).

Reasons for unsuccessful hatching are inadequate humidity levels, improper temperature, infertile eggs, insufficient ventilation, improper turning, and/or poor eggshell quality.

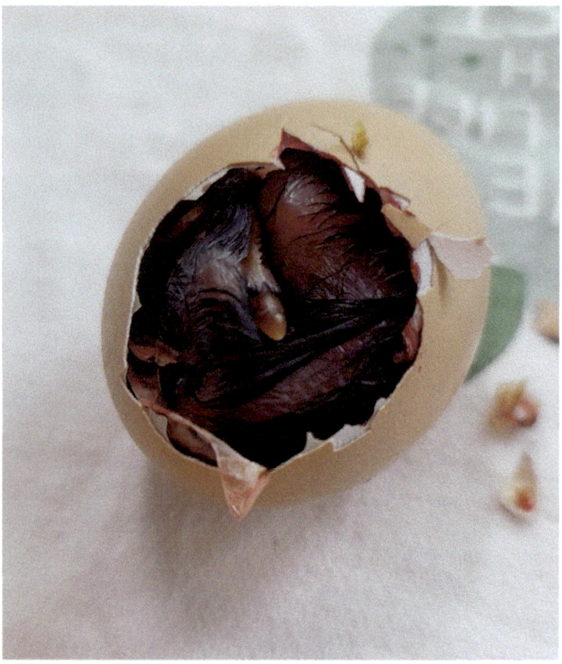

Figure 2.9 A chick emerging from its egg. Courtesy of Sarah Meyer.

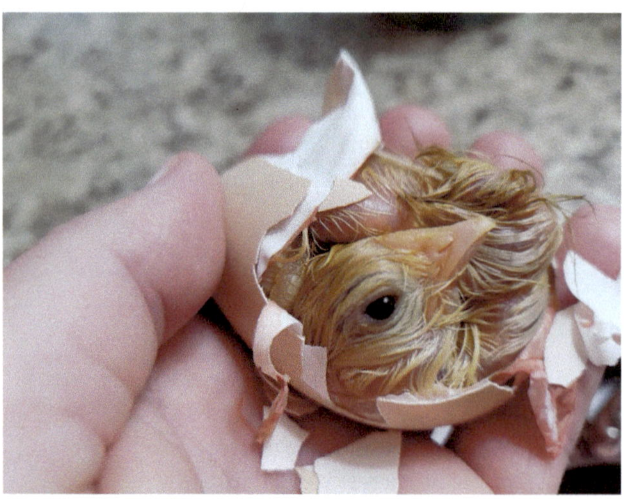

Figure 2.10 Hatching chick. Photo courtesy of Sarah Meyer.

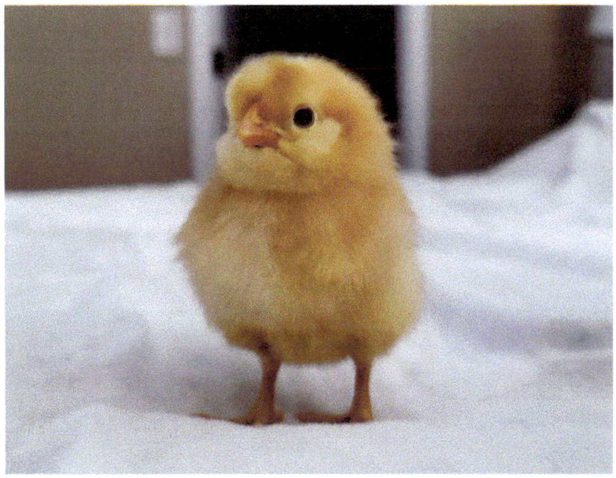

Figure 2.11 Dry chick after hatching. Courtesy of Sarah Meyer.

2.3 Chickhood

The first 6 weeks of life are the fragile neonatal to pediatric chick stage. Chicks require consistent warmth, a safe, clean space, and crumbled grower feed and fresh water. A chick brooder can be purchased from farm supply stores or constructed from safe materials, such as a storage tote adapted to a suitable brooder. These enclosures must be free from drafts and have a sturdy top that allows ventilation. Brooders should be protected from predators, pets, and children. Unintentional harm can result from inexperienced handling (Figures 2.12 and 2.13).

From day one, a chick's environmental temperature must be around 104°F, decreasing by a degree each week until the brooder temperature reaches ambient room temperature and the chicks are fully feathered. A four-legged heating plate is recommended to decrease fire risk compared to a heat lamp. Chicks prefer the security of a heat plate, as they can sleep or play under it while maintaining body temperature. At 3–4 days, chicks begin eating crumble feed, and feathers begin to replace their soft down. The wing feathers will begin to sprout first, and their breed-specific coloring will be evident. Chicks begin exploring and playing with flock mates, becoming braver and stronger as they grow. Even at this young age, they begin establishing a hierarchy. Even before they are fully feathered, chicks will attempt to dust-bathe in bedding. Shallow pans with chick dirt or organic potting soil can be provided for their enrichment. Frequent bedding changes become necessary as the chicks grow and produce more feces/urates (Figure 2.14).

Once fully feathered, chicks can usually be visually identified as a pullet (females) or cockerel (AKA, rooster) by comb development and sex-specific behavior signs. Male chicks tend to posture upright compared to females that "cower" or stand with their bodies in a horizontal posture. Males will play-fight and chest-bump, attempting to establish their place in the flock. This "teenager" stage lasts the next 6–12 weeks of life. They will begin to gain weight, adult feathers will develop, and they will exhibit familiar male or female behaviors (Figure 2.15).

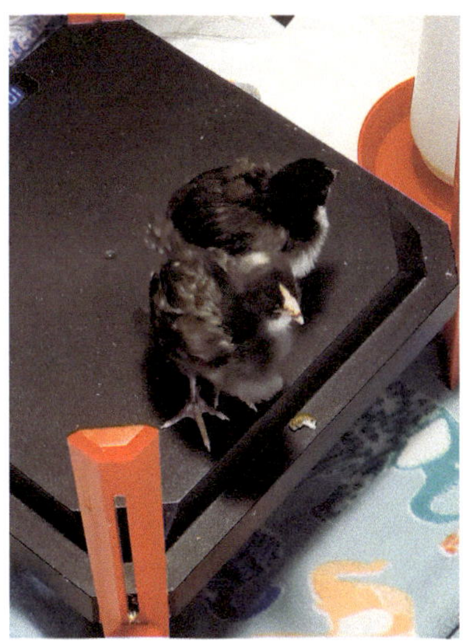

Figure 2.12 Brooder plate with adjustable height and thermostat. Photo courtesy of Sarah Meyer.

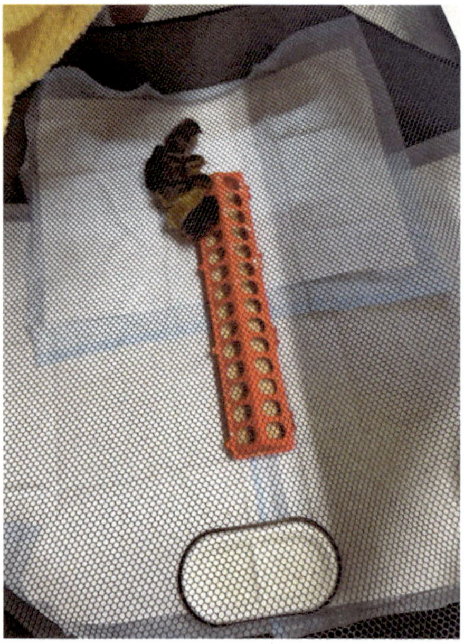

Figure 2.13 Soft-side dog crate used as a brooder. Photo courtesy of Stephanie Freeman.

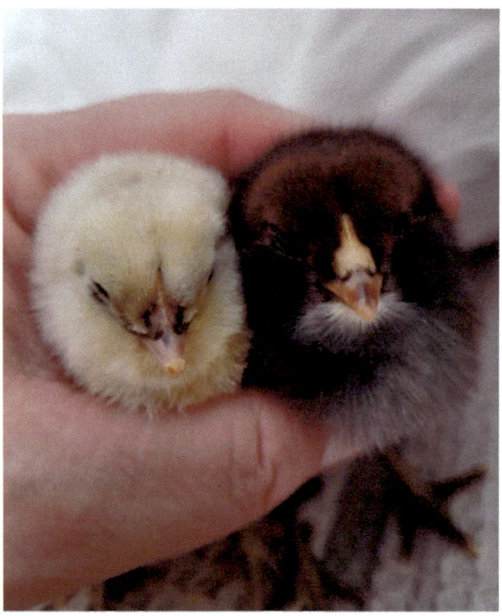

Figure 2.14 Easter Egger chicks. "Egg teeth" noted on beaks. Photo courtesy of Sarah Meyer.

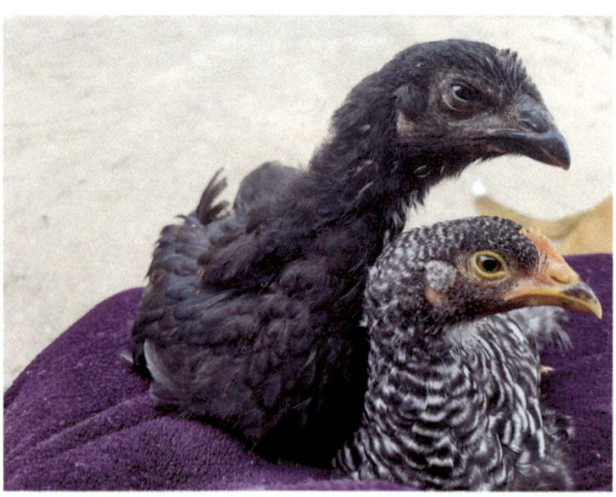

Figure 2.15 Young pullets. Courtesy of Sarah Meyer.

2.4 Youngsters or "Teenagers"

Pullets will begin to show signs of maturity (egg laying) around 18–20 weeks of age. They will begin looking for nesting material and a suitable nest for egg-laying. Submissive squatting with their wings spread indicates receptivity to mounting by roosters. Receptive hens will also display this submissive behavior to caregivers. Once the pullet lays her first egg, she is considered an adult hen. As a hen ages, her egg production slows, but it may never completely stop. Young adult cockerels/roosters will begin practicing their crow, sometimes when still "teenagers," and growing beautiful saddle, neck, and tail feathers to attract females (Figure 2.16).

2.5 Adulthood

Chickens can live an average of 5–10 years (or longer), depending on the mitigation of risk factors, proper healthcare, genetics, and proficient husbandry. If provided with preventive healthcare, including proper nutrition and predator access, chickens can become elderly, requiring age-appropriate care, such as supplements or medicants for osteoarthritis, to add quality to their life (Figure 2.17).

2.6 Elderly and Geriatric Chicken Care

All too often, laying hens are devalued and discarded when their egg production wanes. Hens and roosters can live into their geriatric years (>10 years) and often require adaptations and supplementations to maintain or improve their quality of life. Arthritis development in joints, cognitive function decline, vision and hearing loss, and immunosuppression are typical, just as in other animals and humans. Ambient temperature mindfulness, soft bedding, perch height adjustments, and adequate lighting contribute to the bird's comfort and adaptability to their environment. Feeding with lower protein (unless the hen is still laying eggs or molting) content

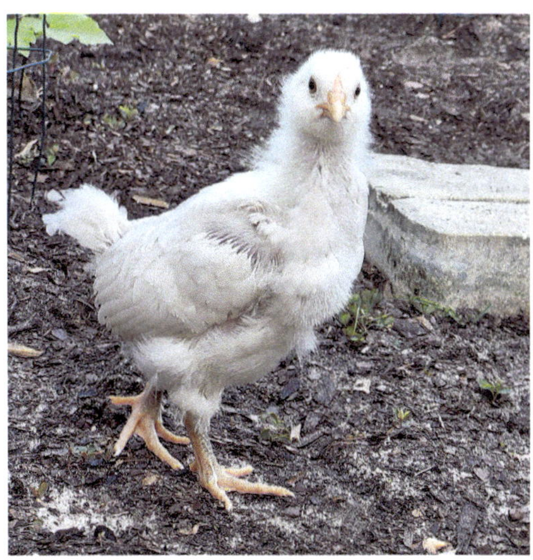

Figure 2.16 Prepubescent Easter Egger rooster. Courtesy of Sarah Meyer.

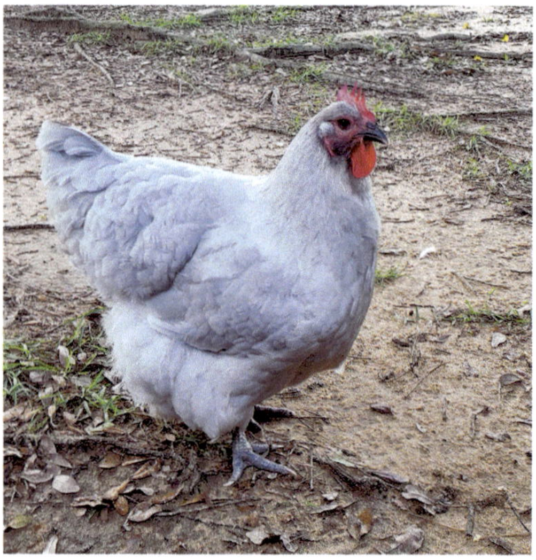

Figure 2.17 Adult Lavendar Orpington hen. Courtesy of Sarah Meyer.

eases renal workload. Reproductive organs and other organ systems are at greater risk of tumor development as the bird ages. Regular veterinary examinations and diagnostic testing can monitor the development of disease and provide treatment options. Guardians can assess their bird's quality of life by using an assessment tool like the HHHHHMM Scale created by Dr. Alice Villalobos. Realistic assessments and discussions with the veterinarian regarding end-of-life options (hospice and euthanasia) are warranted with elderly or terminally ill chickens. Human euthanasia is discussed in Chapter 16.

Further Reading

Fairchild BD. Environmental Factors to Control When Brooding Chicks | CAES Field Report [Internet]. CAES Field Report. 2025. Available from: https://fieldreport.caes.uga.edu/publications/B1287/environmental-factors-to-control-when-brooding-chicks/

Gilbert SF. Early Development in Birds. Developmental Biology 6th Edition [Internet]. 2000; Available from: https://www.ncbi.nlm.nih.gov/books/NBK10070/

Poultry Life Cycle [Internet]. 2025 [cited 2025 Dec 7]. Available from: https://akovet.org/resource-hub/for-animal-owners/backyard-poultry-home/poultry-basics/poultry-life-cycle/

Stages in Chick Embryo Development | Mississippi State University Extension Service [Internet]. Msstate.edu. 2025. Available from: https://extension.msstate.edu/agriculture/livestock/poultry/stages-chick-embryo-development

Stuttgen S. Life Cycle of a Laying Hen [Internet]. [cited 2025 Dec 7]. Available from: https://livestock.extension.wisc.edu/articles/life-cycle-of-a-laying-hen/

3

Husbandry, Housing, and Biosecurity

Proper husbandry is vital to owning healthy chickens. Chickens must receive an appropriate omnivorous diet, have unlimited access to fresh water, and live in a sanitary, safe environment. Many maladies of chickens seen in clinical practice are due to poor husbandry and guardian ignorance about proper chicken husbandry.

3.1 Cleaning and Disinfection

Daily removal of stools is ideal for their living environment, but not always practical. Regular scooping, dusting of all surfaces (removing built-up particulates), and scraping feces from hard surfaces should occur to prevent the accumulation of waste and the attraction of pests. At least once a year, thorough cleaning and disinfection of the enclosures can mitigate disease. Deep cleaning is typically performed in the spring season on warm, sunny days to allow drying of cleansed surfaces. There are many home remedies touted for cleaning hard surfaces, but scrubbing with warm soapy water (dish detergent with or without vinegar) followed by a properly diluted disinfectant spray should be used. Clients/guardians can ask their veterinarian for guidance regarding what disinfectant is appropriate for avian disease prevention. An agent that has broad-spectrum properties (bactericidal, virucidal, sporicidal, and fungicidal) should be selected. When cleaning, the areas should be free of birds, free of soiled bedding/substrate, have organic material removed, be well-ventilated, and be allowed to air dry. Disinfectant dilution per the manufacturer's instructions must be followed to avoid injury to birds and the person using it. Inhaling fumes can damage lungs and air sacs, while chemical burns to feet can occur if the birds are allowed access to recently disinfected, poorly rinsed areas. Avoid using bleach or ammonia-based products, as these can be toxic, especially if improperly diluted (Figure 3.1).

3.2 Substrates

There are plenty of anecdotal opinions on the type of substrate for use in the coop or house and pen. The consensus is to avoid using straw, as it is nonabsorbent and can become moist and harbor mold, thus creating harmful aerosolized spores. Wood (pine or aspen) shavings, hemp, hay, and recycled newspapers seem to be ideal bedding options. Cedar shavings release aromatic hydrocarbons and phenols that will result in respiratory and dermatological irritation.

When choosing wood shavings, select larger flake shavings. Smaller shavings tend to be dustier and more likely to be consumed by chickens, potentially causing a crop obstruction (discussed

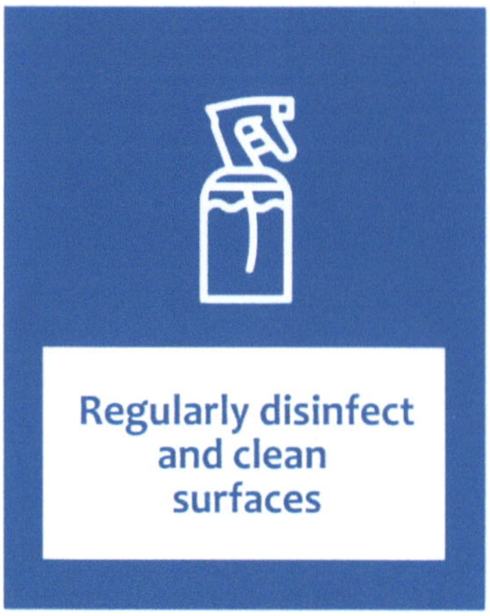

Figure 3.1 Deep clean the coop surfaces at least once a year with a broad-spectrum disinfectant. luca piccini basile / Adobe Stock Photos.

later in Chapter 8). Wood shavings do require regular replacement, as they absorb liquids, which can lead to a malodorous living environment (Figure 3.2).

Hemp is an effective absorbent substrate that reduces odor. This mostly dust-free, compostable material is produced from the shafts of the cannabis plant. It is recommended to replace all the hemp bedding and start fresh every 3–4 months. Daily or regular scooping is still recommended for the reasons previously listed (Figure 3.3).

With any substrate that is not sterile, the risk of mite infestation is a concern. If the guardian has access to a chest freezer, substrate can be placed in the freezer for up to 7 days prior to using in the coop or house. This practice will eradicate potentially harmful mites. An alternative to freezing is to use a permethrin spray or powder on the substrate when it is placed in the coop/house. Some chicken guardians prefer calcium carbonate/citric acid powder or diatomaceous earth sprinkled in the substrate for moisture, odor, and pest control. As with any dust or powder, care must be taken to avoid inhalation and subsequent lung/air sac damage to chickens. Usefulness is readily purported, but clinically, there is little data to prove either product's effectiveness against external parasites or flying insects.

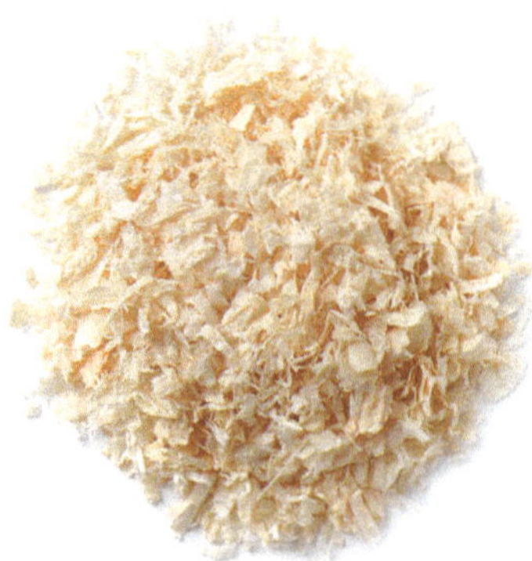

Figure 3.2 Pine shavings. Coprid / Adobe Stock Photos.

For ease of cleanup inside the hen house, some guardians use nonabsorbent materials, such as empty feed sacks under nighttime perches, and sprinkle a layer of granular odor-absorbent products (such as PDZ – a mineral product named zeolite as a result of volcanic activity with odor and moisture absorbent properties) underneath perches and on the floor of the hen house. A cat litter scoop is handy in this situation (Figure 3.4).

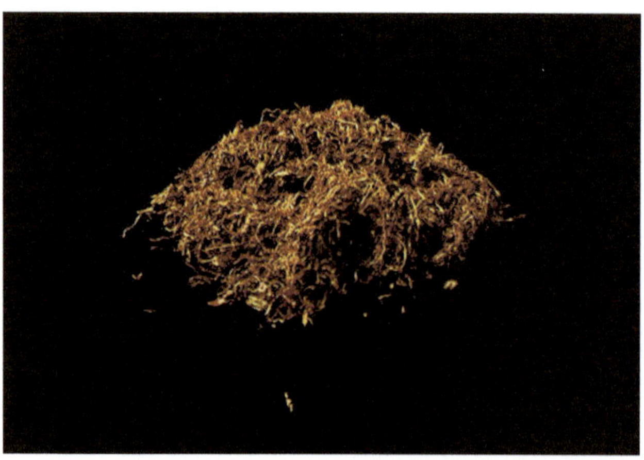

Figure 3.3 Hemp shavings. Dav_782 / Adobe Systems Photos.

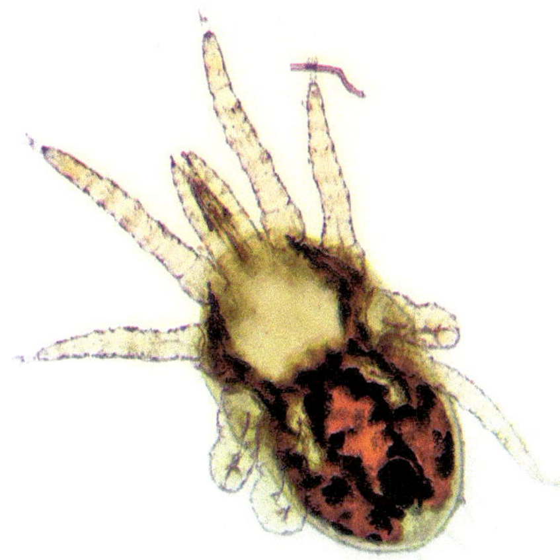

Figure 3.4 Red mite. phototrip.cz / Adobe Stock Photos.

3.3 Housing

Choosing a coop (house) design for chickens will depend on the available or planned space for the house as well as the number of chickens desired. Practicality trumps decor when selecting or building a safe chicken house and pen. Farm supply stores provide attractive pre-made houses that seem perfect, but they are often too small for grown birds. Chicks quickly outgrow these small enclosures, risking their mental and physical health. Materials used in the construction of these prefabricated houses/pens are typically particle board and thin pine, neither of which is made for long-lasting outdoor durability. Mildew growth and rotting often occur quickly. Predators can easily open doors and walls to gain access to birds. While hardware cloth is used on these tiny houses, it is stapled onto the thin wood and easily peeled back. A carefully planned enclosure with ample space and security in mind will provide a long-term housing option for a flock (Figure 3.5).

An ideal house will include a minimum of 4 sq. ft. per chicken inside the enclosed chicken coop. Proper ventilation, like a human dwelling, allows airflow without drafts even in the colder months of the year. Ventilation reduces excess moisture and ammonia production from dropping accumulation. Warm, moist air rises in a coop, so the slats or openings should be located at the top

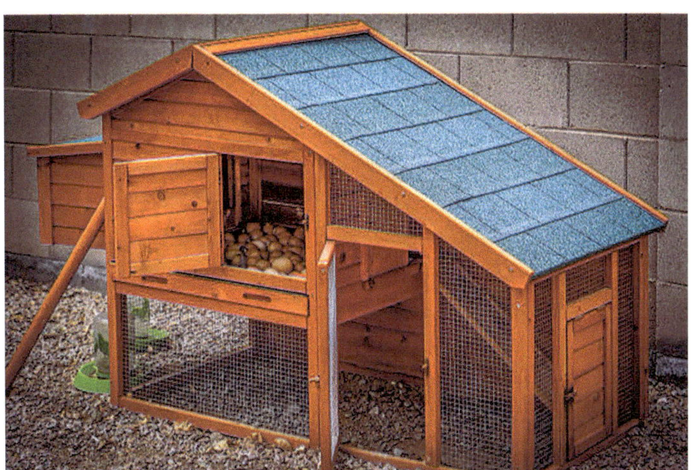

Figure 3.5 Commercially available coop/pen combinations do not provide long-term housing or protection against predators. Xstoria / Adobe Stock Photos.

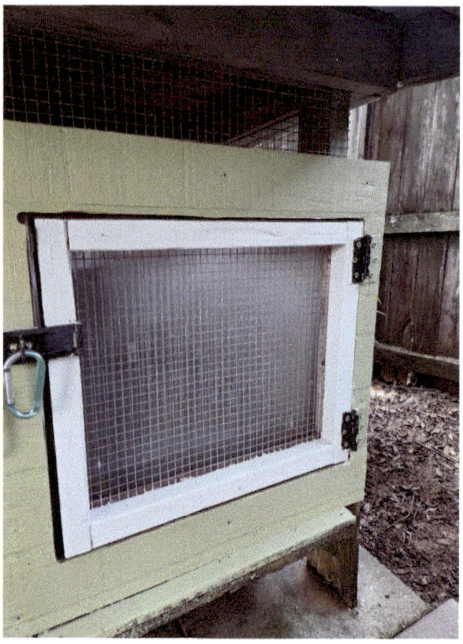

Figure 3.6 Chickens are enclosed in a pen with hardware cloth. Courtesy of Funky Chicken Rescue.

of the house. The coop/house should be insulated, especially in colder climates, to block drafts and provide protection from the elements. Additional predator proofing includes sturdy locks on all doors and windows with hardware cloth securely attached to all openings. Raccoons are intelligent predators who can master a seemingly difficult door or window lock. Small-gauge hardware cloth (not chicken wire) over the windows, doors, and any other openings will block access to chickens and an easy meal for carnivores (Figure 3.6).

3.4 Safe Pen or Run Design

The outdoor space, known as the run or pen, is used for exercise, pecking, socializing, and foraging. Overcrowding can lead to bullying and frustration among the flock. Birds who are lower in the pecking order need space to escape. The standard size of the run is a minimum of 8–10 sq. ft. per chicken and must be completely enclosed on top and sides with hardware cloth to deter flying and climbing predators. Once constructed, regularly inspect the house and pen for possible breaches in safety. Any crack or opening greater than ½ inch can be accessed by hungry or inquisitive animals (Figure 3.7).

To discourage predator digging, bury the hardware cloth "apron" along the sides of the pen and/or place rocks or bricks along the outside and inside. Overhead netting evades hawks, owls, and eagles. One cannot be too careful when protecting their outdoor flock from predators. Carnivorous predators look for easy meals, and enclosed urban and rural chickens are prime targets. Raccoons, minks, and other animals will attempt to locate a weakness in the coop and pen enclosure, so being proactive instead of reactive protects the flock. Allowing birds to be killed by predators is inhumane if preventable (Figure 3.8).

Sand is an effective pen substrate option because it drains well. Construction sand, not play sand, can be useful in both cold and hot temperature climates, but it does require regular cleaning. Construction sand is coarser, which allows for more effective drainage and absorbency. A long-handled cat litter box-type scoop used for sifting droppings is useful. If cleaned daily, the

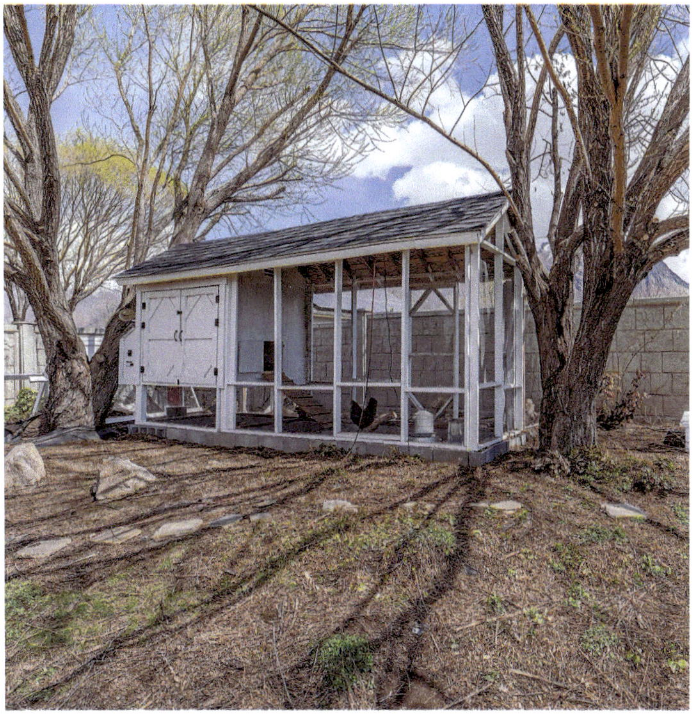

Figure 3.7 Coop with ample space for its flock. Jason / Adobe Stock Photos.

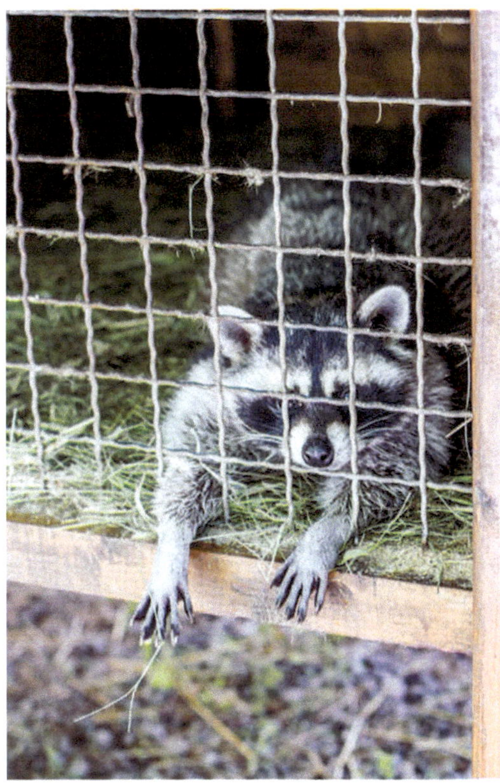

Figure 3.8 Raccoons and other predators can reach through the wire, pulling chicken body parts through. pvector / Adobe Stock Photos.

sand may only need to be replaced every 1–3 years. Sand must be at least 4–5 inches thick to maximize absorbency and drainage. Unfortunately, sand has a tendency to become dusty. Sand is not useful if composting is intended, but the scooped/sifted droppings can be added to compost.

3.5 Inside the Hen House

Inside the enclosed hen house, nesting boxes will be needed for laying hens. One to two nest boxes per 3–4 hens is ideal, as they tend to compete for one "favorite" box/nest. Line the nest boxes with an easily replaceable or washable substrate or pad to avoid broken eggs and increase appeal to the hen. The nesting box(es) are placed in a quiet, dim corner of the coop/house because hens appreciate privacy while laying their eggs. Dried fragrant flowers and herbs can be sprinkled in boxes and litter to detract pests. Using latex paint for the inside and outside walls, ceiling, and floor of the coop seals the wood and enables easier cleaning. Laminate flooring can also be used for this same purpose. Contact paper or wallpaper is not as effective and may have the opposite effect. While these decorations may be aesthetically pleasing for a short period of time, they are not as durable or easily cleaned as one might imagine. Frequent replacing and upgrading adds to the chore of chicken-keeping (Figure 3.9).

Many guardians provide decorative curtains for nesting boxes to increase appeal; however, these curtains must be cleaned or replaced regularly. Raised roosting bars or boards are needed for nightly slumber and enrichment. Chickens are prey animals and like to climb and roost off the ground. Roosts are ideally 2–4 feet off the ground, allowing 8–12 inches of space per bird on bars/boards. Washable padding can be placed on them for comfort, and the bars/boards should not be round (not dowel rods) as this shape places unnecessary strain on the bird's toes and foot pads, resulting in soreness and potential pododermatitis.

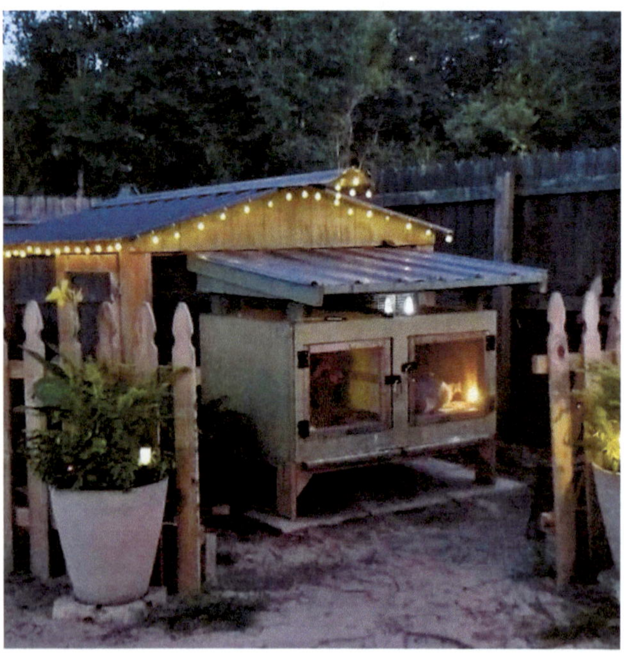

Figure 3.9 Coop with proper ventilation, hardware cloth, concrete paver flooring with a central drain for sanitation. Courtesy of Sarah Meyer.

Another concern for outdoor flocks is flying insects and wild birds that act as disease vectors. Fine-gauge window screen can be placed on the inside of the hardware cloth. Chemical deterrents can also be used for flies and mosquitoes, which carry transmissible avian pathogens. Fly strips can be used only if chickens are not able to encounter them. Fake crows, windsocks, or other moving objects can be used to deter wild birds and flying predators from nearing a chicken pen.

Provide plenty of shade and shelter from inclement weather. A door on the pen, in addition to the house, provides access for cleaning. The height of the pen generally depends on the space available and the desired height of the guardian. In winter, clear plastic sheeting or fiberglass can be placed around the pen to allow light without allowing wind gusts. The edges/bottom of the pen should be connected to the ground or the hardware cloth buried (see explanation above).

Regardless of the type of substrates used in the coop or pen, the guardian should utilize appropriate personal protective equipment (PPE), such as a face mask, while cleaning to avoid inhalation of airborne dust. Goggles, disposable gloves, and designated chicken pen footwear should be worn when cleaning housing and pens. Proper hand sanitation must be conducted after coop and pen cleaning, even if disposable gloves are worn when cleaning enclosures.

3.6 Feeders and Watering Implements, Environmental Enrichment

Clean feeders and waterers are extremely important to reduce pathogens, biofilm, and algae. Chickens are known for indiscriminate defecation, including in feeders and waterers. The chicken guardian will spend a great deal of time cleaning and disinfecting these implements daily to prevent contamination. Waterers should be placed out of direct sunlight to prevent algae growth. The best way to keep the water clean is to thoroughly clean the container every single time it needs to be filled. Keeping a sanitized extra water container on hand and rotating them every day ensures the birds always have clean and fresh water. Wash one container with warm, soapy water and set it out in the sun to air dry. A designated automatic dishwasher can also be used to sanitize water and food implements.

There is no "best" waterer for chickens, as plastic becomes brittle and will break. Caregivers who intend to eat their birds' or their layers' eggs and are concerned about BPA (Bisphenol A) in plastics should avoid this type of waterer unless it specifies that it does not contain this chemical for processing. Metal waterers, even stainless steel, can rust, but tend to be sturdier while also being more expensive. Waterers must be sanitized regularly; therefore, they must be made of a durable material.

The feeder needs to be emptied and cleaned thoroughly with warm, soapy water *at least* every 2 weeks. Make sure to scrub all surfaces of the feeder because any remnants can attract pests and encourage mold growth. The feeder must be thoroughly clean and dry before adding fresh food. A separate feeder or bowl should be used when offering fresh vegetables, fruit, or other foods to avoid contamination of dry feed. Kebab hooks, baskets, or durable chicken snack bags can be used to hang treats off the ground and encourage healthy pecking. Many companies produce chicken-focused feeding implements and puzzle toys, so the guardian has a selection of products to choose from for purchase. A treadle feeder can effectively discourage pests, such as rodents, and is recommended if the flock eats outside in the pen/run. A feeding treadle will require training and patience while ensuring the chickens receive proper nutrition while learning.

3.7 Enrichment and Mental Stimulation

Different types of enrichment (eating stations, perches and roosts of varying heights, and dust bathing tubs) should be provided to prevent boredom among the flock members. If the flock is not allowed regular supervised free-ranging, behavioral conditions will occur and affect the productivity and harmony of the flock or individual chickens. Free-ranging can provide adequate mental stimulation since birds are allowed to express natural behaviors; however, they must be supervised.

Chickens enjoy human companionship, especially if hand-reared as chicks. It is unknown if they consider humans as mothers (foster hens) or guardians (roosters). Oftentimes, chickens will prefer being near "their" humans rather than wandering off and will interact by seeking to be petted or held. High-value treats can strengthen this behavior (Figure 3.10).

3.8 Local Regulations of Backyard Flocks

Prior to purchasing or adopting chicks or adult birds, check local zoning laws or homeowners' association rules for backyard chicken regulations. Chickens are considered livestock in many regions. The number and type of birds are considered. Some counties allow only hens, while others restrict the number of birds allowed to cohabitate within city limits. Construction of a pen and coop may require a permit from the county of residence and may incur fees. Preemptive research will avoid frustration and heartache later. If purchasing straight-run chicks from a hatchery, have a plan for rehoming birds if restrictions exist.

3.9 Ambient Temperature Accommodations

In hot summer months, heavy breeds and those with thick feathering suffer from heat-related maladies, such as heatstroke. Shaded areas, whether they are with a solid roof, tarpaulins, or trees, are vital to keeping birds cool. Water misters and dripping hoses can be provided to reduce body temperatures not only by cooling the air but also by cooling the dirt in the pen. Dry areas should

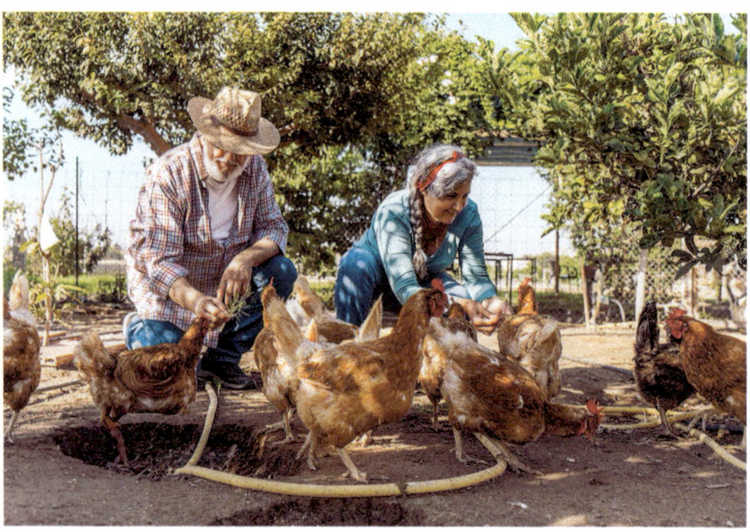

Figure 3.10 Many families enjoy chicken companions, and chickens enjoy treats. Renata Hamuda / Adobe Stock Photos.

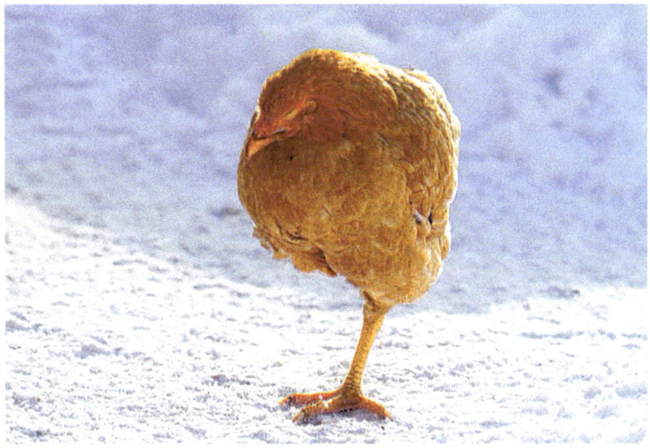

Figure 3.11 Cold hen in snow. drakuliren / Adobe Stock Photos.

be available when the birds want to escape the misting, wet areas. Houses can be built to support climate control modification, such as air conditioning and heating. Overhead or other placement of fans circulates air by forced convection. This air movement also discourages flying pests.

Conversely, in cold winter months, chickens are adept at staying warm by generating body heat. However, in extreme cold weather and frigid wind, they can develop frostbite of the combs, toes, and wattles. Smaller breeds, such as bantams, and breeds with sparse feathering (Naked-necks/Turkens, Silkies, and Frizzles) cannot withstand extremely cold temperatures. Breeds with large combs and wattles and feathered legs and feet easily develop frostbite or hypothermia. Debilitated or ill birds, molting birds, or lower pecking order birds have difficulty regulating body temperature and benefit from warming implements. Prolonged cold temperatures cause undue stress and immunosuppression, leading to illness or death (Figure 3.11).

Plastic or fiberglass sheeting secured around the pen during cold months will prevent wind exposure and moisture from rain and snow. Proper insulation of the house/coop, along with blocking openings to prevent drafts, will help birds stay warmer. Heat lamps are the primary cause of coop fires and bird deaths. Warming panels are a safe method of keeping birds warm if they cannot live in a climate-controlled environment. As mentioned in Chapter 1, some breeds of chickens are bred for hotter climates, while others can better survive colder climates. Regardless of climatic conditions, the caregiver is responsible for providing appropriate, humane protection from the elements.

3.10 Biosecurity and Flock Safety

As a chicken keeper, protecting the flock from predators can never be considered excessive. With that, unintentional harm may occur in the form of fomites. Contaminated shoes or husbandry implements (rakes, litter scoops, hoses, etc.) can expose birds to pathogenic organisms from infected flocks on or off the property. After visiting other properties where chickens live, care must be taken to clean and disinfect shoes or other inanimate objects, as well as wash hands and clothing prior to entering the home property. Limiting chicken-owning visitors to the flock can mitigate disease transmission risks.

Large commercial poultry farms take strict biosecurity measures to prevent lethal outbreaks in their flocks, such as limiting visitors, using full-body disposable PPE (personal protective

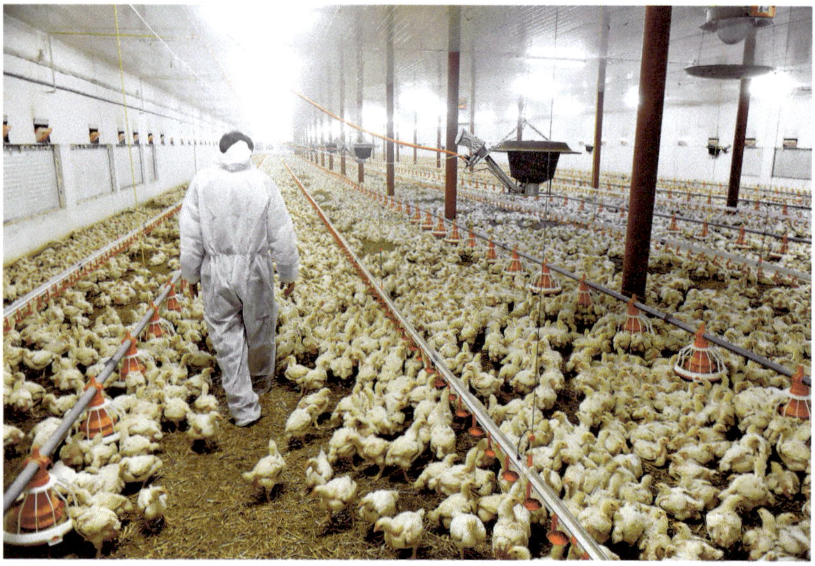

Figure 3.12 Biosecurity measures in a large-scale brooder house. roibu / Adobe Stock Photos.

equipment), and chemical washing vehicles upon entering and exiting the property. Viral influenza and bacteria are the usual culprits that wipe out an entire flock of thousands of birds. Once this occurs, the farms completely remove all carcasses, bedding, implements, and other fomites before disinfecting (incineration and/or chemicals) the large barns. Carcasses are incinerated to eliminate the spread of pathogens (Figure 3.12).

While these steps may seem extreme for a small backyard flock, they can be scaled to a reasonable but effective practice that saves a flock from morbidity or mortality. Proactive biosecurity measures are more cost-effective than veterinary intervention. New birds are quarantined for a minimum of 30 days before slow introduction to the flock. During this time, if the birds remain healthy in appearance and behavior, administration of internal and external antiparasitic agents should commence so as not to introduce new pathogens to the existing flock. The full course of agents should be administered prior to the slow introduction of these new birds.

If new birds exhibit clinical signs, the guardian should alert their veterinarian to discuss identification of the cause and treatment if possible. If the bird's condition worsens, euthanasia and necropsy should be ensued. Many veterinary reference laboratories accept carcasses (or representative specimens) for analysis. In states where commercial flocks are raised, they typically have dedicated veterinary pathologists for the diagnosis of reportable diseases that affect production farms. Many veterinary teaching hospitals and specialty centers have avian veterinary specialists who can provide consultations to referring veterinarians. If new birds do not exhibit illness after 30 days, they can be slowly introduced to the home flock to establish a natural pecking order. For more information about chicken behavior, see Chapter 5.

3.11 Consideration of House Chickens

Many chicken enthusiasts are inviting birds into their domiciles; therefore, certain precautions must be observed to mitigate hazards within the home. Chickens are indiscriminate with their

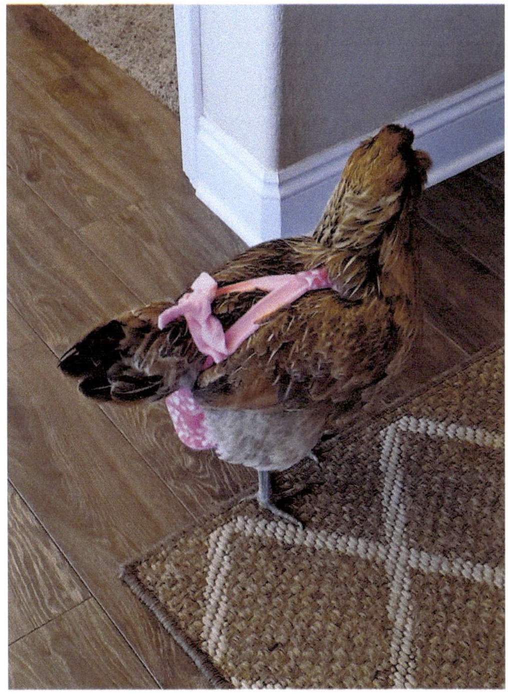

Figure 3.13 Hen with custom made diaper. Courtesy of Sarah Meyer.

droppings, though some caregivers report housetraining their fowl friends. To avoid having droppings littering the shared living quarters, washable diapers are available in many sizes. With diapers in place, the vent and cloaca can become soiled, so regular cleansing of the feathers and skin is necessary to prevent scalding (Figure 3.13).

Despite living in the house, house chickens should have a small hutch or similar enclosure for privacy, rest, and laying eggs. A medium-sized pet carrier, rabbit hutch, or dog crate is suitable for this purpose. Enclosures should be large enough for the bird to stand without its head touching the ceiling and allow for wing-stretching. With the same principle as a companion animal, chickens need their own "space" to retreat from visitors or when the caregiver is completing household tasks that may pose dangerous situations. Chickens are inquisitive and will swallow items thought to be food. Chicken-proofing the household decreases the risks of injury. Birds without clipped wing feathers can risk injury from ceiling fans.

Other household animals can injure chickens unintentionally or intentionally, so all animals must be supervised during interactions. Dogs and cats who resource-guard (food, treats, and toys) can injure or mortally wound a bird. Guardians should also supervise small children and inexperienced adults when they are handling chickens to avoid injury. Learning to read and acknowledge a bird's body language advocates for their welfare and emotional well-being.

House chickens can be fed commercial brands of pellets or crumbles with occasional vegetables and leafy greens. Cohabitating with people increases the chances of food scraps and treats being consumed; thus, monitoring the chicken's intake of such items is important to prevent obesity and obesity-related conditions. Refer to Chapter 4 for more information regarding nutritional requirements for chickens.

Further Reading

Admin A. Poultry Housing: Small Scale [Internet]. 2022 [cited 2025 Dec 8]. Available from: https://www.amerpoultryassn.com/2022/09/poultry-housing-small-scale/

Buy Chicken Coop Kits for Sale | Chicken Coop Enclosures [Internet]. Chickencoopcompany.com. 2024 [cited 2025 Dec 10]. Available from: https://www.chickencoopcompany.com/collections/chicken-coop-designs?srsltid=AfmBOorf8Zi3GTbPGWZjnS6_apjCsaYFJd4ElqrqpWXSqH2c7yb94gwi

IFAS Communications. Backyard Poultry - Escambia County - University of Florida, Institute of Food and Agricultural Sciences - UF/IFAS [Internet]. Ufl.edu. 2025 [cited 2025 Dec 10]. Available from: https://sfyl.ifas.ufl.edu/escambia/commercial-livestock/backyard-poultry/

Legal Protections for Chickens | Animal Legal & Historical Center [Internet]. www.animallaw.info. Available from: https://www.animallaw.info/intro/legal-protections-chickens

LLC P. Predator Proofing [Internet]. [cited 2025 Dec 8]. Available from: https://www.poultrydvm.com/topics/predator-proofing-chickens

Small-scale Poultry Housing [Internet]. 2023 [cited 2025 Dec 8]. Available from: https://www.pubs.ext.vt.edu/2902/2902-1092/2902-1092.html#:~:text=Poultry%20require%20a%20dry%2C%20draft,the%20coop%20and%20outside%20runs.

What Housing Do I Need for My Chickens? [Internet]. RSPCA Knowledgebase. 2023. Available from: https://kb.rspca.org.au/categories/companion-animals/other-pets/birds/backyard-poultry/what-housing-do-i-need-for-my-chickens

4

Nutritional Needs of Backyard Chickens

"You Are What You Eat."

Providing balanced, age-appropriate nutrition is fundamental to avoiding deficiency-related health issues and ensuring proper growth at each life stage of the chicken. Proper nutrition supports egg production, maintains feathering and plumage, functionality of the immune system, and overall health and welfare of backyard chickens. Chickens are omnivorous; therefore, feeding them a vegetarian diet is nonsensical and will cause nutritional deficiencies unless the diet is formulated with a veterinary nutritionist.

Many significant clinical signs, poor progressive growth, neuromuscular conditions, thin or soft eggshells, feather loss, and low egg output, are direct consequences of nutritional imbalances or deficiencies. This chapter examines nutrient categories, life stages (chicks, pullets, adults as layers or meat birds, and senior birds), typical feed types, how to read feed labels, typical state extension service recommendations, practical management of feed, and evaluation of diet via nutritional tools. Veterinary technicians can guide chicken guardians in proper nutrition or, at least, provide credible resources.

4.1 Nutrient Categories and What Healthy Chickens Require

Per the University of Maryland and Penn State Extension Services, the six categories for essential nutrients for poultry are: water, proteins (amino acids), carbohydrates, fats (lipids), vitamins, and minerals.

Water is often overlooked, but it is critical to every living organism, and it must be clean, fresh, and always available. Chickens utilize water in digestion, metabolism, egg production (albumin and yolk), and thermoregulation. Water intake can be 1.5–2× feed by weight in many conditions. If ambient temperatures or humidity are high, chickens will drink more water, so an adequate source must be provided to prevent dehydration and its associated effects. Water temperature can be amended depending on the ambient temperature to reduce the bird's energy needs.

Ensure waterers do not freeze in cold weather and do not get too warm in the warm months. Water warmers can be used in winter. Water coolers can be adapted as drinking implements, and ice blocks can be added to waterers to decrease birds' body temperatures and stress levels. Keep water clean and maintain sufficient waterers for the flock size to reduce competition. Water quality affects absorption and digestion. Supplements added to water are unnecessary if the guardian practices preventive healthcare measures and proper hygiene. If a bird's appetite decreases due to heat/humidity in summer months, electrolytes can be added to water to prevent or correct imbalances. Outdoor birds can easily succumb to hyperthermia, so cool water is essential for drinking and helping them thermoregulate.

4.1.1 Proteins and Amino Acids

Chickens are omnivores and require protein in their diets. Whether the source is animal- or plant-based, they need this nutrient for muscle, bone, skin, and other cell production. Proteins and amino acids are essential nutrients that cannot be synthesized, nor can they be stored in the body for later use. Examples are lysine, methionine, tryptophan, and threonine. Young chicks require higher protein levels to support growth, while pullets and laying hens need slightly lower protein, but higher amino acid balance. Elderly hens require a lower protein intake to support renal health. Roosters can eat "all flock" or shared feed with hens. Attention to breed (meat bird carbohydrate intake must be limited) should be considered when selecting a feed (Figure 4.1).

4.1.2 Carbohydrates

Carbohydrates in the form of grain provide energy. Corn, wheat, barley, and sorghum in scratch feed or a mixture of pellets (or crumbles) are the primary energy providers. A chicken's energy requirements vary with ambient temperature (decreased appetite in warmer weather, increased

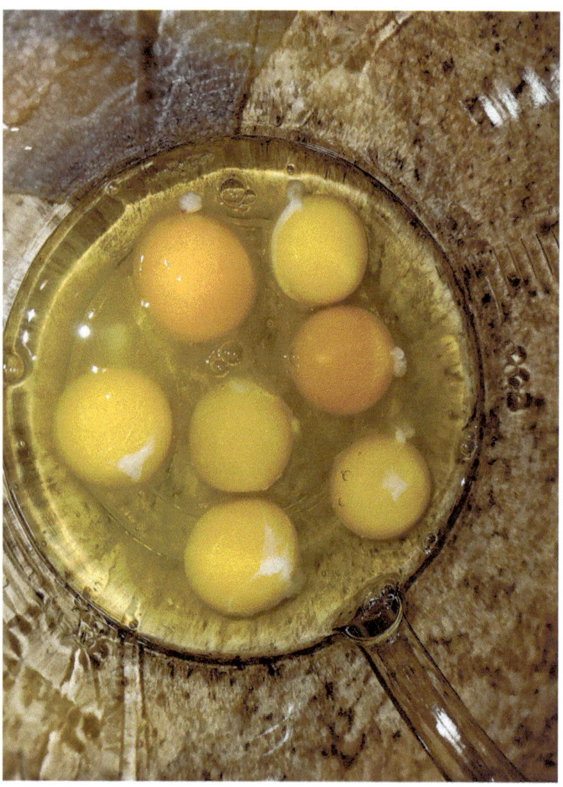

Figure 4.1 Egg yolks from backyard hens (orange yolks) and production layer hens. Courtesy of Sarah Meyer.

appetite in colder months), activity level, growth rate, or egg production. A high-carbohydrate diet with decreased activity results in fat deposition and obesity. These conditions lead to secondary maladies such as osteoarthritis of joints and cardiovascular disease (Figure 4.2).

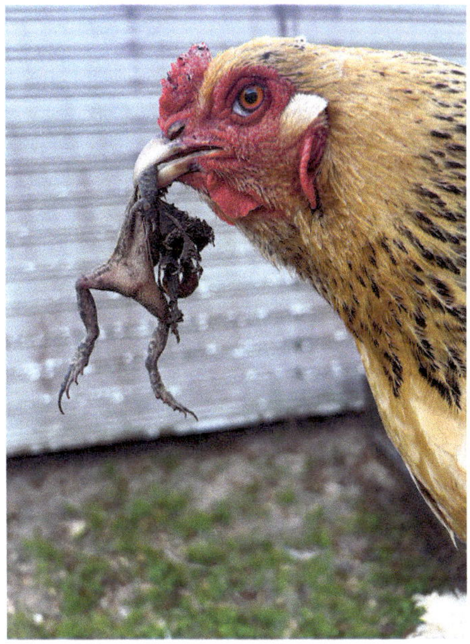

Figure 4.2 Chickens are indiscriminate consumers of protein and, if given the opportunity, will consume their own brethren. Adobe Stock image.

4.1.3 Fats and Lipids

Fats (lipids) are concentrated sources of energy that assist in the absorption of fat-soluble vitamins (A, D, E, and K). Some fatty acids are essential for the central nervous system, but an excess of lipids results in atherosclerosis. Snacks, such as cheese and fatty meats, should be fed sparingly. Cold weather can be better tolerated if fats are provided for energy density.

4.1.4 Microminerals and Macrominerals

Minerals are divided into macrominerals (needed in larger amounts) and microminerals (trace minerals), but all are essential for proper chicken nutrition. Calcium, either included in the feed or supplemented, is especially important in laying hens for eggshell quality and skeletal health. Lack of calcium requires the hen to use skeletal calcium and results in pathological fractures, like osteoporosis in humans. Many chicken guardians wash, crush, and refeed their hens' eggshells to supplement their calcium intake, which is acceptable if they have a constant source. Crushed oyster shells are slower to absorb and require less frequent ingestion. Feeds with high calcium content must be avoided in chicks, as it overloads immature kidneys, leading to damage and ultimately failure.

Along with calcium, phosphorus, magnesium, potassium, and sodium are needed for bone growth, fluid balance, and neuromuscular function. Trace minerals such as zinc, copper, iron, selenium, manganese, and iodine are necessary for enzyme functions, immune system function, feather pigmentation, and metabolic regulation. Vitamins are divided into two categories: fat-soluble and water-soluble. Fat-soluble vitamins include A, D, E, and K. Water-soluble vitamins include B complex and C. Vitamin D is critical for calcium absorption for bone strength and eggshell quality. Vitamin A is necessary for epithelial tissues and immunity. Vitamin E promotes antioxidant function and reproductive system performance. Water-soluble B vitamins support metabolism. Vitamin deficiencies can present in a subtle but acute manner (Figure 4.3). There is another table of nutrients in Chapter 15, Table 15.1.

When recommending chicken feed to a guardian, consultation with a nutritionist at a veterinary college or major feed manufacturer may be time-consuming, so reading feed bag labels is most effective. AAFCO (Association of American Feed Control Officials) is a nonprofit organization of U.S. and Canadian government agencies that sets ingredient definitions, label standards, and laboratory standards for animal feed. AAFCO does not approve or certify individual pet food products; instead, its nutrient profiles and feeding trial protocols are the backbone for most U.S. pet food

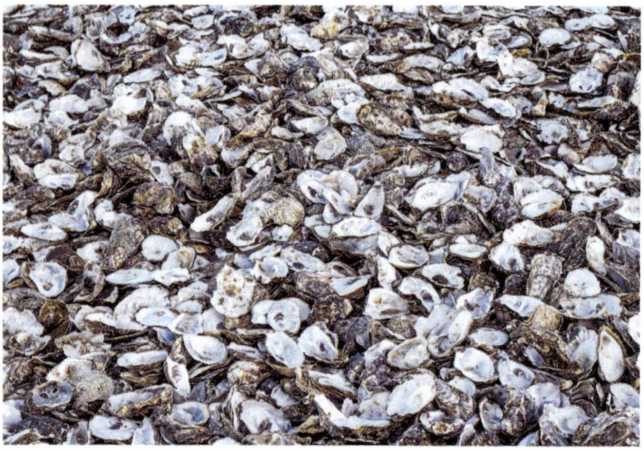

Figure 4.3 Commercially available crushed oyster shells for calcium supplementation. Lucy / Adobe Stock Photos.

labeling that is labeled "complete and balanced" for a specific life stage. Most major manufacturers of chicken feeds are geared toward large production birds, either layers or meat breeds. However, they offer feedstuffs in local farm supply stores and box stores to meet consumer needs for backyard flocks. In a similar fashion to companion animal food, there are boutique makers of chicken feeds. Most of these brands focus their operational budgets on marketing and not balanced nutrition or food trials. Rarely do these companies employ veterinarians with specialties in nutrition or poultry nutritionists.

4.2 Life Stage Nutritional Requirements

The nutritional requirements for the chicken life stages are pronounced. Chicks (0–6 weeks) require high protein (20–24%), high energy/carbohydrates, and modest calcium. Starter crumbles are commercially available in medicated and non-medicated forms. Medicated crumbles are advised for chicks with hens who are not regularly dewormed. Growing pullets require slightly less protein (16–18%), balanced energy/carbohydrates, and an increasing calcium and phosphorus content. Commercial "all flock" feeds are used at this stage. Supplemental fresh fruits and vegetables (washed before offering) can be introduced to this life stage of the bird. When pullets begin laying (now called hens), they are fed a lower protein feed (15–18%), but with a higher calcium, phosphorus, and vitamin D content for eggshell quality. Carbohydrates should be fed based on activity level to prevent obesity. If birds are intended for meat, they are "finished" on a high-protein, high-carbohydrate, and balanced diet to avoid metabolic disorders. Manufacturers create diets specifically for this purpose.

Special circumstances during a bird's life stages will require adjustments to their diet. Molting, cold weather, stress, or recovery from malady/surgery will increase nutritional requirements, such as the amount of protein, vitamins, and minerals provided.

Elderly/geriatric birds require less protein (reducing renal workload) and less calcium (unless hens are continuing to lay eggs) in their diet. Joint supplements for arthritic joint changes aid mobility, and prebiotics/probiotics ensure motility and gut microbiome. Other veterinarian-prescribed therapeutics are discussed in later chapters.

4.3 Feed Types, Reading Labels, and Feeding Tools

Reading and interpreting feed bag labels aids in the selection of a proper diet for chickens. The typical feed types are starter, grower, layer, all-flock or maintenance, and scratch grains. Treats and kitchen scraps are fed sparingly to not promote obesity or feed aversion (Figure 4.4).

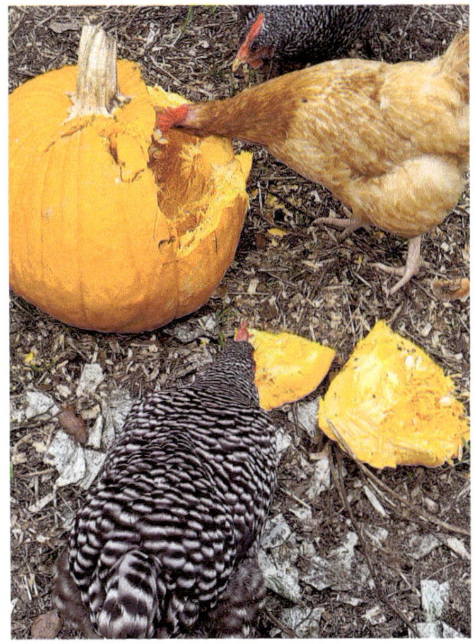

Figure 4.4 Occasional snacks, such as vegetables and leafy greens, are acceptable in a chicken's diet. Image courtesy of Sarah Meyer.

Crude protein should be listed as a percentage. Balanced amino acids are just as important as protein alone. Higher quality feed brands will list these nutrients in order of importance. Calcium/phosphorus is listed as a ratio. These two nutrients, mentioned previously, are vital to hens laying eggs. Fat adds energy, and fiber added to feed is less digestible but aids gut motility. Elevated fiber reduces energy density. Vitamins and minerals may or may not be listed on the label, as well as trace minerals.

The two most common forms of commercial chicken feed are compressed pellets and crumbles. Birds who are only fed a commercial feed (without the ability to free range or given regular treats or other options) tend not to sort through feed and have a more balanced diet. If given an option, chickens will eat the desired foodstuffs rather than pellets or crumbles, leading to nutritional imbalances and secondary effects. Starter crumble feeds are often medicated with a coccidiostat, and, despite what "keyboard warrior chicken experts" tout, virtually all flocks in the United States are exposed to coccidia and should be treated as chicks as if they already have coccidiosis (Figures 4.5 and 4.6).

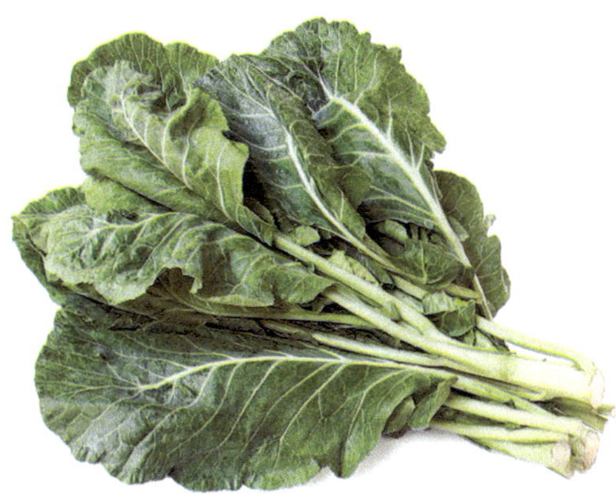

Figure 4.5 Collard and other greens can be fed to chickens. EvergreenPlanet / Adobe Stock Photos.

New, or established, chicken guardians can research credible online sources for "Chicken Feed Comparison Tools" to select a balanced commercial feed for their flock. These allow matching of a bird's nutrition needs, seeing how far from ideal a feed is, or determining whether supplementation is necessary. Boutique feed brands are usually more expensive, but not higher quality. Established manufacturers who employ veterinary nutritionists, conduct food trials, utilize research, and develop chicken feeds guarantee quality and favorable results if fed properly. Cheap "quantity over quality" feeds should be avoided.

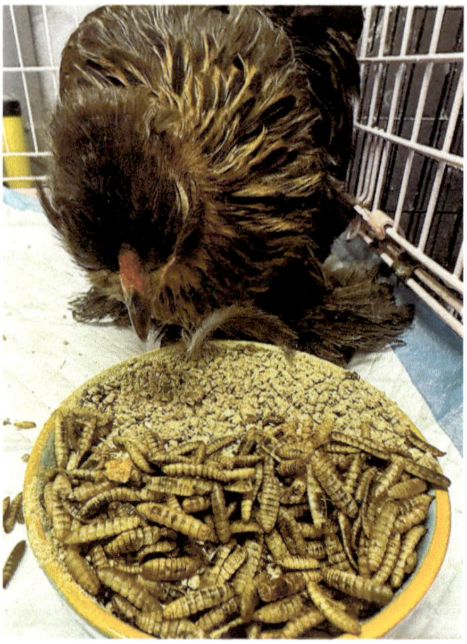

Figure 4.6 A hen enjoys crumbled feed and mealworms. Courtesy of Funky Chicken Rescue.

4.4 Examples of Extension Service Guidelines

Numerous U.S. state extension publications provide target nutrient levels and practical feeding recommendations.

- **Maine Cooperative Extension Bulletin #2222 ("Nutrition for Backyard Chicken Flocks in Maine")**: Gives tables for starter, grower, and layers; warns that feeding an immature chicken a layer diet leads to problems (e.g., kidney damage due to excess calcium); and feeding layers a broiler diet gives poor shell quality.
- **University of Georgia's "Nutrition for the Backyard Flock" (Circular C954)**: Emphasizes that no single ingredient has all nutrients—a well-formulated feed or careful mixing (with premixes) is needed; also, the importance of clean water.
- **Penn State Extension**: Notes that commercial feed must meet safety and quality standards; also gives guidance on estimating water needs and the influence of environmental temperature on feed intake and energy requirements.
- **Mississippi State University**: Points out common deficiencies (e.g., soft or thin eggshells often due to inadequate calcium), suggests that vitamin/mineral premixes are often the weak link in diet.

4.5 Common Deficiencies, Clinical Signs, and Interventions

An excess of one mineral can interfere with the absorption of the other or other minerals (e.g., excess calcium reducing absorption of zinc or magnesium). Recognition of dietary deficiencies or excesses can be remedied by adjusting feed, supplementation, and supportive care.

Concern	Nutrient(s) affected	Clinical signs	Intervention
Soft or thin eggshells	Calcium deficiency and/or vitamin D; phosphorus imbalance	Easily broken shells; deformed eggs; birds eat broken shells	Increase calcium intake by higher quality feed or oyster shell supplementation; sunlight for vitamin D synthesis
Slow growth	Low protein; poor amino acid balance, low phosphorus, or mineral deficiencies	Small egg size; leg abnormalities/ movement/growth; delayed feathering	Use proper starter feed by reading the label to ensure adequate phosphorus, calcium
Feather loss, poor molt recovery	Low protein; possible vitamin A, E, or trace mineral deficiency	Sparse feathers; dull feathers; slow regrowth	Increase protein intake; provide amino acid, vitamin/mineral supplementation; treat underlying stressors or parasites

Concern	Nutrient(s) affected	Clinical signs	Intervention
Reduced or late egg production	Inadequate energy (need more calories, protein)	Fewer eggs; irregular egg-laying; delay in pullet maturity	Increase energy by adjusting feed formulation
Obesity	Excess energy intake	Fat deposition; difficulty ambulating; decreased egg production or reproductive issues	Reduce high-calorie treats; adjust feed energy; encourage foraging and activity

Chart created by Stephanie Freeman.

4.6 Practical Feeding Management

When transitioning to progressive life stage feeds, a slow transition over at least a week (7–10 days mixing 10% more each day) duration is recommended to reduce digestive upset and microbiome disruption. Most flocks are fed ad libitum (free access) unless they are chicks or meat breed birds. Meat breeds benefit from scheduled feedings to promote appropriate growth rates. While tempting, do not mix calcium supplements to feed; allow the birds to choose when to consume calcium, as they inherently know when to add it to their diet. Overabundance of calcium, mentioned previously, causes renal disease in young birds. Place a separate bowl of oyster shells or ground limestone in the flock enclosure for layer hen free access. Grit should be provided for birds that do not have natural access to the ground or who eat whole grains (often included in scratch feeds) for digestion.

Allowance of foraging or free ranging provides a varied diet of protein, carbohydrates, and greens. This activity cannot replace a well-balanced diet of commercial feed. Treats should be less than 10% of the diet to not dilute essential nutrients. Microbiome additives are relatively safe and can be added to water or feed in times of stress or recovery.

With a mixed-age flock, "majority rules" unless accommodations can be made to ensure proper dietary requirements for each age group. A wire dog kennel can be placed inside the house or run for chicks to enter and eat age-appropriate crumbles without compromising laying hens' nutritional needs. Due to hierarchical order, chickens will resource-guard, and attention must be given to lower-level birds to ensure they are eating and drinking adequately (Figure 4.7).

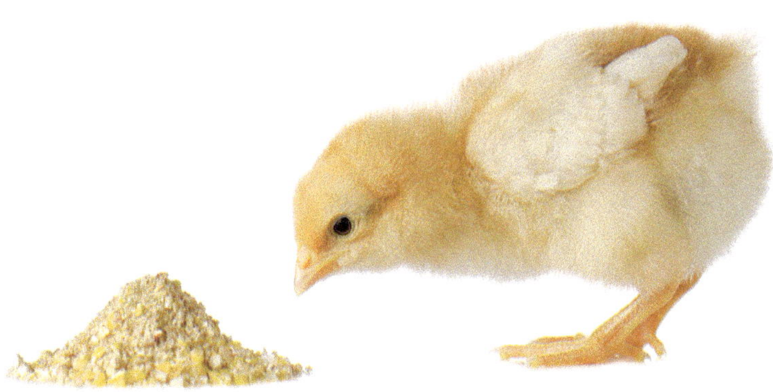

Figure 4.7 Chick feed contains amprolium for treatment of coccidia. Ljupco Smokovski / Adobe Stock Photos.

Chickens will develop a preference for different feeds if available, which can lead to spoilage and waste of undesirable options. This availability leads to the attraction of pests, namely rodents. Feed manufacturers develop sizes, shapes, and colors of feeds that appeal to hens (and caregivers), so finding the right feed that meets all nutritional requirements can be a challenge for the chicken guardian. Unless scratch feed contains balanced nutrition, it should be fed sparingly as a treat, not a main feed source. As mentioned before, selecting a well-established feed producer typically results in healthy birds with nutritional needs met. A quality feed need not be costly to be effective but should be reputable and well-established. Credible resources can aid the veterinary technician to guide the caregiver with the selection of a well-balanced diet for their chicken(s) (Figures 4.8–4.10).

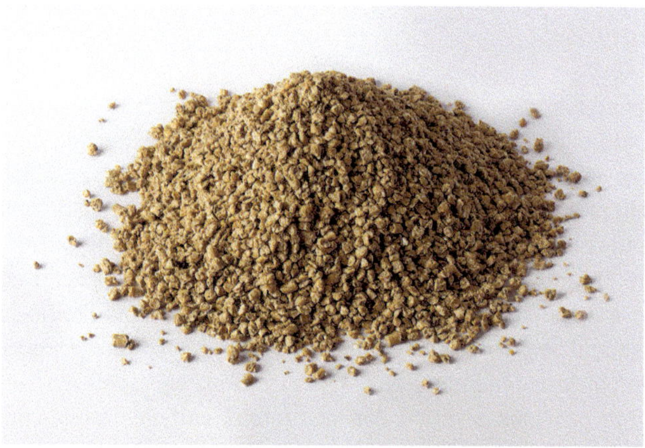

Figure 4.8 Crumbled feed for laying hens. Shamil / Adobe Stock Photos.

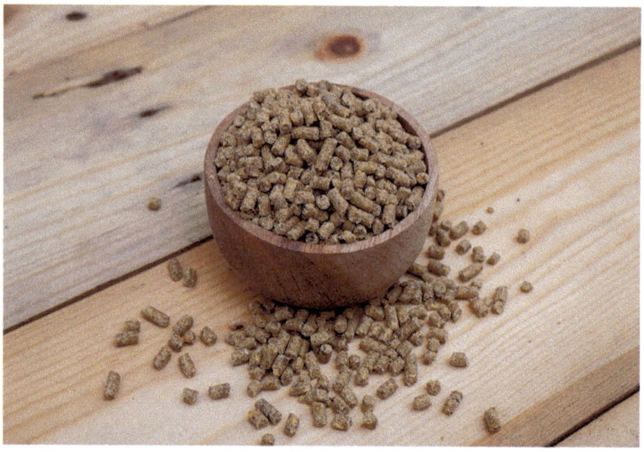

Figure 4.9 Pelleted feed for laying hens. Muhammad / Adobe Stock Photos.

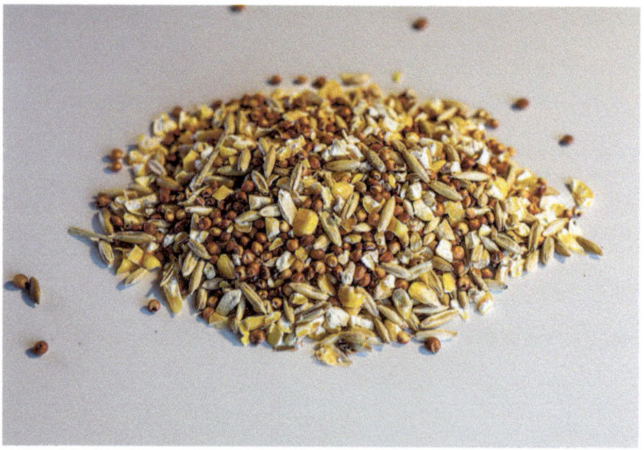

Figure 4.10 Scratch feed for adult chickens. BONNIE C. MARQUETTE / Adobe Stock Photos.

Further Reading

Fowler J. Nutrition for the Backyard Flock [Internet]. 2025 [cited 2025 Dec 7]. Available from: https://fieldreport.caes.uga.edu/publications/C954/nutrition-for-the-backyard-flock/

Bulletin #2222, Nutrition for Backyard Chicken Flocks in Maine - Cooperative Extension Publications University of Maine Cooperative Extension [Internet]. 2024 [cited 2025 Dec 7]. Available from: https://extension.msstate.edu/agriculture/livestock/poultry/feeds-and-nutrition

Successfully Raising a Small Flock of Laying Chickens [Internet]. [cited 2025 Dec 7]. Available from: https://extension.psu.edu/successfully-raising-a-small-flock-of-laying-chickens

5

Behavior, Body Language, and Vocalizations

5.1 Clinical Importance of Chicken Behavior

Behavior is the external expression of the bird's welfare state, health status, and environment. For the veterinary technician, subjective and objective data collection regarding behavior are both a diagnostic clue and an intervention target. Changes in activity, appetite, vocalization, or social interaction are often the first signs of disease or stress. The veterinary healthcare team will determine if the cause of abnormal behavior has a medical cause or is strictly psychological. Behavior also directly affects the success of medical treatments (e.g., broody hens who are anorexic or roosters that continue mating despite injury). Understanding both normal and abnormal behaviors improves triage and treatment, monitoring, client education, and prevention strategies. For a clinical standpoint, see Chapter 6, Physical Examination.

Key clinical uses of behavior observations:

- Early disease detection (lethargy, altered perching, and foraging changes).
- Identifying social stressors that precipitate injuries (fights and pecking).
- Designing environmental changes that prevent recurrence (enrichment and resource distribution).
- Supporting client adherence, owners are more likely to follow recommendations when a veterinary technician gives clear, practical behavior-based instructions.

5.2 Daily Observation Parameters

Teach guardians to perform twice-daily checks and document the following:

- **General Behavior**: Activity level, alertness, and flock interaction
- **Appetite and Water Intake**: Record feed and water consumption
- **Droppings**: Consistency, color, and frequency (note any blood, mucus, or urates)
- **Body Condition**: Assess keel prominence and weight weekly
- **Mobility**: Gait, wing usage, and balance
- **Respiratory Status**: Watch for open-mouth breathing, nasal discharge, and sneezing
- **Skin/Feather Condition**: Examine for new lesions, swelling, and feather loss

5.3 When to Seek Immediate Veterinary Attention

Provide guardians with "red flags" requiring urgent care or necropsy:

- Hemorrhage from wounds and broken blood feathers
- Sudden death or rapid deterioration
- Severe respiratory distress
- Neurological signs (seizures, head tremors, and paralysis)
- Profuse diarrhea, bloody droppings, or persistent anorexia
- Swollen joints, severe lameness, or bone fractures
- Any signs of pain, distress, or unresponsive behavior

5.4 What Is "Normal" Behavior for a Chicken?

- **Foraging and Pecking:** Chickens spend a large portion of daylight hours searching for food, scratching, pecking at soil and objects, and exploring small items that could potentially be edible. Foraging is strongly motivated and satisfies both nutritional and cognitive needs. Chickens are omnivorous, and if allowed to free-range, will consume edible insects, small amphibians, reptiles, rodents, and anything else they can capture. They will also pick grass and growing plants and vegetables.
- **Dustbathing**: A maintenance behavior used for feather hygiene and external parasite control. Dustbathing is highly motivated and social; deprivation leads to frustration and redirected pecking or feather-pulling. Plain soil, with or without dry additives, is desirable for dustbathing. One or more dry, specified containers can be made available in the pen or run.
- **Perching and Roosting:** As a prey species, chickens prefer to roost off the ground at night; perching behavior is a strong, species-typical preference and important to provide for welfare. Perches of various heights serve the hierarchical needs of a flock.
- **Preening and Feather Maintenance:** Frequent grooming with the beak and head-rubbing throughout the day involves the removal of external parasites, dirt, dander, and sheaths; reduced preening is a sign of malaise, which can be of a psychological or physical cause. Molting is discussed in more detail in Chapter 7.
- **Social Interactions and Vocalizations:** Chickens are highly social animals, and companionship provides mental stimulation unless there is bullying amongst flock mates. Cliques can be formed, especially amongst same-breed hens. Communication amongst flock members consists of a repertoire of calls such as alarm calls (predator or intruder), contact calls (varying degrees of greetings), and food purrs. Chickens have a complex social behavior that includes affiliative and agonistic interactions.
- **Reproductive Behaviors:** Roosters show courtship and protective displays, while hens show nesting and, in some breeds, broody behavior (sitting on eggs, reduced food/drink intake, maternal defensive behavior).
- **Hierarchal Behaviors:** Regardless of presence of a rooster, hens will establish a pecking order from most dominant (matriarch) to least dominant. The order may change because of a traumatic event, absence of the matriarch, injury/illness, or for no apparent reason.

Understanding these base chicken behaviors will help the veterinary technician distinguish normal variation (breed differences, age-related change, productivity cycles) from clinical concerns (Figures 5.1 and 5.2).

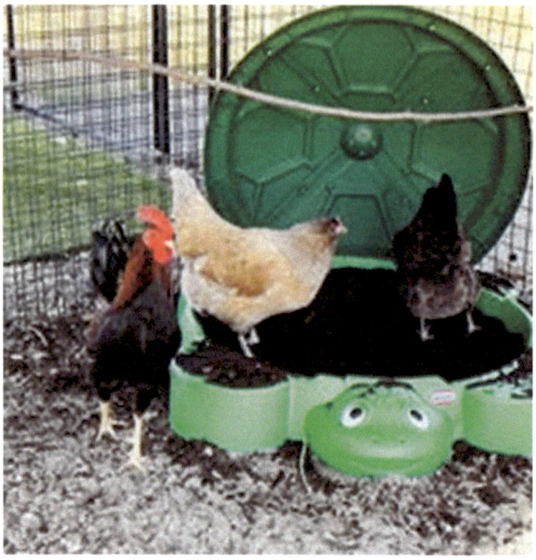

Figure 5.1 Providing an area for dustbathing allows chickens to exhibit natural social and hygiene behaviors. Courtesy of Funky Chicken Rescue.

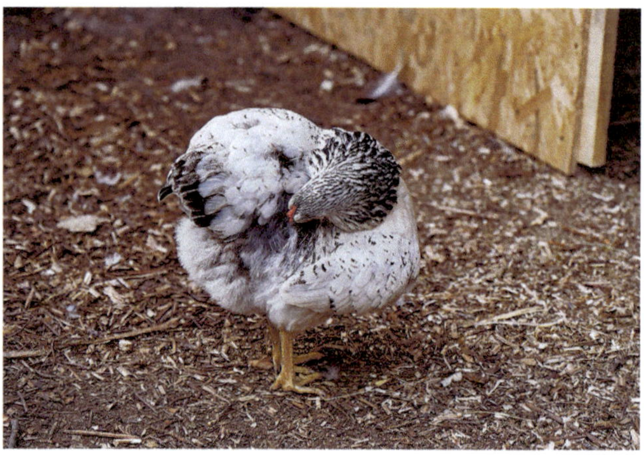

Figure 5.2 Preening is important for hygiene and socialization. Chickens will often preen their companions. Loginova / Adobe Stock Photos.

5.5 Rooster Behavior

Roosters exhibit a wide range of complex behaviors that reflect both their evolutionary origins and their domestication. Understanding rooster behavior is essential for veterinary technicians working with poultry in backyard and clinical settings. Veterinary technicians play a vital role in interpreting behavior during handling, restraint, clinical assessment, and client education. Failure to recognize normal versus abnormal behaviors can lead to misinterpretation, injury risk, or overlooking underlying health problems.

Roosters descend from the red junglefowl of Southeast Asia, which live in social groups led by one or more dominant males. Modern roosters retain many ancestral traits, including vigilance, territorial defense, and hierarchical dominance. Unlike hens, whose maternal behavior focuses on foraging and brooding, roosters primarily serve protective and reproductive roles.

In natural settings, a rooster watches for predators, alerts the flock, directs hens to food resources, and competes with rival males. Domestication has modified the expression of these instincts but not eliminated them. Breed selection also influences behavior; ornamental and game breeds may

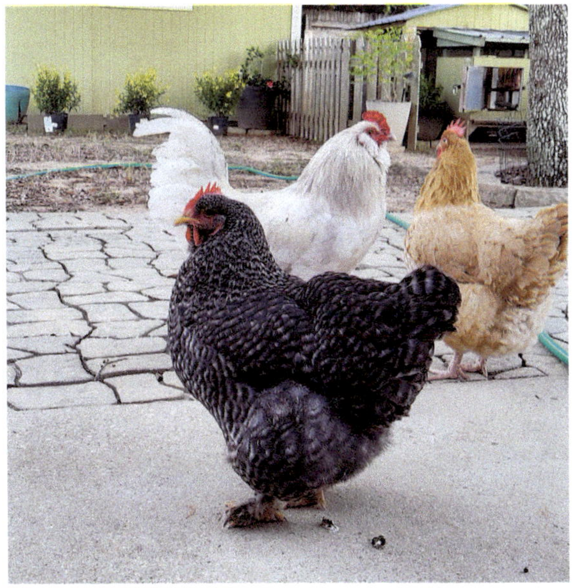

Figure 5.3 White Easter Egger rooster with Cochin-cross and Buff Orpington hens. Courtesy of Sarah Meyer.

show heightened aggression, whereas dual-purpose or production (meat or egg) breeds often display more docility.

Roosters defend defined territories, particularly around food and hens. Encroachment by rival males may trigger aggressive displays, sparring, or sustained combat. Veterinary technicians should recognize that confined environments amplify territorial aggression, increasing injury risk in multi-rooster flocks (Figure 5.3).

5.5.1 Aggression

Aggression is one of the most notable aspects of rooster behavior. It is both hormonally influenced and environmentally modulated. Upright posture, hackle feather raising, wing flapped, and direct eye contact are all visual threats. Pecking, wing beating, flogging, and chasing are all physical attacks. Some notable triggers for these behaviors are the presence of another rooster, perceived intruders (including humans), insufficient space, or lack of environmental enrichment.

Some roosters may over-mate or mate too vigorously, causing feather loss, skin damage, or wounds in hens (especially on the head, back, vent, or dorsal midline). Rooster versus rooster fights can escalate to severe injury or death, especially when subordinate roosters challenge dominant ones. Fights often involve pecking, spur strikes, and loud wing flapping. Some roosters may become aggressive toward caretakers, such as spur attacks, pecking at legs, or trying to mount human hands perceived as "competing" for the hens. This is more likely when roosters regard the handler as part of the flock hierarchy. Recognition of dominant cues by humans (such as picking up hens or moving through the run abruptly) may provoke aggression in some roosters. Sometimes aggression is exhibited, regardless of early handling as chicks.

5.5.1.1 A Side Note About Spurs

Roosters evolved spurs, sharp bony projections on the medial aspect of the legs, for battling rival males. In some online forums, caregivers are encouraged to "remove" their rooster's spurs with pliers. This act is equivalent to removing a human's fingernails without anesthesia. Spurs

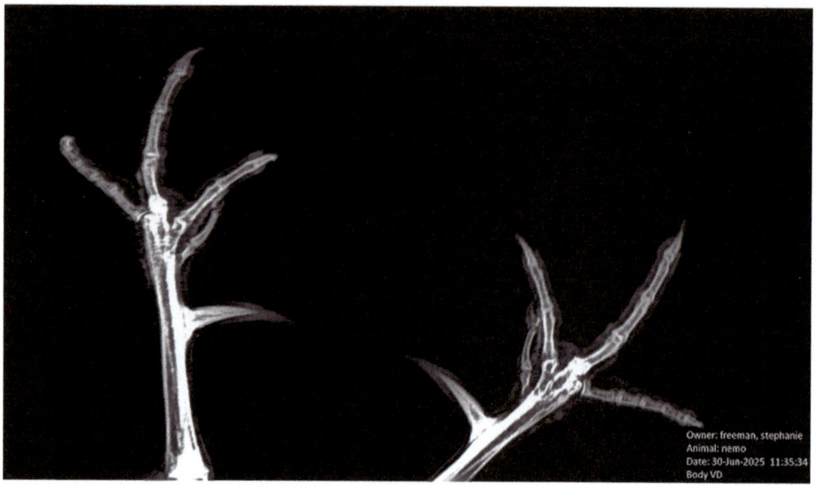

Figure 5.4 Radiographic image of rooster distal limbs and feet. Note the bones within each spur. Removing the cuticle does not result in absolute spur necrosis. The cuticle will regenerate. Clipping and filing of spurs regularly is recommended to prevent injury to caregivers and hens. Photo courtesy of Stephanie Freeman.

are not vestigial and possess a blood supply and nerves. Nerves transmit noxious stimuli (via the pain pathway) to the central nervous system (brain). Not only is this removal painful, but it is also inhumane. Early handling of a male chick does not guarantee a friendly rooster, but restraining and injuring him certainly does not establish a positive relationship or prevent future attacks.

Spurs can be regularly clipped and filed, using an electric sanding tool with a barrel attachment. Rewarding the rooster with tasty treats and soothing words will acclimate him to handling with positive reinforcement, thus making the next interaction less stressful for all involved. Roosters can be sedated by the veterinarian to expedite this procedure if the rooster is anxious or needs other procedures performed.

Reproductively mature hens can develop spurs, seemingly prevalent in breeds with Mediterranean origins. All chickens have rudimentary spur "buds," but not all females will develop spurs of noteworthy length. These hens can also have their spurs clipped and filed regularly (Figure 5.4).

5.5.2 Reproductive and Courtship Behavior

Roosters engage in complex displays to attract and court hens. These behaviors provide insight into hormonal health and social stability.

- **Tid-bitting**: A rooster clucks (chuckles) while pecking at food, offering it to hens. This behavior reinforces his social role and mating success. He may also use this vocalization for deceit.
- **Courtship Dance**: Dropping one wing while circling a hen, often followed by mounting.
- **Crowing**: A signature vocalization used to advertise territory and reproductive status. Frequency and intensity may increase with perceived (or actual) competition.
- **Mating**: Quick copulation involving mounting, clutching of the hen's head feathers, cloacal contact, and sperm transfer (Figure 5.5).

5.5.3 Communication and Vocalizations

Roosters are highly vocal birds, with over 20 recognized call types. Key examples include:

- **Crowing**: Territorial announcements often performed at dawn but also throughout the day
- **Alarm Calls**: Distinct vocalizations for aerial predators (short, sharp clucks) versus ground threats (longer, lower calls or "churtles")
- **Food Calls**: Soft, repetitive clucks to attract hens to discovered food
- **Aggressive Calls**: Harsh, repetitive sounds preceding combat

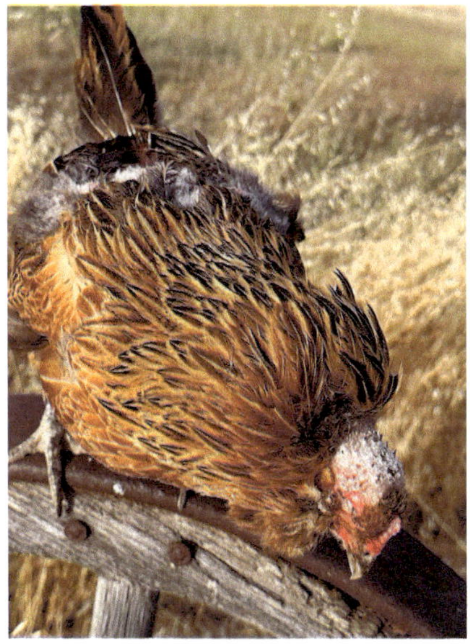

Figure 5.5 Hen with typical feather loss and injuries associated with vigorous over-mating from a rooster. Courtesy of Funky Chicken Rescue.

5.5.4 Environmental and Management Influences

Rooster behavior is strongly shaped by housing, flock composition, and human interaction. Crowding increases aggression and stress. One rooster per 8–12 hens minimizes over-mating and aggression. Access to perches, dust baths, and foraging opportunities reduces undesirable behaviors. Roosters accustomed to calm, consistent handling as juveniles are generally less aggressive toward humans. In contrast, frequent rough handling or inconsistent interaction may heighten fear and aggression.

5.5.5 Client Education

Veterinary technicians are central in helping owners understand rooster behavior and manage expectations, while also teaching owners safe handling protocols (protective clothing, minimal handling, awareness of spur risk). Encourage clients not to treat roosters like pets in the same way as hens; showing dominance (e.g., picking hens up in front of the rooster) may provoke aggression. Emphasize that gentling is gradual; owners must be consistent and patient. Trimming and filing of spurs is also recommended to avoid puncture injuries to the caregiver.

Advise clients to select roosters from flocks with stable social dynamics, or from breeding programs that test temperament. Recommend additional spacing, resource planning, and provision for future rehoming if behavior becomes unmanageable.

5.6 Hen Behavior

Hens are highly social and intelligent animals whose behavior reflects both their evolutionary origins and their adaptation to domestication. Understanding hen behavior is essential for veterinary technicians, since much of the information obtained during a clinical encounter comes from interpreting behavioral cues. Moreover, veterinary technicians often serve as the bridge between scientific knowledge and client management, helping backyard and small-scale poultry owners recognize normal versus abnormal behaviors.

The domestic hen, like the rooster, descends from the red jungle fowl of Southeast Asia. In the wild, junglefowl hens spend most of their time foraging, dust bathing, and nesting. Domesticated hens retain these instinctive behaviors or desires, even under intensive production systems.

Hens establish clear dominance hierarchies, commonly referred to as the "pecking order." This determines the priority of access to food, water, nesting sites, and preferred roosting spots. Dominant hens may peck or chase subordinates to reinforce their position. In the presence or absence of a rooster to a flock, hens will exhibit a matriarchal hierarchy.

5.6.1 Reproductive and Nesting Behavior

Hens display distinct reproductive behaviors, even in the absence of roosters.

- **Pre-laying Restlessness**: Hens vocalize, scratch, and pace before selecting a nest to lay an egg.
- **Nest Site Fidelity**: Once a site is chosen, hens often return repeatedly, reinforcing flock nesting traditions. Often, the entire flock has a preferred nest box despite other available boxes.
- **Cackling**: A loud, distinctive vocalization following egg laying, believed to advertise reproductive success or distract potential predators. Commonly referred to as the "egg song."

5.6.2 Hen Communication and Vocalization

Hens use a rich repertoire of vocalizations and body language to communicate. Certain breeds and birds are more vocal than others.

- **Clucking**: Contentment or maternal contact calls.
- **Alarm Calls**: Distinct vocalizations for aerial versus ground threats.
- **Purring or Trilling**: Indicates relaxation, often during foraging or resting.
- **Distress Calls**: Loud, repetitive cries signaling pain, isolation, or predator presence.
- **Crowing**: Loud vocalizations with similar posturing to rooster behavior

Non-verbal cues, such as feather positioning, crouching, or wing spreading, also convey emotional states. For example, crouching with wings slightly spread (squatting) may signal receptivity to mating or, in a clinical setting, submission to restraint.

5.6.3 Foraging and Enrichment Needs

One of the strongest behavioral drives in hens is foraging. Even when food is freely available, hens spend hours pecking and scratching. The deprivation of this outlet is a major contributor to feather pecking and cannibalism. Veterinary technicians should emphasize to clients that hens require access to litter or soil substrates for scratching, provision of varied diet items or enrichment (scatter feeding, vegetables, insect protein such as mealworms or other larvae), and adequate outdoor access in supervised free range or secure backyard systems. Failure to provide environmental enrichment not only reduces welfare but also predisposes to behavioral/psychological pathologies that may be present in clinical practice.

5.6.4 Human-Hen and Other Species Interactions

Hens are generally less aggressive toward humans than roosters, but individual temperament varies. Birds raised with consistent, gentle handling are calmer and more approachable. Stress behaviors during handling include wing flapping, vocal distress, and attempts to flee.

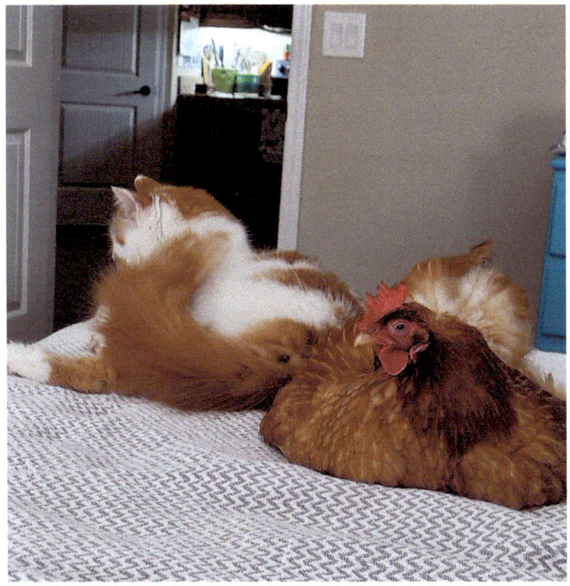

Figure 5.6 Hen and a feline friend. Courtesy of Sarah Meyer.

Regardless of sex, chickens can develop amicable relationships with their human(s) and seek their attention. Hens and roosters alike see "their" humans as flock mates and will ask for affection. Chickens will also occasionally develop bonds with other social species if chickens are not available for same-species socialization (Figure 5.6).

5.6.5 Environmental and Management Influences

Hens' behavior is strongly shaped by their environment. Crowding exacerbates aggression and feather pecking. Recommended spacing varies by system, but backyard hens generally require 8–10 sq. ft. per bird outdoors. Photoperiod manipulation influences egg production and behavior. Excessive light intensity increases aggression, whereas insufficient light can suppress normal activity. One nest per 2–3 hens reduces competition and stress. Elevated roosts satisfy natural roosting instincts and reduce floor aggression.

5.7 Social Structure, Dominance, and the Pecking Order

Social hierarchies (pecking orders) reduce constant conflict by establishing predictable access to resources. Dominance relationships are enforced by pecking, chasing, and postural displays. Disruptions (introducing new birds, reintroducing convalescent birds, and abrupt resource changes) trigger renewed challenges and fights. Aggression and fights commonly occur during hierarchy establishment or when resources (feeders, waterers, nest boxes, and roosts) are limited; veterinary technicians will frequently see injuries from such fights. Practical recognition and management of fights are core skills (separate aggressive birds, inspect injuries, and advise owners on space/resources).

The term "pecking order" was coined by Thorleif Schjelderup-Ebbe (1921) from his observations of domestic hens. It describes a linear dominance hierarchy, where each bird knows its place relative to others. Dominance is established and reinforced through pecking, chasing, feather pulling, or threat displays. The alpha (top hen or rooster) has priority access to food, mates, and preferred perches. Subordinates yield to higher-ranking individuals, reducing the need for constant physical conflict.

Pecking (hierarchical) orders are most actively formed when new birds are introduced or during early life. Chicks start showing dominance behaviors as early as 1–3 weeks old. Challenges to the hierarchy occur, especially when resources are limited or when a top bird is removed. Once established, the pecking order provides social stability. Most interactions become ritualized (threats without actual pecking).

Provide ample feeders and waterers to reduce resource guarding. Ensure adequate space per bird (minimum ~4 sq. ft. indoors, 8–10 sq. ft. outdoors). When introducing new chickens, use gradual methods (see-but-don't-touch enclosures, nighttime introductions). Observe flocks regularly to catch severe bullying (feather loss, wounds, isolation of low-ranking birds).

5.8 Environmental Contributors and Prevention Strategies

Many behavior problems are environmental in origin and thus are among the most modifiable.

Crowding increases aggressive interactions and pecking. Ensure adequate feeder and waterer space, nest boxes, and perches per bird. High light intensity and long photo periods can increase activity and aggression; gradual changes in light and reducing intensity can help mitigate problem pecking. Bare runs without a scratchable substrate elevated redirected pecking; providing litter, scatter feed, or foraging enrichment reduces the risk. Access to perches reduces ground crowding and provides an outlet for normal roosting behavior. Adequate nest boxes reduce competition and associated aggression.

Enrichment addresses cognitive, sensory, social, and foraging motivations. Practical options include puzzle feeders, pecking objects, hanging vegetables or cabbage, varied substrate piles, logs and branches for perching/climbing, and objects that encourage manipulation. Enrichment reduces boredom and many redirected pecking behaviors when implemented thoughtfully.

5.9 Common Abnormal Behaviors

Abnormal behaviors may be the primary reason clients call the veterinary hospital.

5.9.1 Feather Pecking and Severe Feather Pecking (SFP)

Presentation: Vigorous pecking and feather pulling directed at flock mates, leading to feather loss, skin trauma, and sometimes cannibalism.

Causes and Risk Factors: Multifactorial, overcrowding, lack of enrichment/foraging opportunities, poor nutrition, light management (intensity/photoperiod), breed predisposition, stress, and disease. Feather pecking is a redirected foraging behavior in many cases.

Actions: Triage the victims: treat wounds, prevent ongoing pecking (protective jackets, topical wound protection, separation in a calm recovery location). Assess flock/environment: bird density, enrichment availability, feed form/access, light intensity, recent changes (new birds, feed changes). Advice should be shared regarding environmental modifications such as foraging opportunities (scatter scratch grains and treats in deep litter and hang foraging/puzzle toys), reducing light intensity and sudden light changes, and redistribution of resources, and ensuring that food and waterers are adequate for the flock size. Sometimes, either the bully or the victim requires rehoming.

5.9.2 Vent Pecking

Presentation: Targeted pecking at the vent area; can be rapidly fatal if not controlled.

Causes: Any condition exposing red tissue (bleeding, prolapse), or cases where fecal matter around the vent attracts pecking. Hens with prolapse or recent egg-laying trauma are at risk.

Actions: Isolate and treat the victim, clean the wound, apply protective barrier and dressings, and remove or treat the underlying trigger (e.g., reduce prolapse, correct infection). Provide protective gear (no-peck shields or a diaper). Recommend a temporary reduction in light and increase environmental enrichment to redirect pecking (Figure 5.7).

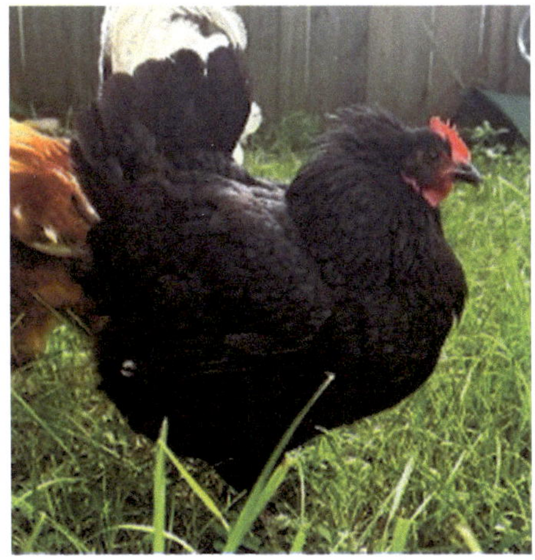

Figure 5.7 Broody hen. Courtesy of Stephanie Freeman.

5.9.3 Excessive or Extreme Broodiness

In some cases, hens may exhibit broodiness, which is persistent nesting behavior coupled with refusal to leave the nest, puffed feathers, and aggressive defense of eggs. While broodiness is natural, it can present husbandry challenges and health risks. Veterinary technicians can educate owners on strategies for managing broodiness, such as removing eggs or providing environmental modifications.

Presentation: Hen sits persistently on a nest or eggs (or even in a nest-box with no eggs), becomes easily agitated and puffs feathers to appear larger, often reduces feed/water intake due to reluctance to leave the nest, aggressive vocalizations and pecking when disturbed, and develops a brood patch (feather loss on breast to incubate eggs).

Clinical Importance: Broodiness can be normal maternal behavior but becomes an owner concern when hens stop laying eggs or lose body condition and body weight due to anorexia. Hens can experience heat stress during the summer months. Eggbinding can occur if laying resumes prematurely. Management can be medical (hormone implantation), environmental (discourage or prevent nest access), or surgical, in refractory cases.

5.9.4 Stereotypic and Redirected Behaviors

These include repetitive pacing, obsessive pecking at non-food objects, or abnormal feather plucking. These behaviors are often linked to inadequate environmental complexity, chronic stress, or restricted foraging opportunities. Birds rescued from production farms often display these behaviors.

5.9.5 Post-Predator Trauma and Fear Responses

Birds surviving predator attacks often display shock, flightiness, hidden wounds, and long-lasting behavioral changes (hypervigilance, separation anxiety, reluctance to roost). Veterinary technicians should evaluate physical injury with the veterinarian and advise the guardian on gradual reconditioning and environmental security.

5.9.6 Egg-Eating

Consumption of a hen's own eggs, or of others, is a sign of boredom, nutritional deficiencies (protein, methionine, or sodium), or opportunistic consumption if the egg is broken. Lack of foraging outlets is also a reason for egg breaking and eating. Collection of eggs soon after lay is recommended, and using a "dummy" egg in each nest is advised.

5.10 Behavior Assessment Checklist for Clinical or Caregiver Use

Activity	Degree
Foraging activity	( )Normal ( )Decreased ( )Absent
Dustbathing	( )Performed ( )Reduced ( )Absent
Perching/roosting	( )Normal ( )Reluctant ( )Abnormal Location
Preening	( )Normal ( )Decreased ( )Excessive
Social interactions	( )Calm ( )Increased Aggression ( )Avoidance ( )Solitary
Vocalization	( )Appropriate ( )Decreased ( )Loud Distress Calls
Feather condition	( )Intact ( )Moderate Loss ( )Severe Loss ( )Wound
Feeding and drinking	( )Normal ( )Reduced ( )Refusal
Locomotion	( )Normal ( )Ataxic ( )Reluctant to Move

Chart courtesy of Stephanie Freeman.

Further Reading

Behavior of Poultry - Behavior [Internet]. [cited 2025 Dec 8]. Available from: https://www.merckvetmanual.com/behavior/behavior-of-poultry/behavior-of-poultry#General-Behaviors_v99417883

Chickens' Startlingly Complex Social and Emotional Lives [Internet]. Sussex Publishers; [cited 2025 Dec 8]. Available from: https://www.psychologytoday.com/us/blog/animal-emotions/202408/chickens-startlingly-complex-social-and-emotional-lives

Marino L. Thinking Chickens: A Review of Cognition, Emotion, and Behavior in the Domestic Chicken [Internet]. U.S. National Library of Medicine; 2017 [cited 2025 Dec 8]. Available from: https://pmc.ncbi.nlm.nih.gov/articles/PMC5306232/

Miller M. Unlocking the Mysteries of the Pecking Order [Internet]. 2022 [cited 2025 Dec 7]. Available from: https://www.uc.edu/news/articles/2022/01/pecking-order--uc-biologist-explains-100-years-of-dominance-hierarchies.html

Posted by: Brigid McCrea and Bethany Baker. Common Backyard Chicken Behaviors [Internet]. 2024 [cited 2025 Dec 8]. Available from: https://www.aces.edu/blog/topics/farming/common-backyard-chicken-behaviors/

6

Physical Exam

The physical examination (PE) is the cornerstone of avian veterinary medicine. In chickens, a thorough and systematic exam provides critical diagnostic information, often before laboratory or imaging results are performed or available. For veterinary technicians, mastering the physical examination is essential not only for supporting the veterinarian but also for triaging emergencies, monitoring hospitalized patients, and educating clients.

Because chickens are prey species, they instinctively mask signs of illness until disease is advanced. Subtle abnormalities in posture, weight, feather condition, or behavior may be the earliest indicators of underlying pathology. A methodical approach to examination ensures that veterinary technicians identify key changes while minimizing stress to the patient.

Before examining the chicken patient, preparation is key. Quiet, dimly lit rooms with nonslip flat surfaces reduce stress. Avoid placing the bird near predator species (cats, dogs, raptors, and wild carnivores). A tabletop scale, stethoscope with pediatric diaphragm, pen light, ophthalmoscope, otoscope, oral speculum, nail clippers, and restraint aids (towels, gloves) are prepared. A dedicated exam room that can be properly disinfected and hand hygiene helps prevent cross-contamination between flocks and other avian patients. Roosters may spur or peck, and hens may flap vigorously in efforts to escape. Long sleeves, gloves, and eye protection are advisable when the risk of injury is high. Birds that have been frequently handled by caregivers are typically collaborative with their handling and treatment.

6.1 Observation Prior to Handling

- **Demeanor:** Alertness, responsiveness, posture. Compromised chickens may appear hunched, with ruffled feathers and closed eyes, and disinterested.
- **Mobility:** Observe gait and wing carriage. Lameness may signal bumblefoot (pododermatitis), arthritis, or neurologic disease. Loose wings may indicate heat stress or lethargy.
- **Respiration:** Watch for open-mouth dyspneic breathing, tail-bobbing, wheezes, sneezes, or discharge from nares or beak.
- **Droppings:** Note consistency, color, and presence of urates or blood, as these are important diagnostic clues (Figure 6.1).

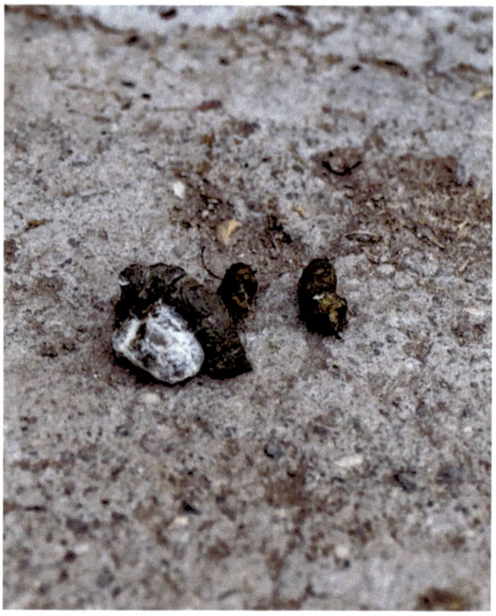

Figure 6.1 Normal droppings. Photo courtesy of Sarah Meyer.

Teach guardians to perform twice-daily checks and document the following:

- **General Behavior:** Activity level, alertness, and flock interaction
- **Appetite and Water Intake:** Record feed and water consumption
- **Droppings:** Consistency, color, frequency (note any blood, mucus, or urates)
- **Body Condition:** Assess keel prominence and weight weekly
- **Mobility:** Gait, wing usage, and balance
- **Respiratory Status:** Observe for open-mouth breathing, nasal discharge, and sneezing
- **Skin/Feather Condition:** Examine for new lesions, swelling, and feather loss

Chart created by Stephanie Freeman.

6.2 Obtaining Subjective Data and History

Asking caregivers open-ended questions about the patient guides the veterinary technician in what diagnostic testing or treatments the veterinarian may want performed. This method of obtaining a history also expedites the appointment to ensure the patient receives adequate examination time.

6.3 Signalment and History

- **Name and Species:** What is the chicken's name, and what is the breed? Even if obvious, the caregiver may not know. Certain breeds are predisposed to diseases.
- **Acquisition:** How long have you owned the bird? Where did you get her/him? Is there a previous owner? Approximate age?
- **Owner's Experience:** What is your previous experience with chickens?

6.4 Presenting Complaint

- **Reason for Visit:** What is the primary complaint or the specific signs you've noticed?
- **Timeline:** How long has the problem been present? Has it been sudden or gradual?
- **Behavioral Changes:** Have the chicken's eating, drinking, or vocalization changed?
- **Other Flock Members:** Are any other birds in the flock showing similar symptoms?
- **Other Household Members:** Have any other pets or humans in the household been ill?

6.5 Health and Management History

- **Past Issues:** What are the chicken's previous medical conditions? Previous veterinary care? Any illness in the flock prior to today?
- **Previous Treatments:** Have any treatments, supplements, or medications been provided recently?
- **Diet:** List everything the flock is fed, including commercial feed brand names and any human foods or scraps. Where and how is the food stored? What water sources are available?
- **Housing:** How often is the coop cleaned? What disinfectants are used? What size is the coop or pen? How is the coop, pen predator-proof?
- **Flock:** How many birds are in the flock? Where is he/she in the pecking order? When was the last bird added to the flock? Are any other birds ill/exhibiting the same signs?
- **Outdoor Access:** Does the chicken free range? If so, is it supervised?
- **For a Hen:** Does she lay eggs? When was the last egg laid? Has she laid any malformed eggs?
- **Prevention:** Is your chicken vaccinated? What, if any, vaccines has she/he received? (Figure 6.2)

6.6 Safe Handling and Restraint for Chickens

Move calmly, quietly, and avoid sudden gestures. Covering the bird's eyes with a towel, or dimming the lights, often reduces struggling. One method of restraint is to gently secure the wings against the bird's body and allow her to stand on the nonslip exam table. Another effective method is to use the handler's body to restrain the bird's closest wing to the handler's body, so the handler's other hand is free to restrain the head or feet. For procedures requiring greater control, one person may hold the wings and keel while another stabilizes the head and/or feet. Avoid excessive body or keel pressure, as birds lack a diaphragm and rely on keel movement for breathing. Compression can cause panic and asphyxiation. Veterinary technicians should monitor for open-mouth breathing, cyanosis, or struggling during restraint, as these are signs that the bird is stressed and becoming compromised.

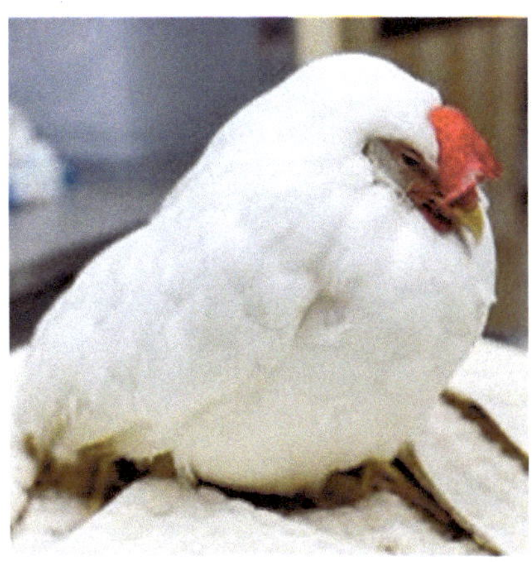

Figure 6.2 Hen displays abnormal posture from reproductive organ disease. Courtesy of Funky Chicken Rescue.

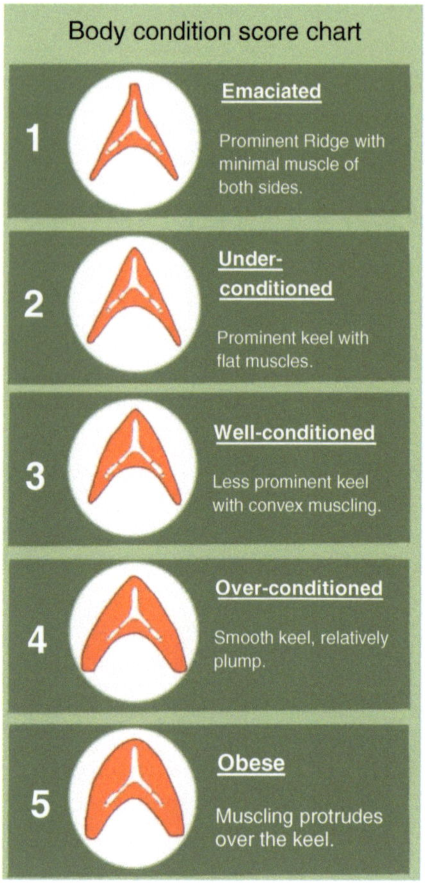

Figure 6.3 Keel scale, 1 being emaciated and 5 being morbidly obese. Original artwork contributed by Rebecca Wood.

6.6.1 Weight and Body Condition

Use a gram scale for small breeds and a digital tabletop scale for medium to large breeds with a nonslip surface or mat. Assess body condition score (BCS) by palpating the keel and pectoral muscles. It is advisable for caregivers to have a scale at home to monitor each bird's body weight on a regular schedule to monitor gains or losses (Figure 6.3).

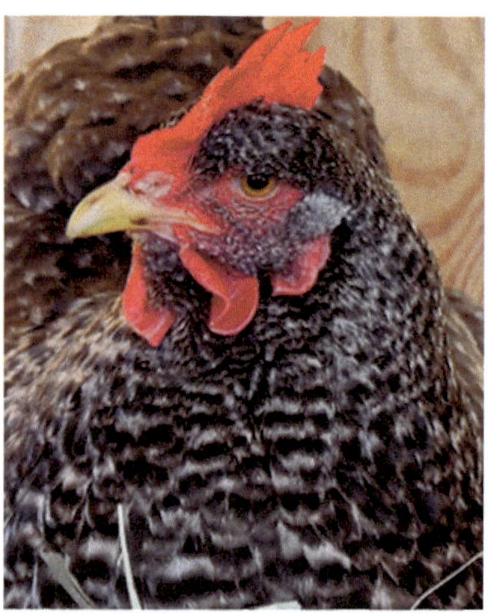

Figure 6.4 Hen with bright eyes, red comb, and wattles. Photo courtesy of Sarah Meyer.

6.6.2 Head and Neck

- **Eyes:** Clear, bright, and free of discharge. Note the absence of pupil movement, conjunctivitis, clouding, blepharospasm, foaming, cataracts, lenticular sclerosis, or ocular parasites.
- **Nares:** Symmetry and patency; discharge suggests respiratory disease.
- **Beak:** Alignment, overgrowth, trauma, or discoloration.

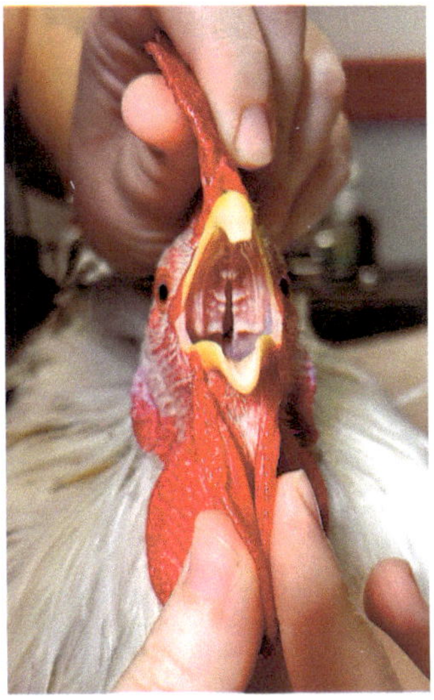

Figure 6.5 Choanal slit and oral examination. Photo courtesy of Stephanie Freeman.

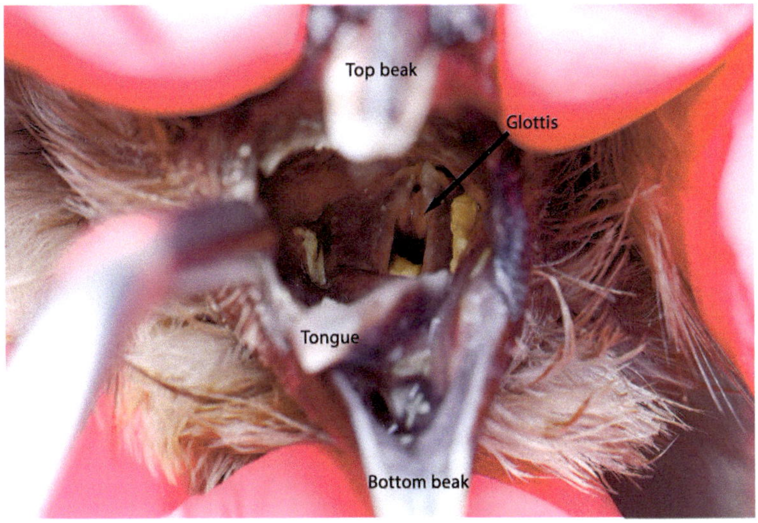

Figure 6.6 Caseous plaques in the pharyngolaryngeal area of a hen. Courtesy of Unusual Pet Vets.

- **Comb and Wattles:** Color, turgor, and symmetry. Pale combs indicate anemia; purple/gray suggests hypoxia or circulatory compromise. Blanching to assess hydration and perfusion.
- **Ears:** Check for swelling, discharge, or presence of parasites.
- **Oral Cavity:** Free of lesions and discharge. Inspect the choanal slit, mucous membranes, and glottis. Mucous membranes should be pink and moist. An avian or reptile oral speculum is recommended; a large paper clip or tongue depressor can also be useful for examining the oral cavity. Caseous plaques of the choana suggest trichomoniasis, candidiasis, or poxvirus (Figures 6.4–6.7).

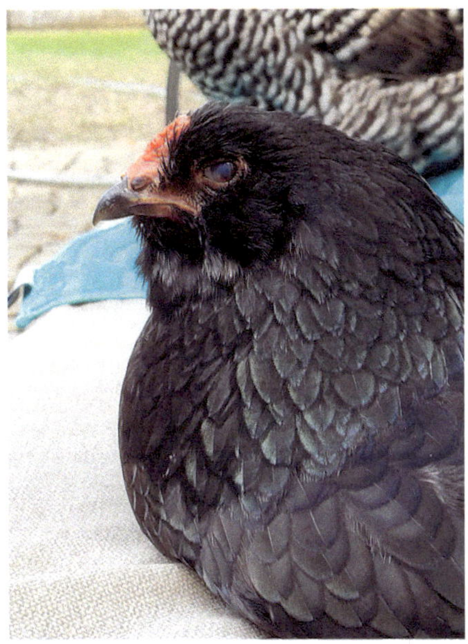

Figure 6.7 Nictitating membrane over the left eye. Courtesy of Sarah Meyer.

6.6.3 Integument and Plumage

Cradle the bird with one hand, and extend each wing gently with the other hand. Inspect the dorsal and ventral aspects of the wing. Evaluate feather quality and molt stage if it is occurring at the time of examination. Molting birds may resist handling due to sensitive pin feathers. Look for ectoparasites (lice and mites), broken feathers, or areas of feather loss. Examine skin (including the comb) for wounds, swelling, or dermatitis, especially around the vent and under wings. Observe the preen (uropygial) gland at the tail base for enlargement or impaction. Inspect dorsal and plantar surfaces of the feet, toes, nails, and spurs. Observe and notate raised scales or crusts on the legs and toes, abrasions, or deformities (Figures 6.8 and 6.9).

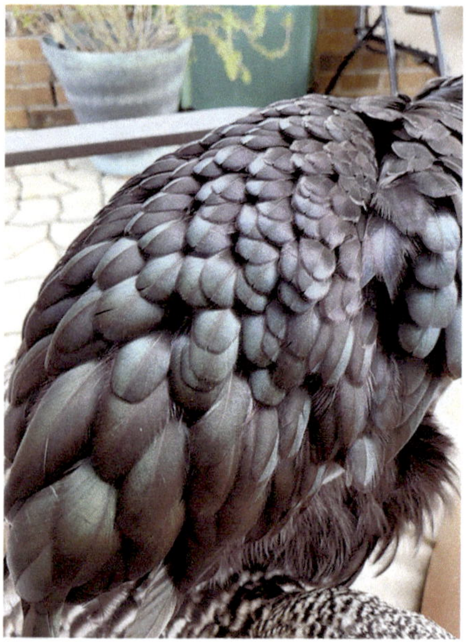

Figure 6.8 Iridescent colors of black hen plumage. Courtesy of Sarah Meyer.

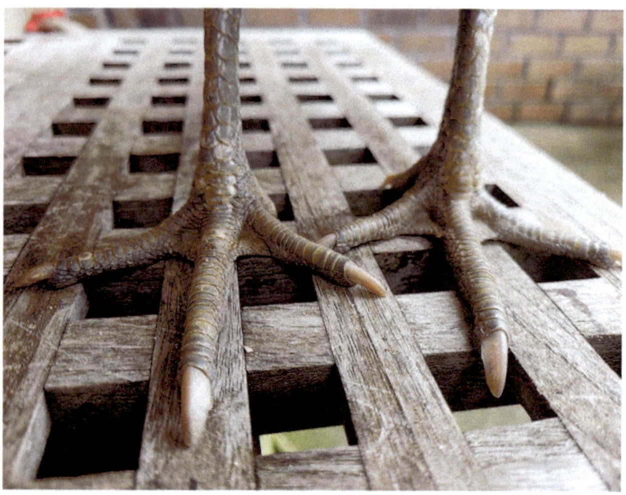

Figure 6.9 Healthy leg and feet scales and toenails. Courtesy of Sarah Meyer.

6.6.4 Musculoskeletal System

Observe symmetry, range of motion, and gait. When examining the legs, palpate each joint, including the coxofemoral joint, stifle, tarsus/hock, and digits. Palpate for swelling or heat. Each joint should move smoothly in both flexion and extension and be free of crepitus. Palpate the musculature of the limbs for symmetry. Evaluate the nonfeathered skin of the lower limbs for scaling and lesions. The nails should be straight, unbroken, and at a comfortable length for the bird to ambulate comfortably (Figure 6.10).

6.6.5 Cardiovascular and Respiratory System

Place the stethoscope over the keel and move left, then right. Normal heart rate ranges from 220 to 360 bpm in adult chickens. A Doppler blood flow monitor can assist with cardiac sound and pulse

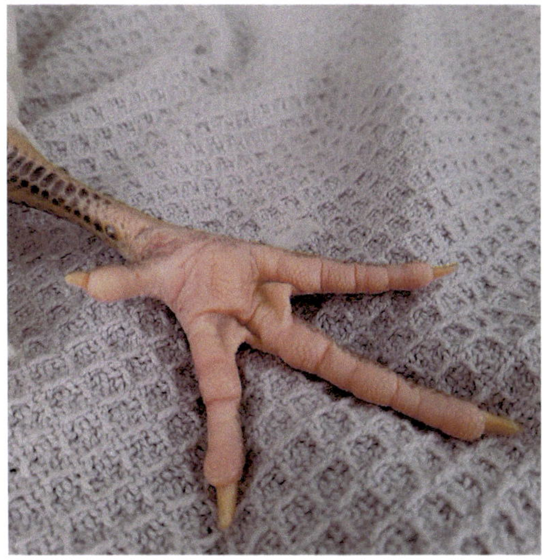

Figure 6.10 Healthy plantar surface of a rooster's foot. Photo courtesy of Sarah Meyer.

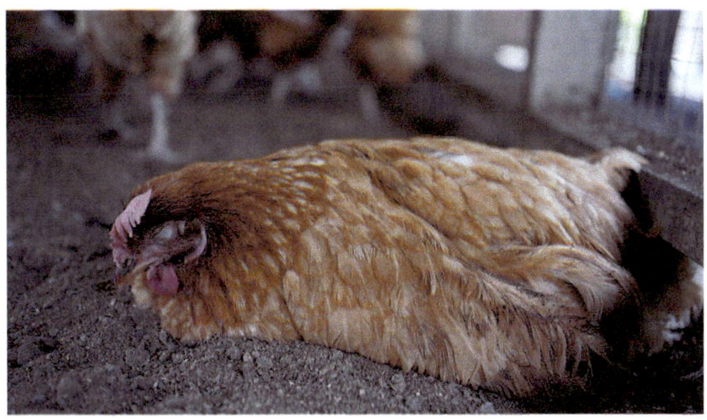

Figure 6.11 Hen exhibiting dyspnea, slight cyanosis of wattles and comb. Chalermphon / Adobe Stock Photos.

quality assessment. Auscultation for murmurs or arrhythmia. Capillary refill time can be assessed when the ventral aspect of the wing is examined by blanching the ulnar wing vein. Blanching of the comb or wattles can also be performed to assess perfusion and hydration.

Lungs and air sacs: normal sounds are minimal and auscultated along the midline dorsum. A respiratory rate is obtained at this location as well. Harsh or wheezy breath sounds may indicate air sacculitis, pneumonia, or aspergillosis. Note discharge from nares, coughing with elicitation, or referred sounds. Tail pumping is indicative of respiratory distress (Figure 6.11).

6.6.6 Coelomic Palpation

Palpate a normally convex coelom, caudal to the sternum/keel gently for distension, masses, fluid, or an enlarged oviduct or retained eggs (left side of the caudal coelom). Organs in this soft space include the ventriculus, the caudal portion of the gastrointestinal system and the spleen, the pancreas, the reproductive system, the adrenal glands, and the kidneys. In hens, enlarged coeloms may suggest egg yolk peritonitis, ascites, neoplasia, or reproductive organ disease. Note asymmetry or pain upon palpation. Diagnostic imaging aids in coelomic evaluation (Figure 6.12).

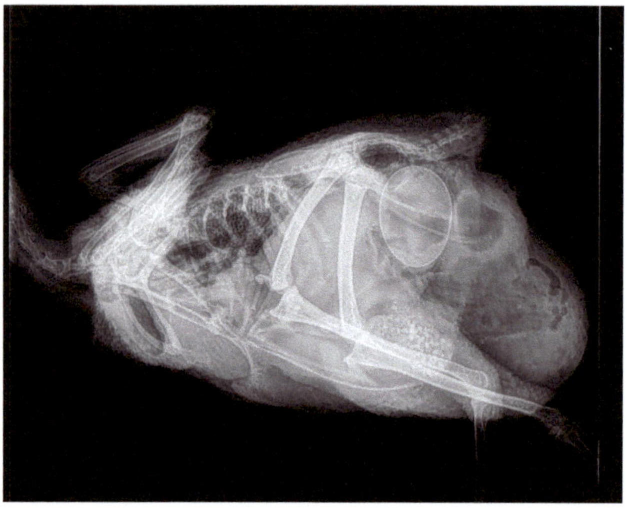

Figure 6.12 Lateral radiograph of a hen with coelomic contents, easily palpated. Courtesy of Sarah Meyer.

6.6.7 Crop

Assess via palpation for fullness, a "doughy" or thickened feel, ability to empty, or foreign bodies. The crop should empty within a few hours and should be empty after fasting. It is abnormal for the crop to have a sour or yeasty odor.

6.6.8 Cloaca and Vent

Check for soiling, prolapse, trauma, or parasites. Surrounding feathers and skin should be clean. If discharge is noted from an ill bird, a sterile swab should be collected for culture and sensitivity. Vent tone should be adequate; relaxed cloacal sphincters may indicate neurologic disease.

The cloaca is the communal chamber of the digestive system, urinary system, and reproductive system. Digital cloacal palpation is performed gently and with water-based lubricant. The healthy cloaca resembles a pink set of lips. Many of the same structures palpated externally may be palpated, including the cloaca itself, oviduct, ventriculus, gastrointestinal tract, and potential free fluid via internal digital palpation. Cloacal palpation may be helpful when assessing a hen for egg binding, as the egg may be felt.

The cloaca of roosters is noticeably smaller and less flaccid than in laying hens. Fresh stool (per bird or a collective flock specimen) should be examined in-house if the veterinary technician is confident in cytology, chicken intestinal parasite identification, or Gram staining. The specimen can be sent to a veterinary reference laboratory for culture and sensitivity if indicated (Figure 6.13).

6.6.9 Neurologic Assessment

Observe mentation, coordination, proprioception, and balance. Assess cranial nerves, pupillary reflexes, palpebral reflexes, and jaw tone. Test limb withdrawal and toe grip strength, as well as foot color and temperature. Head tilt, circling, or ataxia may suggest viral, bacterial, toxic, or nutritional disease.

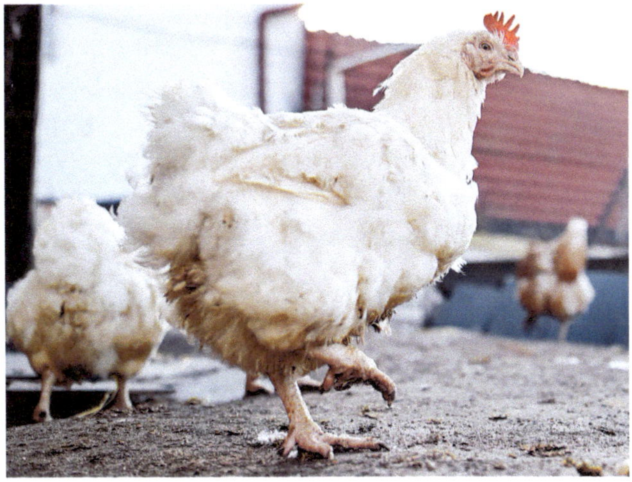

Figure 6.13 Soiled vent feathers from diarrhea. dimik_777 / Adobe Stock Photos.

6.7 Chicken Physical Examination Sample Form

A systematic physical examination is the veterinary technician's most powerful tool when presented with chicken patients. By combining careful observation, gentle handling, and a structured approach, the veterinary technician can detect subtle health changes, support the veterinarian in the diagnosis of patient conditions, and guide caretakers toward improved flock health and welfare. Because chickens are stoic and often hide signs of illness, the veterinary technician's skill in conducting thorough exams may mean the difference between early intervention and advanced disease (Figure 6.14).

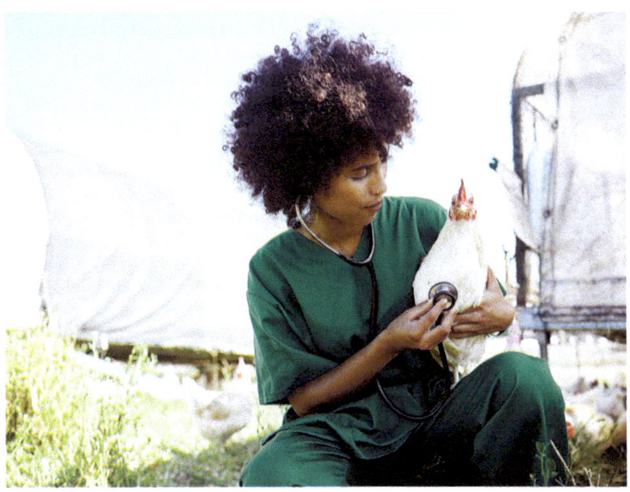

Figure 6.14 Veterinary technician auscultating a hen during physical examination. K Davis/peopleimages.com / Adobe Stock Photos.

Date:________________________
Examiner:________________________
Patient ID:________________________
Owner:________________________
Species / Breed:________________________
Sex: ☐ Male ☐ Female **Age:**____________
Weight:__________g **BCS (1–5):**__________

HR:________**bpm** **RR:** _________ **bpm**

Head & Eyes

Comb / Wattles: ☐ Normal ☐ Pale ☐ Cyanotic ☐ Lesions ☐ Swollen

Eyes: ☐ Clear ☐ Discharge ☐ Cloudy ☐ Swollen ☐ Asymmetrical

Nostrils / Nares: ☐ Clear ☐ Discharge ☐ Crusts

Beak: ☐ Normal ☐ Overgrown ☐ Fractured

Oral Cavity / Crop

Oral mucosa: ☐ Pink ☐ Pale ☐ Lesions ☐ Plaques

Crop: ☐ Empty ☐ Full ☐ Doughy ☐ Sour ☐ Distended

Heart / Circulation

Mucous membrane color: _______________

Capillary refill time: ___________ sec

Rhythm: ☐ Regular ☐ Irregular

Abdomen

Palpation: ☐ Soft ☐ Distended ☐ Firm ☐ Fluid wave

Vent / Cloaca: ☐ Clean ☐ Soiled ☐ Prolapse ☐ Lesions

Musculoskeletal

Wings: ☐ Normal range of motion ☐ Fracture ☐ Drooping

Legs / Feet: ☐ Normal ☐ Swollen joints ☐ Bumblefoot ☐ Lameness

Toe / Nails: ☐ Normal ☐ Overgrown ☐ Missing ☐ Deformities

Integument / Feathers

Feather quality: ☐ Normal ☐ Broken ☐ Missing ☐ Mites / Lice present

Skin: ☐ Intact ☐ Lesions ☐ Scabs ☐ Discoloration

Neurologic

Mentation: ☐ Normal ☐ Dull ☐ Ataxic

Reflexes: ☐ Wing / leg withdrawal ☐ Righting reflex

Tremors / Head tilt / Nystagmus: ☐ Present ☐ Absent

Physical examination sheet created by Stephanie Freeman.

Further Reading

Delamarter M. Performing an Avian Physical Examination in Practice [Internet]. 2024 [cited 2025 Dec 7]. Available from: https://todaysveterinarypractice.com/exotic-medicine/performing-an-avian-physical-examination-in-practice/

[Internet]. [cited 2025 Dec 7]. Available from: https://onlinelibrary.wiley.com/doi/abs/10.1002/9781119511816.ch8

7

Integumentary Diseases and External Parasites

7.1 Why Does the Integumentary System Matter?

The integumentary system in chickens comprises the skin, feathers, beak, claws, and uropygial (preen) gland. The integumentary system is crucial to thermoregulation, waterproofing, flight/locomotion, balance, barrier immunity, and social signaling. Unlike many mammals, avian skin is thin, relatively inelastic in bare areas, and highly specialized with feathers that arise in pterylae (feather tracts) separated by apteria (bare skin); these anatomic realities shape how ectoparasites colonize, where lesions develop, and how birds are examined and treated.

The uropygial gland at the dorsal tail base secretes lipids that are spread through preening; together with epidermal lipids, these secretions support feather condition and surface antimicrobial activity. Therefore, disease of this gland or extensive feather/skin pathology can multiply the impact of ectoparasites on barrier function and performance.

Clinically, integument disease often presents first as "poor doer" phenotypes: weight stagnation, ragged plumage, reduced laying, and restlessness. For the veterinary healthcare team, a structured approach (history, environment, flock exam, targeted skin/feather exam, point-of-care diagnostics) is essential.

7.2 Where and How to Examine

- **Vent and Under the Tail:** Backward ruffling of feathers at the base of the tail and vent can reveal visible external parasites such as lice or mites. Clear cellophane tape can also aid in this dermatologic examination and treatment, regardless of species, consistently. Concentrate on the vent, breast, and thighs for lice/mites; part feathers to the skin and look for moving specks, clumped eggs (nits), and blackish debris. Check the underwings (axillary), neck base, and saddle feathers on roosters.
- **Legs and Feet:** Inspect scales for lifting, honeycomb crusts, hyperkeratosis, and pain; these are all classic for scaly leg mites.
- **Face, Wattles, Comb, Eyelids:** Look for embedded stick-tight fleas (sessile, firmly attached) and excoriations.
- **Roosts, Cracks, Nest Boxes (Night):** For red mites and other temporary blood feeders that hide by day, inspect housing at night with a headlamp (Figure 7.1).

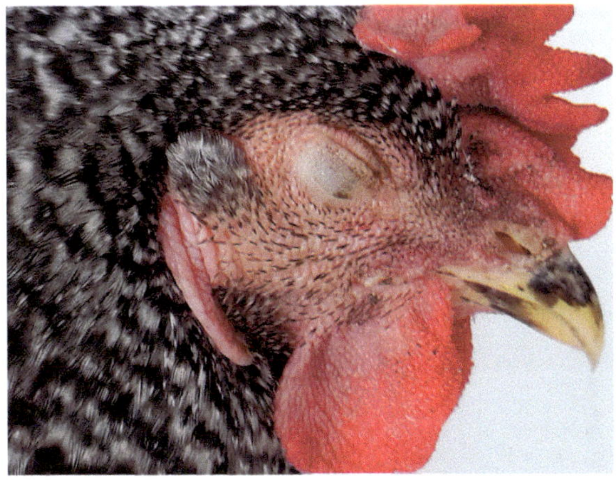

Figure 7.1 Healthy Barred Rock hen's facial skin, comb, earlobes, and wattles. Courtesy of Sarah Meyer.

7.3 External Parasites of Clinical Importance

Below are the ectoparasites encountered most often in backyard and small-flock practice, with practical notes for veterinary recognition, triage, and sampling (Taxonomy and common names vary regionally) (Figure 7.2).

Quick reference chart

Parasite/group	Common name	Primary location on bird	Transmission/ source	Key clinical signs	Pathology/key lesions
Dermanyssus gallinae	Red mite (roost mite)	Feeds on birds at night; hides in crevices during day	Infested housing, perches, litter	Restlessness at night, anemia, decreased egg production	Pale combs/ wattles, blood loss, feather loss, visible mites on inspection
Ornithonyssus sylviarum	Northern fowl mite	Feathers around vent, back, neck (remains on bird full time)	Bird-to-bird contact, contaminated housing	Dirty, soiled feathers, irritation, reduced productivity	Dermatitis, anemia, scabbing, visible mites on feathers/skin
Knemidocoptes mutans	Scaly leg mite	Beneath leg scales	Direct contact, contaminated perches	Lameness, raised/crusty leg scales, pain	Thickened, crusty legs; deformity in chronic cases
Knemidocoptes gallinae	Depluming/ face mite	Feather shafts, facial areas	Direct contact	Feather pulling, irritation, bald patches	Broken feathers, inflamed skin
Echidnophaga gallinacea	Sticktight flea	Face, comb, wattles	Contact with infested soil/ hosts	Black specks on head, anemia, weakness	Embedded fleas in skin, local irritation, anemia
Argas persicus	Fowl tick	Night feeding, hides in cracks during day	Infested housing, wild bird exposure	Weakness, decreased egg production, death in heavy infestations	Blood loss anemia, toxemia, tick-borne disease transmission

Chart created by Stephanie Freeman.

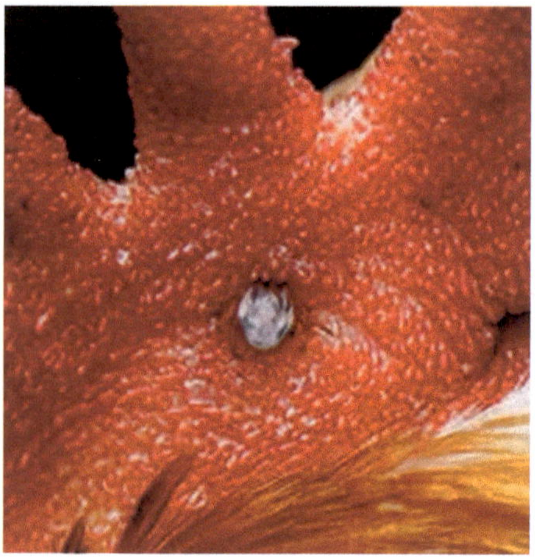

Figure 7.2 Tick on a rooster's comb. Courtesy of Unusual Pet Vets.

7.3.1 Lice (*Phthiraptera*; Chewing Lice)

7.3.1.1 Overview

Lice are one of the most common external parasites affecting chickens worldwide. They are ectoparasitic insects that live exclusively on the host, feeding on skin debris, feathers, and occasionally blood. Unlike fleas or mites, chicken lice are highly host-specific, meaning they spend their entire life cycle on poultry and do not survive long in the environment. Understanding their biology and epidemiology is essential for effective control and prevention in both backyard and commercial flocks.

- **Size:** 1–6 mm, dorsoventrally flattened.
- **Color:** Typically, yellowish to brown.
- **Mouthparts:** Chewing (mandibulate), adapted for feeding on keratin, feather debris, and epidermal scales.
- **Legs:** Equipped with claws for clinging tightly to feathers.
- **Egg Stage:** Nits are oval, whitish, and firmly cemented to feather shafts.

Entire life cycle occurs on the host. Female lice lay eggs (nits) directly on feather shafts, especially around the vent, breast, and thighs. Incubation is 4–7 days. Nymphal development is 2–3 weeks, passing through three nymphal stages. Adults live 3–6 weeks. Transmission is primarily by direct contact between birds, rarely via contaminated equipment. Off-host survival is very limited, usually less than 7 days, as lice require host body heat and constant access to feathers.

7.3.1.2 Epidemiology

Chicken lice species are host-specific and typically do not infest humans or mammals. Wild birds can occasionally carry similar lice but generally do not contribute significantly to infestations in domestic chickens. Lice infestations are common worldwide in both backyards and small-scale flocks. Prevalence may exceed 80% in poorly managed or untreated flocks. Outbreaks are most frequent in warm, humid climates where ectoparasite survival is optimized.

7.3.1.3 Pathogenesis

Lice feed primarily on feather debris and epidermal scales, but heavy infestations may cause irritation, feather damage, and mild anemia. Lice themselves are not major disease vectors, but feather damage predisposes birds to secondary infections and hypothermia.

7.3.1.4 Clinical Signs

Birds may appear uncomfortable, constantly moving or shifting and frequently picking at feathers, sometimes leading to self-trauma. Feathers look dirty, broken, or frayed. Patchy feather loss especially around the vent, breast, thighs, and under wings. Small yellowish-brown lice are crawling, or white egg clusters are glued to feather shafts.

7.3.2 Northern Fowl Mite (*Ornithonyssus sylviarum*)

7.3.2.1 Overview

The northern fowl mite (NFM), *Ornithonyssus sylviarum*, is one of the most important external parasites of poultry worldwide, particularly in temperate regions. Unlike lice (which remain on feathers and eat keratin debris), NFM are blood-feeding mites that spend their entire life cycle on the host, causing irritation, feather damage, anemia, and reduced productivity. Heavy infestations are associated with significant economic losses in both commercial and backyard flocks.

- **Size:** Adults ~0.7–1.1 mm long, barely visible to the naked eye.
- **Color:** Dark red to black when engorged with blood; pale gray/white when unfed.
- **Body:** Oval, flattened dorsoventrally, with long legs adapted for crawling.
- **Mouthparts:** Piercing-sucking, specialized for blood feeding.

The entire life cycle occurs on the host (unlike the Red Poultry Mite, *Dermanyssus gallinae*, which hides off the host during the day). Development involves eggs, larva, protonymph, deutonymph, and adult. Developmental duration is as short as 5–7 days under favorable conditions (warmth, humidity, continuous host access). Female mites lay eggs directly on feathers near the skin (especially around the vent). Adults live up to 3 weeks on host. Transmission is primarily by direct bird-to-bird contact; it can also spread via fomites (contaminated equipment, personnel, or wild birds). Off-host survival is typically only 2–3 weeks.

7.3.2.2 Epidemiology

Affects chickens, turkeys, pigeons, and wild birds (e.g., sparrows, starlings). Chickens are the preferred host. Not a zoonotic parasite, but mites may transiently bite humans, causing minor irritation. In untreated flocks, prevalence can exceed 70–90%. Mite populations build rapidly, with thousands of mites found on a single bird. Outbreaks tend to spread quickly through the flock, especially in crowded conditions.

7.3.2.3 Pathogenesis

NFMs are obligate hematophagous mites. Their repeated blood feeding causes skin irritation, pruritus, feather soiling and breakage, blood loss, reduced egg production, and weight loss. Severe infestations may cause death in young or debilitated chickens due to anemia.

7.3.2.4 Clinical Signs

Restlessness, agitation, excessive preening, decreased activity, and reluctance to move. Dirty, matted feathers around the vent, thighs, and tail base (mite feces and dried blood). Blackened or darkened appearance at feather bases ("mite dirt"). Broken or missing feathers near infested sites. Skin irritation such as erythema, scabs, or crusting at feeding sites.

7.3.3 Red Poultry Mite (*Dermanyssus gallinae*)

7.3.3.1 Overview

The red poultry mite (RPM), *Dermanyssus gallinae*, is one of the most significant ectoparasites in chickens worldwide. Unlike lice or the Northern Fowl Mite, *D. gallinae* is a nocturnal, blood-feeding mite that lives off the host during the day and feeds on chickens at night. It has a rapid life cycle and is not known for causing severe infestations that can lead to production losses, anemia, and even mortality. Its ability to survive long periods without a host makes it a persistent and difficult-to-control parasite.

- **Size:** 0.6–1 mm in length, just visible to the naked eye.
- **Color:** Grayish-white when unfed; bright red when engorged with blood; turns black after digestion.
- **Body:** Oval, flattened, long legs adapted for rapid crawling.
- **Mouthparts:** Piercing-sucking stylets specialized in hematophagy.

Development involves eggs, larva, protonymph, deutonymph, and adult. Developmental duration can be completed in 7–10 days under optimal conditions. Nymphs and adults feed on blood, typically at night for 30–60 minutes. Off-host survival is up to 5–8 months without feeding, hiding in cracks, crevices, roosts, and nest boxes. Female mites lay eggs in the environment, not on the bird. Transmission is by movement of infested equipment, workers, wild birds, rodents, and direct bird-to-bird transfer in shared housing.

7.3.3.2 Epidemiology

Particularly common in Europe and Asia, and increasing in prevalence in North America. The primary host is chickens. Wild birds act as reservoirs. Can reach high infestation rates in poorly managed flocks. Infestations often go unnoticed at first due to mite feeding only at night.

7.3.3.3 Pathogenesis

Blood feeding leads to severe irritation and restlessness (especially at night), feather damage, anemia, weight loss, and decreased egg production.

7.3.3.4 Clinical Signs

Birds are reluctant to enter coops at night due to irritation. Feather damage and poor plumage from excessive preening and scratching. Reduced egg production (fewer eggs, smaller size, thinner shells). Pale combs and wattles, weakness, and lethargy. Feather loss, scabs, and dermatitis around vent, breast, and under wings. Mites are visible at night on skin and feathers (but are rarely seen during the day). Dark specks (mite feces and crushed mites) in nest boxes, perch ends, and cracks. Blood-stained eggshells from crushed, engorged mites.

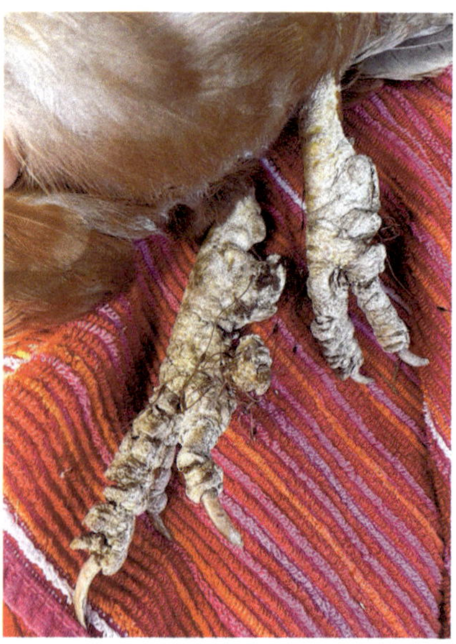

Figure 7.3 Severe case of Scaly Leg Mites. Courtesy of Darcy Dickinson Smith, Funky Chicken Rescue.

7.3.4 Scaly Leg Mite (*Knemidocoptes mutans*)

Figure 7.3.

7.3.4.1 Overview

The Scaly Leg Mite (*Knemidocoptes mutans*) is a microscopic burrowing mite that primarily infests the legs and feet of chickens. Unlike lice or surface-dwelling mites, *K. mutans* live under the scales of the shanks and toes, tunneling into the skin, where it causes chronic irritation, thickened crusts, and distortion of the legs. Infestation is highly contagious within flocks and may persist for years if untreated.

- **Size:** ~0.2–0.4 mm (microscopic, round-bodied).
- **Color:** Transparent to pale white.
- **Shape:** Short legs, round body, adapted for burrowing.
- **Microscopy:** Difficult to detect without skin scrapings, but lesions are highly suggestive.

The entire life cycle occurs on the bird, within the skin of the legs. A life cycle consists of egg, larva, nymph, and adult. Life duration is 10–14 days under optimal conditions. Females burrow under the leg scales to lay eggs. Mites consume keratin and tissue fluids. Transmission is by direct contact between birds; mites can also spread indirectly via contaminated perches and housing.

7.3.4.2 Epidemiology

Especially prevalent in older, neglected, or poorly managed flocks. Chickens are the primary host. It can become highly endemic in small backyard flocks if untreated.

7.3.4.3 Pathogenesis

Female mites burrow beneath the keratinized scales of the legs and feet. Chronic irritation stimulates hyperkeratosis, scale lifting, and deformity of the shank. Unlike red mites or NFMs, scaly leg mites do not suck blood, but they cause progressive disfigurement.

7.3.4.4 Clinical Signs

Raised, thickened scales on shanks and toes. Birds may scratch their legs more frequently or rub them against perches. Slight enlargement or swelling of the shank. Thick crusts may merge to form large plaques. Chronic cases may result in permanent leg deformity. Chronic discomfort may reduce activity and feeding efficiency.

7.3.5 Depluming Mite (*Knemidocoptes gallinae*)

7.3.5.1 Overview

The Depluming Mite (*Knemidocoptes gallinae*) is a burrowing mite that primarily affects the skin at the base of feathers, especially on the head, neck, back, and vent regions of chickens. Unlike surface-feeding ectoparasites, these mites tunnel into feather follicles, causing feather loss (depluming), thickened skin, and irritation. Infestations are highly contagious and can spread rapidly in flocks, particularly in overcrowded or poorly managed conditions.

- **Size:** 0.2–0.4 mm (microscopic).
- **Color:** Transparent to pale white.
- **Body:** Round, short legs adapted for burrowing.
- Adapted for intracutaneous habitation in feather follicles.

The entire life cycle occurs on the host in the skin at the base of feathers. Life consists of eggs, larva, nymph, and adult. Life duration is 10–14 days under optimal conditions. Female mites burrow into the skin, lay eggs, and continue feeding on epidermal tissue and follicular debris. Transmission by direct bird-to-bird contact; indirect transmission is possible via contaminated equipment, perches, and housing.

7.3.5.2 Epidemiology

Primarily chickens, but also affects turkeys, pheasants, canaries, pigeons, and other gallinaceous or ornamental birds. Transmission is direct contact between birds, indirect spread via contaminated housing, equipment, or caretakers' clothing/hands. Infestations often begin with the introduction of new infested birds. Tends to worsen in warm weather when mite activity is higher.

7.3.5.3 Pathogenesis

Burrow into feather follicles and skin at feather bases. Feed on tissue fluids, causing intense irritation and pruritus. Birds respond by pulling out their own feathers ("depluming"). Chronic infestations lead to thickened, inflamed skin and secondary bacterial infections.

7.3.5.4 Clinical Signs

Birds are restless and scratch and peck persistently at affected areas. Self-inflicted wounds due to irritation; mites burrow into feather follicles, prompting birds to pull out feathers. Lesions are commonly around the back, breast, vent, thighs, and sometimes the neck. Inflamed, thickened, scabby, or crusty skin at feather bases. Small papules or nodules may form where mites burrow. Broken or damaged feathers; regrowth may be poor. Excoriations can lead to bacterial dermatitis or pyoderma.

7.3.6 Stick-Tight Flea (*Echidnophaga gallinacea*)

7.3.6.1 Overview

The stick-tight flea is a small, dark brown flea that parasitizes a wide range of domestic and wild birds, including chickens. Unlike most fleas, which move freely through the host's feathers or fur, the stick-tight flea attaches firmly to the skin around the comb, wattles, eyelids, and vent. Its feeding behavior leads to irritation, dermatitis, and severe infestations, debilitation, blindness, or even death in young birds. It is also a potential vector for pathogenic agents.

- **Size:** 1–2 mm in length (smaller than most fleas).
- **Color:** Dark brown to black.
- Females embed their mouthparts deeply into the host's skin, remaining attached for long periods.
- Unlike jumping fleas, stick-tight fleas have reduced ctenidia (spines) and less developed legs, adapted for remaining fixed to the host.

Complete metamorphosis involves egg, larva, pupa, and adult. It can be completed in 4–5 weeks under favorable conditions. Eggs are laid in the environment (litter, soil, cracks), not on the host. Larvae are free living, feeding on organic matter (e.g., skin debris, dried blood, and flea feces). The pupae develop in the soil, litter, and cracks, not on the host. Adults seek hosts for blood meals. Females firmly attach to the host's skin, often for several days to weeks. Males are more mobile but also feed on blood.

7.3.6.2 Epidemiology

Primarily affects chickens and turkeys. Also infests a wide range of domestic animals (dogs, cats, and goats) and wildlife. Found worldwide, especially in warm, humid, subtropical, and tropical regions. Transmission is by adult fleas actively jumping onto birds from the environment. Infestation spreads when birds encounter contaminated soil, bedding, or perches. No host-specific, infestations often spread between poultry and other animals.

7.3.6.3 Pathogenesis

Adult fleas attach firmly to the host's comb, wattles, eyelids, and vent-skin. Persistent feeding causes inflammation and ulceration at attachment sites, dermatitis, scab formation, and secondary bacterial infections.

7.3.6.4 Clinical Signs

Small, dark brown fleas are embedded tightly around the comb, wattles, eyelids, earlobes, and sometimes the vent area. They appear as blackish crusty spots. Birds show scratching, head shaking, and rubbing against objects. Localized dermatitis, erythema, and crusty scabs where fleas are attached. Swelling of eyelids, tearing, impaired vision, or even blindness if fleas cluster around the eyes. Heavy infestations can cause significant blood loss, leading to pale combs, lethargy, weight loss, and decreased egg production. Flea bites may predispose to bacterial infections at the attachment sites. In severe cases, debilitation, stunted growth in young birds, and occasionally death due to anemia, starvation (inability to see/feed), or secondary complications.

7.4 Diagnostic Testing

7.4.1 History and Risk Mapping

- Time of year, housing type and sanitation routine, dust-bathing access, introduction of new birds, proximity to wild birds, show attendance, and multi-species on premises for flea risk.

7.4.2 Point-of-care Tests

- **Clear tape preps** of impressions of moving ectoparasites, eggs, and debris.
- **Skin scrapings** (deep for burrowers—*Knemidocoptes*) around raised leg scales; pluck broken feathers for depluming mite inspection.
- **Environmental swabs** of crevices/roosts for red mites; place tape into a sealable bag and label with location/time (night versus day).
- **CBC/PCV** in anemic birds with heavy mite load.

7.4.3 Differentials to Consider

- Bacterial dermatitis (*Staphylococcus*), fungal dermatitis, nutritional feathering issues (methionine/biotin deficits), self-mutilation from stress, viral (pox—cutaneous), and environmental irritants (ammonia, caustics).

7.4.4 When to Escalate

- Severe anemia or collapse, periocular flea burdens in chicks, suspected blackhead co-risk when chickens cohabit with turkeys.

7.5 Treatment

The "Three Pillars" of ectoparasite control in chickens are:

- **Treat the bird** (topical/on-bird-directed therapy).
- **Treat the environment** (roosts, nest boxes, cracks/crevices; break life cycles).
- **Treat the flock** (all birds, with repeat treatments synced to life cycles).

Always follow the specific product label and regional regulations and document any extra-label uses under a veterinarian's direction, especially for egg or meat withdrawal. Refer to FARAD (Food Animal Residue Avoidance Databank).

7.5.1 Pyrethrins/Pyrethroids (e.g., Permethrin)

Bird-directed

- **Permethrin Dust (≈0.25%):** Apply to each bird (vent, underwings, neck base), typically around 1 pound per 100 birds; repeat in 7–10 days. Practical for lice and NFM; ensure the product is labeled for poultry.
- **Permethrin Spray:** Label examples include dilution rates for bird spray and house/roost treatment; fine mist to skin contact (avoid face). Treat roosts, walls, and nest boxes as well.

Environment-directed

- Use permethrin solutions per label on roosts, cracks, nest boxes, and litter areas after removing bedding and organic matter; allow to dry before birds' return.

7.5.2 Spinosyns (Spinosad)

- **Label Indication:** Effective against NFMs on birds and for premise control; approved for direct bird application per manufacturer. Particularly useful in resistance management rotations.
- **Premise Directions:** Manufacturer tech sheet instructs thorough application to cracks/crevices for red mites (environmental), with re-treat after sanitation cycles.
- **Clinical Advantages:** Effective, flexible, and widely used in poultry practice; favored because of efficacy and safety when used as labeled. Brand name—Elector PSP.

7.6 Nursing Care and Veterinary Team-led Prevention

7.6.1 Husbandry Interventions that Make-or-Break Outcomes

- **Litter and Dryness:** Keep litter dry and friable; fix leaks in housing; improve drainage/ventilation. Wet litter accelerates parasite success and skin maceration.

- **Dust Baths:** Ensure access to dry dust baths (sand/soil). Birds use dust to groom and control ectoparasites; lack of dust baths correlates with higher lice and mite loads.
- **Roost and Nest Design:** Smooth, cleanable roosts; nest boxes that can be removed and pressure-washed; eliminate deep cracks where red mites hide.
- **Wild-bird Exclusion:** Install screens and repair holes; many mites are mechanically spread by wild birds.
- **Quarantine and Show Biosecurity:** Isolate new additions for 30 days; post-show inspection and treatment if needed.

7.6.2 Client Communication and Documentation Tips

- **Set Expectations**: "This takes **at least two treatments** and **house sanitation;** a single dusting or spray won't do it."
- **Demonstrate** feather parting and leg scale checks.
- **Provide** exact product, dilution, dates, and **when to repeat**; include any **withdrawal instructions** if applicable.
- **Encourage routine checks** (every **2–4 weeks**) during warm, humid, or high-wild-bird seasons.

7.7 Integumentary Diseases

7.7.1 Avian Cellulitis

7.7.1.1 Overview and Pathogenesis

Avian cellulitis in chickens is a condition characterized by diffuse inflammation and infection of the subcutaneous tissue, most often associated with bacterial invasion following minor skin trauma, scratches, or feather follicle damage. It is a common cause of carcass condemnation in commercial poultry, making it both a health and economic concern. The condition is most frequently caused by *Escherichia coli*, though other opportunistic bacteria such as *Staphylococcus* and *Enterococcus* may also be involved.

Pathogenesis begins when the skin barrier is compromised, allowing bacteria from the environment or intestinal tract to enter subcutaneous tissues. Once established, these bacteria trigger an inflammatory response with exudation of fibrin, accumulation of heterophils, and tissue edema. The lesions often develop as yellowish to greenish gelatinous exudates under the skin, most commonly in the abdominal and thigh regions. Chronic cases may progress to abscess formation, fibrosis, or systemic spread, potentially leading to septicemia. Factors such as poor litter quality, high stocking density, skin injuries, and immunosuppression predispose flocks to cellulitis. The disease not only affects bird welfare but also significantly impacts carcass quality and food safety in poultry production.

7.7.1.2 Risk Factors

- **Environmental and Housing Factors**

  Wet, caked, or soiled litter harbors bacteria and predisposes to skin infections. Sharp edges, coarse flooring, or wire floors cause skin trauma that serves as bacterial entry points. Overcrowding increases stress, feather picking, and mechanical injury.

- **Host-Related Factors**
  Broilers (meat birds) are more prone due to mechanical trauma from excessive pressure and poor mobility. Older birds are more likely to develop chronic cellulitis lesions. Feather pecking, scratches, and vent trauma provide portals for bacteria.
- **Nutritional Factors**
  Vitamin A deficiency weakens skin integrity. Vitamin E and selenium deficiency can impair immune response and tissue repair. Poor protein and mineral content affect skin resilience and wound healing.
- **Management and Behavioral Factors**
  Rough catching or transport causes skin abrasions. With vaccination or injection trauma, improper techniques can cause local abscesses that progress to cellulitis.
- **Pathogen-Related Factors**
  Virulent strains of *S. aureus* or *E. coli* are more likely to cause deep or systemic infections. Bacteria exploit wounds, feather follicles, or vent trauma to colonize subcutaneous tissue.

7.7.1.3 Clinical Signs and Pathology

- **External Findings**
  Localized swelling under the skin, often in the back, thighs, or abdominal areas. Warm, firm, or fluctuant nodules, indicating abscess formation. Redness or discoloration of overlying skin. Skin ulceration or scabs in chronic cases. Lameness or reluctance to move if lesions are near joints.
- **Necropsy Findings**
  Yellow to green subcutaneous abscesses, often with a caseous center. May extend to deep fascia and muscles in severe cases. Skin over lesions may be thickened, necrotic, or ulcerated.

7.7.1.4 Diagnostic Testing

- **Culture**
  Aspirated pus or excised tissue. Isolate *S. aureus* or other causative bacteria. Antimicrobial sensitivity testing guides treatment.

7.7.1.5 Treatment and Therapeutic Interventions

- **Supportive Care**
  Isolation of affected birds prevents pecking or secondary trauma and reduces environmental contamination. Soft bedding, reduced crowding, and easy access to feed and water. A nonsteroidal anti-inflammatory agent and opioid analgesic may be used. Prevent self-injury.
- **Wound Management**
  Remove scabs and debris; clean lesions with properly diluted antiseptic solutions (e.g., iodine, chlorhexidine). If the lesion fluctuates, abscesses may be incised and drained under aseptic conditions. Apply antibacterial ointments to reduce local infection and promote healing.
- **Medication**
  Amoxicillin/Clavulanate: 125–250 mg/kg by mouth every 8–12 hours for 5–7 days.
  Amoxicillin Sodium: 50–250 mg/kg intramuscularly every 8–12 hours for 5–7 days.
  Amoxicillin Trihydrate: 55–200 mg/kg by mouth, subcutaneous, or intramuscularly every 4–12 hours for 5–7 days.
  Trimethoprim-Sulfamethoxazole: 100 mg/kg by mouth every 12 hours for 5–7 days.

7.7.1.6 Prevention and Control

- **Environmental Management**
  Maintain dry, clean litter, and avoid wet or caked bedding. Prevent overcrowding and reduce rough or abrasive surfaces. Control ammonia levels in housing.
- **Nutritional Management**
  Provide adequate protein, vitamins (A, E), and minerals (selenium, zinc) to support skin and immune health.
- **Management Practices**
  Minimize handling trauma and avoid poorly administered injections. Reduce feather pecking through enrichment and appropriate lighting.

7.7.1.7 Nursing Considerations

Nursing care for chickens with avian cellulitis emphasizes infection control, supportive management, and prevention of recurrence. Affected birds should be carefully examined and, if practical, isolated to prevent further stress and allow close monitoring. Wound areas must be kept clean and dry, with gentle cleansing to minimize bacterial load, and veterinary-directed antibiotic therapy may be required for systemic or severe cases. Supportive care includes ensuring birds have easy access to feed and water, supplementing vitamins and electrolytes to boost immune response, and reducing handling stress to encourage recovery. Since cellulitis often arises from environmental and management-related factors, nursing staff must also ensure good litter management, proper ventilation, and reduction of skin trauma risks, such as sharp equipment or overcrowding. Close monitoring for signs of systemic infection, including lethargy, decreased feed intake, or septicemia, is essential to detect worsening disease early. Preventive nursing measures focus on maintaining flock hygiene, minimizing injury, and supporting overall health through biosecurity and nutritional balance.

7.7.2 Biotin Deficiency

7.7.2.1 Overview and Pathogenesis

Biotin deficiency in chickens is a nutritional disorder that arises when dietary levels of biotin, a water-soluble B-complex vitamin, are inadequate to meet metabolic needs. Biotin plays a vital role as a coenzyme in carboxylation reactions essential for carbohydrate, fat, and protein metabolism, as well as for maintaining the health of skin and keratinized tissues. In poultry, the deficiency most often results from feeding rations lacking sufficient biotin or containing high levels of raw egg whites, which contain avidin, a glycoprotein that binds biotin and prevents its absorption.

Pathogenesis involves impaired enzymatic activity, leading to defective lipid and amino acid metabolism, resulting in poor feathering, dermatitis, reduced growth, and decreased hatchability in breeders. Lesions are most prominent on the skin and appendages, with signs including hyperkeratosis, foot pad dermatitis, fissures at the corners of the beak and eyes, and necrosis of the foot skin. In severe cases, leg deformities and paralysis may occur due to compromised connective tissue and cartilage development. The deficiency negatively impacts both welfare and productivity, particularly in young, fast-growing birds and in breeding flocks where embryonic development depends heavily on adequate biotin supply.

7.7.2.2 Risk Factors

- **Nutritional Factors**
  Diets that do not supplement adequate biotin, especially in corn- or wheat-based rations. Raw egg consumption: raw eggs contain avidin, a protein that binds biotin and prevents absorption. Excessive heat during pelleting or storage can destroy biotin. Low protein, poor amino acid content, or high levels of avidin-containing ingredients.
- **Management and Environmental Factors**
  Long storage, moisture, and mold can reduce biotin availability. Inadequate premix inclusion or failure to adjust for life stage requirements. Overcrowding, heat stress, or illness can increase biotin requirements.
- **Host-Related Factors**
  Higher metabolic rates increase biotin demand. Young chicks are more susceptible because stores of biotin are low at hatch. Some breeds may have higher requirements for proper leg and skin development.

7.7.2.3 Clinical Signs and Pathology

- **External Findings**
  Thickened, dry, scaly skin, especially on footpads, hocks, and legs. Red, inflamed, sometimes ulcerated footpads. Poor feathering, broken or brittle feathers, delayed feather development in chicks. Malalignment of the gastrocnemius tendon, leading to hock deviation and splayed legs. Bowed legs, twisted tarsometatarsus, or valgus/varus deformities. Slow weight gain and poor feed conversion in young birds. Lameness or reluctance to move due to painful legs and feet. Reduced activity and exercise.
- **Necropsy Findings**
  Footpads and hocks show thickened scaly skin, sometimes with hemorrhages or ulceration. Hock deviation and tendon misalignment in perosis (seen in rapidly growing chicks). Muscle waste in severe, chronic cases.

7.7.2.4 Diagnostic Testing

- **Feed Analysis**
  Measures biotin content to confirm inadequate dietary supply.
- **Response to Treatment**
  Rapid improvement in skin, feathering, and leg function after biotin supplementation supports the diagnosis.

7.7.2.5 Treatment and Therapeutic Interventions

- **Immediate Biotin Supplementation**
  Add 0.5–1 mg/kg feed for corrective treatment. Water-soluble biotin can be added to drinking water in acute cases. Usually for 2–4 weeks, or until signs improve.
- **Supportive Care**
  Footpad protection, soft and clean bedding to reduce trauma. Leg support for severe perosis, splints, or restricted movement.

7.7.2.6 Prevention and Control

- **Nutritional Prevention**
  Provide adequate dietary biotin, including 0.1–0.2 mg/kg feed for growing chicks; adjust based on age, breed, and production type. Use a balanced commercial feed or vitamin premix to ensure

all essential vitamins and trace minerals are included. Avoid raw eggs in feed as they contain avidin, which binds biotin and prevents absorption. Avoid excessive heat during storage, which may destroy biotin.

- **Management Practices**
  Keep feed dry, protected from mold, and free of contaminants. Early detection of footpad lesions, poor feathering, or leg deformities allows timely intervention. Overcrowding or poor husbandry increases metabolic demand and susceptibility. Encourage movement to promote proper skeletal and muscular development.

7.7.2.7 Nursing Considerations

Nursing care for chickens with biotin deficiency focuses on nutritional correction, supportive management, and prevention of secondary complications. Affected birds should be provided with a balanced diet containing adequate biotin, either through high-quality commercial rations or supplementation with feed ingredients rich in biotin, such as soybean meal, alfalfa, or fish meal. In individual birds or flocks showing clinical signs, biotin supplementation in feed or water may be required under veterinary or nutritionist guidance to restore normal metabolic function. Nursing staff should carefully monitor birds for skin lesions, footpad dermatitis, poor feathering, or leg weakness, and provide supportive care such as clean, dry litter and padded perches to minimize discomfort from dermatitis or lameness. Close attention should be given to breeder flocks, since deficiency can cause reduced hatchability and embryonic deformities. Preventive nursing considerations include avoiding feeding raw egg whites, ensuring feed quality is not compromised by mold or spoilage, and maintaining overall flock nutrition with proper vitamin balance. Regular monitoring of flock condition, growth performance, and feather quality helps detect deficiencies early, allowing for prompt corrective measures that safeguard both bird health and productivity.

7.7.3 Broken Blood Feather

Figure 7.4.

7.7.3.1 Overview and Pathogenesis

A broken blood feather in chickens is a traumatic injury involving a developing feather that is still supplied with blood through the feather shaft, also known as the calamus or quill. Blood feathers typically occur during the molting or growth phase when new feathers are actively developing and remain vascularized to support keratin production. When these feathers are damaged by trauma, pecking, or accidental impact against equipment, the shaft can fracture and lead to continuous bleeding, as the blood vessel within the quill is exposed.

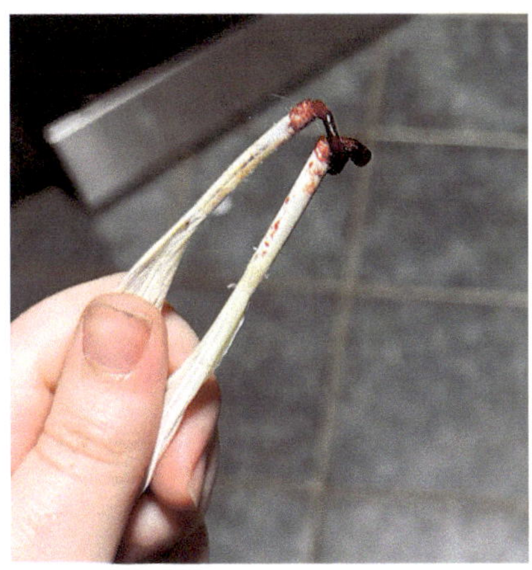

Figure 7.4 Broken blood feathers. Courtesy of Stephanie Freeman.

The pathogenesis is mechanical in nature, with hemorrhage resulting from the disruption of the vascular supply inside the shaft. If not managed promptly, the feather may continue to bleed significantly due to its direct connection to the bird's circulatory system, leading to hypovolemia, anemia, or even death in small birds. Additionally, the open shaft creates a potential entry point for bacterial contamination, which may predispose to localized infection or folliculitis. Broken blood feathers, therefore, represent not only a welfare concern due to pain and blood loss but also a management issue requiring rapid intervention.

7.7.3.2 Risk Factors

- **Host-Related Factors**
  Molting periods are when higher numbers of new blood feathers make birds more vulnerable. Young and growing birds have more developing feathers at risk. Birds with ornamental plumage are more prone to breakage. Birds that flap excessively, fight, or are restless have a higher risk of feather trauma.
- **Environmental and Housing Factors**
  Small or overcrowded enclosures increase feather breakage due to contact with walls, perches, or other birds. Wire cages, rough fencing, or poorly sanded perches can damage feathers.
- **Social and Behavioral Factors**
  Feather pecking or aggression as other birds may bite or pull at feathers, especially in stressful or crowded flocks. Submissive birds chased or cornered are at high risk of feather damage.
- **Management Factors**
  Improper wing clipping, cutting developing blood feathers by accident.

7.7.3.3 Clinical Signs and Pathology

- **External Findings**
  Visible bleeding from the feather shaft. Blood on surrounding feathers, coop, or perch. The feather shaft appears dark or red due to the blood vessel inside. If bleeding is severe or prolonged, pale comb/wattles, lethargy, and weakness occur.
- **Necropsy Findings**
  Clot formation at broken blood feather.

7.7.3.4 Diagnostic Testing

- **Clinical Examination**
  Inspect the bird for active bleeding, broken feather shafts, and surrounding trauma.

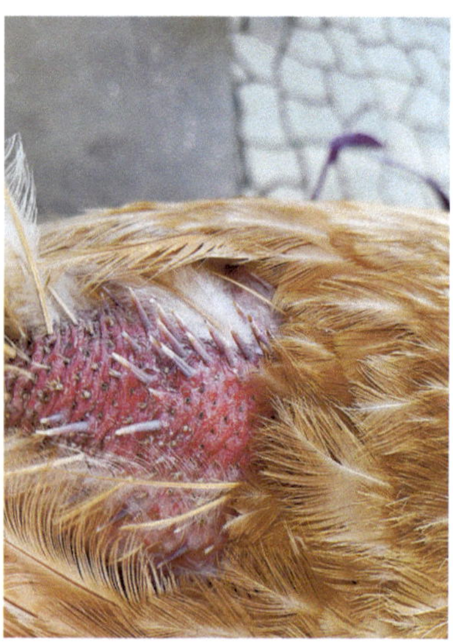

Figure 7.5 Emerging feathers. Courtesy of Sarah Meyer.

7.7.3.5 Treatment and Therapeutic Interventions

- **Feather Removal**
  If bleeding persists, pluck the entire blood feather from its follicle. Use sterile hemostats to apply steady traction in the direction of feather growth. Once removed, follicle seals and bleeding will usually stop. Clean with an appropriate antiseptic and apply antibiotic ointment to the follicle opening. Prevent further injury by self or other birds.

7.7.3.6 Prevention and Control

- **Housing Factors**
  Eliminate sharp edges, rough wire, or overcrowding.
- **Management Factors**
  Handle carefully during molt, and avoid wing clipping of blood feathers.
- **Social Factors**
  Reduce aggression and feather pecking through space, enrichment, and a balanced diet (Figure 7.5).

7.7.3.7 Nursing Considerations

Nursing care for a chicken with a broken blood feather emphasizes rapid bleeding control, wound management, and prevention of complications. Affected birds should be gently restrained in a calm, quiet environment to minimize stress and movement that could worsen blood loss. If the feather continues to bleed, the standard intervention is to remove the damaged feather shaft at its base using sterile forceps or hemostats, which seals off the blood vessel within the follicle. Direct pressure with sterile gauze may also be applied to aid clot formation. After bleeding is controlled, the site should be cleaned with a mild antiseptic to prevent infection, and the bird should be monitored for any recurrence of hemorrhage. Supportive nursing care includes providing the bird with rest, easy access to food and water, and a clean, dry environment to promote healing. Close observation is essential for signs of anemia, weakness, or secondary infection. To prevent recurrence, nursing considerations include monitoring flock behavior to reduce feather pecking, removing sharp equipment hazards, and providing adequate nutrition to support healthy feather development during molting.

7.7.4 Cutaneous Mucinosis

7.7.4.1 Overview and Pathogenesis

Cutaneous mucinosis in chickens is a rare integumentary condition characterized by the abnormal accumulation of mucin, a glycosaminoglycan-rich substance, within the dermis and subcutaneous tissues. This leads to the formation of localized or diffuse gelatinous swellings under the skin, most often observed in the comb, wattles, or other featherless areas. The exact etiology in poultry is not fully understood, but it is thought to involve dermal fibroblast dysfunction, where excessive mucin production or impaired degradation disrupts normal skin architecture.

Pathogenesis centers on the infiltration of mucopolysaccharides into the connective tissue, resulting in thickened, edematous, and translucent lesions that may interfere with normal blood circulation in the affected tissues. While cutaneous mucinosis in chickens is generally considered a benign and noncontagious condition, secondary complications such as skin trauma, impaired thermoregulation, or bacterial invasion may occur. In some cases, the lesions may resemble infectious processes, making accurate diagnosis important to rule out other dermatologic or systemic diseases.

7.7.4.2 Risk Factors

- **Host-Related Factors**
  Certain chicken lines or breeds may carry genetic tendencies for abnormal connective tissue metabolism. Heavy-breed birds (meat birds) may be more susceptible due to high metabolic demand.
- **Metabolic and Nutritional Factors**
  Abnormal collagen or glycosaminoglycan synthesis can lead to mucin buildup. Particularly, deficiencies affecting skin/connective tissue integrity (e.g., biotin, zinc, vitamin A). Overfeeding or rapid growth promotes connective tissue disorders.
- **Environmental and Management Factors**
  Chronic irritation or trauma to the skin may trigger mucin deposition in response to repeated injury. Moist, dirty litter can predispose to skin inflammation, encouraging abnormal dermal responses. High stocking density increases skin injury from crowding and pecking.
- **Immune and Infectious Factors**
  Long-term immune stimulation may promote mucin deposition in connective tissues. Secondary bacterial infections can complicate lesions and accelerate tissue changes.

7.7.4.3 Clinical Signs and Pathology

- **External Findings**
  Localized or diffuse skin swellings with a soft, gelatinous feel. Lesions may appear translucent or thickened, sometimes resembling tumors. Non-painful masses under the skin, often on the breast, back, or thighs. Feather loss over affected areas due to skin changes. Reduced mobility if lesions are extensive, interfering with locomotion.
- **Necropsy Findings**
  Skin appears thickened, gelatinous, and may exude a slimy or mucinous fluid when cut. Masses are poorly circumscribed and infiltrate the dermis/subcutis. Dermis infiltrated by pale blue, amorphous mucin deposits (staining with Alcian blue or PAS).

7.7.4.4 Diagnostic Testing

- **Histopathology**
  The tissue biopsy examined microscopically. Alcian blue or PAS staining demonstrates mucin (glycosaminoglycan) accumulation in the dermis. Confirms diagnosis and rules out neoplastic conditions.
- **Cytology**
  Smears may show a mucinous, clear to bluish background with sparse cells.

7.7.4.5 Treatment and Therapeutic Interventions

No specific curative therapy exists; management focuses on supportive care and reducing risk factors.

- **Supportive Care**
  Supplement diet with biotin, zinc, and vitamin A, and ensure adequate protein balance. Maintain clean, dry litter, and reduce trauma and skin irritation.
- **Surgical Interventions**
  Surgical excision of localized lesions may be attempted (though recurrence is possible).

7.7.4.6 Prevention and Control

- **Genetic Management**
  Avoid breeding birds with a history of mucinosis (possible hereditary predisposition).
- **Nutritional Balance**
  Provide adequate protein, essential amino acids, biotin, zinc, and vitamin A to support skin/connective tissue health.
- **Environmental Control**
  Keep litter clean, dry, and well-ventilated to prevent skin irritation. Avoid overcrowding and reduce the risk of trauma or pecking injuries.

7.7.4.7 Nursing Considerations

Nursing care for chickens with cutaneous mucinosis focuses on supportive management, monitoring, and prevention of secondary complications. Since the condition is generally benign and noncontagious, affected birds should be observed closely for changes in lesion size, skin trauma, or signs of discomfort. If swellings interfere with normal activity, such as feeding or thermoregulation, supportive adjustments—like ensuring easy access to food and water and maintaining a stable, stress-free environment—are essential. The affected skin should be kept clean and free from injury, as mucin-rich swellings are prone to abrasion and secondary bacterial infection. In cases where lesions become damaged, gentle cleansing and topical antiseptics may be applied under veterinary guidance. Regular monitoring of flock mates is advised to rule out other causes of dermal swelling that may mimic mucinosis, such as infectious conditions or neoplasia. Preventive considerations include maintaining good flock nutrition, minimizing environmental stressors, and providing safe housing that reduces the risk of skin trauma. Nursing efforts therefore prioritize observation, wound prevention, and supportive care while collaborating with veterinarians for diagnosis and long-term management.

7.7.5 Fly Strike (Myiasis)

7.7.5.1 Overview and Pathogenesis

Fly strike, or myiasis, in chickens is a parasitic condition caused by the infestation of fly larvae (maggots) in wounds, soiled feathers, or damaged skin. It is most associated with blowflies (*Calliphoridae*), which are attracted to moist, contaminated areas such as the vent, wounds, or necrotic skin (Figure 7.6).

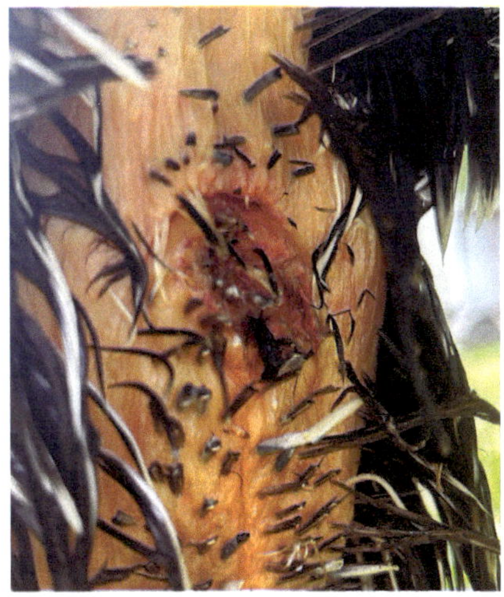

Figure 7.6 Post-procedure image; maggots were removed from the lesion. Courtesy of Stephanie Freeman.

Pathogenesis begins when adult flies lay eggs on compromised or dirty skin, often around sites of fecal contamination, trauma, or integumental disease. Within hours, the eggs hatch into larvae that burrow into the compromised skin and underlying tissues, feeding on necrotic and, in severe cases, healthy tissue. This invasion results in progressive tissue destruction, intense inflammation, pain, and foul-smelling lesions. The breakdown of skin integrity facilitates secondary bacterial infections, leading to cellulitis, septicemia, and toxemia if untreated. Severe infestations can rapidly debilitate the bird, causing anorexia, weakness, shock, and potentially death. Fly strike is therefore both a welfare issue and a management concern, strongly linked to environmental hygiene, wound care, and fly control practices.

7.7.5.2 Risk Factors

- **Environmental and Management Factors**
  Accumulation of manure, wet litter, and spilled feed attracts flies. Lack of fly control programs increases risk.
- **Host-Related Factors**
  Birds with fecal soiling, wet feathers, or caked litter near the vent are highly attractive to flies. Cuts, abrasions, or pecking injuries serve as egg-laying sites. Soiling around the cloaca provides moisture and odor that attract flies. Prolapse of the vent as exposed tissue is particularly vulnerable. Skin infections, bumblefoot, or abscesses predispose to strike.
- **Physiological and Health Factors**
  Obesity or poor mobility in birds makes them unable to preen effectively and making them more likely to have soiled feathers. Birds weakened by disease (e.g., coccidiosis, parasitism) may be less able to resist infestation.

7.7.5.3 Clinical Signs and Pathology

- **External Findings**

  Restlessness, agitation, or excessive preening. Foul odor near the affected area. Dirty, moist, or discolored feathers, often around the vent, wounds, or under wings. Visible maggots (fly larvae) in wounds or under feathers. Painful swelling and reddened or inflamed skin. Birds may become lethargic, depressed, or stop eating/drinking. Reluctance to move due to pain, especially if lesions are on the legs, feet, or vent area. Necrosis of tissue with ulcerated or open wounds. Strong, putrid odor from decaying tissue and bacterial growth. Death if untreated.
- **Necropsy Findings**

  Presence of larvae feeding on skin and subcutaneous tissue. Affected areas are moist, necrotic, and ulcerated, often with extensive tissue destruction. Hemorrhage and tissue liquefaction due to larval secretions (proteolytic enzymes). In severe cases, larvae may penetrate deep tissues, exposing muscles or even bones.

7.7.5.4 Diagnostic Testing

- **Clinical Examination**

  Primary method of diagnosis.

7.7.5.5 Treatment and Therapeutic Interventions

- **Immediate Wound Management**

  Isolate affected birds to reduce stress and prevent further fly exposure. Provide analgesia. Carefully remove larvae manually with sterile forceps and/or warm water from a sprayer. Clip feathers around the wound, flush and irrigate wounds with warm saline or dilute antiseptic solution (e.g., chlorhexidine, povidone-iodine). Ensure fly egg casings are also removed from feathers and skin.
- **Local Wound Therapy**

  Debridement of necrotic tissue to promote healing. Apply antiseptic ointments or sprays. Maintain wound cleanliness with daily flushing and reapplication. Apply insecticides to intact skin/feathers. Avoid spraying on compromised skin.
- **Medication**

  Amoxicillin

  Amoxicillin/Clavulanate: 125–250 mg/kg by mouth every 8–12 hours for 5–7 days.

  Amoxicillin Sodium: 50–250 mg/kg intramuscularly every 8–12 hours for 5–7 days.

  Amoxicillin Trihydrate: 55–200 mg/kg by mouth, subcutaneous, or intramuscularly every 4–12 hours for 5–7 days.

  Trimethoprim-Sulfamethoxazole

  100 mg/kg by mouth every 12 hours for 5–7 days.

  Meloxicam

  0.5 mg/kg by mouth or intramuscularly every 12–24 hours.

  or

  Carprofen

  5–10 mg/kg by mouth or intramuscularly once daily.
- **Supportive Care**

  Hydration and nutrition support offer electrolytes and vitamin supplements (esp. A, C, E, and zinc to aid skin healing). Reduce stress by keeping birds in a quiet, clean, fly-free environment. Prevent self-injury.

7.7.5.6 Prevention and Control

- **Environmental Management**
  Remove wet, caked litter and fecal buildup regularly. Maintain dry, well-ventilated housing to discourage fly breeding. Dispose of carcasses and spilled feed promptly, as they attract flies. Good airflow and dry flooring reduce fly density.
- **Fly Population Control**
  Predatory wasps (*Muscidifurax*, *Spalangia*) can reduce fly larvae. Fly traps, sticky tapes, bait stations in and around poultry houses. Residual sprays or dust in housing, not directly on birds unless poultry-safe. Rotation of products to prevent resistance.
- **Flock Health and Hygiene**
  Regular inspection of birds, especially around vent and under wings. Control and treat diarrheal causes, vent gleet, and cloacal prolapse. Treat wounds and pododermatitis early to avoid fly attractions. Birds with soiled vents or matted feathers should be cleaned promptly. Bathing and/or trimming of feathers surrounding vent.

7.7.5.7 Nursing Considerations

Nursing care for chickens affected by fly strike focuses on immediate removal of larvae, wound management, and prevention of recurrence. Affected birds should be isolated in a clean, dry environment to reduce stress and prevent further contamination. Larvae must be carefully removed manually or with veterinary-approved larvicidal treatments, and the wound should be thoroughly cleaned with antiseptic solutions to remove necrotic tissue and reduce bacterial load. Supportive care includes veterinarian-directed pain management, prescribed antibiotic, fluid therapy if necessary, and ensuring easy access to feed and water to support recovery. Environmental management is critical: clean, dry litter, prompt removal of feces, and control of fly populations through traps, screens, or insecticides help prevent recurrence. Regular inspection of the flock, especially the vent area and any wounds, is essential for early detection. Nursing also involves monitoring for systemic infection, administering antibiotics if prescribed, and maintaining overall flock hygiene. Overall, nursing considerations emphasize wound care, infection prevention, environmental sanitation, and supportive care to protect both bird welfare and flock health.

7.7.6 Hemangiomas and Hemangiosarcoma

7.7.6.1 Overview and Pathogenesis

Hemangiomas are benign vascular tumors arising from endothelial cells, commonly observed in older chickens, often manifesting as solitary, well-circumscribed nodules in the skin, comb, wattle, or occasionally internal organs. Hemangiosarcomas, by contrast, are malignant endothelial neoplasms that demonstrate aggressive local invasion and a high potential for metastasis, frequently affecting the liver, spleen, or lungs.

The pathogenesis of both tumor types involves the proliferation of endothelial cells forming irregular vascular channels. While the exact etiology remains unclear, chronic trauma, ultraviolet light exposure, and possibly viral factors have been implicated in tumor development. Hemangiomas generally grow slowly and rarely metastasize, whereas hemangiosarcoma's exhibit rapid growth, necrosis, hemorrhage, and disruption of normal organ architecture, leading to systemic clinical signs such as anemia, weakness, or sudden death in severe cases. Histologically, hemangiomas show well-formed, endothelial-lined vascular spaces, while hemangiosarcomas display cellular atypia, mitotic figures, and poorly organized vascular channels.

7.7.6.2 Risk Factors

- **Host-Related Factors**
  Most observed in older laying hens. Incidence increases with age due to cumulative cellular damage and chronic exposure to environmental stressors. Some studies suggest certain commercial layer breeds may be more prone, possibly due to genetic factors related to rapid growth or high egg production.
- **Environmental and Management Factors**
  Chronic trauma or irritation (e.g., from perches, overcrowding) may contribute to localized vascular proliferation. UV exposure in outdoor flocks has been implicated in rare cases of cutaneous vascular lesions. Poor husbandry leading to immunosuppression can indirectly increase tumor risk. Limited evidence exists in poultry, but exposure to carcinogens or toxic compounds in feed or environment could theoretically promote endothelial cell malignancy.
- **Chronic Irritation or Trauma**
  Persistent injury to the integument or subcutaneous tissue may create an environment conducive to malignant transformation.

7.7.6.3 Clinical Signs and Pathology

- **External Findings**
  Often asymptomatic, especially when small. May present as raised, red to purple nodules on the skin, comb, wattles, or sometimes on internal organs. Nodules are usually soft, compressible, and non-ulcerated. Rarely, if large or ulcerated, they may cause secondary bleeding or local irritation. Birds generally remain active and feed normally unless lesions interfere with movement or cause discomfort.
- **Necropsy Findings**
  Hemangioma
  Well-circumscribed, reddish blue to purple masses, often subcutaneous. Nodules may vary in size from a few millimeters to several centimeters. Surrounded by fibrous connective tissue capsules in some cases.

  Hemangiosarcoma
  Poorly circumscribed, dark red to black masses, often with areas of hemorrhage and necrosis. Internal organ involvement is common; the liver and spleen are frequently affected.

7.7.6.4 Diagnostic Testing

- **Cytology**
  Fine needle aspirates may show blood-filled vascular spaces, but distinction from hemangiosarcoma can be difficult. Limited utility due to risk of hemorrhage.
- **Radiographs**
  May detect masses in liver, spleen, or lungs.
- **Ultrasound**
  Useful for evaluating organ involvement, internal hemorrhage, or metastasis.

7.7.6.5 Treatment and Therapeutic Interventions

- **Surgical Interventions**
  Hemangioma
  Preferred treatment for accessible cutaneous lesions. Excisional surgery with clean margins is usually curative. Minimal risk of recurrence if completely removed. Local anesthesia or light sedation may be used.

Hemangiosarcoma

Excision of cutaneous tumors may be attempted if localized, but recurrence is common due to the malignant nature. Internal tumors are usually not amenable to surgery in poultry.

7.7.6.6 Prevention and Control

- **Genetic and Breeding Considerations**
  Use lines with a low incidence of vascular tumors, especially in commercial layers. Avoid breeding birds with a history of hemangiomas or hemangiosarcomas. Maintain genetic diversity to reduce predisposition to neoplasia.
- **Husbandry and Environmental Management**
  Ensure perches, feeders, and housing structures are safe and minimize injury. Avoid overcrowding, which increases fighting and irritation. Balanced diets supporting immune function may indirectly reduce tumor risk. Avoid exposure to mycotoxins or contaminants that could contribute to cellular damage. Outdoor flocks should have shaded areas to minimize excessive UV exposure that may trigger cutaneous lesions.
- **Health Management**
  Minimize stressors (handling, transportation, temperature extremes). Early detection of cutaneous nodules allows prompt removal of benign lesions before malignant transformation occurs.

7.7.6.7 Nursing Considerations

Nursing care of chickens with hemangiomas or hemangiosarcomas focuses on supportive care, early detection, and minimizing stress and trauma. For benign hemangiomas, surgical excision may be warranted if the lesion interferes with feeding, mobility, or is prone to bleeding, and post-operative care should include monitoring for hemorrhage, infection, and proper wound healing. In cases of hemangiosarcoma, supportive care aims to maintain hydration, nutrition, and comfort, as surgical removal is often limited by the tumor's invasiveness and potential for metastasis. The healthcare team should handle affected birds gently to prevent hemorrhage from friable tumor tissue. Environmental management, including soft bedding and reduced overcrowding, can reduce the risk of trauma and secondary infection. Monitoring systemic signs such as anemia, lethargy, or sudden weakness is essential, and decisions regarding humane euthanasia should be made promptly when quality of life is severely compromised.

7.7.7 Lipomas and Liposarcomas

7.7.7.1 Overview and Pathogenesis

Lipomas are benign tumors of adipose tissue commonly found in older chickens, often presenting as soft, slow-growing, well-circumscribed masses beneath the skin or in the subcutaneous tissue of the abdominal or ventral regions. Liposarcomas, in contrast, are malignant adipose tissue tumors that are rare in poultry but may demonstrate invasive growth, local tissue destruction, and potential for metastasis.

The pathogenesis of both tumor types involves the proliferation of adipocytes, with liposarcomas exhibiting cellular atypia, increased mitotic activity, and variable differentiation. Etiology is poorly understood, but age, obesity, chronic trauma, and possibly genetic predisposition are considered contributing factors. While lipomas are generally asymptomatic unless they interfere with movement or feeding, liposarcomas can compromise organ function, induce systemic illness, and occasionally lead to sudden deterioration. Histologically, lipomas consist of mature adipocytes arranged in lobules, whereas liposarcomas show pleomorphic cells, irregular fat vacuoles, and infiltrative growth patterns.

7.7.7.2 Risk Factors

- **Host-Related Factors**
  Most frequently seen in older birds, often >2 years. Some high-production layer lines may have increased susceptibility. Birds with high body fat may be at greater risk for malignant adipose tumors.

7.7.7.3 Clinical Signs and Pathology

- **External Findings**
  Lipomas
  Usually asymptomatic, especially when small. Subcutaneous, soft, slow-growing masses, often mobile under the skin. Common locations are abdomen, ventral thorax, near the keel, or along the back. Generally, birds maintain normal activity, appetite, and egg production. It may become problematic if large, interfering with mobility or causing pressure on adjacent structures.
  Liposarcomas
  Often slowly growing initially but may become rapid and infiltrative. Masses may feel firm, irregular, or lobulated, sometimes attached to deeper tissues. May ulcerate or cause secondary infection if near the skin surface. Birds may show lethargy, reduced feed intake, or weight loss if tumors interfere with organ function. Internal liposarcomas may remain subclinical until large or metastatic.
- **Necropsy Findings**
  Lipomas
  Well-circumscribed, soft, yellowish nodules composed of fat. They may be encapsulated and range from a few millimeters to several centimeters.

  Liposarcomas
  Poor circumscribed, yellow to pale tan masses with firm, irregular borders. May infiltrate surrounding muscles or internal organs. Necrosis or hemorrhage can occur in larger lesions.

7.7.7.4 Diagnostic Testing

- **Cytology**
  Lipomas
  Can identify mature adipocytes. Cells appear large, vacuolated, with small peripheral nuclei.

  Liposarcomas
  Can identify atypical adipocytes, pleomorphism, and mitotic figures.
- **Histopathology**
  Lipomas
  Excisional or incisional biopsy is the gold standard. Confirms diagnosis and rules out malignancy. Shows well-differentiated adipocytes, lobular arrangement, and minimal mitoses.

  Liposarcomas
  Excisional or incisional biopsy is the gold standard. Shows malignant adipocytes with nuclear pleomorphism, hyperchromasia, and increased mitotic activity.

7.7.7.5 Treatment and Therapeutic Interventions

- **Surgical Excision**

  Lipomas

  Preferred treatment for accessible or large masses. Complete removal is usually curative, with low-risk recurrence. Small lipomas may be left under observation if asymptomatic and not interfering with mobility. Local anesthesia and light sedation are typically sufficient.

  Liposarcomas

  Attempt a wide excision if the tumor is superficial and localized. Margins should be generous, as incomplete removal often results in recurrence. Surgery is usually not feasible for internal or infiltrative tumors.
- **Supportive Care**

  Monitor the surgical site for infection or delayed healing. Apply topical antiseptics as needed post-surgery. Ensure adequate nutrition, hydration, and comfort. Monitor for anemia, weight loss, or secondary infections. Prevent self-injury.

7.7.7.6 Prevention and Control

- **Genetic and Breeding Management**

  Avoid breeding birds with a history of lipomas or liposarcomas. Select lines with low predisposition to adipose tumors, particularly in commercial layers and broilers. Maintain genetic diversity to reduce susceptibility to neoplasia.
- **Nutrition and Body Condition**

  Provide a balanced diet to prevent excessive fat deposition. Avoid overfeeding high-calorie diets, particularly in layers with low activity. Promote exercise and mobility with housing to reduce obesity.
- **Husbandry and Environmental Management**

  Minimize chronic trauma by ensuring safe housing, perching, and equipment. Avoid overcrowding, which can contribute to stress and injury. Maintain clean and dry environments to reduce secondary infections associated with tumors.
- **Health Management**

  Prevent immunosuppression through vaccination programs (e.g., Marek's disease, IBD). Reduce stress handling, transportation, and extreme temperatures. Monitor flocks regularly for subcutaneous masses, especially in older birds.

7.7.7.7 Nursing Considerations

Nursing care of chickens with lipomas or liposarcomas focuses on supportive care, monitoring, and minimizing stress. Lipomas are usually benign and require intervention only if they interfere with mobility, feeding, or become traumatized; surgical excision may be performed, with careful post-operative monitoring for hemorrhage, infection, and proper wound healing. Liposarcomas, being malignant, often limit treatment options, so care emphasizes maintaining hydration, nutrition, and comfort while monitoring for systemic signs such as weight loss, lethargy, or sudden decline. Gentle handling is essential to prevent trauma to tumor masses. Environmental management, including soft bedding and adequate space, can reduce injury risk. Decisions regarding humane euthanasia should be made promptly if the bird's quality of life deteriorates due to tumor progression.

7.7.8 Melanoma

7.7.8.1 Overview and Pathogenesis

Melanomas are neoplasms of melanocytes, the pigment-producing cells, and are relatively rare in chickens. These tumors can be benign or malignant, with malignant forms demonstrating aggressive local invasion, tissue destruction, and potential for metastasis to internal organs such as the liver, spleen, and lungs.

Pathogenesis involves uncontrolled proliferation of melanocytes, often producing variably pigmented (black, brown, or gray) lesions in the skin, feather follicles, or occasionally internal tissues. Etiological factors are not fully understood, but genetic predisposition, chronic irritation, and ultraviolet light exposure have been suggested as contributing factors. Clinically, melanomas may present as raised, firm, pigmented masses that can ulcerate or interfere with normal feathering and skin integrity. Histologically, benign melanomas display well-differentiated melanocytes with minimal atypia, while malignant melanomas exhibit cellular pleomorphism, increased mitotic activity, invasiveness, and variable melanin production.

7.7.8.2 Risk Factors

- **Host-Related Factors**
  Dark-feathered breeds (e.g., Black Australorp, Ayam Cemani) appear more susceptible. Genetic factors influencing melanocyte distribution and activity may predispose certain lines. More common in older birds, typically layers over 2–3 years. Cumulative genetic and cellular damage increases risk.
- **Environmental Factors**
  Prolonged or intense sunlight exposure may trigger melanocyte proliferation, particularly in lightly pigmented skin areas. Repeated injury to feather follicles or skin may stimulate aberrant melanocyte activity. Exposure to chemical carcinogens, mycotoxins, or feed contaminants could theoretically contribute, though documented cases in poultry are limited.

7.7.8.3 Clinical Signs and Pathology

- **External Findings**
  Often appear as darkly pigmented nodules (black, brown, or gray). May be raised, firm, and irregularly shaped. They are commonly found on the comb, wattles, beak, eyelids, and feathered skin. Slow growing initially, it may become rapidly enlarging. Ulceration or secondary infection can occur in advanced lesions.
- **Necropsy Findings**
  Cutaneous Melanomas
  Darkly pigmented, firm nodules, sometimes multifocal. May ulcerate or bleed in advanced cases.

  Internal Melanomas
  Dark nodules in liver, spleen, heart, or lungs. Often poorly circumscribed with areas of necrosis or hemorrhage.

7.7.8.4 Diagnostic Testing

- **Cytology**
  It can reveal pigmented melanocytes, cellular pleomorphism, and variable nuclear-cytoplasmic ratios. Cytology alone may not definitively distinguish benign and malignant melanocytic tumors.

- **Histopathology**
  Excisional or incisional biopsy is the gold standard. Atypical melanocytes with pleomorphic nuclei, variable melanin pigmentation, mitotic activity, and invasion into surrounding tissue.

7.7.8.5 Treatment and Therapeutic Interventions

- **Surgical Excision**
  Primary treatment for accessible cutaneous melanomas. Wide excision with clean margins is recommended due to invasive potential. Small, localized tumors often respond well to complete removal. Local anesthesia and light sedation are generally sufficient.
- **Supportive and Palliative Care**
  Monitor for secondary infection at surgical sites. Provide adequate nutrition, hydration, and comfort, especially for older birds. Pain management and wound care as needed.
- **Advanced/Internal Tumors**
  Surgery is often not feasible for internal melanomas. Palliative care or euthanasia may be indicated for birds with extensive internal disease or systemic compromise.
- **Prognosis**
  Cutaneous, small, localized tumors are fair to good if completely excised. Large, invasive, or internal tumors have a poor prognosis due to aggressive behavior and potential metastasis.

7.7.8.6 Prevention and Control

- **Genetic and Breeding Management**
  Avoid breeding birds with a history of melanomas, especially in line prone to pigmentation-related tumors. Select breeds or lines with a lower incidence of melanocytic tumors, particularly in dark-feathered or high-value ornamental breeds. Maintain genetic diversity to reduce susceptibility.
- **Environmental Management**
  Provide shaded areas on outdoor flocks to reduce excessive sunlight, which may trigger melanocyte proliferation. Reduce chronic trauma or irritation to feathered skin and combs. Maintain clean, safe environments to minimize secondary infections.
- **Health Management**
  Early detection of cutaneous lesions allows timely surgical excision before tumors become invasive.

7.7.8.7 Nursing Considerations

Nursing care for chickens with melanomas emphasizes monitoring, supportive management, and minimizing trauma. Benign lesions may require little intervention unless they interfere with movement, feeding, or become ulcerated, in which case surgical removal can be considered, with attention to post-operative care to prevent infection and ensure proper healing. Malignant melanomas are often challenging to treat due to invasiveness and potential metastasis, so supportive care focuses on maintaining hydration, nutrition, and overall comfort. Birds should be handled gently to avoid damaging tumor tissue, and housing should be safe, with soft bedding and sufficient space to prevent injury. Regular observation for systemic signs such as lethargy, weight loss, or sudden decline is critical, and humane euthanasia should be considered if the bird's condition worsens or quality of life is severely compromised.

7.7.9 Molting

Figure 7.7.

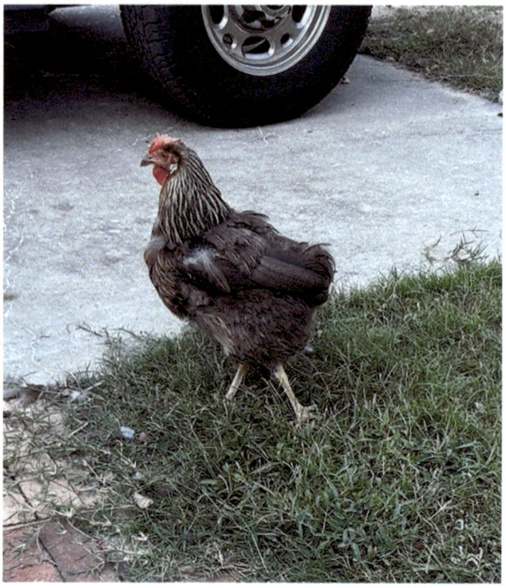

Figure 7.7 Brown Leghorn Hen Molting. Courtesy of Stephanie Freeman.

7.7.9.1 Overview and Pathogenesis

Molting is a natural, physiological process in chickens characterized by the periodic shedding and replacement of feathers, typically occurring annually or in response to environmental and nutritional factors. The process is hormonally regulated, primarily by fluctuations in thyroid hormones, prolactin, and corticosteroids, which influence feather follicle activity and feather keratin synthesis. Molting can be partial (light molt) or complete (hard molt), with the most noticeable feather loss occurring on the body, wings, and tail, often accompanied by a temporary reduction in egg production due to the redirection of nutrients toward feather regeneration. Chickens can also have two light molts in one season. Stressors such as changes in photoperiod, nutritional deficiencies, disease, or environmental challenges can accelerate or exacerbate the molting process.

Physiologically speaking, molting involves the regression of old feather follicles, apoptosis of follicular epithelial cells, and initiation of new feather germ development, culminating in the emergence of replacement feathers. While typically a normal and reversible process, prolonged or abnormal molting may indicate underlying health issues or suboptimal husbandry. A hen may also have a light molt after hormone pellet implantation. Hens of laying age will not simultaneously molt and lay eggs, as these two processes utilize great amounts of energy.

7.7.9.2 Risk Factors

- **Host-Related Factors**
  Most chickens undergo a post-laying molt at 18–24 months. Older layers may experience more pronounced or prolonged molting due to cumulative stress and physiological wear. Some commercial layer lines are more prone to stress-induced or partial molts. Breeds selected for high egg production may experience more pronounced egg-laying cessation during molt.
- **Light Factors**
  Decreasing daylight hours in fall can trigger molting in laying hens. Sudden changes in lighting schedule (too short or inconsistent photoperiods) may induce stress-related molting.

- **Nutrition and Body Condition**
  Protein deficiency is a major contributor, as feather regrowth requires high-quality protein. Deficiencies in methionine, cysteine, zinc, and vitamins (A, E, biotin) can delay or impair feather regeneration. Energy deficits can exacerbate weight loss during molts.
- **Stress and Environmental Factors**
  Overcrowding, poor ventilation, heat or cold stress, or rough handling may induce premature molt. Disease or parasitic infestations can also contribute by diverting nutrients and energy from feather regrowth (Figure 7.8).

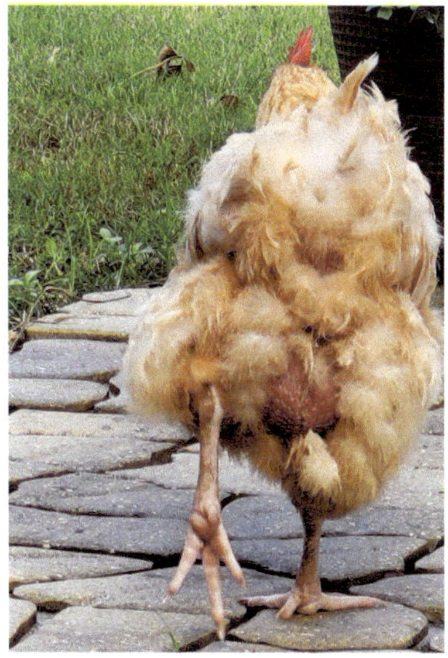

Figure 7.8 Normal molting of a Buff Orpington hen. Courtesy of Sarah Meyer.

7.7.9.3 Clinical Signs and Pathology

- **External Findings**
  Symmetrical or patterned shedding of body and wing feathers. Old, worn feathers are replaced by new growth. Initial shedding often occurs on the neck, back, and ventral body, followed by wings and tail. Egg-laying slows or ceases temporarily during molt. Pecking or aggression may increase due to discomfort from feather loss. Temporary weight loss may occur due to energy redirected to feather regrowth. Comb and wattles may pale as blood flow and reproductive activity decrease. Decreased activity level from diverted energy for feather regrowth (Figure 7.9).
- **Necropsy Findings**
  Skin appears thinner and paler under featherless areas. Follicular pores may be more prominent temporarily.

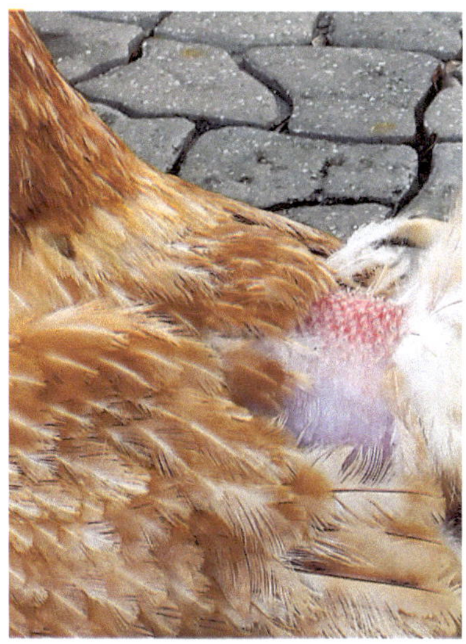

Figure 7.9 Feather loss due to self-trauma and bullying. New growth appears at each follicle. Courtesy of Stephanie Freeman.

7.7.9.4 Diagnostic Testing

- **Clinical History and Observation**
  Natural molts usually occur at 18–24 months and seasonally with shorter daylight hours. A predictable drop or cessation of lay is associated with molt. Symmetrical, staged feather replacement. Client reports lethargy in the bird and refusal to handle.

7.7.9.5 Treatment and Therapeutic Interventions

- **Supportive Care**
  Increase dietary protein (16–20%) to support feather regrowth. Ensure adequate levels of methionine, cysteine, zinc, vitamin A, vitamin E, and biotin. Provide balanced energy to prevent excessive weight loss. Analgesics should be considered on a case-by-case basis.

7.7.9.6 Prevention and Control

- **Management of Natural Molt**
  Provide consistent 14–16 hours of light per day for layers to maintain production. Avoid abrupt changes in light intensity or duration, which can trigger an early molt. Maintain a balanced diet with adequate protein, amino acids, and micronutrients.
- **Prevention of Stress-Induced or Abnormal Molt**
  Maintain stable temperatures; avoid sudden cold or heat stress. Prevent overcrowding; allow enough space per bird. Provide shaded, quiet areas in outdoor flocks. Control ectoparasites and endoparasites. Gentle handling to avoid feather breakage. Minimize loud noises, predators, or other stress triggers.

7.7.9.7 Nursing Considerations

Nursing care during molting: chickens require supportive care to maintain health and minimize stress. Nutritional support is critical, as feather regrowth demands higher levels of protein, vitamins (particularly A, D, and E), and minerals such as zinc and sulfur-containing amino acids. Ensuring access to clean water and a balanced diet helps prevent weight loss and supports immune function. Environmental management, including adequate lighting, comfortable housing, and reduced stressors, can promote a smoother molting process. Egg production may temporarily decline, which is normal and does not require intervention. Monitoring birds for secondary issues such as feather pecking, skin irritation, or signs of illness is important, and adjustments to flock management or diet should be made if molting is prolonged or unusually severe.

7.7.10 Severe Feather-Picking

7.7.10.1 Overview and Pathogenesis

Severe feather picking, also referred to as feather pecking or cannibalistic behavior, is a behavioral disorder in chickens characterized by repetitive pecking, plucking, or pulling of feathers, often leading to skin injury, stress, and secondary infections. The condition is multifactorial, with both environmental and physiological contributors.

Pathogenesis involves a combination of social hierarchy dynamics, boredom or stress due to overcrowding, nutritional deficiencies (particularly protein, methionine, and salt imbalances), and genetic predisposition. Feather pecking may begin as gentle preening but can escalate to severe damage as the behavior becomes habitual and reinforced within the flock. Neuroendocrine factors, including serotonin and corticosterone levels, influence aggression and stress responses, which can exacerbate the behavior. Chronic feather picking disrupts the integumentary system, resulting in inflammation, ulceration, hemorrhage, and increased susceptibility to parasites and opportunistic bacterial infections. Left unmanaged, it can lead to decreased productivity, poor welfare, and mortality in affected flocks.

7.7.10.2 Risk Factors

- **Environmental and Management Factors**
  Overcrowding increases aggression and competition. Limited access to feeders, drinkers, or nest boxes. Too bright or intense light stimulates aggression. Erratic light schedules disrupt normal behavior. Birds without foraging opportunities redirect pecking behavior toward flock mates.
- **Nutritional Factors**
  Inadequate dietary protein or amino acids increases feather eating. Especially sodium, calcium, magnesium, and vitamins A, D, and E. Leads to frustration and abnormal foraging behavior.

- **Social and Behavioral Factors**
  Introduction of new birds increases pecking order disputes. Mixed-age or mixed-breed flocks, differences in size, feather color, or maturity increase targeting.
- **Genetic and Breed Predisposition**
  Some commercial layer strains (particularly white egg laying lines) are more prone to feather pecking. Selective breeding for high productivity has been associated with increased behavioral vices.
- **Health and Physical Condition**
  Skin irritation or parasites as birds may peck themselves or others. Exposed skin and emerging pinfeathers attract pecking. Red lesions, the red color, or blood triggers further pecking.

7.7.10.3 Clinical Signs and Pathology

- **External Findings**
  Feather loss is localized at first typically to the tail, back, vent, wings, or neck. Progresses to generalize feather loss in severe cases. Exposed skin may appear red, inflamed, or irritated. Broken feathers, scratches, abrasions, or bleeding wounds. Raw areas may attract more pecking, escalating to cannibalism. Increased aggression in dominant birds. Submissive, stressed behavior in victims. Birds may show restlessness or preoccupation with pecking activity. Reduced egg production due to stress.
- **Necropsy Findings**
  Feather loss with exposed, erythematous skin. Excoriations, scabs, ulcerations, or hemorrhages where pecking is severe. Severe pecking may penetrate the abdominal cavity (coelom), especially around the vent.

7.7.10.4 Diagnostic Testing

- **Clinical History**
  Onset patterns often begin with a few birds and spread through the flock. Careful observation of flock behavior may reveal aggressive peckers targeting victims.

7.7.10.5 Treatment and Therapeutic Interventions

- **Immediate Management Interventions**
  Remove dominant birds initiating the behavior to protect the victims. Isolate injured birds for recovery, reducing the risk of cannibalism. Lower stocking density, provide adequate feeder and waterer space, and maintain proper ventilation and temperature.
- **Wound Care for Affected Birds**
  Clean with antiseptics (iodine, chlorhexidine) and apply topical antibiotic ointment to wounds. Use bitter-tasting sprays to discourage further pecking. A "onesie" can be placed on a bird to prevent further pecking while feathers are regrown. In cases of severe infection, systemic antibiotics may be administered under veterinary supervision.

7.7.10.6 Prevention and Control

- **Environmental Management**
  Maintain recommended space allowances. Use low- to moderate-intensity lighting and avoid sudden changes in light intensity or duration. Prevent overheating, humidity buildup, and poor air quality that increase restlessness. Provide foraging materials (pecking blocks, hanging vegetables, straw bales, puzzle toys). Ensure dust bathing opportunities. Scatter feed or grains to stimulate natural pecking behaviors.

7.7.10.7 Nursing Considerations

Nursing care of severe feather picking focuses on reducing stress, preventing injury, and addressing underlying causes. Environmental enrichment, including adequate space, perches, dust baths, and foraging opportunities, can reduce boredom and aggression. Nutritional support is critical; ensure diets meet protein, amino acid, and mineral requirements. Affected birds should be monitored closely for skin trauma, infection, and feather loss. Physical barriers or protective devices (e.g., collars or modified beak devices) may be used temporarily to prevent further damage. Prompt removal of severely injured birds and isolation of aggressive individuals can help prevent escalation. Maintaining proper flock management, minimizing overcrowding, and ensuring consistent lighting and temperature conditions are essential. In chronic or severe cases, consultation with a veterinarian for behavioral or medical interventions may be necessary to safeguard bird welfare (Figure 7.10).

7.7.11 Squamous Cell Carcinoma

7.7.11.1 Overview and Pathogenesis

Squamous cell carcinoma (SCC) is a malignant epithelial tumor arising from keratinizing cells of the skin or mucous membranes in chickens. It most commonly affects areas exposed to chronic irritation, ultraviolet light, or previous injury, such as the comb, wattles, eyelids, or oral cavity.

Pathogenesis involves the uncontrolled proliferation of atypical squamous epithelial cells, which invade underlying tissues and can metastasize regional lymph nodes or internal organs. Chronic trauma, viral infections (such as avian papillomavirus), and ultraviolet exposure are considered predisposing factors. Histologically, SCC is characterized by keratin pearls, cellular pleomorphism, and evidence of local invasiveness. Clinically, lesions may present as firm, ulcerated, or nodular masses that bleed easily, compromise normal tissue function, and, in advanced cases, can lead to systemic illness due to metastasis or secondary infections.

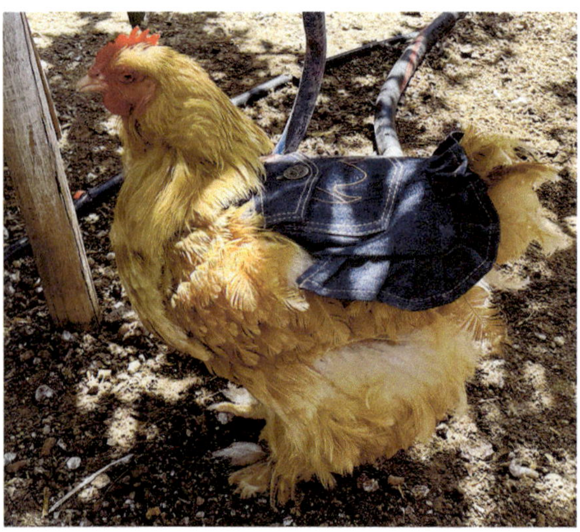

Figure 7.10 Hen wearing a cloth "saddle" to protect her back from a vigorous rooster. Courtesy of Funky Chicken Rescue.

7.7.11.2 Risk Factors

- **Environmental and Physical Factors**
  Chronic irritation or trauma to skin or mucous membranes (e.g., from pecking, injury, or poorly fitting equipment). UV radiation exposure, especially in areas of sparse feathering (e.g., comb, wattles, eyelids). Poor ventilation or high ammonia levels in housing, which cause chronic irritation of mucosal surfaces.
- **Infectious Agents**
  Oncogenic viruses (retroviruses, papillomaviruses) are implicated in SCC development in birds. Chronic infections (bacterial, fungal, or parasitic dermatitis) may predispose to malignant transformation due to sustained inflammation.
- **Genetic and Host-Related Factors**
  More common in older chickens, reflecting accumulation of genetic damage. Some evidence suggests certain genetic lines may be predisposed, though this is less defined in poultry than in mammals. Birds with underlying immunosuppression may have higher neoplastic risk.
- **Chemical and Dietary Factors**
  Prolonged exposure to toxins (e.g., polycyclic aromatic hydrocarbons, nitrosamines) may increase risk. Chronic deficiencies in vitamins A and E can impair epithelial integrity, predisposing to neoplasia.

7.7.11.3 Clinical Signs and Pathology

- **External Findings**
  Firm, raised, ulcerated masses on comb, wattles, eyelids, or featherless skin. Nonhealing wounds or ulcers that bleed easily. Progressive enlargement, sometimes with crusting or keratinized "horn-like" growths. Localized pain, pruritus, or irritation may cause pecking/self-trauma. Proliferative, ulcerated growth around cloaca. May cause straining, secondary infections, or bleeding. In advanced cases, there is evidence of metastasis (dyspnea, lameness, or visceral organ dysfunction depending on spread).
- **Necropsy Findings**
  Nodular, proliferative, or ulcerated masses arising from squamous epithelium. Often irregular, with necrotic centers and keratinized surfaces. Tumors may infiltrate underlying muscle, connective tissue, and bone. Frequently solitary but can be multiple. Most common on comb, wattles, skin, eyelids, oral cavity, esophagus, and cloaca.

7.7.11.4 Diagnostic Testing

- **Cytology**
  Fine needle aspiration (FNA) or impression smears of lesions. May reveal pleomorphic squamous epithelial cells, keratin debris, and inflammatory cells. It is useful for screening, but cannot definitively distinguish SCC from other epithelial tumors.
- **Histopathology**
  Biopsy samples submitted for histology. Confirm SCC by identifying invasive nest/cords of squamous epithelial cells, keratin pearls, cellular atypia, and loss of normal tissue architecture. Essential for differentiating SCC from fowlpox, papilloma, or granulomatous dermatitis.

7.7.11.5 Treatment and Therapeutic Interventions

- **Surgical Management**
  Excision of localized tumors may be attempted for small, accessible lesions. Wide margins are required to prevent recurrence but are difficult due to limited skin availability and tumor invasiveness. Recurrence is common if the tumor is not completely excised.

7.7.11.6 Prevention and Control

- **Environmental Management**
  Provide shaded areas in outdoor systems to limit solar radiation exposure, especially for light-skinned or sparsely feathered areas (comb, wattles). Reduce skin trauma from pecking, poorly designed cages, or sharp housing structures. Maintain proper flooring to avoid repeated injury to feet or vent area. Control ammonia and dust levels to reduce chronic mucosal irritation.
- **Infectious Disease Control**
  Limit exposure to oncogenic viruses (retroviruses and papillomaviruses) through biosecurity and good breeding stock management. Control bacterial, fungal, and parasitic dermatitis to prevent chronic inflammation that predisposes to neoplastic transformation.

7.7.11.7 Nursing Considerations

Nursing care for chickens with SCC focuses on supportive management, minimizing trauma, and monitoring for complications. Surgical excision is often the primary treatment for localized lesions, with careful postoperative care to prevent hemorrhage, infection, and delayed wound healing. Malignant or advanced tumors may limit treatment options, so supportive care emphasizing hydration, nutrition, and overall comfort is essential. Birds should be handled gently to avoid disrupting fragile tumor tissue, and housing should provide soft bedding and adequate space to reduce injury risk. Regular monitoring for systemic signs such as lethargy, weight loss, or worsening lesions is critical. Humane euthanasia should be considered when the tumor compromises the bird's quality of life or when metastasis causes significant systemic illness.

7.7.12 Uropygial Gland Infection

7.7.12.1 Overview and Pathogenesis

Uropygial gland infection, also referred to as preen gland infection or adenitis, is an inflammatory condition affecting the sebaceous uropygial gland located at the dorsal base of the tail. The condition may be caused by bacterial, fungal, or mixed microbial infections, such as those from *Staphylococcus spp.*, *E. coli*, and *Candida spp.* commonly implicated.

Pathogenesis involves obstruction of the gland duct or trauma to the gland, leading to accumulation of glandular secretions, secondary microbial proliferation, and subsequent inflammation. Clinical lesions include swelling, redness, pain, and, in chronic cases, abscess formation or necrosis of glandular tissue. Infected secretions can alter feather condition and predispose the bird to skin irritation, feather damage, and opportunistic infections. Predisposing factors include poor hygiene, feather-picking, nutritional deficiencies, or immunosuppression. Histologically, affected glands show ductal dilation, epithelial hyperplasia, infiltration with heterophils and lymphocytes, and necrotic debris within the lumen.

7.7.12.2 Risk Factors

- **Environmental and Management Factors**
  Dirty litter or soiled housing increased bacterial and fungal exposure. Wet bedding or high humidity favors microbial proliferation. Overcrowding increases stress-induced pecking and the risk of trauma to the gland. Rough surfaces can traumatize the gland or surrounding skin.
- **Trauma and Mechanical Factors**
  Injury to the uropygial gland (pecking, abrasion, or catching on perches) creates an entry point for pathogens. Over-preening or self-trauma causes irritation of the gland, which may predispose it to infection.

7.7.12.3 Clinical Signs and Pathology

- **External Findings**
  Swelling at the base of the tail where the uropygial gland is located. Redness, heat, and pain on palpation. Discharge may be watery, creamy, or purulent, sometimes with a foul odor. Crust formation around the gland or feathers coated with exudate. Birds may peck or scratch at the affected area. Reduced activity, fever-like lethargy in severe cases. Reluctance to roost or preen due to discomfort. Feather matting or loss around the gland due to discharge or self-trauma. Reduced egg production in laying hens due to systemic stress.
- **Necropsy Findings**
  Enlarged gland, firm, swollen, may feel fluctuant if abscessed. Surrounding tissues may show erythema, edema, and feather matting.

7.7.12.4 Diagnostic Testing

- **Culture**
  Sterile swab of exudate or aspirate from the gland. Identifies bacterial pathogens (commonly *Staphylococcus* spp., *E. coli,* and *Pseudomonas* spp.) and informs antibiotic choice.

7.7.12.5 Treatment and Therapeutic Interventions

- **Medication**
  Trimethoprim-Sulfamethoxazole
  100 mg/kg by mouth every 12 hours for 5–7 days.

  Amoxicillin
  Amoxicillin/Clavulanate: 125–250 mg/kg by mouth every 8–12 hours for 5–7 days.
  Amoxicillin Sodium: 50–250 mg/kg intramuscularly every 8–12 hours for 5–7 days.
  Amoxicillin Trihydrate: 55–200 mg/kg by mouth, subcutaneous, or intramuscularly every 4–12 hours for 5–7 days.

  Meloxicam
  0.5 mg/kg by mouth or intramuscularly every 12–24 hours.

  Carprofen
  5–10 mg/kg by mouth or intramuscularly once daily.
- **Local Therapy**
  Gland flushing with sterile saline or antiseptic irrigation to remove debris and pus. Clean with antiseptics, such as iodine and chlorhexidine, and apply a topical like silver sulfadiazine or triple antibiotic ointment. Keep feathers trimmed or matting removed to allow drainage and healing.
- **Surgical Intervention**
  Indicated for abscesses or chronic, nonresponsive infections. Excision or drainage of the gland under local or general anesthesia. Post-operative care includes antibiotics, analgesics, and bandaging if needed.

7.7.12.6 Prevention and Control

- **Environmental Management**
  Keep litter clean and dry to reduce bacterial and fungal loads. Regular removal of feces and wet bedding. Maintain good airflow to minimize moisture accumulation. Avoid sharp edges and overcrowding that could injure the gland.

- **Trauma Prevention**
  Prevent pecking or fighting within the flock by maintaining stable social groups. Minimize feather damage around the uropygial gland to prevent secondary infection. Ensure gentle handling during management procedures. A hen saddle may be used.

7.7.12.7 Nursing Considerations

Nursing care of uropygial gland infections focuses on reducing inflammation, controlling infection, and preventing recurrence. Birds should be handled gently to avoid exacerbating pain or gland damage. Local care may include cleaning the gland with antiseptic solutions and applying topical antimicrobial or antifungal agents as indicated by veterinary guidance. Systemic antibiotic therapy may be necessary for severe or deep infections. Environmental management, including maintaining clean housing, reducing moisture, and minimizing trauma to the tail region, is essential to prevent reinfection. Monitoring for signs of systemic illness, such as lethargy or decreased feed intake, is important. In chronic or severe cases with abscess formation or necrosis, surgical drainage or excision of the gland may be required. Supportive care, including ensuring easy access to feed and water and reducing stress, helps optimize recovery.

Further Reading

Common Poultry Diseases [Internet]. [cited 2025 Dec 7]. Available from: https://poultry.extension.org/articles/poultry-health/common-poultry-diseases/

LLC P. Skin & Feathers [Internet]. [cited 2025 Dec 7]. Available from: https://poultrydvm.com/system/skin

8

Gastrointestinal Diseases and Internal Parasites

"The worms crawl in, the worms crawl out ... "

Gastrointestinal (GI) diseases are among the most common health concerns encountered in chickens, regardless of whether they are raised in commercial facilities, small flocks, or backyard settings. Because chickens rely on an efficient digestive system for nutrient absorption and overall productivity, disruptions to GI health quickly translate into reduced growth, decreased egg production, poor feed conversion, and in severe cases, mortality.

Veterinary technicians often serve as the first point of contact in identifying subtle early warning signs of GI disorders. Their role encompasses observation, fecal sample collection, assistance in necropsy, treatment administration, and client education. Intestinal and crop diseases frequently present with nonspecific clinical signs, requiring careful assessment of flock history, environment, and diet for accurate diagnosis.

This chapter provides a comprehensive review of GI diseases and crop disorders in chickens, with emphasis on clinical signs, diagnostic testing, therapeutic strategies—including both pharmacological and supportive care—and nursing considerations.

8.1 Anatomy and Physiology of the Digestive Tract

Understanding the structure and function of the avian digestive system is essential to recognizing disease processes. Unlike mammals, birds lack teeth; instead, their digestive system is adapted to process ingested feed efficiently through a series of specialized organs (Figure 8.1).

1) **Beak and Oral Cavity,** feed enters via the beak. The oral cavity contains the tongue and salivary glands that moisten feed. Saliva contains amylase to begin the digestion of starch.
2) **Esophagus and Crop,** the esophagus is a muscular tube leading from the pharynx to the crop, a thin-walled outpouching located at the thoracic inlet. The crop serves as a temporary storage organ and softens ingested material before it passes into the proventriculus.
3) **Proventriculus and Gizzard,** the proventriculus (glandular stomach) secretes hydrochloric acid and pepsin. The gizzard (ventriculus) mechanically grinds feed, aided by grit.
4) **Intestines,** the small intestines, are divided into the duodenum, jejunum, and ileum, where most digestion and absorption occur. Paired ceca at the ileocecal junction serve as fermentation chambers. The large intestine is short and leads to the cloaca, where waste products mix before excretion.
5) **Microbiota and Immunity,** the avian gut contains a diverse microbiome critical for nutrient absorption, pathogen exclusion, and immune modulation. Disturbances to this microbiota—through antibiotics, diet changes, stress, or parasitism—can predispose chickens to GI disease.

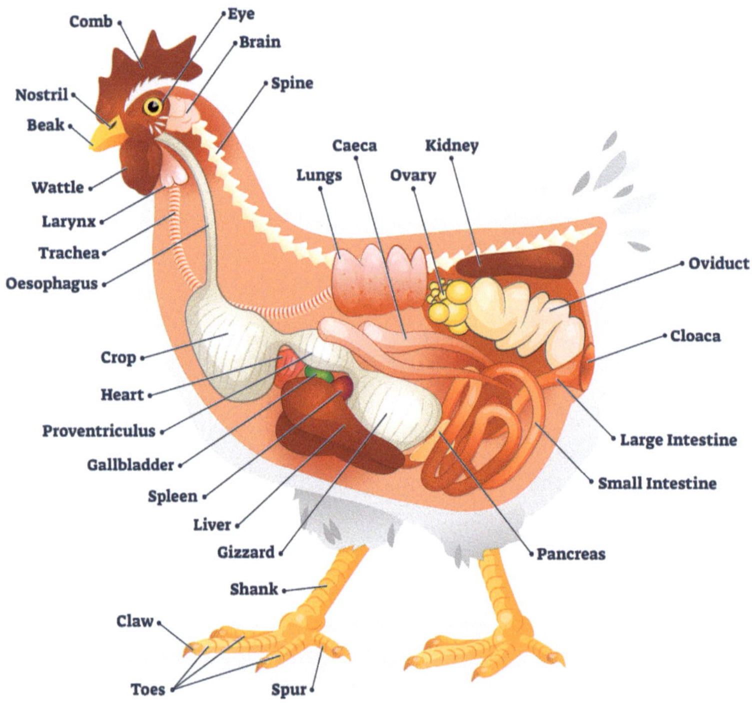

Figure 8.1 Internal anatomy of the hen. VectorMine / Adobe Stock Photos.

8.2 General Clinical Signs of Gastrointestinal Disease

Clinical signs of GI disease are often nonspecific and may overlap with systemic conditions.
The veterinary technician should be observant for:

- Weight loss or poor growth despite adequate feed.
- Ruffled feathers (unthriftiness) and general malaise.
- Changes in droppings: watery, mucoid, bloody, or containing undigested feed.
- Crop abnormalities: distension, delayed emptying, foul odor from the mouth.
- Decreased egg production or poor shell quality.
- Soiling of vent feathers with fecal material.
- Dehydration (sunken eyes, reduced skin elasticity, tacky mucous membranes).

Because many diseases produce overlapping signs, diagnostic testing is critical to confirm the etiology.

8.3 Crop Disorders

The crop is a frequent place of disease because of its role as a storage organ. Disorders may be primary or secondary to systemic illness.

Quick reference chart

Disorder/ condition	Etiology/cause	Clinical signs	Diagnosis	Treatment/management
Impacted crop (crop stasis)	Ingestion of long fibrous material (grass, straw, feathers); dehydration; foreign body; poor grit access	Firm, non-emptying crop; reduced appetite; lethargy; weight loss	Palpation of firm crop; history; radiography (if needed)	Withhold feed, provide fluids; gentle crop massage; crop lavage; surgical emptying if severe; correct underlying cause
Sour crop (candidiasis/ crop mycosis)	*Candida albicans* overgrowth due to prolonged antibiotics, stress, or feed stasis	Foul-smelling fluid in crop; soft, doughy crop; regurgitation; depression	Cytology (yeast, pseudohyphae); culture	Empty and flush crop; antifungal (nystatin, fluconazole); correct diet and hygiene; probiotics post-antibiotic use
Pendulous crop	Overeating, chronic impaction, loss of crop muscle tone, nerve damage	Crop hangs low and fails to empty overnight; soft, sagging sac	Physical exam, history	Supportive bra to elevate crop; manage feed intake; treat underlying infection or impaction; may require surgical correction if chronic
Crop burn (thermal injury)	Feeding overheated formula or fluids (common in hand-reared chicks)	Pain, swelling, visible necrosis of crop skin; lethargy; anorexia	History, clinical signs	Supportive care, antibiotics, surgical repair if perforated; prevent by checking feed temperature (<41°C/105°F)
Crop necrosis/ rupture	Secondary to severe impaction, burn, trauma, or infection	Open wound or leakage of feed through skin; inflammation	Visual inspection	Surgical debridement and closure; antibiotics; supportive care
Foreign body ingestion	Ingestion of nondigestible material (plastic, string, metal)	Inappetence, palpable mass in crop, stasis	Palpation, radiography	Crop lavage or surgical removal; prevent access to foreign material.
Bacterial crop infection	Secondary to trauma, foreign body, or impaction; *E. coli*, *Staphylococcus* spp.	Foul odor, inflammation, possible abscess	Culture and sensitivity	Broad-spectrum antibiotics; crop lavage; treat predisposing cause

Chart created by Stephanie Freeman.

8.3.1 Crop Impaction

8.3.1.1 Overview and Pathogenesis

Crop impaction is a digestive disorder in chickens characterized by physical obstruction of the crop, preventing normal passage of ingested feed into the proventriculus and gizzard. The condition primarily affects adult birds, particularly those in flocks fed fibrous, coarse, or indigestible materials, and is of significance due to reduced feed intake, poor growth, decreased egg production, and increased risk of secondary infections. Predisposing factors include ingestion of long grasses, straw, hair, feathers, plastic, or other foreign materials, dehydration, improper feed particle size, and underlying motility disorders. Clinically affected birds may present visible crop distension, firm or doughy crop contents, regurgitation, anorexia, lethargy, weight loss, and sometimes dehydration or weakness.

The pathogenesis of crop impaction begins with the accumulation of indigestible feed or foreign material in the crop, which physically obstructs the normal flow of ingesta. The retained material can absorb moisture, swell, and further distend the crop, leading to mechanical stretching of the crop wall and interference with muscular motility. Prolonged retention may result in mucosal irritation, local inflammation, secondary microbial overgrowth, and souring of crop contents, compounding the obstruction. Severe or chronic impaction can compromise nutrient absorption, cause systemic weakness, and predispose the bird to secondary infections or starvation. Overall, crop impaction is a mechanical digestive disorder in which physical obstruction, impaired motility, and secondary microbial changes converge to impair feed passage, growth, and productivity in affected chickens.

8.3.1.2 Risk Factors

- **Dietary Factors**
  Consumption of long grass, straw, hay, pine needles, or tough plant matter can clump together and block the crop. Bedding material (wood shavings, straw), feathers (self- or flock-plucked), string, plastic, or other debris. Grit (small stones) helps grind food in the gizzard. Without it, larger food particles may accumulate in the crop. Diets low in digestible nutrients or poorly balanced feeds can slow GI motility, encouraging stasis.
- **Environmental and Management Factors**
  Access to contaminated litter, feathers, or trash increases the chances of ingesting foreign material. Overcrowding leads to stress and feather pecking/ingestion. Bored birds may eat nonfood items (pica behavior). Sudden changes in feed type or feeding schedule can disrupt normal digestive rhythm and crop emptying.
- **Individual Bird Factor**
  Young or inexperienced birds may be more prone to eating inappropriate materials. Diseases that reduce crop motility, such as Marek's disease, Candidiasis, or systemic infections, can predispose to impact. Lack of water intake causes food material to become dry and compact, making it harder to pass. Poor general condition can weaken crop muscles and reduce motility.

8.3.1.3 Clinical Signs and Pathology

- **External Findings**
  The crop remains full and hard even after an overnight fast, often feels like a solid lump or mass when palpated. Birds may stop eating or pick at food. Decrease in water consumption. Weight loss and poor body condition. Lethargy and depression. Decreased or absent fecal output. Foul-smelling breath may occur if stagnant material ferments, leading to secondary infection (often Candidiasis or bacterial overgrowth).
- **Necropsy Findings**
  Proventriculus and gizzard are empty due to obstruction. Emaciation and muscle atrophy are common in prolonged anorexia. Mucosal hyperplasia, ulceration, or necrosis of the crop lining. Yeast hyphae or bacterial colonies, if secondary infection is present.

8.3.1.4 Diagnostic Testing

Diagnosing crop impaction is primarily clinical, but additional tests may be used to confirm the severity, rule out other conditions, or identify secondary infections.

- **Diagnostic Imaging**
  Useful to visualize foreign objects, large fibrous masses, or impacted material. Help differentiate crop impaction from tumors, abscesses, or other obstructive lesions. Ultrasonography can assess crop wall thickness, mucosal integrity, and fluid content. Less commonly used in backyard practice but helpful in complicated cases.
- **Crop Lavage/Cytology**
  Samples of crop contents can identify yeast or bacterial overgrowth.

8.3.1.5 Treatment and Therapeutic Interventions

- **Supportive Care**
  For severe dehydration, subcutaneous, intravenous, or intraosseous fluids may be necessary in a clinical setting. Withhold feed temporarily if the crop is severely impacted. After resolution, reintroduce softened or easily digestible feed gradually (e.g., moistened pellets, cooked grains, or scrambled egg). Reduce stress to support recovery. Maintain comfortable temperatures (75–80°F) to aid gut motility. Pre- and probiotics can be introduced for a healthy microbiome.
- **Crop Emptying Techniques**
  For soft impactions, gently massage the crop to help move contents toward the proventriculus. A supportive crop "bra" can be applied to the bird. Monitor closely for pain or rupture risk. Administer vegetable oil, mineral oil, or poultry-safe laxatives orally to soften fibrous masses. In cases where manual methods fail, a crop tube can be used to gently flush out the impacted material with warm water. Perform under veterinary supervision to prevent trauma or aspiration, rarely required, reserved for severe, chronic impactions with necrotic or obstructive material. Ingluviotomy, an incision into the crop to remove impacted material (Figures 8.2 and 8.3).

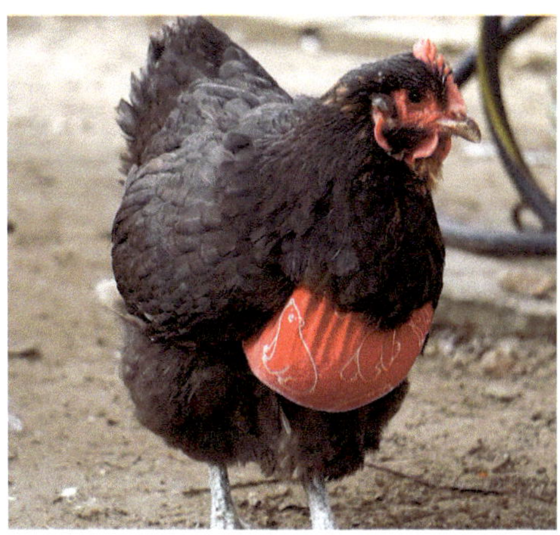

Figure 8.2 "Bra" apparatus for crop support. Courtesy of Cindy Justice Liles.

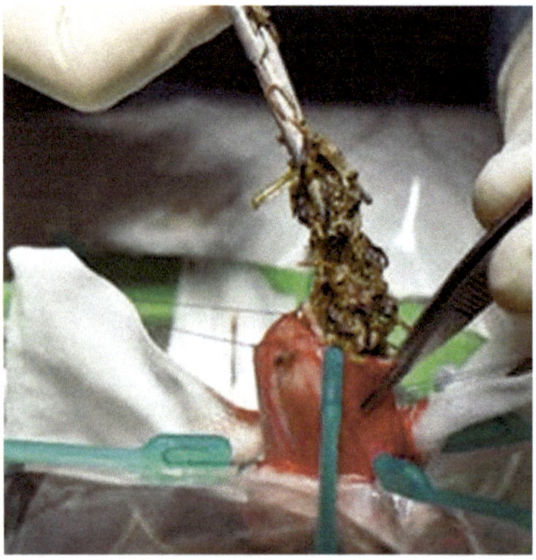

Figure 8.3 Surgical removal of impacted crop contents. Courtesy of Unusual Pet Vets.

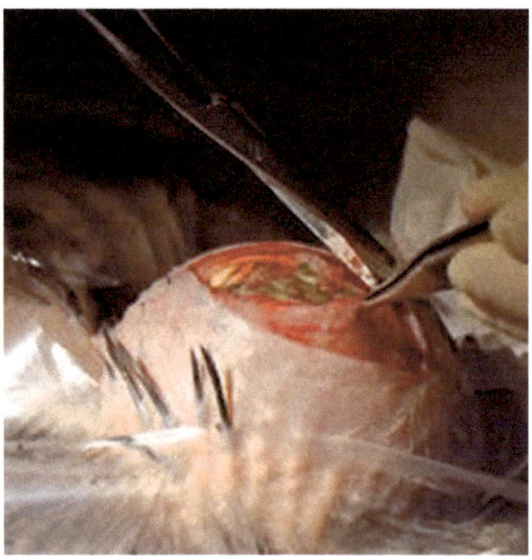

Figure 8.4 Incision made into the crop. Courtesy of Unusual Pet Vets.

8.3.1.6 Nursing Considerations

Nursing care for chickens with crop impaction focuses on relieving the obstruction, providing supportive care, and preventing recurrence. Affected birds should be monitored closely for signs of discomfort, dehydration, lethargy, and poor appetite, and offered easy-to-digest feed or softened mash to reduce strain on the crop. Ensuring access to clean, fresh water is critical, as hydration aids in softening impacted material and maintaining overall health. Nursing interventions may include gentle massage of the crop or careful manual removal of obstructive material under veterinary guidance. Environmental management is equally important: maintain clean litter, avoid overcrowding, and remove access to indigestible or fibrous materials that may contribute to recurrence. Observation for secondary complications, such as sour crop, microbial overgrowth, or systemic weakness, is essential, and birds showing persistent signs should receive veterinary evaluation and supportive treatment, including fluids or probiotics if indicated. Overall, nursing considerations for crop impaction emphasize monitoring, supportive feeding and hydration, environmental management, and timely intervention to restore normal crop function and prevent further morbidity (Figures 8.4–8.6).

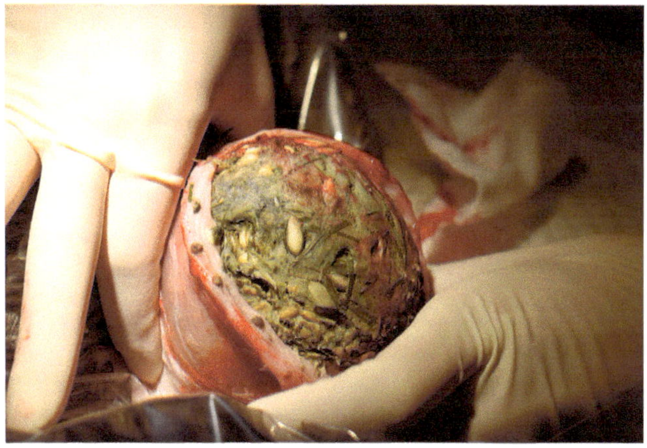

Figure 8.5 Extrication of impacted crop contents. Courtesy of Unusual Pet Vets.

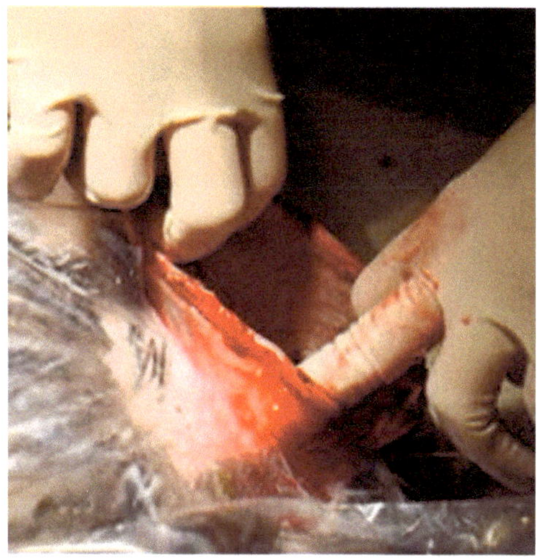

Figure 8.6 Empty crop after extraction of crop contents. Courtesy of Unusual Pet Vets.

8.3.2 Sour Crop (Candidiasis, "Crop Mycosis")

8.3.2.1 Overview and Pathogenesis

Sour crop, also referred to as candidiasis or crop mycosis, is a fungal disease of chickens caused primarily by *Candida albicans*, which colonizes the crop and upper digestive tract. The condition predominantly affects young chicks, immunocompromised birds, or birds subjected to prolonged antibiotic therapy, and is of economic significance due to reduced feed intake, poor growth, decreased egg production, and potential secondary infections. Predisposing factors include high-moisture feed, poor sanitation, overuse of antibiotics, immunosuppression, or underlying GI disorders. Clinically, affected birds may present with a distended and flaccid crop, regurgitation of foul-smelling feed, whitish plaques or pseudomembranes in the oral cavity and crop, lethargy, decreased appetite, and in severe cases, weight loss and poor body condition.

The pathogenesis of sour crop begins with overgrowth of *C. albicans* in the crop, usually following disruption of normal microbial flora or immune suppression. The yeast adheres to the epithelial lining of the crop and esophagus, proliferates, and forms pseudomembranes composed of fungal cells, desquamated epithelium, and inflammatory exudate, which interfere with normal crop motility and feed passage. Local inflammation leads to mucosal irritation, edema, and in severe cases, ulceration, which can predispose the bird to secondary bacterial infections. Prolonged crop stasis exacerbates microbial fermentation, causing further distension and souring of crop contents. Overall, sour crop is a fungal and secondary digestive disorder in which microbial overgrowth, mucosal damage, and impaired crop function combine to reduce feed efficiency, growth, and productivity in affected poultry.

8.3.2.2 Risk Factors

- **Nutritional and Dietary Factors**
  Diets high in indigestible fiber or long grass/stringy materials slow crop emptying and increase the chance of feed stagnation. Spoiled or moldy feed can irritate the crop lining and disrupt normal flora. Abrupt dietary changes can disturb gut and crop motility. Lack of insoluble grit impairs the mechanical grinding of feed, leading to retention in the crop.
- **Management and Environmental Factors**
  Dirty feeders and waterers allow yeast and bacterial contamination. Stress from competition increases susceptibility to digestive disorders. Heat stress or chilling slows crop motility.
- **Health and Physiological Factors**
  Antibiotics kill beneficial bacteria, allowing yeast overgrowth. Immunosuppression from illness, transport, handling, or parasitism. A concurrent illness or crop impaction slows the crop from emptying and creates an ideal environment for yeast proliferation. Immature immune systems make birds more prone to yeast infections.

8.3.2.3 Clinical Signs and Pathology

- **External Findings**
  - **Crop-Related Signs**
    Distended, squishy, doughy crop that remains full even after overnight fasting. Foul, sour, or yeasty odor from the beak. Regurgitation of foul-smelling fluid when the crop is gently palpated. Slow or absent crop emptying.
  - **General Systemic Signs**
    Decreased appetite or anorexia, weight loss/poor growth, depression, lethargy, dehydration, reduced egg production, ruffled feathers, and poor feather condition.
- **Necropsy Findings**
  Sour-smelling, fermented, often liquid or mushy feed material in the crop. The crop may also have gas bubbles from fermentation. Crop walls may be thickened, inflamed, or have erythemic mucosa. May also have white plaques or pseudomembranes on the mucosal surface from *C. albicans* overgrowth. Esophagus and proventriculus may also be inflamed in severe or chronic cases.

8.3.2.4 Diagnostic Testing

- **Crop Content Evaluation**
  Use a soft feeding tube or gentle massage to collect crop contents. Assess odor, consistency, and presence of bubbles or gas. Wet mount cytology can be used to identify budding yeast cells or pseudohyphae of *C. albicans*.

- **Culture**
  Crop content or swabs can be cultured on Sabouraud dextrose agar to confirm *Candida* spp. growth. Reference laboratories can perform culture and sensitivity.
- **Imaging**
  Radiographs may be used to help rule out foreign bodies, impaction, or masses compressing the crop.
- **Bloodwork**
  May be used to evaluate systemic effects such as dehydration, electrolyte imbalances, and secondary infections.

8.3.2.5 Treatment and Therapeutic Interventions

- **Initial Crop Emptying and Supportive Care**
  Crop Flushing (if needed)
  Ensure proper placement of the pliable esophageal tube to prevent aspiration of saline and/or crop contents. Use a soft feeding tube or catheter and warm saline (~5–10 mL at a time for bantams, 20–30 mL for large hens) to flush and remove contents.

  Crop Rest
  Withhold food for 12–24 hours while offering only clean, fresh water and electrolyte solution.

  Hydration
  Provide subcutaneous fluids (30–50 mL/kg every 8–12 hours) if dehydrated.
- **Antifungal Therapy**
  Because sour crop is often caused by *C. albicans*, antifungal treatment is the mainstay.

  Nystatin
  300,000–600,000 U/kg by mouth every 8–12 hours for 5–7 days

  Fluconazole
  2–5 mg/kg by mouth every 24 hours for 7–10 days
  Use if nystatin is unavailable or infection is recurrent/severe.
- **Optional Antibacterial Therapy**
  Use only if bacterial secondary infection is suspected (e.g., foul odor, thick mucoid crop contents, systemic illness) or diagnosed via culture/sensitivity.

  Clindamycin
  25–50 mg/kg by mouth every 8–12 hours for 5 days.
- **Reintroduction of Diet**
  After the crop clears and begins contracting, start with easily digestible foods (softened pellets, scrambled egg, hand-feeding formula). Feed small frequent meals. Gradually return to normal feed over several days.
- **Prokinetics (If Crop Motility Is Sluggish)**
  Metoclopramide
  0.3–0.5 mg/kg by mouth or intramuscularly every 8–12 hours
  Helps stimulate crop contractions; only use if no impaction is present.
- **Surgical Intervention**
  Crop surgery (ingluviotomy) is rarely needed but may be considered if:
  - There is recurrent severe sour crop with thick fungal plaques.
  - Crop wall is chronically atonic or distended and not responding to medical therapy.

8.3.2.6 Prevention and Control

- **Nutritional Management**
  Provide a balanced commercial poultry ration appropriate for the bird's age and production stage. Avoid overuse of treats or table scraps such as excessive carbohydrates, sugary fruits, or bread, which can disrupt normal crop flora and slow emptying. Ensure adequate dietary fiber and grit to promote normal grinding and movement of feed. Avoid moldy or spoiled feed, which can introduce fungal spores. Prebiotics and probiotic use are encouraged.
- **Water Quality and Hygiene**
  Provide fresh, clean water daily. Clean waterers and feeders frequently (at least weekly, more often in hot or humid weather). Disinfect with a mild bleach solution (1:32 dilution) or poultry-safe disinfectants, then rinse thoroughly.
- **Environmental Sanitation**
  Maintain clean, dry, well-ventilated housing to reduce fungal spore buildup. Remove wet bedding, spilled feed, or droppings promptly. Avoid overcrowding, which increases stress and promotes the spread of pathogens.

8.3.2.7 Nursing Considerations

Nursing care for chickens affected by sour crop focuses on supportive management, hygiene, and correction of underlying predisposing factors. Affected birds should be monitored closely for feed intake, hydration status, body condition, and signs of secondary bacterial infections, and provided with softened or easily digestible feed to reduce strain on the crop. Ensuring access to clean, fresh water is essential, as hydration helps flush the crop and maintain overall health. Environmental management is critical: maintain clean litter and feeders, minimize overcrowding, and eliminate contaminated feed or water sources to prevent reinfection and spread. Nursing may also involve gently massaging the crop to aid emptying and administering probiotics to restore normal microbial balance, always under veterinary guidance. Observation for progression to systemic illness, dehydration, or severe malnutrition is necessary, and birds showing persistent or severe symptoms should receive prompt veterinary intervention, including antifungal therapy if indicated. Overall, nursing considerations for sour crop emphasize supportive feeding and hydration, hygiene, environmental management, and timely veterinary care to restore crop function, reduce microbial overgrowth, and promote recovery in affected poultry.

8.3.3 Pendulous Crop

8.3.3.1 Overview and Pathogenesis

Pendulous crop, also known as sour crop or crop stasis, is a condition in chickens characterized by distension and impaired emptying of the crop, resulting in a pendulous, flaccid, and often malodorous crop. The disorder primarily affects adult layers and broilers, and is of economic significance due to reduced feed intake, poor growth, decreased egg production, and increased susceptibility to secondary infections. Predisposing factors include ingestion of indigestible material (fibrous feed, bedding), sudden dietary changes, fungal or bacterial overgrowth (*Candida* spp., Lactobacillus imbalance), motility disorders, nerve damage, or systemic illness. Clinically, affected birds may present with visible crop distension, regurgitation, foul-smelling crop contents, decreased appetite, lethargy, and poor body condition.

The pathogenesis of pendulous crop begins with impaired crop motility or obstruction, which prevents normal passage of ingested feed into the proventriculus and gizzard. This stagnation allows for overgrowth of fermentative microbes, such as bacteria and yeasts, leading to fermentation, souring of crop contents, and gas accumulation, which further distends the crop. Chronic stagnation may result in mucosal inflammation, ulceration, and secondary systemic effects due to malnutrition and toxin absorption. In severe or prolonged cases, pendulous crop can predispose birds to starvation, dehydration, and secondary infections, further compromising health and productivity. Overall, pendulous crop is a functional and secondary infectious digestive disorder in which impaired crop motility, microbial overgrowth, and fermentation converge to cause abdominal distension, reduced feed efficiency, and decreased performance in affected chickens.

8.3.3.2 Risk Factors

- **Dietary and Feeding-Related Factors**
  Overconsumption of feed or water in one sitting, especially after periods of starvation or water restriction. Ingestion of long, fibrous, tough, or indigestible material (e.g., straw, long grass, feathers, string, foreign bodies) that can cause initial crop impaction. High-carbohydrate or highly fermentable diets that expand in the crop and slow motility. Feeding spoiled or moldy feed that contributes to microbial overgrowth and crop inflammation.
- **Husbandry and Management Factors**
  Inadequate access to grit (needed to mechanically grind fibrous feed and promote normal crop emptying). Poor environmental sanitation that increases exposure to pathogens like *C. albicans* (leading to secondary Candidiasis/sour crop). Housing designs that allow birds to gorge (e.g., sudden introduction to free-choice feed after restriction).
- **Disease and Health-Related Factors**
  Chronic or recurrent crop impaction causing overstretching and progressive atony. Previous episodes of Candidiasis (sour crop), which inflame and weaken crop tissues. Nerve damage affecting the vagus nerve or crop innervation (can occur with systemic illness or trauma). Concurrent systemic illness or debilitation that reduces gut motility and appetite regulation.
- **Individual and Genetic Factors**
  Older birds with naturally reduced muscle tone and slower digestive motility. Heavy or large-breed chickens (especially high-production breeds) that are prone to overeating. Individual predisposition to crop motility disorders.

8.3.3.3 Clinical Signs and Pathology

- **External Findings**
  Visible sagging enlarged crop that hangs down below the normal breast contour, especially when standing. Soft, fluid-filled, or doughy crop upon palpation, often swinging or sloshing when the bird moves. Delayed or absent crop emptying overnight (crop still full in the morning before feeding). Weight loss and poor body condition despite having access to feed. Decreased appetite or selective eating. Regurgitation of feed or sour-smelling liquid from the beak (especially if secondary *Candidiasis* or fermentation is present). Lethargy, decreased activity, and ruffled feathers. Diarrhea or abnormal droppings, due to reduced feed passage and gut function.
- **Necropsy Findings**
  Elongation and weakening of the crop's smooth muscle fibers and supportive connective tissue. Thinned, stretched crop wall. Possible fungal hyphae on mucosa if secondary *Candidiasis*.

8.3.3.4 Diagnostic Testing

- **Crop Content Evaluation**
  Crop aspiration or swab for cytology and culture to detect secondary *C. albicans* (yeast), *Escherichia coli*, or other bacterial overgrowth. Gram stain or wet mount reveals budding yeast or bacterial rods/cocci.
- **Diagnostic Imaging**
  Plain radiographs can confirm markedly distended crop and rule out foreign bodies or masses. Contrast radiographs show delayed or absent passage of contrast into the proventriculus/gizzard over time.

8.3.3.5 Treatment and Therapeutic Interventions

Supportive care and surgical correction have variable success. Feed soft, easily digestible diets in small frequent amounts and monitor hydration and body weight closely. For birds with recurrent or chronic pendulous crop, a "bra" can be placed to provide support, allowing proper emptying of the organ (Figure 8.7).

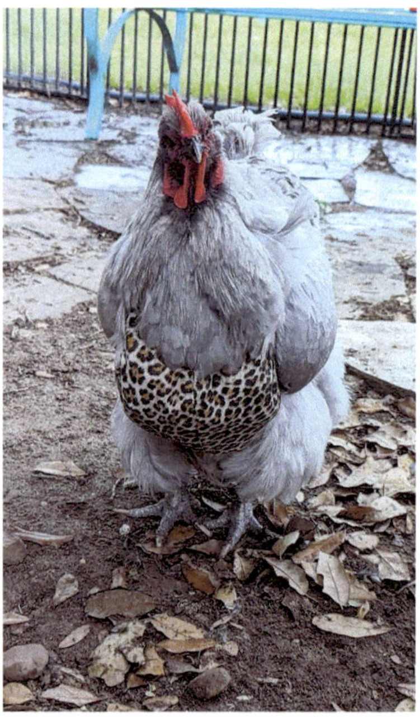

Figure 8.7 Lavender Orpington hen with crop "bra." Courtesy of Cindy Justice Liles.

8.3.3.6 Prevention and Control

- **Nutritional Management**
  Avoid excessive indigestible fibers or foods that slow crop emptying. Offer frequent, small meals to prevent overeating and chronic crop distention. Supports mechanical breakdown of feed and proper crop motility. Reduces risk of fungal overgrowth (e.g.,) and secondary sour crop.
- **Environmental and Management Measures**
  Prevent overcrowding by reducing stress and competition at feeders. Promptly remove wet bedding and spilled feed to prevent fungal growth. Avoid abrupt feed changes that could disrupt crop function or microbial balance.

8.3.3.7 Nursing Considerations

Nursing care for chickens with pendulous crop focuses on supportive management, promoting crop emptying, and preventing secondary infections. Affected birds should be closely monitored for feed intake, hydration status, body condition, and signs of discomfort or lethargy. Providing softened or easily digestible feed, as well as fresh clean water, helps reduce fermentation and encourages crop motility. Gentle crop massage or expressing crop contents may be necessary under veterinary guidance to relieve stagnation and prevent further distension. Environmental management is important: maintain clean litter, proper ventilation, and minimize stressors such as overcrowding or sudden handling. Nursing care also includes monitoring for secondary bacterial or fungal infections, correcting underlying nutritional deficiencies, and adjusting diet to prevent recurrence. Overall, nursing considerations for pendulous crop emphasize supportive feeding, hydration, environmental hygiene, and timely intervention to restore normal crop function and maintain health and productivity in affected chickens.

8.3.4 Crop Burn

8.3.4.1 Overview and Pathogenesis

Crop burn, also known as thermal or chemical crop injury, is a condition in which the inner lining of the crop (ingluvies) becomes damaged due to exposure to excessively hot, caustic, or irritant substances. This injury commonly occurs in young chicks that are hand-fed or given liquid feeds or medications that are too hot, improperly mixed, or overly concentrated. The crop's mucosa is delicate and highly sensitive to temperature and chemical irritation; when exposed to injurious agents, tissue necrosis and inflammation rapidly develop.

Pathogenesis begins with direct thermal or chemical damage to the stratified squamous epithelial lining of the crop. This results in coagulative necrosis, edema, and sloughing of mucosa. In severe cases, the necrotic process extends through the submucosa and muscular layers, leading to ulceration and, ultimately, full-thickness perforation of the crop wall. Secondary bacterial invasion, typically involving *E. coli*, *Staphylococcus aureus*, or other opportunistic pathogens, exacerbates inflammation and may lead to abscess formation or cellulitis. Leakage of ingesta through perforated tissue causes localized infection and cellulitis in the surrounding skin and subcutaneous tissue, sometimes progressing to systemic septicemia. If not promptly treated, the injury impairs crop motility and healing, leading to chronic crop dysfunction, scarring, and in some cases, death.

8.3.4.2 Risk Factors

- **Overheated Feeding Formula or Liquids**
  Feeding formulas, liquid diets, or water above 105°F is the most common cause. Hot liquids cause thermal necrosis of the crop wall within minutes. Risk increases when food temperature is not tested before feeding.
- **Improper Mixing of Formula**
  Uneven heating (e.g., microwave warming) can create hot spots in the formula. Incomplete mixing may result in concentrated "pockets" that burn tissue upon contact. Incomplete mixing may result in concentrated "pockets" that burn tissue upon contact.
- **Overfeeding or Rapid Feeding**
  Overfilling the crop can stretch and thin the crop wall, making it more susceptible to heat damage. Rapid syringe or tube feeding increases the risk of spillage and localized scalding.
- **Young Age**
  Chicks under 2 weeks old have very delicate crop mucosa and minimal feather insulation, increasing susceptibility to heat damage.

8.3.4.3 Clinical Signs and Pathology

- **External Findings**

  First Few Hours

  Visible distension or swelling of the crop. Chick may flinch, shake its head, or gasp after feeding. Crop feels warm or tender on palpation. Mild redness or discoloration of skin over crop area.

  12–24 Hours Post-Injury

  Depression and lethargy. Crop stasis and discolored or darkened skin over crop. Moist scab or blister formation. Possible leakage of fluid through damaged crop wall.

  24+ Hours Post-Injury

  Necrosis and perforation of the crop wall. Feed leakage through skin, foul odor, and signs of infection or cellulitis. Anorexia, dehydration, and weakness.

- **Necropsy Findings**
  Focal or diffuse necrosis of the crop wall, often on the ventral aspect. Discolored tissue (gray, brown, or black) with possible ulceration. In severe cases, full-thickness perforation with feed leakage into subcutaneous tissue. Surrounding cellulitis or abscessation in chronic cases.

8.3.4.4 Diagnostic Testing

- **Visual Inspection and Palpation**
  Examine crop region for skin discoloration, moist/necrotic patches or blisters, and feed leakage through an opening or scab. Gently palpate to assess crop contents and integrity of the crop wall.
- **Cytology**
  If discharge or fluid is present, prepare smears from the crop exudate to detect bacteria, yeast, or fungal overgrowth. Helps identify secondary infections such as Candida or *E. coli*.
- **Culture and Sensitivity**
  Sample from crop fluid or necrotic tissue if infection is suspected. Guides appropriate selection post-debridement or surgery.

8.3.4.5 Treatment and Therapeutic Interventions

- **Initial Stabilization**
  Isolate the affected bird to minimize stress and prevent contamination of the wound. Withhold food of 12–24 hours if the crop is leaking or necrotic to prevent further irritation. Oral or subcutaneous (if no perforation) to correct dehydration. Warm electrolyte solutions.
- **Wound Care and Local Care**
  Gently clean the crop and surrounding skin. Use warm saline, dilute chlorhexidine, or dilute povidone-iodine. Remove necrotic tissue or feed material. Do not use harsh antiseptics such as alcohol or hydrogen peroxide, as they impede cellular growth and healing.
- **Surgical Management (If Perforation or Necrosis Is Present)**
  Aseptically, debride necrotic tissue. Flush crop lumen with warm sterile saline. Suture the crop wall into two layers (inner continuous absorbable suture, outer interrupted layer). Close the skin separately to prevent fistula formation.
- **Medication**
  Optional antibacterial therapy only if bacterial secondary infection is suspected (e.g., foul odor, thick mucoid crop contents, systemic illness) or diagnosed via culture/sensitivity.
- **Nutritional and Supportive Care**
  Start with lukewarm, soft, easily digestible feeds once the crop healing begins. Avoid solid feed until the crop empties normally. Ensure all feeds and fluids are below 105°F before administration. Probiotics may help restore normal crop flora after antibiotic use. Vitamin A and E aid in mucosal and epithelial healing.

8.3.4.6 Prevention and Control

- **Temperature Control**
  Always check formula temperature before feeding. Use a reliable digital food/meat thermometer for accuracy. Never microwave formulas, as it heats unevenly and can create hot spots that burn the crop. Instead, warm formula by placing the container in warm water (or on the stovetop) and stir thoroughly before use. Allow formulas to cool and mix evenly before feeding.

- **Proper Feeding Technique**
  Feed slowly and gently to avoid overfilling or forcing hot liquid into the crop. Use appropriately sized syringes or feeding tubes designed for chicks (or adults). Ensure the chick or adult bird is in a natural upright position when feeding; improper positioning can cause aspiration or localized injury. Do not overfill the crop; allow time for digestion between feedings. Avoid feeding if the crop from the previous meal has not emptied fully. This can be determined by palpation of the crop prior to feeding the next meal.
- **Formula Preparation and Handling**
  Prepare fresh formula for each feeding. Discard any leftover or reheated feed to avoid bacterial or fungal growth. Stir continuously while warming to maintain an even temperature. Use a digital food/meat thermometer. If formula sits for any period, recheck the temperature before feeding. Ensure consistent texture, with no thick clumps or sediment that could retain heat.

8.3.4.7 Nursing Considerations

Nursing care for chickens with crop burn focuses on stabilizing the patient, supporting healing, and preventing secondary infections or complications. Birds should be isolated in a warm, clean, and stress-free environment to minimize energy expenditure and contamination of the affected area. Feeding should be withheld initially if the crop is severely damaged, allowing time for inflammation to subside. Once healing begins, soft, easily digestible feeds or rehydration solutions at room temperature can be gradually reintroduced, avoiding any hot or chemically irritating substances. Wound care is critical; if the burn has resulted in necrotic tissue or perforation, gentle cleansing with sterile saline and topical antimicrobial application may be needed under veterinary supervision. Bandaging or protective coverings can help prevent contamination and self-trauma. Systemic antibiotics and anti-inflammatory medications may be prescribed to control infection and pain. Crop flushing or surgical debridement may be necessary in severe cases with necrosis or leakage. Ongoing monitoring includes checking crop emptying efficiency, hydration status, appetite, and any signs of infection such as swelling, discharge, or foul odor. The veterinary nurse or caretaker should record feeding tolerance and crop motility daily. Client education is important—emphasizing correct feed preparation temperature, proper dilution of medications or supplements, and gentle feeding techniques to prevent recurrence.

8.3.5 Crop Necrosis

8.3.5.1 Overview and Pathogenesis

Crop necrosis in chickens refers to the death and breakdown of the crop tissue, particularly the mucosal and muscular layers, resulting from compromised blood supply, severe infection, chemical injury, or prolonged inflammation. It can occur secondary to conditions such as crop burns, impaction, foreign body trauma, or chronic infection. The necrotic process disrupts the normal function of the crop, which serves as a temporary storage and softening chamber for ingested feed, leading to impaired digestion, feed retention, and systemic illness if untreated.

The pathogenesis of crop necrosis begins with injury to the crop's lining or underlying vasculature. Thermal, chemical, mechanical, or infectious insults cause cellular damage and inflammation, leading to edema, vascular compromise, and hypoxia of the tissue. As blood flow becomes restricted, the affected tissue undergoes ischemic degeneration and eventually necrosis. In bacterial-associated cases, toxins from invading pathogens such as *S. aureus*, *E. coli*, or *Clostridium* species further damage the tissue and exacerbate necrosis through enzymatic destruction and liquefaction. As necrotic tissue accumulates, it sloughs off, leaving ulcerated or perforated areas in the crop wall. This allows leakage of ingesta into surrounding tissues, predispose to cellulitis, abscess formation, and septicemia. Chronic cases may result in fibrosis and scarring, which impair crop motility and elasticity, leading to persistent crop stasis or distension. Without timely intervention, crop necrosis can progress to systemic infection and death due to endotoxemia or starvation.

8.3.5.2 Risk Factors

- **Thermal Injury**
  Feeding overheated formula or fluids causing initial mucosal damage leading to full-thickness necrosis if untreated. Most common cause in hand-reared, young, or anorexic birds.
- **Crop Impaction or Overdistension**
  Chronic impaction (due to long grass, string, or indigestible material) stretches the crop wall. Reduced blood circulation leads to ischemia, resulting in necrosis of crop tissue. Overfeeding or lack of grit exacerbates risk.
- **Foreign Body Injury**
  Sharp or abrasive materials (plastic, wire, hay, feathers) lodged in the crop can cause mechanical trauma leading to localized necrosis and ulceration.
- **Infectious Causes**
  Secondary bacterial infection (especially *E. coli, S. aureus*, and *Pseudomonas*) after trauma or burn. Fungal overgrowth (*C. albicans*) may worsen mucosal damage and delay healing.
- **Chemical or Caustic Injury**
  Accidental ingestion of chemical disinfectants, concentrated cleaning agents, or improperly diluted medications. Direct mucosal corrosion results in necrosis.
- **Post-Surgical Complications**
  Inadequate asepsis or tension at suture sites following crop surgery (crop burn repair or impaction removal) can lead to localized necrosis and dehiscence.

8.3.5.3 Clinical Signs and Pathology

- **External Findings**
  Early Stage
  Reluctance to eat or drink. Palpable crop distension that fails to empty overnight. Crop feels firm or doughy, may be painful on palpation. Lethargy and reduced activity. Mild redness or heat over crop region.

  Progressive Stage
  Crop wall thinning or dark discoloration (gray, brown, or black) is visible through skin. Foul-smelling discharge or seepage from the crop. Wet feathers or crusts over the crop region (indicating leakage). Regurgitation or dripping of feed or fluid from the wound. Anorexia, dehydration, and weight loss.

  Advanced/Ruptured Stage
  Visible hole or tear in the crop wall. Feed material leaking from the crop onto the skin or feathers. Surrounding cellulitis, swelling, and inflammation. Foul odor and possible maggot infestation in neglected cases. Sign of toxemia or septicemia in severe infections.
- **Necropsy Findings**
  Mucosal Lesions
  Necrotic, discolored, or sloughed mucosa. Thickened, roughened inner lining with patches of ulceration or caseous debris. Coagulative necrosis of mucosal and submucosal layers. Loss of

epithelial continuity. Inflammatory infiltrate (heterophils, macrophages, lymphocytes) around necrotic tissue.

Full-Thickness Lesions

Perforation of the crop wall with leakage of feed into subcutaneous tissues. Surrounding edema and hemorrhage. Fibrinous or purulent exudates under the skin. Suppurative inflammation with bacterial colonies. Fungal hyphae may be present in chronic Candida-associated cases. Granulation tissue or fibrosis in healing or chronic stages.

Chronic/Healed Lesions

Thickened, fibrotic crop wall. Reduced elasticity leading to functional stasis or "pendulous crop." Fibrosis and scarring, minimal inflammation.

8.3.5.4 Diagnostic Testing

- **Cytology**
  Detects bacteria (Gram-positive or -negative overgrowth), fungal hyphae (e.g., *Candida* spp.), or inflammatory cells. Necrotic debris and desquamated epithelium may be evident.
- **Culture and Sensitivity**
  Identifies opportunistic or pathogenic bacteria (e.g., *E. coli*, *Staphylococcus* spp., *Pseudomonas* spp.). Guides appropriate antimicrobial selection.
- **Endoscopy**
  If available, crop endoscopy allows direct visualization of necrotic mucosa, ulceration, or perforation.
- **Diagnostic Imaging**
  Radiographs may show gas accumulation, soft tissue swelling, or foreign bodies. Contrast studies reveal crop wall integrity, filling defects, delayed emptying, or perforations. It is useful to differentiate necrosis from simple impaction or dilation. Avoid contrast if perforation is suspected to prevent coelom contamination.

8.3.5.5 Treatment and Therapeutic Interventions

- **Supportive Care and Stabilization**
  Before initiating definitive treatment, the bird should be stabilized to improve prognosis. Correct dehydration and electrolyte imbalances using warmed fluids (e.g., lactated Ringer's solution). Route depends on patient status, oral (if GI tract is functional), subcutaneous, or intravenous/intraosseous. Provide supplemental heat to maintain body temperature. Withhold solid feed temporarily if severe crop stasis or necrosis is present. Parenteral or easily digestible liquid diets may be introduced after stabilization. Pain control improves recovery and welfare. Options may include meloxicam and/or butorphanol or buprenorphine.
- **Crop Lavage and Debridement**
  Gentle crop lavage is performed to remove retained feed, necrotic debris, and microorganisms. Use warm sterile saline administered through a soft feeding tube, followed by gentle aspiration. Avoid excessive pressure to prevent perforation. Repeat lavage as needed over 24–48 hours. If necrotic sloughing or perforation is present, surgical exploration may be indicated.
- **Medication**
  Empirical therapy should begin promptly, then adjusted based on culture and sensitivity results. Antifungal therapy is indicated when cytology or culture reveals *Candida* spp. or other fungi. Duration typically ranges from 7–14 days, adjusted for severity and response.

- **Nutritional and Dietary Modifications**
  Feed soft, easily digestible diets during recovery to minimize trauma to the crop wall. Avoid dry grains or fibrous feeds until normal motility resumes. Gradually reintroduce regular feed once crop emptying is restored. Probiotics may support the restoration of normal crop microflora after antimicrobial therapy.

8.3.5.6 Prevention and Control

- **Husbandry and Environmental Management**
  Prevent thermal injuries to the crop by ensuring that heating elements or feeding solutions are not excessively hot. Always check temperatures of gavage or hand-feeding formulas. Avoid feeding overheated mash or liquid feeds that can scald the mucosa. Reduce environmental pathogen load that can predispose to secondary bacterial or fungal infections. Overcrowding increases stress and risk of injury during feeding or crop impaction episodes. Provide adequate feeder space and avoid sudden diet changes.
- **Feeding Practices**
  Train veterinary staff and caretakers in proper crop-tube placement to avoid perforation or chemical burns. Use soft, rounded feeding tubes and gentle technique; avoid forcing fluids. Ensure proper bird positioning to minimize aspiration or trauma. Provide balanced, fresh feed free of contaminants, molds, or sharp particles that could irritate the crop mucosa. Avoid stale or fermented feed, which predisposes to sour crop and mucosal damage. Avoid stale or fermented feed, which predisposes to sour crop and mucosal damage. Overfilling the crop, particularly in neonates or sick birds, can cause stretching, stasis, and eventual ischemic injury. Feed small, frequent meals appropriate for age and species.
- **Biosecurity and Disease Control**
  Keep feed storage areas dry and well-ventilated to prevent fungal growth (*Candida, Aspergillus*). Use antifungal disinfectants for feeders and water lines as appropriate. Clean feeding equipment between uses. Avoid reusing gavage syringes or tubes without proper sterilization. Use treated or clean water sources to minimize bacterial introduction. Implement routine crop checks, especially in hand-reared chicks, to detect stasis early. Address impactions, sour crop, or infectious crop conditions promptly before necrosis develops.
- **Management of Predisposing Factors**
  Avoid caustic medications or food additives that can irritate the crop lining. Monitor birds on prolonged antibiotic therapy for secondary fungal overgrowth that can damage the crop mucosa. Promptly treat parasitic, nutritional, or systemic illnesses that can impair crop emptying and predispose to necrosis.
- **Isolation and Quarantine**
  Birds with suspected crop infections or necrosis should be isolated to prevent the spread of opportunistic pathogens. New additions to the flock should undergo quarantine to minimize the introduction of infectious agents that could contribute to crop disease.

8.3.5.7 Nursing Considerations

Nursing care of crop necrosis centers on stabilizing the bird, supporting tissue healing, preventing systemic infection, and maintaining nutrition and hydration. Affected birds should be isolated in a quiet, warm, and clean environment to reduce stress and contamination risk. Initially, withholding feed and water by mouth may be necessary if the crop wall is perforated or necrotic to prevent leakage of ingesta into surrounding tissues. Parenteral or subcutaneous fluid therapy should be provided to correct dehydration and support circulation during the recovery phase. Close observation of the crop region is essential. The veterinary nurse or guardian should monitor for swelling, discoloration, odor, or discharge that may indicate infection or tissue breakdown. If necrotic debris or purulent material is present, gentle wound cleansing with sterile saline and application of topical antiseptics or antimicrobials may be performed under veterinary supervision. In severe cases, surgical debridement or crop resection may be required, followed by careful postoperative care to ensure healing and prevent recurrence. Nutritional support is critical once feeding can safely resume. Soft, easily digestible feeds or hand-fed formulas at body temperature should be introduced gradually, ensuring that the crop empties appropriately. Antibiotic therapy, anti-inflammatory medication, and pain relief are typically part of the treatment regimen as prescribed by a veterinarian. Thorough documentation of the bird's appetite, crop motility, weight, and wound healing progress helps evaluate recovery.

8.3.6 Bacterial Crop Infection

8.3.6.1 Overview and Pathogenesis

Bacterial crop infections in chickens are typically secondary conditions that arise when the normal defenses of the crop are compromised. The crop is a thin-walled, distensible outpouching of the esophagus that serves as a temporary storage organ for ingested feed and water. Under normal conditions, the crop maintains a balanced microbial flora and mildly acidic environment that help suppress pathogenic bacterial growth. However, factors such as improper diet, prolonged feed retention (crop stasis), unsanitary water or feed sources, injury to the mucosa, immunosuppression, or concurrent diseases can disrupt this balance and create an environment favorable to opportunistic bacterial proliferation. Common bacterial agents include *E. coli*, *Staphylococcus* spp., *Streptococcus* spp., *Pseudomonas* spp., and occasionally anaerobes like *Clostridium* species.

Pathogenesis begins when pathogenic or opportunistic bacteria colonize the crop mucosa, often facilitated by retained feed material and impaired peristalsis. The organisms adhere to the mucosal surface, multiply, and release toxins or enzymes that damage the epithelial lining. This leads to inflammation (cropitis), edema, and sometimes ulceration or necrosis of the mucosa. In acute infections, birds may show crop distension, foul-smelling fluid, delayed crop emptying, and regurgitation. In chronic or severe cases, bacterial invasion can breach the mucosal barrier, allowing pathogens to spread into deeper tissues or the bloodstream, potentially resulting in septicemia. Toxin production and inflammatory mediators further disrupt local motility and worsen feed stasis, perpetuating a cycle of infection and dysfunction. If left untreated, bacterial crop infections can lead to significant weight loss, dehydration, systemic illness, and death.

8.3.6.2 Risk Factors

- **Husbandry and Environmental Factors**
  Accumulation of feed residues in feeders and waterers supports bacterial growth (*E. coli*, *Staphylococcus* spp., *Pseudomonas* spp.). Contaminated drinking water systems are a common source of bacterial introduction to the crop. Infrequent cleaning of crop-tubes, gavage syringes, and feeding utensils allows biofilm formation and pathogen persistence. Moist, fermenting feed promotes bacterial proliferation. Birds consuming spoiled or moldy feed are at increased risk of mucosal irritation and secondary infection. Overcrowding, poor ventilation, and damp litter increase exposure to environmental bacteria. Birds in dirty environments may ingest bacteria while preening or feeding.
- **Feeding and Iatrogenic Factors**
  Use of contaminated feeding tubes or poor hygiene introduces bacteria directly into the crop. Repeated feeding with inadequately disinfected or sterilized equipment can lead to colonization

by opportunistic bacteria. Thermal or chemical injury to the crop mucosa compromises its protective barrier, allowing bacteria to invade underlying tissues. Large feeding volumes stretch the crop and slow emptying, creating a warm, moist environment ideal for bacterial overgrowth. Irregular feeding schedules may lead to prolonged feed retention, predisposing to fermentation and bacterial proliferation.

- **Physiological and Anatomical Factors**
  Any condition that impairs crop motility (e.g., impaction, foreign bodies, systemic illness, dehydration) promotes bacterial growth by allowing feed to remain stagnant. Over time, this leads to bacterial fermentation, acid production, and mucosal irritation. Chicks and neonates have underdeveloped immune defenses, making them more susceptible to opportunistic bacterial colonization. In hand-reared chicks, inadequate maternal antibody transfer further increases vulnerability. Mechanical trauma (e.g., from sharp feed particles, foreign bodies, or rough handling) disrupts the crop lining, facilitating bacterial invasion.
- **Underlying Disease and Immunosuppression**
  Respiratory or enteric diseases can weaken birds and slow crop function, increasing susceptibility to bacterial infections. Viral infections such as infectious bursal disease or chicken infectious anemia reduce immune competence, predisposing birds to secondary crop infections. Disruption of normal crop microflora allows opportunistic bacteria, including resistant strains, to proliferate unchecked.
- **Environmental Stressors**
  Heat stress causes dehydration and slows crop emptying; cold stress reduces immune response. Both scenarios increase infection risk. Stress impairs local immunity and digestive function, facilitating bacterial establishment in the crop. Overcrowding, poor ventilation, and inadequate feeder space increase competition and stress, indirectly predisposing birds to crop infections.

8.3.6.3 Clinical Signs and Pathology

- **External Findings**

  Early/Mild Infection

  The crop may feel soft, fluid-filled, or doughy on palpation. Feed may remain in the crop for >12 hours, indicating impaired clearance. Foul odor from the crop is caused by bacterial fermentation of feed and tissue breakdown. Mild regurgitation or crop "overflow" noticeable after handling or feeding. Decreased appetite and slower weight gain, particularly in chicks or growing birds.

  Moderate to Severe Infection

  Marked crop enlargement with palpable thickening of the crop wall. Birds may flinch, struggle, or vocalize when the crop area is touched. Regurgitation of foul-smelling fluid, sometimes containing feed or mucus. Halitosis (bad breath), indicating advanced bacterial overgrowth. Reduced feed intake, lethargy, depression, and poor body condition. Crop "sloshing" on auscultation or gentle manipulation due to fluid accumulation. Feather fluffing, huddling, or decreased activity in chicks.

  Advanced/Complicated Infection

  Signs of systemic infection or septicemia, such as marked lethargy, dehydration, sunken eyes, tachypnea, open-mouth breathing, and cyanosis of comb/wattles in severe cases. Fistula formation at the crop if necrosis and perforation occur, with leakage of crop contents through the skin. Sudden death in neonates or immunocompromised birds, particularly if septicemia develops rapidly.

- **Necropsy Findings**

  Crop Lesions

  Mucosal hyperemia and edema are typical early findings. Thickened crop wall, with variable degrees of fibrinous or caseous exudate adherence to the mucosa. Foul-smelling fluid or semi-liquid contents often accumulate in the lumen. Necrosis and ulceration of the mucosal surface may develop in more advanced cases. In severe infections, mural perforation may be observed, sometimes with localized cellulitis or subcutaneous abscessation at the cervical region.

  Systemic Lesions

  Mild hepatosplenomegaly may occur with systemic bacterial spread. Fibrinous peritonitis or septicemia may be present if the infection has extended beyond the crop. Dehydration and poor body condition are common in chronic infections.

8.3.6.4 Diagnostic Testing

- **Wet Mount**

  Identifies motile bacteria and inflammatory cells. Differentiates bacterial overgrowth from fungal infections (e.g., absence of budding yeast or hyphae).
- **Gram Stain**

  Reveals bacterial morphology and Gram reaction. Numerous mixed bacteria with inflammatory cells suggest infection rather than normal transient flora. Intracellular bacteria in heterophils support active infection. Chronic infections may show necrotic debris and reduced cellularity.
- **Culture and Sensitivity**

  This is the gold standard for identifying causative organisms and selecting appropriate antimicrobial therapy. Samples should be plated on standard media (e.g., blood agar, MacConkey) under aerobic conditions. Sensitivity testing guides target antimicrobial selection and help detect resistant strains. Culture is also useful to rule out mixed infections with fungi.
- **Diagnostic Imaging**

  Radiographic evaluation is useful when mechanical obstruction, impaction, or perforation is suspected. Show crop enlargement, abnormal gas patterns, or foreign bodies. Contrast studies can assess crop wall integrity and emptying time. Delayed passage of contrast indicates stasis or infection-induced motility impairment. Focal mural defects or leakage may indicate necrosis or perforation. Use contrast cautiously if perforation is suspected to avoid leakage into the cervical tissues or coelom.

8.3.6.5 Treatment and Therapeutic Interventions

- **Stabilization and Supportive Care**

  Many affected birds are debilitated, dehydrated, or malnourished, requiring immediate supportive measures prior to or alongside specific therapy. Correct dehydration and electrolyte imbalances using warmed fluids (e.g., Lactated Ringer's solution, Normosol-R). Routes: subcutaneous (most common), intravenous, or intraosseous in severe cases. Provide a warm, quiet, draft-free environment (ambient 84–90°F) to reduce metabolic stress. Avoid overheating; monitor closely. Withhold food for 12–24 hours in birds with severe crop stasis, while maintaining hydration. Once crop motility improves, offer small, frequent, easily digestible meals (e.g., warm formulated gruel, soft pellets, or scrambled eggs).
- **Crop Emptying and Lavage**

  Manual emptying of the crop removes stagnant, fermenting material and reduces bacterial load. Gently restrain the bird in an upright position. Use a soft feeding tube attached to a syringe to aspirate the contents. Avoid excessive pressure to prevent regurgitation or aspiration. Crop lavage may be indicated if significant debris remains. Use warm sterile saline or Lactated Ringer's solution. Instill gently, massage crop to loosen contents, then aspirate. Repeat until lavage fluid is clear. Birds must be fully conscious and positioned correctly to minimize aspiration risk.

- **Medication**

  Antibiotic selection should ideally be guided by culture and sensitivity results. Empirical therapy may be initiated while awaiting results.

  Trimethoprim-sulfamethoxazole 100 mg/kg by mouth every 12 hours for 5 days.

  Amoxicillin/Clavulanate 125–250 mg/kg by mouth every 8–12 hours for 5–7 days.

  Oral is most common for localized crop infections. Injectable therapy is indicated if systemic signs (e.g., septicemia) are present. Typically, 7–14 days, adjusted based on clinical response and culture results. Chronic or necrotizing infections may require extended courses.

  Crop motility may be impaired by inflammation and infection. Prokinetic agents help restore normal function.

  Metoclopramide 0.3–0.5 mg/kg by mouth or intramuscularly every 8–12 hours.

  - Stimulates crop contractions; only use if no impaction is present.

  Probiotics (avian-specific) may help restore normal crop microflora after antibiotic therapy. Activated charcoal or kaolin-pectin can be used if toxins or fermentation products are suspected, but only after the crop is emptied.

- **Surgical Intervention**

  In severe cases, particularly those with necrosis, foreign bodies, or abscesses—medical management alone is insufficient. Surgical cropotomy may be required.

8.3.6.6 Prevention and Control

- **Optimal Feeding Practices**

  Improper feeding techniques are among the most common risk factors, especially in hand-reared chicks and impaired adult birds. Use commercially formulated diets designed for the species and age. Prepare formula with fresh, clean water; avoid using water that has been sitting out. Maintain correct temperature (102–105°F) cold formula delays crop emptying; overheated formula can damage mucosa. Mix the formula to proper consistency; overly thick mixtures can slow crop transit. Use appropriately sized, clean feeding equipment (pliable tubes, and syringes). Avoid overfilling the crop, feed to normal fullness, allowing complete emptying between feedings. Feed at regular intervals to maintain crop motility. Do not feed if the crop is full of a previous meal. Disinfect or sterilize feeding equipment between uses. Residual formula is an excellent bacterial growth medium. Discard unused formula after 20–30 minutes; never reheat or reuse old formula. Clean preparation surfaces and utensils before each feeding.

- **Environmental Hygiene and Biosecurity**

  Maintain dry, clean, and well-ventilated enclosures. Remove feces and spilled feed promptly to reduce bacterial proliferation. Prevent contamination of water sources with droppings or debris. Provide fresh, clean drinking water daily. Regularly scrub and disinfect drinkers and feeding containers to prevent biofilm formation. Avoid standing water or stagnant sources. Avoid overcrowding to reduce stress and bacterial load. Separate age groups, especially young chicks (more susceptible) from adults, to reduce transmission risk. Quarantine new arrivals for at least 30 days to prevent the introduction of pathogenic bacteria.

- **Promoting Normal Crop Function**
  Maintaining normal crop motility and mucosal integrity is critical to preventing bacterial overgrowth. Ensure that birds empty their crops at least once daily. Monitor chicks closely to ensure complete emptying overnight. Address delayed emptying promptly to prevent fermentation and bacterial proliferation. Provide nutritionally balanced feed to support mucosal health and immune function. Avoid excessive sugary treats or inappropriate human foods that may alter crop flora. Use gentle feeding techniques to prevent mucosal injury, which predisposes to infection. Inspect feeding tubes and syringes for rough edges or damage.
- **Stress Reduction and Immunity Support**
  Stress impairs immunity and slows crop motility, increasing infection risk. Minimize sudden environmental changes (temperature fluctuations, loud noises). Avoid overhandling or improper restraint, especially in young or sick birds. Provide species-appropriate social interactions and enrichment to support overall health. Ensure adequate lighting and rest periods to prevent chronic stress.
- **Early Detection and Prompt Intervention**
  Routine monitoring allows early identification of crop issues before infection becomes established. Daily crop checks in hand-fed chicks for emptying time, distension, and odor. Observe adult birds for changes in appetite, weight loss, or regurgitation. Address delayed emptying, mild crop stasis, or sour odors early with crop emptying and supportive care. Isolate affected birds to prevent spread to flock mates.

8.3.6.7 Nursing Considerations

Nursing care plays a critical role in the successful management and recovery of birds with bacterial crop infections. The priority is to stabilize the patient by assessing hydration status, crop distension, and overall condition. Birds with delayed crop emptying may require gentle crop massage and withholding of feed for a short period while maintaining hydration through oral or parenteral fluids, depending on severity. Crop flushing with warm (body temperature) sterile saline may be performed to remove impacted or fermenting material, but this must be done carefully to prevent aspiration. After the crop is cleared, easily digestible, soft, and clean food should be reintroduced gradually to support recovery and prevent further irritation. Strict hygiene and biosecurity measures are essential to prevent reinfection and limit spread to flock mates. Feeding equipment, waterers, and housing should be thoroughly cleaned and disinfected, and contaminated feed should be discarded. Monitoring the bird's crop emptying overnight is an important daily nursing task; a normally functioning crop should be empty by morning. Supportive care may include providing warmth, minimizing stress, and isolating affected birds to reduce competition and prevent transmission. If systemic antibiotics are prescribed based on culture and sensitivity testing or empirical therapy, proper dosing and duration must be adhered to, and withdrawal times observed if the bird is planned to be consumed. Probiotics may be administered after antibiotic treatment to help restore normal crop flora. Close observation for recurrence of crop stasis, worsening clinical signs, or complications such as aspiration pneumonia or systemic infection is critical. Clear documentation of fluid therapy, crop interventions, medication administration, and the bird's response to care helps ensure coordinated and effective treatment.

8.4 Protozoal Gastrointestinal Diseases

Protozoal diseases represent some of the most economically significant and clinically impactful conditions in chickens.

Quick reference chart

Disease/ pathogen	Common name	Primary site in GI tract	Transmission/ source	Key clinical signs	Pathology/key lesions
Eimeria spp.	Coccidiosis	Intestine and ceca (species-dependent)	Ingestion of sporulated oocysts in litter/feed/ water	Bloody or watery diarrhea, poor growth, ruffled feathers, dehydration, mortality (young birds)	Thickened mucosa, hemorrhage, necrotic cores, species-specific lesion sites
Histomonas meleagridis	Blackhead disease	Cecum and liver	Ingestion of *Heterakis gallinarum* eggs carrying parasite	Sulfur-yellow droppings, depression, anorexia, drooping wings, high mortality in turkeys (chickens often carriers)	Necrotic cecal cores, circular "target" liver lesions
Trichomonas gallinae	Trichomoniasis ("canker")	Crop, esophagus, oropharynx	Direct transmission via contaminated water/feed or carrier birds	Dysphagia, weight loss, drooling, caseous oral/crop lesions	Yellow-white caseous plaques in mouth, throat, crop; necrotic lesions
Giardia spp.	Giardiasis	Small intestine	Ingestion of cysts in contaminated water	Diarrhea, malabsorption, poor weight gain, lethargy	Catarrhal enteritis, villous atrophy, malabsorption syndrome
Cryptosporidium spp.	Cryptosporidiosis	Intestine (esp. ileum, ceca)	Ingestion of oocysts (water, litter contamination)	Watery diarrhea, dehydration, poor growth, reduced feed efficiency	Villous atrophy, enteritis, oocysts on mucosal surface

Chart created by Stephanie Freeman.

8.4.1 Coccidiosis (*Eimeria* spp.)

8.4.1.1 Overview and Pathogenesis

Coccidiosis is an enteric disease of poultry caused by protozoan parasites of the genus *Eimeria*, which infect the epithelial cells of the intestine. The disease primarily affects young birds, with significance due to reduced weight gain, poor feed conversion, diarrhea, decreased egg production, increased susceptibility to secondary infections, and occasional mortality. Transmission occurs via the fecal-oral route, through ingestion of sporulated oocysts present in contaminated litter, feed, water, or equipment. Clinically, affected birds may exhibit diarrhea (often bloody), lethargy, ruffled feathers, anorexia, poor growth, and dehydration, with subclinical infections contributing to reduced productivity without overt clinical signs.

The pathogenesis of coccidiosis begins when ingested sporulated oocysts release sporozoites in the intestinal lumen, which invade enterocytes and replicate intracellularly through both asexual (schizogony) and sexual (gametogonia) stages. This replication causes destruction of intestinal epithelial cells, villus atrophy, mucosal inflammation, and hemorrhage, leading to impaired nutrient absorption and diarrhea. The degree of tissue damage varies depending on the *Eimeria* species involved, parasite load, and host immune status. Secondary bacterial infections may exacerbate intestinal pathology and reduce flock performance. Overall, coccidiosis is a protozoal enteric disease in which intracellular replication, epithelial destruction, and inflammatory responses lead to intestinal dysfunction, poor growth, and significant economic losses in poultry operations.

8.4.1.2 Risk Factors

- **Environmental and Management Factors**
  Wet, damp, or caked litter provides the ideal environment for *Eimeria* oocysts to sporulate and survive. Accumulation of feces increases oocyst load and environmental contamination. Increased bird-to-bird contact facilitates rapid horizontal transmission of oocysts. Higher stress levels lower immunity and allow heavier parasite burdens. Warm, humid conditions favor sporulation of oocysts and prolong their survival. Dusty or ammonia-rich environments compromise birds' respiratory and immune defenses. Infrequent or ineffective cleaning and disinfection allows build-up of infective oocysts between production cycles. Oocysts are highly resistant to many disinfectants if not physically removed.
- **Host-Related Factors**
  Diseases such as infectious bursal disease, Marek's disease, or malnutrition can reduce immune responsiveness. Allows more severe coccidial replication and tissue damage. At a young age, immune system is immature, making them more susceptible to heavy infections.
- **Production and Management System Factors**
  Deep litter or floor-reared systems have a higher risk than cage systems due to greater fecal-oral exposure. Litter recycling between flocks increases oocyst accumulation. Handling, transport, vaccination, or environmental stressors can predispose to outbreaks by suppressing immunity. Absence or improper use of anticoccidials or coccidiosis vaccines can allow rapid buildup of parasite load in susceptible flocks.

8.4.1.3 Clinical Signs and Pathology

- **External Findings**
  Birds appear fluffed up, listless, and reluctant to move. Rapid weight loss and poor growth rates. Pale combs and wattles. Watery, mucoid, or bloody diarrhea.
- **Necropsy Findings**
  Lesions vary by the intestinal location and species of *Eimeria*, as each species has a preferred site of infection within the gut. Intestinal thickening, congestion, and hemorrhage are most marked in the ceca (*Eimeria tenella*) and lower small intestine (*Eimeria necatrix*). Petechial to ecchymotic hemorrhages on intestinal serosa and mucosa. Coagulated blood or blood clots in ceca (*E. tenella*). Creamy or caseous core plugs in ceca. Ballooning, distension, and excess mucus in the small intestine (*Eimeria acervulina, Eimeria maxima*).

8.4.1.4 Diagnostic Testing

- **Fecal Float for Ova**
- **PCR**
  Can identify specific *Eimeria* species. Used mostly in research or commercial diagnostic labs, not routine clinic/field use.

8.4.1.5 Treatment and Therapeutic Interventions

- **Supportive Care**
  Provide electrolyte-enriched water to prevent dehydration and shock. Offer vitamins A, D3, E, and B-complex, especially vitamin K to reduce hemorrhage. Recolonize the gut and help restore intestinal integrity post-infection with prebiotics and probiotics. Easily digestible, high-protein feed aids intestinal mucosal repair.
- **Medications**
  Amprolium 13–30 mg/kg by mouth for 5–7 days.
  Toltrazuril 6–25 mg/kg once and repeat in 5 days.

8.4.1.6 Prevention and Control

- **Biosecurity and Sanitation**
  Keep bedding dry and frequently replaced; moisture promotes oocyst sporulation and survival. Remove manure, clean feeders and waterers, and disinfect housing between flocks. Use disinfectants effective against oocysts (e.g., ammonia-based products or heat treatment). Limit movement of people, equipment, and other animals between flocks to prevent spreading.
- **Vaccination**
  Live oocyst vaccines are widely used, especially in broilers and breeder/layer pullets. Given at 1 day old (spray or feed gel droplets) to induce controlled immunity. Must be combined with careful early management to allow mild exposure and immunity development. This is not typically an option for backyard birds/flocks.
- **Prophylactic Anticoccidial Programs**
  Incorporate coccidiostats (e.g., monensin, lasalocid, salinomycin, amprolium) into starter and grower feeds. Use rotation or shuttle programs (changing drug class partway through grow-out) to prevent resistance development.
- **General Flock Health and Stress Reduction**
  Provide balanced nutrition to strengthen immunity. Maintain good ventilation to reduce humidity and ammonia. Minimize other concurrent diseases (e.g., infectious bursal disease) that lower immunity. Reduce stressors such as abrupt feed changes, chilling, or overcrowding.

8.4.1.7 Nursing Considerations

Nursing care for chickens affected by coccidiosis focuses on supportive management, environmental hygiene, and prevention of secondary infections. Affected birds should be closely monitored for diarrhea, dehydration, feed intake, body condition, and overall behavior, with early detection of severe cases improving outcomes. Providing easily digestible, high-quality feed and access to clean water helps maintain hydration and nutrient balance, supporting recovery. Environmental management is critical: maintain dry, clean litter, reduce overcrowding, and implement strict biosecurity to limit oocyst contamination and spread. Nursing may also involve reducing stress, managing concurrent infections, and supplementing electrolytes or vitamins to aid in recovery. In severe cases, birds should receive veterinary intervention with appropriate anticoccidial medication. Overall, nursing considerations for coccidiosis emphasize monitoring clinical signs, maintaining hydration and nutrition, optimizing hygiene, and supporting immunity to minimize morbidity and mortality while enhancing flock recovery and productivity.

8.4.2 Histomoniasis (Blackhead Disease)

8.4.2.1 Overview and Pathogenesis

Histomoniasis, commonly known as blackhead disease, is a protozoal infection of poultry caused by *Histomonas meleagridis*, which primarily affects the ceca and liver. Although turkeys are highly susceptible, chickens, particularly young or immunocompromised birds, can also be affected, with significance due to mortality, decreased growth, poor feed conversion, and reduced egg production. Transmission occurs via the ingestion of infective *Heterakis gallinarum* eggs containing the protozoan or through direct contact with contaminated litter, feed, or water, and earthworms, which may serve as paratenic hosts. Clinically, affected chickens may present with depression, lethargy, sulfur-colored diarrhea, reduced appetite, ruffled feathers, drooping wings, and occasionally sudden death, although disease severity is generally lower than in turkeys.

The pathogenesis of histomoniasis begins when *H. meleagridis* is released in the gut from ingested *Heterakis* eggs or paratenic hosts and invades the cecal mucosa, causing necrosis, ulceration, and inflammation. The protozoa then reach the liver via the portal circulation, where they induce hepatocellular necrosis, inflammatory infiltration, and characteristic circular lesions. Infection leads to impaired nutrient absorption, diarrhea, dehydration, and systemic illness. Concurrent infections, such as coccidiosis or enteric bacterial pathogens, exacerbate intestinal damage and increase morbidity. Overall, histomoniasis is a protozoal enteric and hepatic disease in which cecal colonization, hepatic invasion, and tissue necrosis combine to cause GI and systemic pathology, reduced productivity, and potential mortality in affected poultry.

8.4.2.2 Risk Factors

Several factors increase the likelihood of chickens becoming infected with or spreading *H. meleagridis*. While chickens often show mild or subclinical signs, they are critical reservoirs for the parasite and can transmit infection to other flock members and to more susceptible species like turkeys. Understanding these risk factors helps guide prevention strategies. If a flock is known to be carriers, the caretaker should avoid the integration of turkeys.

- **Presence of *Heterakis gallinarum* (Cecal Worms)**
  Primary vector for *H. meleagridis* transmission. *H. meleagridis* survives within embryonated *Heterakis* eggs for months in the environment. Flocks with high *Heterakis* burdens are at significantly higher risk of Histomoniasis.
- **Co-housing or Proximity to Turkeys**
  Chickens can serve as asymptomatic carriers. If chickens and turkeys share pasture, litter, or housing, the risk of spreading to turkeys (which are highly susceptible) increases dramatically.
- **Contaminated Environment**
  Soil, litter, and dust contaminated with *Heterakis* eggs can serve as long-term reservoirs. Poor sanitation and infrequent litter changes allow eggs to accumulate and persist.
- **Presence of *Lumbricus terrestris* (Earthworms)**
  Act as paratenic hosts for *Heterakis* eggs containing *H. meleagridis*. Outdoor or free-range birds are more likely to ingest earthworms during foraging.

- **Age and Immune Status of Birds**
  Young birds (especially <12 weeks) are more susceptible to severe disease. Immunocompromised birds are at higher risk for clinical disease and complications.
- **Concurrent Parasitic or Bacterial Infections**
  Infections such as coccidiosis or heavy nematode burdens can damage the gut lining. This creates an environment more favorable for *H. meleagridis* invasion and multiplication.

8.4.2.3 Clinical Signs and Pathology

- **External Findings**
  Mild depression and lethargy. Reduced feed and water intake. Poor growth or stunted development in young birds. Soft or watery droppings; occasionally yellow-green cecal diarrhea. Some birds may show ruffled feathers or huddling behavior. Mortality is usually low in chickens but can increase with heavy infection or concurrent disease.
- **Necropsy Findings**
  The hallmark of histomoniasis is necrotic lesions in the ceca and liver. Cecal enlargement and thickening of the wall. Caseous, sulfur-yellow cores or plugs in the lumen. Inflammatory infiltrates in the lamina propria. Focal circular areas of necrosis with depressed gray centers and hyperemic borders on the liver.

8.4.2.4 Diagnostic Testing

- **Microscopic Examination**
  Direct smears of cecal contents may show flagellated forms, though sensitivity is low. Usually requires fresh material and skilled observation.
- **PCR Assays**
  Can detect *H. meleagridis* DNA from cecal or liver tissues. Used primarily for epidemiological studies or confirmation of subclinical infections.

8.4.2.5 Treatment and Therapeutic Interventions

Histomoniasis in chickens is often subclinical, so treatment is not always necessary. However, intervention may be needed in cases of clinical disease or to prevent spreading to more susceptible birds (e.g., turkeys). Currently, there are no drugs specifically labeled for histomoniasis in many countries, so treatment is often off-label under veterinary supervision, and emphasis is placed on prevention and management.

- **Supportive Care**
  Provide electrolyte-enriched water for birds with diarrhea. Offer high-quality, easily digestible food to support growth and recovery. Minimize handling and maintain optimal temperature and ventilation.

8.4.2.6 Prevention and Control

- **Control of the Cecal Worm Vector**
  The protozoan *H. meleagridis* is carried inside the eggs of *H. gallinarum* (cecal worm). Routine deworming with approved anthelmintics helps break the cycle. Conduct regular fecal exams to monitor worm burden.
- **Separation of Species and Age Groups**
  Avoid co-housing chickens and turkeys, as turkeys are highly susceptible, and chickens can serve as asymptomatic carriers. If turkeys and chickens are residing on the same property, the turkeys should be cleaned, fed, and watered before the chicken flock chores are performed.

- **Environmental Management**
  Remove and replace old litter between flocks to reduce infective *Heterakis* eggs. Keep litter dry; moisture promotes egg and worm survival. Clean and disinfect housing, feeders, and waterers thoroughly between flocks.
- **Control of Paratenic Hosts**
  Limit access to earthworms and other insects that can carry infected *Heterakis* eggs. Maintain well-drained, fenced outdoor runs to minimize contact with soil-dwelling hosts.
- **Biosecurity Practices**
  Restrict movement of people and equipment between flocks. Quarantine new or returning birds for at least 30 days. Use footbaths, clean clothing, and dedicated tools in flock areas.

8.4.2.7 Nursing Considerations

Nursing care for chickens affected by histomoniasis focuses on supportive management, prevention of secondary infections, and minimizing stressors. Affected birds should be closely monitored for lethargy, reduced feed and water intake, diarrhea, and signs of systemic illness, as early recognition of disease can help improve outcomes. Providing easy access to clean water and high-quality, easily digestible feed supports hydration and nutritional status, which is critical during recovery. Environmental management is essential: maintain clean, dry litter, limit contact with intermediate hosts such as earthworms, and implement strict biosecurity to prevent further transmission. Nursing care also involves reducing flock stress, isolating severely affected birds, and monitoring concurrent infections, as immunosuppressed or young birds are more susceptible to complications. Overall, nursing considerations for histomoniasis emphasize supportive care, environmental hygiene, biosecurity, and vigilant monitoring to reduce morbidity, support recovery, and maintain health.

8.4.3 Trichomoniasis (Canker)

8.4.3.1 Overview and Pathogenesis

Trichomoniasis, commonly referred to as canker in chickens, is a protozoal disease caused by *Trichomonas gallinae*, a flagellated protozoan parasite. The disease primarily affects young chicks and pigeons but can also infect adult chickens, with significance due to reduced growth, poor feed conversion, decreased egg production, and increased mortality in severe cases. Transmission occurs primarily via the oral route, through ingestion of infected crop milk, contaminated water, feed, or direct contact with infected birds. Clinically, affected chickens may present with yellowish or whitish oral plaques, caseous lesions in the mouth, throat, and esophagus, difficulty swallowing, lethargy, decreased feed intake, and weight loss, with severe infections potentially leading to death.

The pathogenesis of trichomoniasis begins when ingested trophozoites colonize the upper digestive tract, particularly the oral cavity, crop, and esophagus. The parasites adhere to the epithelial surface, multiply by binary fission, and release cytotoxic factors that induce localized necrosis and caseous lesion formation. Inflammation results in edema, heterophilic infiltration, and mucosal thickening, which can obstruct normal feeding and swallowing. Secondary bacterial infections may exacerbate tissue damage, particularly in immunocompromised or stressed birds. Chronic infections may lead to persistent lesions, impaired growth, and decreased productivity. Overall, trichomoniasis is a protozoal upper digestive tract disease in which epithelial colonization, cytotoxic activity, and local inflammation converge to impair feeding, growth, and overall health in affected poultry.

8.4.3.2 Risk Factors

Although *T. gallinae* primarily affects pigeons and doves, chickens can become infected under certain predisposing conditions. The main risk factors include:

- **Exposure to Carrier Birds**
  Direct or indirect contact with infected pigeons, doves, or wild birds is the most significant risk factor. Shared water, feeders, or housing with carrier birds increases the chance of transmission.
- **Contaminated Environment**
  Use of contaminated water sources (ponds, standing water, shared troughs). Dirty or unsanitized feeders/drinkers that allow the organism to persist and spread between birds.
- **Age and Immune Status**
  Young chicks or juveniles are more susceptible due to immature immune systems. Immunocompromised or stressed birds (from illness, transport, or poor nutrition) have a higher risk of infection and severe disease. No natural immunity develops in flocks that have never been exposed, making them vulnerable if the parasite is introduced. Mixed-species housing (e.g., chickens kept with pigeons or turkeys) can introduce the parasite into naïve chicken populations.

8.4.3.3 Clinical Signs and Pathology

- **External Findings**
  Clinical presentation can vary depending on the severity of infection, age, and species of bird. In chickens, the disease is usually less common and often milder than in pigeons or doves, but signs can still be significant in young or immunocompromised birds.
  - Early to moderate Infection
    - Lethargy and depression
    - Decreased appetite (anorexia)
    - Drooling or wet feathers around the beak
    - Dysphagia (difficulty swallowing)
    - Weight loss and poor growth
    - Ruffled feathers and general unthriftiness
  - Advanced or severe infection
    - Swelling of the throat or crop area
    - Dyspnea (labored breathing) due to obstructive plaques
    - Regurgitation of feed or water
    - Open-mouth breathing or gaping
    - Sudden death in severe, acute systemic cases
- **Necropsy Findings**
  Presence of yellow-white, firm, caseous plaques or nodules firmly attached to the mucosa in the oral cavity, pharynx, esophagus, and crop. Lesions may coalesce to form large masses, partially or completely obstructing the lumen. Surrounding mucosa is thickened, inflamed, and ulcerated. Extension of necrotic lesions to the liver, lungs, or other visceral organs. Foci of necrosis surrounded by inflammatory cells. Firm, caseous masses in the upper digestive tract are considered pathognomonic for trichomoniasis (especially in pigeons and doves but can also be seen in chickens).

8.4.3.4 Diagnostic Testing

- **Direct Wet Mount Microscopy**
  Rapid, first-line diagnostic method. Collect fresh exudate or scrapings from oral/crop lesions using a sterile cotton swab. Place a drop of warm saline on a glass slide, cover with coverslip, and examine under a microscope immediately (within 20 minutes). Motile pear-shaped *T. gallinae* trophozoites showing jerky, rolling movement. Organisms lose motility quickly outside the host; prompt examination is critical.
- **Cytology**
  Visualize morphology if motility has ceased. Prepare air-dried smears from lesion material. Stain with Giemsa, Wright's stain, or Diff-Quik. Pear-shaped organisms with pale blue cytoplasm and a central nucleus.
- **Culture**
  Increases sensitivity when organism numbers are low. InPouch TF culture system or other selective trichomonad media. Growth within 2–5 days; confirmed by observing motile trophozoites microscopically.
- **PCR**
  Highly sensitive and specific detection of *T. gallinae* DNA. Lesion swabs, crop content, or tissue samples. Confirms species identity, especially important in mixed infections or when organisms are few.

8.4.3.5 Treatment and Therapeutic Intervention

- **Supportive and Adjunctive Care**
  Gently remove necrotic plaques in the mouth/crop under veterinary supervision. Avoid bleeding; excessive trauma can worsen infection. Hand-feed soft, easily digestible foods (moistened feed, egg yolk mash, or recovery formula).
- **Environmental and Flock Management**
  Thoroughly clean and disinfect drinkers, feeders, and housing to reduce environmental contamination. Prevent contact between chickens and wild birds or pigeons, which are common carriers of *T. gallinae.*
- **Monitoring and Follow-up**
  Recheck affected birds after treatment to ensure lesions have resolved and appetite has returned. Repeat wet-mount examination if birds remain symptomatic. Consider a second course of therapy if organisms are still present after initial treatment.
- **Antiprotozoal Medications**
  Metronidazole 10–50 mg/kg by mouth once daily for 5–7 days.

8.4.3.6 Prevention and Control

- **Biosecurity and Flock Management**
  Preventing contact with wild birds (especially pigeons, doves, and turkeys), these species are natural reservoirs of *T. gallinae* and commonly spread the protozoa via saliva and regurgitated feed. Exclude wild birds from housing, feeders, and waterers with netting or covered runs. Isolate and quarantine new birds for at least 30 days before introducing them to the flock.
- **Environmental Sanitation**
  Daily cleaning of feeders and waterers: scrub and disinfect with a dilute bleach solution (1:32 or 1/2 cup per gallon of water) and rinse thoroughly. Keep feed and water sources elevated and dry

to prevent contamination with saliva, feces, or debris. Use absorbent bedding (pine shavings) and replace regularly.

- **Nutritional and Health Management**
  Provide balanced nutrition and clean water to maintain immune function and resistance. Avoid overcrowding, which increases stress and facilitates spread. Minimize concurrent infections (respiratory or parasitic diseases) that can lower immunity and predispose birds to trichomoniasis.

8.4.3.7 Nursing Considerations

Nursing care for chickens affected by trichomoniasis focuses on supportive management, maintaining hydration and nutrition, and preventing secondary infections. Affected birds should be closely monitored for oral lesions, difficulty swallowing, reduced feed and water intake, lethargy, and weight loss, as early intervention can improve recovery. Providing softened or easily digestible feed and ensuring constant access to clean water helps minimize discomfort and maintain hydration. Environmental management is crucial: maintain clean feeders, water, and litter, reduce overcrowding, and isolate infected birds to prevent transmission within the flock. Nursing may also involve gentle cleaning of oral lesions if advised by a veterinarian, stress reduction, and monitoring for secondary bacterial infections that may complicate recovery. Overall, nursing considerations for trichomoniasis emphasize supportive feeding and hydration, hygiene, isolation, and careful monitoring to reduce morbidity, promote healing of oral lesions, and maintain flock health and productivity.

8.4.4 Giardiasis

8.4.4.1 Overview and Pathogenesis

Giardiasis in chickens is an intestinal parasitic disease caused by *Giardia* spp., flagellated protozoan parasites that colonize the small intestine. The disease predominantly affects young birds and immunocompromised individuals, with significance arising from reduced growth, poor feed conversion, diarrhea, and decreased egg production in severe cases. Transmission occurs via the fecal-oral route, through ingestion of cysts shed in the feces of infected birds, often contaminating litter, water, or feed. Clinically affected chickens may exhibit diarrhea, weight loss, poor body condition, lethargy, and occasionally malabsorption-related stunting, while light infections are often subclinical.

The pathogenesis of giardiasis begins when ingested cysts excyst in the duodenum and jejunum, releasing trophozoites that attach to the intestinal epithelium using a ventral adhesive disc. The parasites interfere with nutrient absorption and intestinal function, inducing villus blunting, epithelial damage, and mild inflammation. These changes lead to malabsorption, diarrhea, and poor weight gain, particularly in young or stressed birds. Although *Giardia* infection rarely causes severe systemic disease, it predisposes the host to secondary bacterial infections and can exacerbate the effects of other intestinal pathogens. Overall, giardiasis is a protozoal enteric disease in which epithelial attachment, nutrient competition, and mucosal damage result in intestinal dysfunction, reduced growth, and decreased productivity in poultry flocks.

8.4.4.2 Risk Factors

- **Host Factors**
  Young chicks are the most susceptible due to immature immune systems and higher nutritional demands. Older birds may become asymptomatic carriers, shedding cysts without clinical

disease. Birds that are immunocompromised (due to concurrent infections, stress, or poor nutrition) are at increased risk of developing clinical disease. Malnourished or poorly fed birds are more likely to develop symptomatic infections because of weakened immunity and compromised intestinal integrity.

- **Environmental and Management Factors**
  Accumulation of fecal matter allows cysts to persist in litter and water sources, increasing exposure. Overcrowding increases contact between birds and contaminated fecal material, accelerating transmission. Wet or soiled bedding fosters cyst survival and increases the risk of ingestion.

8.4.4.3 Clinical Signs and Pathology

- **External Findings**
  Diarrhea, poor weight gain, failure to thrive, unthriftiness, dehydration, and mild lethargy.
- **Necropsy Findings**
  Necropsy findings in giardiasis are often mild, nonspecific, or even absent, especially in subclinical cases. When present, changes reflect chronic malabsorption and enteritis rather than overt tissue destruction. Pale, thin, and flaccid intestinal walls. Mild distension of the duodenum and proximal jejunum. Mild catarrhal enteritis (excess mucus on mucosal surfaces).

8.4.4.4 Diagnostic Testing

- **Wet Mount Examination**
  Collect fresh intestinal content or fecal material, preferably from the duodenum or proximal jejunum at necropsy or from freshly voided feces. Examine under light microscopy (40× objective) using saline wet mounts. Look for motile trophozoites—pear-shaped, bilaterally symmetrical, with flagella and a ventral adhesive disc. Motility is rapid, "falling leaf"–like but trophozoites are fragile and degrade quickly after sample collection.
- **Fecal Float**
  Can detect cysts in feces, though sensitivity is often low due to intermittent shedding.
- **ELISA Testing**
  Developed for mammals may cross-react with *Giardia* antigens in birds, though their use in avian species is less validated. Useful for flock screening if confirmed by microscopy.

8.4.4.5 Treatment and Therapeutic Interventions

- **Supportive Therapy**
  Rehydration and electrolyte therapy for birds with diarrhea and dehydration. Improved nutrition ensures high-quality, balanced food to support recovery and immune function. Vitamin A and B complex supplementation to aid mucosal healing.
- **Antiprotozoal Medications**
  Metronidazole 50–100 mg/kg by mouth once daily for 5–7 days.

8.4.4.6 Prevention and Control

- **Biosecurity Measures**
  Quarantine and screen new birds before introducing them to the flock. Disinfect boots, tools, and clothing before entering poultry areas. Seal feed storage, maintain structural barriers, and eliminate standing water to deter wildlife vectors.

- **Environmental Sanitation**
  Daily removal of feces and soiled litter. For routine disinfection of housing and equipment, use effective disinfectants (e.g., quaternary ammonium compounds, chlorine-based solutions) after thorough cleaning. Moisture prolongs cyst survival; good ventilation reduces humidity.
- **Water and Feed Hygiene**
  Provide clean, potable water to avoid surface or stagnant water sources that can harbor cysts. Clean and disinfect drinkers and feeders daily. Prevent fecal contamination of feed and water lines.
- **Flock Management**
  Avoid overcrowding to reduce stress and fecal-oral exposure. Promptly isolate clinically affected birds to reduce environmental contamination. Rotate pens or pastures if birds are on the ground to reduce environmental buildup.

8.4.4.7 Nursing Considerations

Nursing care for chickens affected by giardiasis focuses on supportive management such as maintaining hydration and nutrition and minimizing stressors to aid recovery and prevent secondary infections. Affected birds should be closely monitored for diarrhea, poor weight gain, decreased feed intake, lethargy, and signs of dehydration, with early detection helping reduce complications. Providing clean, fresh water and easily digestible, nutrient-rich feed supports hydration and nutrient absorption while reducing intestinal irritation. Environmental management is essential: maintain clean litter, prevent overcrowding, and ensure proper sanitation of feeders and waterers to limit reinfection and spread of *Giardia* cysts. Nursing may also involve reducing stress, managing concurrent intestinal infections, and consulting a veterinarian for appropriate antiparasitic therapy if indicated. Overall, nursing considerations for giardiasis emphasize monitoring clinical signs, supporting hydration and nutrition, maintaining hygiene, and controlling environmental contamination to promote intestinal health, reduce morbidity, and enhance flock productivity.

8.4.5 Cryptosporidiosis

8.4.5.1 Overview and Pathogenesis

Cryptosporidiosis in chickens is a parasitic disease caused by *Cryptosporidium* spp., intracellular protozoan parasites that primarily infect the epithelial cells of the GI tract, particularly the small intestine, bursa of Fabricius, and sometimes the respiratory tract. The disease predominantly affects young chicks, although birds of all ages can be infected, and is of economic significance due to diarrhea, poor growth, reduced feed efficiency, and increased susceptibility to secondary infections. Transmission occurs via the fecal-oral route through ingestion of sporulated oocysts present in contaminated litter, feed, water, or equipment. Clinically, infected birds may present with watery or pasty diarrhea, dehydration, weight loss, ruffled feathers, lethargy, and in severe cases, mortality, while subclinical infections can result in chronic poor performance.

The pathogenesis of cryptosporidiosis begins when ingested oocysts excyst in the GI tract, releasing sporozoites that invade the microvillus epithelium of the small intestine or other target tissues. The parasites undergo intracellular yet extracytoplasmic replication, forming trophozoites and meronts that cause epithelial cell damage, villus atrophy, and disruption of nutrient absorption. The resulting intestinal dysfunction manifests diarrhea, malabsorption, and weight loss. Cryptosporidium infection may also impair local immune responses, predisposing birds to secondary bacterial or viral infections. Overall, cryptosporidiosis is a protozoal enteric disease in which epithelial invasion, intracellular replication, and mucosal damage lead to diarrhea, impaired growth, and reduced productivity in affected poultry flocks.

8.4.5.2 Risk Factors

- **Age and Immune Status**
  Young chicks (especially 1–4 weeks old) are the most susceptible due to immature immune systems and underdeveloped gut microflora. Immunocompromised or stressed birds (due to concurrent disease, malnutrition, or environmental stressors) are at increased risk.
- **Environmental Contamination**
  High stocking density and overcrowding increase fecal-oral exposure to oocysts. Poor litter management (wet, soiled bedding) enhances oocyst survival and transmission. Inadequate cleaning and disinfection of housing and equipment allow persistent environmental contamination.
- **Water and Feed Contamination**
  Contaminated drinking water is a significant source of infection, especially in open or shared water systems. Fecal contamination of feed and feeders contributes to oral exposure.
- **Biosecurity Factors**
  Introduction of infected birds without quarantine can seed the parasite into a naïve flock. Lack of control of rodents, wild birds, and insects can facilitate mechanical transmission. Shared equipment or footwear can spread oocysts between pens or flocks.

8.4.5.3 Clinical Signs and Pathology

- **External Findings**
  Clinical presentation varies depending on age, immune status, and the site of infection. Many older birds may be subclinical carriers, whereas young or immunocompromised chicks often develop noticeable illness.
  - Enteric Form (Intestinal Infection)
    Diarrhea, weight loss, poor growth, unthriftiness, dehydration, and occasional mortality.
  - Respiratory Form (*C. baileyi*)
    Respiratory distress, sneezing, nasal discharge, swollen infraorbital sinuses, and reduced growth.
  - Proventricular Form (*C. galli*)
    Regurgitation, vomiting, crop distension, reduced feed intake, and poor weight gain.
- **Necropsy Findings**
  Necropsy findings may be subtle, particularly in mild infections, but typical observations include:
  - Enteric Form: Watery to mucoid intestinal contents, mildly distended, pale, or thin-walled intestines, and occasionally visible mucosal thickening or inflammation.
  - Respiratory Form: Thickened tracheal mucosa, mucus accumulation in the trachea or bronchi, and swelling of the infraorbital sinuses.
  - Proventricular Form: Hyperplastic or thickened proventricular mucosa and retained or undigested feed in proventriculus.

8.4.5.4 Diagnostic Testing

- **Fecal or Intestinal Examination**
  Sample Types
  Fresh feces, post-mortem intestinal scrapings (duodenum, jejunum), or proventricular tissue.

  Staining Techniques
  Modified acid-fast stain (most used) highlights oocysts as red or pink, round to oval bodies against a blue or green background. Giemsa or hematoxylin-eosin (H&E) may also demonstrate trophozoites on tissue sections.

- **Respiratory Samples**
  Tracheal or nasal swabs may be used in cases of *C. baileyi* infection. Oocysts can be visualized using acid-fast or immunofluorescent staining.
- **PCR**
  High sensitivity and specificity, species or genotype identification (e.g., *C. baileyi*, *C. meleagridis*, *C. galli*), useful for research, epidemiology, and outbreak investigation.

8.4.5.5 Treatment and Therapeutic Interventions

- **Supportive Therapy**
  Hydration and electrolytes for birds with diarrhea. High-quality, easily digestible feed; supplemental A, B-complex, and E vitamins to promote mucosal repair. Ensure proper ventilation, minimize dust, and maintain optimal temperature and humidity. Avoid overcrowding and sudden environmental changes.
- **Environmental Management**
  Because oocysts are highly resistant and immediately infective, treatment must be combined with strict hygiene and biosecurity:
  - Daily removal of feces and soiled litter.
  - Thorough cleaning and disinfection of pens, feeders, and waterers (e.g., with quaternary ammonium or chlorine-based solutions).
  - Clean drinking water and prevent stagnant water sources.
  - Quarantine new or affected birds to prevent spread.
- **Medications**
  No drugs are specifically approved for Cryptosporidium in poultry; treatment is primarily supportive, and some agents are used off-label under veterinary supervision.

8.4.5.6 Prevention and Control

Effective prevention of cryptosporidiosis relies on biosecurity, environmental management, and flock health due to the parasite's high environmental resilience and fecal-oral transmission.

- **Biosecurity**
  Quarantine new birds for at least 30 days and monitor for signs of infection. Limit exposure to wild birds, rodents, and insects, which may act as mechanical vectors. Restrict movement of equipment and personnel between flocks; disinfect clothing, footwear, and tools.
- **Environmental Management**
  Regular cleaning and disinfection of housing, feeders, and drinkers. Daily removal of wet or soiled litter. Maintain dry, well-ventilated housing to reduce oocyst survival. Clean water supply is essential; avoid surface or stagnant water.
- **Flock Management**
  Avoid overcrowding to reduce stress and fecal-oral transmission. Rotate pens or pastures if birds are kept on the ground. Isolate clinically affected birds when it is feasible to minimize environmental contamination.
- **Nutrition and Immunity**
  Ensure balanced feed to support immune system development. Provide vitamin supplementation, particularly A, E, and B-complex, to enhance mucosal defenses.

8.4.5.7 Nursing Considerations

Nursing care for chickens affected by *Cryptosporidiosis* focuses on supportive management by maintaining hydration and nutrition and preventing secondary infections. There is no specific

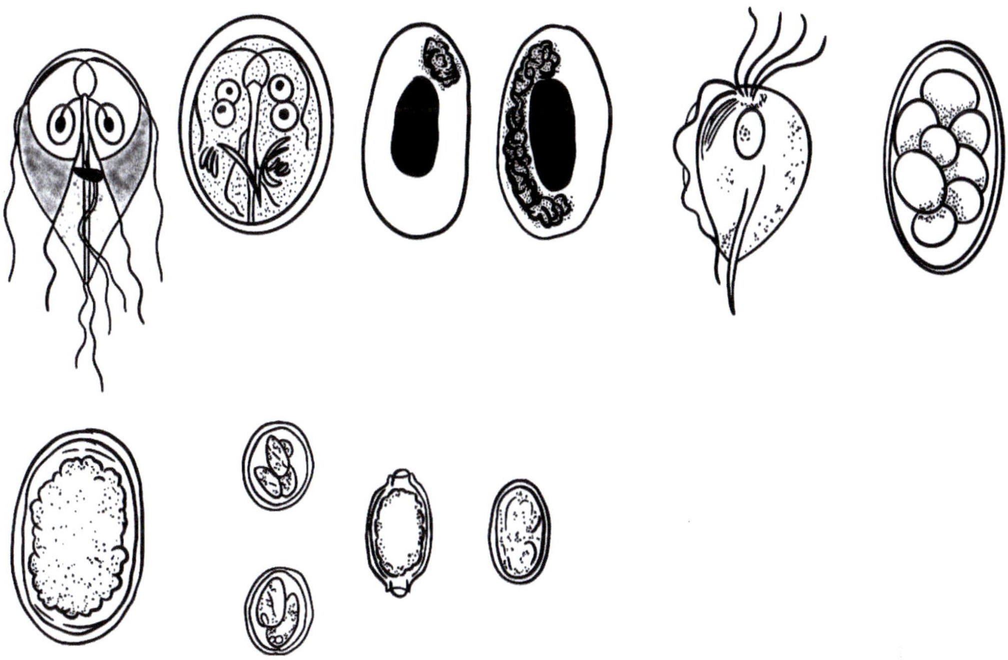

Figure 8.8 Left to right. *Giardia sp. Trophozoite, Giardia sp. Cyst, Plasmodium sp., Haemoproteus sp., Trichomonas gallinae, Syngamus trachea, Ascaridia sp., Sporulated coccidia, and Dispharynx sp.* Drawing by Rebecca Wood.

curative treatment for the protozoal infection. Affected birds should be closely monitored for diarrhea, weight loss, reduced feed intake, lethargy, and signs of dehydration, with early recognition helping to minimize morbidity. Providing clean, fresh water and easily digestible, nutrient-rich feed supports hydration, nutrient absorption, and overall health. Environmental management is critical: maintain dry, clean litter, minimize overcrowding, and implement strict biosecurity measures to prevent oocyst contamination and spread. Nursing may also involve reducing stress, isolating severely affected birds, and monitoring for secondary bacterial or viral infections that can worsen clinical outcomes. Overall, nursing considerations for cryptosporidiosis emphasize supportive care, hygiene, biosecurity, and careful monitoring to sustain intestinal function, reduce disease impact, and maintain flock productivity (Figure 8.8).

8.5 GI Disorders

8.5.1 Intestinal Volvulus

8.5.1.1 Overview and Pathogenesis

Intestinal volvulus is an acute GI disorder in chickens characterized by the abnormal twisting of a segment of the intestine around its mesenteric axis, leading to obstruction of the intestinal lumen and compromise of blood flow. This condition can occur in any intestinal segment but is most observed in the duodenum or jejunum.

Pathogenesis involves a combination of predisposing factors, including rapid growth, high-energy diets, sudden feed changes, excessive gut motility, or anatomical variations that increase intestinal mobility. Twisting of the intestine results in vascular compromise, ischemia, and necrosis of the affected intestinal segment. Clinically, affected birds may exhibit sudden depression, abdominal distention, anorexia, diarrhea, and rapid deterioration, often leading to death if untreated. Histopathological findings include congestion, hemorrhage, necrosis of the intestinal wall, and secondary bacterial translocation contributing to systemic sepsis.

8.5.1.2 Risk Factors

- **Host-Related Factors**
  Fast-growing meat bird breeds are particularly prone due to disproportionate gut size relative to body cavity. Excessive fat can alter intestinal positioning and mobility. It is most commonly occurs in rapidly growing meat birds between 3–6 weeks of age, when body mass and intestinal length increase rapidly. Rare in adult egg layers or slower-growing large breeds.
- **Management and Environmental Factors**
  Overcrowding increases stress and activity, which may contribute to intestinal displacement. Sudden temperature changes, heat stress, or fright can expedite volvulus. Very slippery or uneven floors may lead to sudden movements and gut torsion.
- **Physiological and Behavioral Factors**
  Vigorous wing flapping or struggling during handling may increase risk. Any underlying enteric pathology slowing transit may predispose to twisting. Abnormal feeding behavior such as overeating, rapid intake, or gorging may increase risk of volvulus.

8.5.1.3 Clinical Signs and Pathology

- **External Findings**
  Sudden weakness or collapse, sometimes without warning. Lethargy and reluctance to move. Abdominal distension is often pronounced and asymmetric. Sudden death is common in severe volvulus with vascular compromise. Pale comb and wattles if shock or circulatory compromise occurs.
- **Necropsy Findings**
  Twisting of the intestine around the mesenteric axis, usually involving the duodenum, jejunum, or mid-intestine. Intestinal distension is proximal to twist due to gas and fluid accumulation. Hemorrhage and congestion in the affected segment. Necrosis of the intestinal wall if blood flow is compromised. Serosal congestion and petechiae may be present. Mesenteric torsion, twisting blood vessels, leading to rapid ischemia.

8.5.1.4 Diagnostic Imaging

- Radiographs may reveal gas-filled, distended intestinal loops or abnormal positioning. Ultrasound can help visualize torsion and assess vascular compromise in live birds.

8.5.1.5 Treatment and Therapeutic Interventions

- **Emergency Surgical Intervention**
  Exploratory laparotomy may be attempted. Untwist the affected intestinal segment, assess for viability of intestinal tissue, and resect necrotic portions if feasible and perform anastomosis.

8.5.1.6 Prevention and Control

- **Host-Related Factors**
  Select meat bird breeds with moderate growth rates to reduce disproportionate gut length and abdominal mass.

- **Nutritional Management**
  Provide appropriate energy, protein, fiber, and mineral content. Avoid sudden diet changes; introduce new food gradually to prevent hypermotility. Prevent gorging or overeating, especially in broilers. Adequate fiber supports normal gut motility and prevents twisting.
- **Environmental and Husbandry Measures**
  Maintain stable temperatures, avoid overcrowding, and proper ventilation. Avoid slippery or uneven flooring that could trigger sudden activity leading to torsion. Minimize fright or sudden disturbances, especially in fast-growing breeds.

8.5.1.7 Nursing Considerations

Nursing care focuses primarily on prevention and supportive care, as surgical intervention is rarely feasible in chickens. Birds should be monitored closely for early signs such as depression, anorexia, abdominal distention, or diarrhea. Rapid deterioration and pain require prompt veterinary assessment, and humane euthanasia is often necessary to prevent prolonged suffering. Prevention strategies include providing a balanced diet, avoiding sudden changes in feed, controlling rapid growth in meat-type birds, and minimizing stressors that may increase gut motility. Environmental management, including adequate space and reduced overcrowding, can reduce the risk of sudden intestinal torsion. Supportive care prior to intervention involves maintaining hydration, electrolyte balance, and reducing stress, although the prognosis is generally poor once volvulus has occurred.

8.5.2 Malabsorption Syndrome

8.5.2.1 Overview and Pathogenesis

Malabsorption syndrome (MAS), also known as "runting–stunting" syndrome, is a multifactorial condition in chickens characterized by impaired nutrient digestion and absorption, leading to poor growth, uneven flock performance, and increased susceptibility to other diseases. The syndrome is most frequently observed in young meat chickens, particularly during the first weeks of life, when rapid growth demands efficient intestinal function. Affected birds often display stunted growth, poor feathering, diarrhea, and variable morbidity within a flock. The condition is not caused by a single agent but is instead associated with a complex interplay of infectious agents, nutritional imbalances, and environmental stressors.

Viruses such as reoviruses, astroviruses, adenoviruses, and rotaviruses have been implicated, often acting synergistically with bacterial pathogens (e.g., *E. coli*, *Clostridium* spp.) and coccidial infections. These agents damage the intestinal epithelium, reduce villus height, and alter enzyme activity, leading to impaired digestion of fats, carbohydrates, and proteins. The resulting malabsorption causes undigested feed particles and excess fat to appear in the feces, contributing to wet litter and further welfare concerns. Secondary nutritional deficiencies, including fat-soluble vitamin malabsorption, exacerbate poor growth and skeletal abnormalities. Environmental factors such as poor litter quality, overcrowding, and suboptimal brooding conditions increase the severity of the syndrome.

The pathogenesis of MAS involves direct viral or bacterial injury to enterocytes, villus atrophy, crypt hyperplasia, and disruption of the intestinal microbiota, ultimately compromising nutrient uptake and immune competence. This cascade not only limits growth potential but also predisposes birds to additional enteric and systemic diseases, resulting in significant economic losses in poultry production.

8.5.2.2 Risk Factors

- **Infectious Risk Factors**
  Enteric viruses such as reoviruses, astroviruses, rotaviruses, and adenoviruses. Bacterial involvement such as *E. coli*, *Clostridium perfringens*, *Enterococcus* spp. Co-infection with coccidia (*Eimeria* spp.) exacerbates intestinal damage.
- **Nutritional Risk Factors**
  Diets high in indigestible carbohydrates or poorly digestible fats. Imbalances in essential amino acids or micronutrients. Oxidized or rancid fats impairing nutrient absorption. Poor pellet quality or feed dust reduces feed intake. Mycotoxins (e.g., aflatoxin, ochratoxin, T-2 toxin) damage intestinal mucosa.
- **Management and Environmental Factors**
  Suboptimal temperature, humidity, or ventilation during the first week of life. High stocking density, increasing pathogen load and stress. Inadequate litter management leading to buildup of pathogens. Inconsistent feed or water supply, especially in young chicks. Poor biosecurity, exposure to contaminated equipment, people, or other flocks.
- **Host-Related Factors**
  Disease is most severe in chicks <2–4 weeks old. Some commercial broiler strains are more prone. Immunosuppression due to infectious bursal disease virus (IBDV), chicken anemia virus (CAV), or stress. Chicks from poor-quality hatching eggs or parent stock in poor health.

8.5.2.3 Clinical Signs and Pathology

- **External Findings**
  Stunted growth with poor muscle development. Chronic diarrhea or wet, pasty droppings. Distended abdomen, ruffled feathers, poor feathering, sometimes with twisted or brittle shafts. Lameness or poor skeletal development, including valgus/varus deformities. Signs of weakness, lethargy, and reduced activity.
- **Necropsy Findings**
  Pale, thin-walled intestines. Excessive fluid and undigested feed in the lumen. Sometimes ballooning or dilatation of the small intestine. Atrophy or fibrosis of the pancreas. Soft or brittle bones, growth plate abnormalities, especially in long bones.

8.5.2.4 Diagnostic Testing

MAS is a syndrome, not a single disease; testing is aimed at identifying contributing factors (viruses, nutrition, environment).

- **PCR or RT-PCR**
  Detect associated enteric viruses such as reoviruses, astroviruses, rotaviruses, and adenoviruses.
- **Differential Diagnosis**
  Conditions to rule out are coccidiosis, necrotic enteritis (NE), nutritional deficiencies, and primary viral disease-causing immunosuppression.

8.5.2.5 Treatment and Therapeutic Interventions

- **Supportive Care**
  Provide a balanced, high-quality commercial feed formulated for age/production stage. Supplement diet with easily digestible proteins (soy protein concentrate, fishmeal), medium-chain fatty acids (MCFAs) or vegetable oils (improved energy absorption). Enzyme supplements (proteases, lipases, carbohydrases) may improve digestion and nutrient uptake. Ensure clean,

fresh water free of contamination. Electrolytes and glucose for weak or dehydrated birds. Probiotics/prebiotics to support gut microbiota balance. Organic acids (formic, lactic, citric) to lower gut pH and suppress pathogens.

8.5.2.6 Prevention and Control

- **Biosecurity and Husbandry**
  Prevent introduction of enteric viruses and secondary pathogens. Limit visitor access and require clean boots/clothing. Quarantine new birds for at least 30 days. Disinfect equipment, feeders, drinkers, and housing routinely.
- **Housing and Environment**
  Maintain dry litter to reduce bacterial growth and parasite burden. Provide adequate ventilation and avoid overcrowding. Use all-in, all-out systems when possible. Allow a downtime period (minimum 10–14 days) between flocks to clean and disinfect.
- **Nutrition and Feed Management**
  Purchase feed from reputable mills with quality control programs. Store feed in cool, dry areas to reduce mold growth and mycotoxin contamination. Ensure adequate levels of vitamins A, D3, E, and B-complex. Monitor feed particle size (too coarse or fine can impair digestion).

8.5.2.7 Nursing Considerations

Nursing care in cases of MAS centers on maintaining hydration, nutrition, and comfort while minimizing environmental stressors. Affected chicks are often stunted, weak, and prone to secondary infections, so technicians should closely monitor body weight, crop fill, fecal consistency, and feather quality to track flock response to interventions. Technicians should implement enhanced biosecurity measures to limit the spread of enteric pathogens and monitor for concurrent diseases such as coccidiosis or bacterial enteritis, initiating diagnostic sampling when warranted. Client education is also an important role; technicians should advise on the importance of balanced nutrition, proper brooding, and vigilant observation of young chicks. By focusing on supportive husbandry, early detection, and preventive management, veterinary technicians can reduce the impact of MAS and improve flock performance.

8.5.3 Ulcerative Enteritis

8.5.3.1 Overview and Pathogenesis

Ulcerative enteritis (UE), also called "quail disease," is a rapidly progressive bacterial disease of chickens, quail, and other game birds caused by *Clostridium colinum*. It is most common in young, stressed, or immunocompromised birds, and frequently occurs in association with coccidiosis or other enteric disturbances. The disease is characterized by sudden onset, high morbidity, and potentially severe mortality, with affected birds showing depression, anorexia, diarrhea, ruffled feathers, and rapid weight loss before death.

Pathogenesis begins with ingestion of *C. colinum* spores, which germinate in the intestine when gut integrity is compromised. The organism proliferates in the ceca and lower intestine, releasing toxins that damage the mucosa and cause sharply demarcated ulcers. These lesions disrupt absorption, lead to hemorrhage, and allow bacterial toxins and necrotic debris to enter the bloodstream. In severe cases, the infection spreads to the liver, producing characteristic necrotic foci. The combined effects of intestinal ulceration, impaired nutrient absorption, systemic toxemia, and concurrent stressors overwhelm the bird's defenses, resulting in rapid clinical decline and death.

8.5.3.2 Risk Factors

- **Pathogen Exposure**
  C. colinum, the causative bacterium, spreads via the fecal–oral route. Contaminated feed, water, soil, or litter are major sources. Infected carrier birds (especially quail, turkeys, pigeons, and game birds) can transmit the organism to chickens.
- **Immune and Physiological Status**
  Young birds (4–12 weeks old) are more susceptible, especially pullets in transition from starter to grower diets. Immunosuppressed birds (from Marek's disease, infectious bursal disease, or stressors) are at greater risk. Concurrent coccidiosis damages intestinal lining and predisposes birds to UE. Nutritional deficiencies (poor-quality feed, lack of vitamins A and E) reduce gut integrity and immunity.
- **Environmental and Husbandry Factors**
  Poor sanitation and wet litter favor the survival and spread of *C. colinum*. Overcrowding increases stress and fecal contamination. Poor ventilation raises humidity and bacterial growth. Mixed-species housing (quail, turkeys, pigeons, chickens) increases exposure risk.
- **Stress Factors**
  Transport, handling, or environmental stress (sudden temperature changes, poor brooding conditions). Feed changes or diet inconsistency can disrupt gut flora. Predator pressure or high noise levels can suppress immunity.

8.5.3.3 Clinical Signs and Pathology

- **External Findings**
  Ruffled feathers and poor grooming. Watery or bloody diarrhea; vent feathers stained with feces. Weight loss and emaciation, despite feed availability. Pale combs and wattles (signs of anemia). Hunched posture and reluctance to move.
- **Necropsy Findings**
  Small, button-like ulcers in the small intestine and ceca. Severe cases may show perforation of the intestinal wall causing peritonitis. Enlarged, friable, mottled liver. White to gray necrotic foci are scattered throughout the parenchyma. The spleen may be enlarged and mottled.

8.5.3.4 Diagnostic Testing

- **PCR**
  Can detect *C. colinum* directly from intestinal content or tissue.

8.5.3.5 Treatment and Therapeutic Interventions

- **Medication**
  Tylosin 50 mg/kg by mouth once daily for 5–7 days or 15–30 mg/kg intramuscularly every 6–12 hours for 5–7 days.
  Lincomycin 25–50 mg/kg by mouth every 12 hours.
- **Supportive Care**
  Provide clean, fresh water, possibly with electrolytes or glucose to support weak birds. Minimize stress by reducing handling during acute outbreaks. Ensure high-quality food, easily digestible to minimize further gut irritation. Offer small frequent meals if birds are depressed or weak. Assisted feeding if indicated.

8.5.3.6 Prevention and Control

- **Biosecurity Measures**
  Quarantine new birds (especially quail, turkeys, or pigeons) for at least 30 days. Limit access of wild birds and other animals to poultry housing. Clean and disinfect feeders, waterers, and housing between

flocks. Remove and replace soiled litter promptly. Technicians and guardians should wear clean clothing and footwear when entering houses. Avoid cross-contamination between houses or farms.

- **Environmental Management**
  Maintain dry, friable litter to minimize bacterial growth. Regularly remove wet or caked areas. Prevent damp, humid conditions that favor bacterial proliferation. Avoid overcrowding, sudden temperature changes, or excessive handling.
- **Nutrition and Feed Management**
  Ensure appropriate protein, vitamin, and mineral levels. Store feed in dry, pest-free areas. Avoid moldy or spoiled feed that can compromise immunity. Provide clean, fresh water at all times; disinfect drinkers periodically.

8.5.3.7 Nursing Considerations

Nursing care for chickens affected by UE focuses on reducing stress, maintaining hydration, and preventing secondary infections. Affected birds often appear weak, dehydrated, and lethargic, so technicians should ensure easy access to clean water and easily digestible feed, potentially supplemented with electrolytes and vitamins to support recovery. Because UE often occurs in conjunction with other enteric disturbances, technicians should observe for concurrent coccidiosis or other intestinal infections and report abnormalities to the supervising veterinarian. Pain and discomfort management, as well as minimizing stress, are important to prevent worsening of the disease. Finally, veterinary technicians play a key role in educating caretakers on prevention measures, including reducing flock stress, avoiding overcrowding, and ensuring adequate nutrition, to minimize recurrence and maintain overall flock health.

8.5.4 Vent Gleet

8.5.4.1 Overview and Pathogenesis

Vent gleet, also known as cloacitis or fungal vent infection, is a chronic inflammatory condition of the vent and cloaca in chickens, characterized by foul-smelling, mucous-laden discharge, feather matting around the vent, and irritation. It is most seen in laying hens or birds with poor hygiene, prolonged moisture exposure, or compromised immunity.

Pathogenesis involves disruption of the normal cloacal microflora and mucosal integrity, often allowing opportunistic organisms such as *Candida* spp., *Saccharomyces*, or mixed bacterial populations to colonize the vent. Moisture accumulation from diarrhea, poor perching, or prolonged contact with wet litter promotes fungal overgrowth, while mechanical irritation from fecal material or vent prolapse exacerbates mucosal inflammation. Chronic inflammation leads to thickening of the cloacal mucosa, hyperkeratosis, and excessive mucus production. Secondary bacterial infections can further aggravate the condition, causing pain, decreased egg-laying, and general malaise. Stressors such as overcrowding, nutritional deficiencies, and poor sanitation increase susceptibility and prolong the course of disease, making proper husbandry critical for prevention and management.

8.5.4.2 Risk Factors

- **Immunosuppression and Stress**
  Young or newly hatched chicks are more susceptible due to immature immune systems. Stressful conditions increase susceptibility. Concurrent diseases that suppress immunity (e.g., Marek's disease, infectious bursal disease) increase risk.
- **Nutritional Factors**
  High-carbohydrate or high-sugar diets can promote overgrowth of yeast in the gut. Vitamins or mineral deficiencies, particularly vitamin A and B-complex. Poor-quality feed, moldy feed, or feed contaminated with mycotoxins may predispose birds.

- **Gastrointestinal Dysbiosis**
  Disruption of normal gut flora encourages yeast proliferation. Prolonged antibiotic use can kill beneficial bacteria, allowing *Candida* overgrowth. Improper water quality or inconsistent feeding can also upset gut microbiota.
- **Environmental and Husbandry Factors**
  Poor sanitation around the vent and housing. Inadequate ventilation leads to high humidity and moist conditions. Shared housing with other species or birds with chronic infections.

8.5.4.3 Clinical Signs and Pathology

- **External Findings**
  Soiling around the vent with white to yellow cheesy or pasty exudate. Reddening and inflammation of the vent mucosa. Foul odor due to secondary bacterial contamination. Feather loss around the vent from chronic irritation. Straining or discomfort during defecation. Reduced feed intake and growth in affected chicks.
- **Necropsy Findings**
  Swollen, reddened, or inflamed vent tissue. Accumulation of yellow-white, pasty exudate adhering to feathers and skin. In chronic cases, thickening of vent mucosa may be visible. Feather matting, crusts, and dermatitis from persistent irritation. Fecal contamination may lead to cutaneous bacterial infection.

8.5.4.4 Diagnostic Testing

- **Culture**
  Sabouraud dextrose agar or other fungal media. Confirms presence of *Candida* spp. and allows antifungal sensitivity testing if needed.

8.5.4.5 Treatment and Therapeutic Interventions

- **Medication**
  Nystatin 100,000 U/L in drinking water or 300,000–600,000 U/kg by mouth every 8–12 hours.
- **Supportive Care**
  Clean the vent and surrounding feathers daily to remove exudate. Soak affected feathers in warm water and gently remove debris. Apply diaper rash cream to clean, dry affected skin. Keep litter or bedding dry and clean to minimize reinfection. Prevent self-injury and fly strike.

8.5.4.6 Prevention and Control

- **Biosecurity and Hygiene**
  Remove soiled litter, droppings, and wet areas promptly. Clean feeders, waterers, perches, and surrounding areas regularly. Veterinary technicians and owners should wear clean clothing and gloves when handling birds and change them before handling/visiting the flock. Isolate for at least 30 days to prevent introducing yeast or other pathogens.
- **Environmental Management**
  Maintain dry litter to prevent persistent moisture around the vent. Ensure adequate ventilation to reduce humidity. Minimize overcrowding to lower stress and fecal contamination. Avoid sudden temperature or environmental changes, which can stress birds and compromise gut health.
- **Nutritional and Feed Management**
  Provide balanced, high-quality food appropriate for age and production stage. Limit high-sugar or high-starch treats that promote yeast growth. Ensure fresh, clean water, disinfect drinkers

regularly. Use probiotics or fermented feed additives to support healthy gut microbiota, especially after antibiotic therapy.

- **Stress Reduction**
  Reduce handling and transport stress, especially in young birds or laying hens during peak production. Minimize environmental stressors such as noise, predator exposure, or overcrowding.

8.5.4.7 Nursing Considerations

Nursing care of chickens affected by vent gleet focuses on improving hygiene, reducing irritation, and supporting recovery while minimizing stress. Veterinary technicians should regularly clean the vent area, carefully removing accumulated fecal matter and matted feathers to reduce moisture and bacterial or fungal overgrowth. In flocks with multiple affected birds, isolation of severely affected individuals can limit the spread of opportunistic infections. Stress reduction through gentle handling, adequate space, and proper lighting is important, as stress can exacerbate the condition. Veterinary technicians should also educate caretakers on preventive husbandry practices, including routine vent inspection, proper litter management, and prompt attention to fecal soiling, to maintain long-term flock health and productivity.

8.6 Helminthic Gastrointestinal Diseases

Helminth parasites are common in backyards and free-range flocks. They cause disease by competing for nutrients, damaging mucosa, and predisposing birds to secondary infections. Many infections are subclinical, making veterinary awareness critical.

Quick reference chart

Parasite/ disease	Common name	Primary site in GI tract	Transmission/ source	Key clinical signs	Pathology/key lesions
Ascaridia galli	Roundworm	Small intestine	Ingestion of infective eggs in litter, soil, or feed	Weight loss, diarrhea, anorexia, poor growth; intestinal blockage in heavy infections	Large white worms in intestine, thickened mucosa, possible impaction
Heterakis gallinarum	Cecal worm	Cecum	Ingestion of embryonated eggs from litter/ soil	Usually subclinical; diarrhea, weight loss; vector of *Histomonas meleagridis* (blackhead)	Cecal inflammation, carrier role more significant than direct damage
Capillaria spp.	Hairworm	Crop, esophagus, intestine	Direct ingestion of eggs or via intermediate hosts (earthworms)	Weight loss, anemia, diarrhea, ruffled feathers, droopiness	Thread-like worms embedded in mucosa; catarrhal inflammation

(Continued)

Quick reference chart

Parasite/ disease	Common name	Primary site in GI tract	Transmission/ source	Key clinical signs	Pathology/key lesions
Raillietina spp.	Tapeworm	Intestine	Ingestion of intermediate hosts (ants, beetles, flies)	Diarrhea, stunting, reduced egg production, cachexia	Nodules at attachment sites, mucosal irritation, visible proglottids
Strongyloides avium	Threadworm	Small intestine	Skin penetration or ingestion of larvae	Weakness, diarrhea, poor weight gain, debilitation	Enteritis with mucosal irritation; villous damage

Chart created by Stephanie Freeman.

8.6.1 *Ascaridia galli* (Large Roundworm)

8.6.1.1 Overview and Pathogenesis

Ascaridiosis in chickens is caused by *Ascaridia galli*, a large, white nematode that inhabits the small intestine of domestic fowl. The parasite primarily affects young chickens and pullets, although birds of all ages can be infected, and is of economic significance due to reduced growth, poor feed conversion, decreased egg production, intestinal obstruction, and increased susceptibility to secondary infections in heavy infestations. Transmission occurs via the ingestion of embryonated eggs from contaminated litter, soil, feed, or water, with the eggs highly resistant to environmental conditions, facilitating long-term persistence. Clinically, affected birds may exhibit diarrhea, poor weight gain, emaciation, lethargy, reduced egg production, and in severe cases, intestinal obstruction or sudden death, while light infections are often subclinical.

The pathogenesis of *A. galli* begins with ingestion of embryonated eggs, which hatch in the small intestine, releasing larvae that mature into adult worms. Adult worms attach loosely to the intestinal mucosa, causing mechanical irritation, mucosal inflammation, and epithelial damage, which leads to malabsorption and diarrhea. Heavy infestations can physically obstruct the intestinal lumen, leading to severe distension, impaired nutrient uptake, and increased mortality. The intestinal damage caused by the worms also predisposes birds to secondary bacterial infections, further compromising health and productivity. Overall, *A. galli* infection is a parasitic enteric disease in which larval development, adult colonization, mechanical irritation, and mucosal damage collectively impair intestinal function, growth, and egg production in affected poultry flocks.

8.6.1.2 Risk Factors

- **Age and Host Susceptibility**
  Young chicks (1–12 weeks) are most susceptible due to immature immune system and higher exposure to contaminated litter or soil. Older birds may be subclinical carriers, shedding eggs into the environment and maintaining the parasite life cycle.
- **Environmental and Management Factors**
  Accumulation of feces in pens or runs facilitates egg survival and transmission. Birds foraging in soil have increased exposure to infective eggs. Eggs survive longer in humid, warm environments, increasing infection risk.

- **Nutrition and Health Status**
  Malnourished birds are more susceptible due to weaker immune defenses. Concurrent diseases or immunosuppression (e.g., coccidiosis, viral infections) exacerbate susceptibility and disease severity.

8.6.1.3 Clinical Signs and Pathology

- **External Findings**
  The clinical presentation of *A. galli* infection depends on age, worm burden, and host immune status. Low-intensity infections are often subclinical, while high-intensity infections produce noticeable disease. Poor growth or stunted development in young birds, reduced feed efficiency and weight gain, diarrhea, and unthriftiness. Severe or heavy infections may cause distended abdomen, intestinal obstruction, anorexia, dehydration, and mortality in young chicks.
- **Necropsy Findings**
  Necropsy may reveal visible adult worms in the intestinal tract, duodenum, and jejunum primarily. Mild to moderate catarrhal enteritis, distended intestinal loops filled with worms and digesta, and occasional hemorrhagic foci on mucosa in heavy infestations.

8.6.1.4 Diagnostic Testing

Early detection is important to prevent heavy parasitic burdens that can impair growth or cause mortality.

- **Direct Fecal Smear**
  Fresh fecal samples are examined under a microscope for Ascaridia eggs. Eggs are ellipsoidal, thick-shelled, and contain a single-cell embryo when freshly passed. It is useful for confirming active infection, especially in live birds.
- **Fecal Flotation**
  Concentration techniques such as Sheather's sugar solution or zinc sulfate flotation increase egg detection. It is most sensitive when multiple fecal samples are collected over several days due to intermittent shedding.

8.6.1.5 Treatment and Therapeutic Interventions

- **Supportive Therapy**
  Provide high-quality feed to compensate for nutrient loss due to worm infestation. Ensure access to clean water; electrolyte solutions may be needed in cases of diarrhea. Avoid overcrowding and environmental extremes during recovery.
- **Medications**
  Several drugs are commonly used to treat *A. galli*, usually administered orally. Dosages must follow veterinary guidance, particularly in food-producing birds.
  Fenbendazole 20–25 mg/kg by mouth daily for 3–5 days, repeated for another 3–5 days in 10 days.
  Ivermectin 0.2–0.4 mg/kg by mouth or subcutaneously once can be repeated in 10–14 days.

8.6.1.6 Prevention and Control

- **Biosecurity Measures**
  Quarantine new birds for at least 30 days before introducing them to the flock. Restrict access of wild birds, rodents, and insects, which can mechanically transmit eggs. Limit shared equipment and personnel between birds and flocks; disinfect footwear, clothing, and tools.

- **Environmental Sanitation**
  Regular removal of feces and soiled litter to reduce egg accumulation. Thorough cleaning and disinfection of housing, feeders, and waterers. Dry, well-ventilated housing reduces egg survival. Pasture rotation for free-range flocks to allow natural egg degradation. Provide clean, uncontaminated drinking water. Keep feed off the ground to prevent fecal contamination.
- **Flock Management**
  Avoid overcrowding, which increases exposure to infective eggs. Separate age groups to reduce infection pressure on young, susceptible chicks. Monitor flock health regularly to identify early signs of infection.

8.6.1.7 Nursing Considerations

Nursing care for chickens affected by *A. galli* focuses on supportive management, maintaining nutrition and hydration, and preventing secondary infections. Affected birds should be closely monitored for signs of diarrhea, weight loss, poor body condition, reduced feed intake, lethargy, and possible intestinal obstruction, with early detection reducing the risk of severe complications. Providing clean water and easily digestible, nutrient-rich feed supports hydration and growth while minimizing GI stress. Environmental management is crucial: maintain clean litter, control intermediate hosts such as earthworms, and implement strict sanitation and biosecurity measures to reduce egg contamination and reinfection. Nursing may also involve reducing flock stress, isolating heavily infested birds, and consulting a veterinarian for appropriate anthelmintic therapy. Overall, nursing considerations for *A. galli* emphasize monitoring clinical signs, supporting nutrition and hydration, maintaining hygiene, and implementing preventive measures to reduce parasite load, improve health, and maintain productivity in affected flocks.

8.6.2 *Heterakis gallinarum* (Cecal Worm)

8.6.2.1 Overview and Pathogenesis

Heterakiasis in chickens is caused by *H. gallinarum*, a small nematode commonly referred to as the cecal worm, which inhabits the ceca of domestic fowl. The parasite primarily affects free-range and backyard chickens, with economic significance arising indirectly due to its role as a vector for *H. meleagridis*, the causative agent of blackhead disease, rather than through direct pathogenicity in most cases. Transmission occurs via the ingestion of embryonated eggs from contaminated litter, soil, or water, or through paratenic hosts such as earthworms, which harbor infective larvae. Clinically, H. gallinarum infections are often subclinical; however, heavy infestations may cause cecal irritation, diarrhea, weight loss, decreased feed efficiency, and occasional lethargy.

The pathogenesis of *H. gallinarum* begins with ingestion of infective eggs or larvae, which migrate to the ceca and mature into adults. Adult worms attach superficially to the cecal mucosa, causing mild mechanical irritation and localized inflammatory responses, including infiltration by heterophils and lymphocytes. While the worms themselves rarely cause severe disease, they can create a favorable environment for secondary pathogens and facilitate transmission of *H. meleagridis*, which invades the cecal mucosa and liver, leading to blackhead disease. Chronic heavy infestations may contribute to malabsorption, poor growth, and reduced egg production, particularly in young or immunocompromised birds. Overall, *H. gallinarum* is a parasitic cecal nematode in which mucosal colonization and vector potential contribute to intestinal irritation, secondary infections, and indirect economic impact in poultry flocks.

8.6.2.2 Risk Factors

- **Environmental Factors**

  Eggs are highly resistant, surviving for months in moist, shaded litter and soil. Infrequent cleaning or accumulation of organic matter increases environmental load. Birds with a higher risk of contact with paratenic hosts (earthworms) that carry infective larvae.
- **Host-Related Factors**

  Young birds lack protective immunity, making them more susceptible to initial infections. Chickens act as reservoir hosts, shedding eggs that transmit *H. meleagridis* to turkeys. Overcrowding increases fecal contamination of the environment and the rate of egg ingestion.
- **Management Factors**

  Lack of regular deworming programs allows gradual buildup of worms and eggs in the flock. Shared equipment, boots, or tools can transfer eggs between pens or flocks. Accumulation of moist litter creates ideal conditions for egg survival and transmission.

8.6.2.3 Clinical Signs and Pathology

- **External Findings**

  In most cases, heterakiasis is subclinical to chickens. Clinical disease is uncommon unless birds carry heavy worm burdens or have concurrent infection with *H. meleagridis*. When present, signs are typically nonspecific and mild. Reduced weight gain or poor growth performance in young birds, mild diarrhea, decreased feed intake, mild depression, and slight reduction in egg production.
- **Necropsy Findings**

  Mild cecal inflammation and visible small white worms in the cecal lumen.

8.6.2.4 Diagnostic Testing

- **Fecal Float**

  Fecal flotation using saturated salt or sugar solutions, concentration techniques improve sensitivity, especially with low burdens. Eggs are indistinguishable from *A. galli* eggs under routine microscopy; differentiation requires location of adult worms at necropsy.

8.6.2.5 Treatment and Therapeutic Interventions

- **Supportive Care**

  Treat the entire flock simultaneously to prevent reinfection from untreated carriers. Repeat treatments at 3–4-week intervals if environmental contamination is high. Monitor fecal egg counts post-treatment to assess efficacy and detect potential resistance.
- **Medication**

  Fenbendazole

  20–50 mg/kg by mouth daily for 3–5 days, repeated for another 3–5 days in 10 days.

8.6.2.6 Prevention and Control

- **Biosecurity and Management Practices**

  Maintain dry, clean litter to reduce egg survival. Regularly remove and replace soiled litter, especially in brooder and grow-out areas. Clean and disinfect floors, walls, feeders, and drinkers between flocks. Rotate birds between clean pastures to disrupt the parasite's life cycle. Allow contaminated outdoor areas to rest for several months; *Heterakis* eggs are resistant and can survive for long periods in soil. Limit foraging in heavily contaminated soil or use raised pens with wire floors to prevent access to earthworms. Avoid co-housing chickens and turkeys or rotating turkeys into areas previously used by chickens since chickens can carry and shed *H. gallinarum* eggs infected with *H. meleagridis*.

- **Strategic Anthelmintic Use**
  Treat entire flocks with effective anthelmintics on a preventive schedule if infection is endemic. Rotate drug classes periodically to reduce the risk of resistance. Always observe appropriate withdrawal times for eggs and meat.

8.6.2.7 Nursing Considerations

Nursing care for chickens affected by *H. gallinarum* focuses on supportive management, maintaining flock hygiene, and preventing secondary infections, as the parasite itself is often subclinical but serves as a vector for *H. meleagridis*. Affected birds should be monitored for diarrhea, weight loss, lethargy, and decreased feed intake, with attention to early signs of blackhead disease in susceptible flocks. Providing clean, fresh water and easily digestible feed helps maintain hydration and nutritional status. Environmental management is critical: maintain clean litter, prevent access to contaminated soil or intermediate hosts such as earthworms, and implement strict biosecurity to reduce the risk of reinfection and *Histomonas* transmission. Nursing may also involve isolating birds showing clinical signs, reducing stressors, and consulting a veterinarian for appropriate anthelmintic therapy if indicated. Overall, nursing considerations for *H. gallinarum* emphasize monitoring clinical signs, maintaining nutrition and hydration, controlling environmental contamination, and implementing preventive strategies to support flock health and minimize indirect disease impact.

8.6.3 *Capillaria* spp. (Hairworms)

8.6.3.1 Overview and Pathogenesis

Capillariasis in chickens is caused by *Capillaria* spp., commonly referred to as hairworms, which are slender, thread-like nematodes that inhabit the small intestine, ceca, and occasionally the crop or esophagus. The disease predominantly affects free-range, backyard, or poorly managed flocks, and is of economic significance due to reduced growth, poor feed efficiency, decreased egg production, and increased susceptibility to secondary infections in heavy infestations. Transmission occurs via the ingestion of embryonated eggs from contaminated litter, soil, feed, water, or intermediate hosts such as earthworms, which may harbor infective larvae. Clinically, affected birds may exhibit diarrhea, poor body condition, emaciation, decreased feed intake, anemia, and, in severe infestations, sudden death, although light infections are often subclinical.

The pathogenesis of capillariasis begins with ingestion of embryonated eggs or larvae, which hatch and mature within the GI tract. Adult worms attach to the mucosa using their slender anterior ends, causing mechanical irritation, epithelial damage, and inflammation. This leads to malabsorption, mucosal erosion, and disruption of intestinal integrity, which can result in diarrhea, poor nutrient uptake, and weight loss. Heavy infestations may predispose birds to secondary bacterial infections, further exacerbating morbidity. Chronic infections can contribute to stunted growth, reduced egg production, and overall decline in flock performance. Overall, *Capillaria* spp. infections are parasitic enteric diseases in which mucosal attachment, tissue irritation, and nutrient competition lead to intestinal pathology, decreased productivity, and compromised health in affected chickens (Figure 8.9).

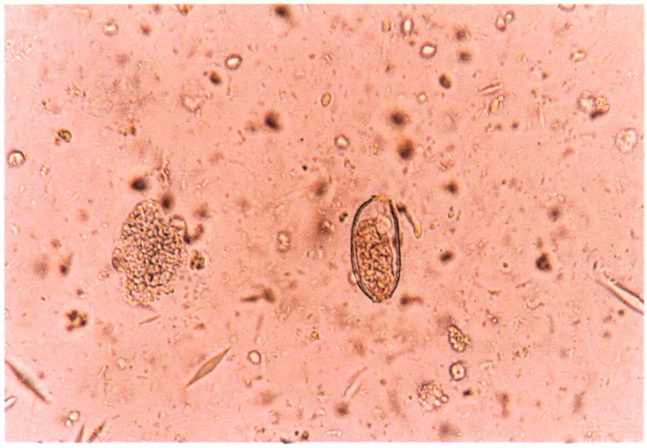

Figure 8.9 *Capillaria* spp. ova. Chatsikan / Adobe Stock Photos.

8.6.3.2 Risk Factors

- **Environmental Factors**
  Moist, wet litter or soil promotes the survival and development of infective eggs. Humidity allows eggs to embryonate more rapidly and persists longer. Birds are exposed to contaminated soil and intermediate hosts (earthworms), which can carry infective larvae. Accumulation of fecal matter increases environmental contamination with eggs. Warm, humid climates accelerate egg development and increase transmission potential.
- **Host-Related Factors**
  Young age, immature immune systems make them more susceptible to heavy burdens. Concurrent disease, overcrowding, or nutritional deficiencies can lower resistance. High stocking densities increase exposure to infective eggs through contaminated litter and feed/water.

8.6.3.3 Clinical Signs and Pathology

- **External Findings**
  Clinical disease due to *Capillaria* spp. infection depends on the worm burden, the species involved, and the overall health status of the host. Light infections may be subclinical, while heavy infestations can cause significant illness. Common clinical signs include:
  - Poor growth and weight loss—particularly in young birds
  - Decreased feed efficiency and egg production
  - Ruffled feathers and general unthriftiness
  - Diarrhea, which may be mucoid or occasionally bloody
  - Anorexia and depression
  - Pale combs and wattles from chronic anemia and debilitation
  - Emaciation in advanced infections
  - Gagging or difficulty swallowing (particularly with species affecting the crop and esophagus such as *Capillaria annulata* and *Capillaria contorta*)
  - Sudden death in severe cases, especially in young or immunocompromised birds
- **Necropsy Findings**
  - Crop and esophagus (*C. annulata, C. contorta*)
    Thickened, inflamed mucosa, hyperkeratosis and hyperplasia of the epithelium, and caseous or mucoid exudate may be present.

- Intestines and ceca (*C. obsignata, C. caudinflata*)
  Congested, thickened intestinal wall, catarrhal or hemorrhagic enteritis, focal necrosis of mucosa, adult worms or larvae visible in mucosal scrapings, and reduced intestinal contents and emaciated carcass.

8.6.3.4 Diagnostic Testing

Because light infections are often subclinical, laboratory confirmation is usually necessary for accurate detection and management.

- **Direct Fecal Smear**
  Fresh fecal samples examined microscopically can reveal Capillaria eggs. Useful for detecting active infections in live birds.
- **Fecal Flotation**
  Concentration techniques (e.g., Sheather's sugar solution or zinc sulfate flotation) improve detection sensitivity. Multiple samples over several days may be required due to intermittent egg shedding.

8.6.3.5 Treatment and Therapeutic Interventions

- **Treatment Considerations**
  Treat entire flock simultaneously to prevent reinfection from untreated carriers. Repeating treatments may be necessary in heavily contaminated environments. Monitor for efficacy via follow-up fecal exams or observation of flock performance. Avoid underdosing to reduce the risk of resistance development.
- **Medications**
  Fenbendazole 20–50 mg/kg by mouth daily for 3–5 days, repeated for another 3–5 days in 10 days.

8.6.3.6 Prevention and Control

- **Biosecurity Measures**
  Quarantine new birds for 30 days before introducing them to the flock. Restrict access of wild birds, rodents, and insects, which may mechanically transfer eggs. Avoid co-housing birds of different ages to reduce transmission from older, chronically infected birds.
- **Environmental Management**
  Remove soiled litter and fecal matter regularly to prevent egg buildup. Disinfect housing, feeders, and drinkers between flocks. Maintain dry and well-ventilated housing to reduce egg survival. Pasture rotation or pen resting in free-range systems to limit exposure to contaminated soil. Control intermediate hosts (earthworms) in outdoor runs when possible.
- **Flock Monitoring**
  Perform routine fecal examinations to detect early infections. Conduct necropsies on representative birds to monitor worm burdens. Implement scheduled deworming programs based on risk assessment and diagnostics.

8.6.3.7 Nursing Considerations

Nursing care for chickens affected by *Capillaria* spp. focuses on supportive management, maintaining hydration and nutrition, and preventing secondary infections. Affected birds should be closely monitored for diarrhea, poor weight gain, lethargy, reduced feed intake, anemia, and signs of GI discomfort, as early recognition can reduce morbidity and prevent severe infestations. Providing clean, fresh water and easily digestible, nutrient-rich feed supports hydration, nutrient absorption, and overall recovery. Environmental management is essential: maintain clean litter, control intermediate hosts such as earthworms, and implement strict biosecurity and sanitation measures to minimize reinfection and spread of eggs. Nursing may also involve reducing stress, isolating heavily affected birds, and consulting a veterinarian for appropriate anthelmintic treatment. Overall, nursing considerations for capillariasis emphasize monitoring clinical signs, supporting hydration and nutrition, maintaining environmental hygiene, and implementing preventive strategies to reduce parasite burden, improve health, and maintain productivity in affected flocks.

8.6.4 Cestodes (Tapeworms: *Raillietina, Davainea* spp.)

8.6.4.1 Overview and Pathogenesis

Cestode infections in chickens are caused by tapeworms such as *Raillietina* spp. and *Davainea* spp., which inhabit the small intestine and occasionally the ceca. These parasites predominantly affect free-range and backyard poultry, with significance arising from reduced weight gain, poor feed conversion, anemia, and decreased egg production in heavy infestations. Transmission occurs via the ingestion of intermediate hosts, such as beetles, ants, or slugs, which harbor the larval cysticercoid stage of the tapeworm. Clinically, infected birds may exhibit weight loss, reduced growth, diarrhea, lethargy, poor feather condition, and in severe infestations, intestinal obstruction or sudden death, although light infections are often subclinical.

The pathogenesis of cestode infection begins with ingestion of infected intermediate hosts, allowing the larval cysticercoids to attach to the intestinal mucosa using their scolex and hooks or suckers. The adult tapeworms mature within the intestine and absorb nutrients directly through their tegument, competing with the host for essential nutrients. Heavy infestations can cause mechanical irritation, mucosal damage, and enteritis, leading to malabsorption and impaired growth. Secondary bacterial infections may develop due to mucosal compromise, exacerbating disease severity. Chronic infections may contribute to emaciation, anemia, and decreased productivity in affected flocks. Overall, cestode infections are parasitic enteric diseases in which attachment, nutrient competition, and mucosal irritation combine to impair growth, health, and production efficiency in chickens.

8.6.4.2 Risk Factors

- **Environmental Factors**
  Presence of intermediate hosts, free-range or outdoor flocks are more likely to ingest infected hosts. Birds foraging in soil are at higher risk of encountering infected arthropods or mollusks. Warm and humid climates favor the survival and activity of intermediate hosts and increase transmission potential.
- **Host-Related Factors**
  Immature immune systems make them more susceptible to heavy infestations. *Davainea* spp. infections can be particularly severe and even fatal in chicks. Stress from overcrowding, poor nutrition, or concurrent disease may enhance susceptibility. Overcrowding increases the likelihood of birds encountering contaminated intermediate hosts.
- **Management and Flock Factors**
  Free-range and backyard flocks have increased contact with intermediate hosts in soil or vegetation. Poor control of insects and snails. Lack of routine anthelmintic prophylaxis.

8.6.4.3 Clinical Signs and Pathology

- **External Findings**

  Affected birds often exhibit poor growth, reduced weight gain, and a rough or ruffled feather coat. Noticeable drop in egg production and overall performance. Diarrhea may be intermittent, sometimes containing visible tapeworm segments (especially with heavy *Raillietina* infections). Weakness and lethargy especially in young birds or heavily infected birds. In severe infestations due to chronic nutrient malabsorption and mild blood loss. Heavy *Davainea proglottina* infections have occasionally been associated with ataxia or tremors due to severe intestinal inflammation and toxemia.

- **Necropsy Findings**

  Numerous tapeworms visible in the intestinal lumen, sometimes forming dense masses. Mucosal thickening and congestion at sites of attachment. Pinpoint hemorrhages, erosions, or ulcerations at the sites where the scolices embed. Catarrhal enteritis (mucus-laden intestinal content). *Davainea* infections, nodular enteritis with small raised whitish nodules on the intestinal mucosa due to deep mucosal invasion.

8.6.4.4 Diagnostic Testing

- **Fecal Float**

  Detects tapeworm eggs or proglottids shed in droppings. *Raillietina* eggs are found in egg capsules within proglottids, while *Davainea* eggs are single and small. Often, whole or partial segments (proglottids) are more readily detected than individual eggs.

- **Wet Mount**

  It is useless for detecting motile segments or eggs in fresh feces, especially in young birds with heavy burdens.

8.6.4.5 Treatment and Therapeutic Interventions

- **Medications**

  Praziquantel is highly effective against both *Raillietina* and *Davainea* species.
  10–20 mg/kg body weight orally, single dose (may repeat in 10–14 days if reinfection risk is high). Always verify withdrawal periods for eggs and meat before using these drugs in food-producing birds. Many products are used extra-label in poultry and should be administered under veterinary supervision.

- **Supportive Care**

  Provide balanced nutrition to address malabsorption and weight loss caused by tapeworms. Correct dehydration or electrolyte imbalances if diarrhea is present. Offer vitamin and mineral supplements, particularly B-complex and iron, if birds are anemic.

8.6.4.6 Prevention and Control

- **Biosecurity and Management Practices**

  Strict biosecurity measures to prevent the introduction and spread of tapeworms into flocks. Quarantine and fecal screening of new birds before integrating them into the existing flock to prevent introducing infected individuals. Segregate age groups; younger birds are more susceptible and should be housed separately from older birds to reduce exposure risk.

- **Control of Intermediate Hosts**

  Raillietina and *Davainea* require arthropod intermediate hosts (e.g., ants, beetles, flies, slugs). Implement insect control programs. Remove spilled feed, wet litter, and manure promptly to reduce breeding sites for insects. Good ventilation and low humidity make the environment less favorable for intermediate hosts.

- **Strategic Deworming**
  Implement routine flock deworming schedules in endemic areas. Use effective cestocidal anthelmintics at recommended intervals.

8.6.4.7 Nursing Considerations

Nursing care for chickens affected by cestode infections focuses on supportive management, maintaining flock hygiene, and minimizing reinfection. Affected birds should be monitored for weight loss, diarrhea, poor growth, lethargy, and reduced feed intake, with early detection helping to prevent severe infestations and production losses. Providing clean, fresh water and easily digestible, nutrient-rich feed supports hydration and nutrient absorption while alleviating GI stress. Environmental management is essential: maintain clean litter, remove intermediate hosts such as beetles, ants, or slugs from the environment, and implement strict biosecurity measures to reduce exposure to infective cysticercoids. Nursing may also involve reducing stress, isolating heavily infested birds, and consulting a veterinarian for appropriate anthelmintic therapy. Overall, nursing considerations for cestode infections emphasize monitoring clinical signs, supporting hydration and nutrition, maintaining environmental hygiene, and controlling intermediate hosts to reduce parasite burden, enhance recovery, and maintain productivity in affected flocks.

8.6.5 *Strongyloides* sp. (Threadworm)

8.6.5.1 Overview and Pathogenesis

Strongyloides avium, commonly referred to as threadworm, is a small intestinal nematode that infects chickens and other avian species. The parasite has both free-living and parasitic life cycles, with infection occurring primarily through ingestion of infective larvae or skin penetration. Once inside the host, the larvae migrate to the small intestine, where they develop into adult females that reproduce parthenogenetically, producing embryonated eggs. These eggs hatch into larvae within the intestinal tract, perpetuating autoinfection or being shed into the environment to continue the cycle. Pathogenesis results from the combined effects of mucosal invasion, irritation, and disruption of normal nutrient absorption. Infected birds often develop enteritis characterized by villous atrophy, increased mucosal permeability, and localized inflammatory reactions. Clinically, this may manifest as diarrhea, weight loss, stunted growth, and reduced feed conversion. In heavy infestations, severe malabsorption and dehydration may occur, predisposing birds to secondary infections and increased mortality in young or immunocompromised flocks.

8.6.5.2 Risk Factors

- **Host-Related Factors**
  Young birds, especially chicks and pullets, are more susceptible due to immature immune systems. Birds with compromised immunity (stress, concurrent diseases, poor nutrition) are at higher risk.
- **Environmental Factors**
  Crowded housing increases contact with contaminated litter or soil, facilitating transmission. Accumulated feces and damp litter harbor infective larvae. *Strongyloides* larvae thrive in moist, warm environments, increasing infective potential.
- **Management Factors**
  Birds with access to soil are more likely to ingest larvae from contaminated ground. Rare litter changes or improper drying can allow larvae to persist. Contaminated feeders or drinkers can spread larvae among flock members (Figure 8.10).

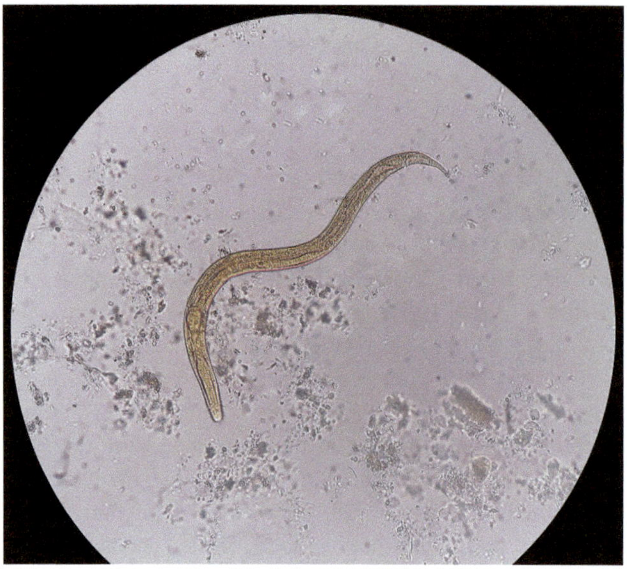

Figure 8.10 Strongyloides. Sirikwan / Adobe Stock Photos.

8.6.5.3 Clinical Signs and Pathology

- **External Findings**
  Young chicks are most severely affected; adults are often subclinical carriers. Diarrhea, poor growth, anorexia, weight loss, dehydration, weakness, lethargy, pale comb and wattles.
- **Necropsy Findings**
  Catarrhal enteritis with hyperemia (reddening) of the intestinal lining. Intestinal villi damage, atrophy, and blunting due to larval invasion of mucosa. Sticky intestinal content with mucoid exudate. Pinpoint hemorrhages may be present in severe cases. Adult worms (slender, threadlike, only a few millimeters long) may be visible in mucosal scrapings. Carcasses are thin with empty or fluid-filled intestines.

8.6.5.4 Diagnostic Testing

- **Fecal Flotation or Direct Smear**
  Detects embryonated eggs (oval, thin-shelled) or occasionally larvae. Eggs are smaller and thinner-walled than those of other nematodes.
- **Baermann Technique**
  Concentrates and recovers motile larvae from fresh fecal samples or intestinal contents. Considered more sensitive than flotation in early infections.

8.6.5.5 Treatment and Therapeutic Interventions

- **Medication**
  Fenbendazole 20 mg/kg by mouth every 24 hours for 3–5 days, repeat in 10 days.
  Ivermectin 0.2–0.4 mg/kg by mouth or topically once and repeat in 10–14 days.
- **Supportive Care**
  Provide electrolytes and fluids in drinking water to combat dehydration in chicks. Ensure nutritionally balanced food to counteract malabsorption and weight loss. Improve chick brooding conditions (temperature, ventilation, overcrowding) to reduce stress and mortality.

8.6.5.6 Prevention and Control

- **Biosecurity Measures**
  Restrict introduction of infected birds; quarantine new stock before mixing with the main flock. Limit exposure of young chicks to contaminated litter, runs, or pens. Control access of wild birds that may act as mechanical carriers of infective larvae.
- **Litter and Housing Management**
  Keep litter clean and dry, as moisture favors the development of infective larvae. Regularly replace or compost litter to destroy parasite stages. Ensure proper drainage and ventilation in poultry houses to reduce humidity. Periodically clean hard surfaces and perches with hot water and appropriate disinfectants. Rotate pastures or rest runs regularly to allow time for natural die-off of larvae in the environment.

8.6.5.7 Nursing Considerations

Nursing care for chickens infected with *S. avium* focuses on reducing parasite burden, minimizing complications of diarrhea and malabsorption, and promoting recovery through nutritional and environmental management. Technicians should monitor affected birds for weight loss, dehydration, weakness, and poor feather condition, providing supplemental fluids and easily digestible feeds as needed. Good sanitation is critical since infective larvae develop rapidly in moist litter; housing should be kept dry, clean, and well-ventilated, with frequent bedding replacement to break the parasite cycle. Severely affected or young birds may require isolation to ensure they receive adequate nutrition and are protected from bullying. After deworming treatments, monitoring droppings and bird condition helps assess therapeutic success. Technicians should also educate caretakers on preventive strategies, such as regular fecal checks, rotational use of dewormers under veterinary guidance, and pasture or litter management to reduce reinfection risk. By combining direct supportive care with environmental hygiene, the long-term health and productivity of the flock can be safeguarded.

8.7 Bacterial Gastrointestinal Diseases

8.7.1 Necrotic Enteritis

8.7.1.1 Overview and Pathogenesis

NE is an acute to subacute enteric disease of poultry caused primarily by C. *perfringens*, a Gram-positive, anaerobic, spore-forming bacterium. The disease predominantly affects meat chickens and occasionally egg layers, particularly during periods of rapid growth, dietary changes, or immunosuppression, and is significant due to mortality, reduced weight gain, poor feed conversion, and secondary infections. Transmission occurs via ingestion of spores from contaminated litter, feed, or the environment, with predisposing factors including high-protein diets, coccidial infections, stress, and intestinal dysbiosis. Clinically affected birds may exhibit diarrhea, depression, ruffled feathers, reduced feed intake, sudden mortality, and in chronic cases, poor growth and uneven flock uniformity.

The pathogenesis of NE begins with overgrowth of *C. perfringens* in the small intestine, typically following disruption of normal gut flora or damage to the intestinal mucosa caused by coccidial infection or dietary factors. The bacteria produce exotoxins, including alpha-toxin and NetB toxin, which induce epithelial necrosis, villus atrophy, and mucosal inflammation, leading to malabsorption, fluid loss, and diarrhea. The local inflammatory response involves heterophilic infiltration, edema, and fibrin deposition, which exacerbate mucosal damage. In severe cases, extensive intestinal necrosis may lead to systemic bacterial translocation, septicemia, and death. Overall, NE is an opportunistic enteric disease in which bacterial overgrowth, toxin production, and predisposing factors converge to cause intestinal necrosis, impaired nutrient absorption, and significant economic losses in poultry production.

8.7.1.2 Risk Factors

- **Host-Related Factors**
  Young age (2–6 weeks old), especially in rapidly growing broilers, whose immune systems are still developing. Viral (e.g., infectious bursal disease, Marek's disease) or bacterial infections weaken immunity and increase susceptibility. High feed intake and metabolic rate can predispose to gut disturbances.
- **Nutritional and Dietary Factors**
  High dietary protein content, especially animal-based proteins (fish meal, meat meal), provides a substrate for *C. perfringens* proliferation. High levels of indigestible carbohydrates (non-starch polysaccharides) promote intestinal viscosity and reduce gut motility, favoring bacterial overgrowth. Sudden dietary changes disrupt gut flora and epithelial integrity. Vitamin/mineral deficiencies (especially vitamins A, E, selenium) impair gut mucosal integrity and immune function.
- **Environmental and Management Factors**
  Poor litter quality (wet, caked litter) increases bacterial load and stress, promoting dysbiosis. Overcrowding causes stress and facilitates the rapid spread of enteric pathogens. Inadequate ventilation raises humidity and ammonia, which indirectly impair immunity and gut health.
- **Pathogen-Related Factors**
  Concurrent coccidiosis infection is the most significant risk factor as it damages the intestinal mucosa, providing attachment sites and nutrients for *C. perfringens*. Abrupt withdrawal of in-feed antimicrobial growth promoters may allow rapid overgrowth of *C. perfringens* in the gut.

8.7.1.3 Clinical Signs and Pathology

- **External Findings**
  Clinical presentation varies with the form of the disease: peracute, acute, or subclinical.

  Peracute Form
  Sudden death in apparently healthy birds. Often the first and only sign noticed during an outbreak. Mortality can be high (up to 50%).

  Acute Form
  Rapid onset with depression, decreased appetite and reluctance to move, diarrhea, dehydration, and weight loss. Mortality is typically 5–15% but can escalate rapidly without intervention.

  Subclinical Form
  No overt clinical signs.
- **Necropsy Findings**
  Intestinal loops are distended and friable, filled with foul-smelling brown fluid and gas. Mucosa covered by diphtheritic, tan-to-yellow necrotic plaques (pseudomembranes). Segmental or diffuse thickening of the intestinal wall. In severe cases, complete sloughing of the mucosa with hemorrhage. Concurrent lesions of coccidiosis may also be present (petechiae, mucosal erosions).

8.7.1.4 Diagnostic Testing

- **Culture**
  Anaerobic culture of intestinal content in selective media (e.g., blood agar under anaerobic conditions). Isolation of large numbers of *C. perfringens* from affected intestinal segments. Quantitative cultures are important since low numbers alone are not diagnostic.
- **Toxin Detection**
  Detection of NetB toxin (and occasionally α-toxin) from isolates or intestinal contents via PCR assays (for NetB gene detection) and ELISA or Western blot (for NetB protein). The presence of NetB-positive *C. perfringens* strongly supports diagnosis.

8.7.1.5 Treatment and Therapeutic Intervention

- **Supportive Care**
  Fluids and electrolytes for dehydrated birds. High-quality, easily digestible feed to reduce gut stress. Vitamin and mineral supplementation (especially vitamin E and selenium) to support mucosal healing.
- **Medications**
  NE is primarily managed with antibiotics, ideally guided by sensitivity testing.
  Amoxicillin/Clavulanate 125–250 mg/kg by mouth every 8–12 hours for 5–7 days.
  Amoxicillin sodium 50–250 mg/kg intramuscular every 8–12 hours for 5–7 days.
  Amoxicillin trihydrate 55–200 mg/kg by mouth, subcutaneous, or intramuscularly every 4–12 hours for 5–7 days.
  Tylosin 50 mg/kg by mouth once daily for 5–7 days or 15–30 mg/kg intramuscularly every 6–12 hours for 5–7 days.
  Always follow withdrawal periods for meat and eggs; use antimicrobials judiciously to reduce resistance risk.

8.7.1.6 Prevention and Control

- **Biosecurity and Management**
  Quarantine new birds and monitor for intestinal disease before introducing them to the flock. Segregate age groups to reduce stress and pathogen transmission. Avoid overcrowding. Ensure good ventilation to reduce humidity and ammonia buildup in housing. Regular litter management keeps bedding dry, clean, and free of caked feces.
- **Dietary Management**
  Gradual dietary changes to prevent gut upset. Avoid excessive animal protein or indigestible feed components that predispose to *C. perfringens* proliferation. Include prebiotics, probiotics, and fiber to maintain healthy gut microbiota. Ensure balanced vitamin and mineral supplementation, especially vitamins A, D, E, and selenium.
- **Coccidiosis Control**
  Vaccination against coccidiosis or use of anticoccidial feed additives. Minimizes mucosal damage, which is the key predisposing factor for NE. Reduces intestinal lesions and bacterial overgrowth.
- **Environmental Control**
  Control of wet litter and water spillage, which creates favorable anaerobic conditions. Frequent cleaning of feeders and drinkers to reduce bacterial contamination. Disinfection of housing between flocks to limit environmental spores.

8.7.1.7 Nursing Considerations

Nursing care for chickens affected by NE focuses on supportive management, maintaining hydration and nutrition, and preventing secondary infections. Affected birds should be closely monitored for diarrhea, lethargy, reduced feed intake, weight loss, ruffled feathers, and signs of systemic illness, as early recognition can improve outcomes. Providing clean, fresh water and easily digestible, high-quality food helps maintain hydration and nutrient balance while minimizing GI stress. Environmental management is critical: maintain clean, dry litter, reduce overcrowding, and implement strict biosecurity measures to limit exposure to *C. perfringens* and predisposing factors such as coccidial infection. Nursing care may also involve reducing stress, isolating severely affected birds, and administering veterinary-prescribed supportive treatments, including probiotics or antibiotics if indicated. Overall, nursing considerations for NE emphasize monitoring clinical signs, supporting hydration and nutrition, maintaining environmental hygiene, and minimizing stress to enhance recovery, prevent complications, and maintain flock health and productivity.

8.7.2 Colibacillosis (Enteric *E. coli*)

8.7.2.1 Overview and Pathogenesis

Colibacillosis, caused by pathogenic strains of *E. coli*, is a common bacterial disease in poultry that can present as respiratory, systemic, or enteric forms, with the enteric form primarily affecting the GI tract. The disease affects chickens of all ages, although young, immunocompromised, or stressed birds are most susceptible, and is significant due to poor growth, reduced feed efficiency, decreased egg production, diarrhea, and increased mortality. Transmission occurs via the fecal-oral route, contaminated feed, water, litter, and equipment, with environmental contamination and concurrent infections predisposing birds to disease. Clinically, enteric colibacillosis manifests as diarrhea, pasty vents, dehydration, reduced weight gain, lethargy, and occasionally sudden death, while subclinical infections may lead to chronic production losses.

The pathogenesis of enteric bacillosis begins with colonization of the intestinal epithelium by pathogenic *E. coli* strains, which adhere to enterocytes using fimbrial adhesins and other surface structures. These bacteria produce enterotoxins, cytotoxins, and other virulence factors that disrupt epithelial integrity, impair nutrient absorption, and induce local inflammation. Host responses include heterophilic and lymphocytic infiltration, mucosal edema, and mucus hypersecretion, which contribute to diarrhea and malabsorption. Environmental stressors, immunosuppression, and co-infections with viruses or other bacteria exacerbate disease severity. Chronic or severe infections may lead to systemic dissemination, resulting in septicemia and multi-organ involvement. Overall, enteric colibacillosis is an opportunistic bacterial disease in which intestinal colonization, toxin production, and host inflammatory responses combine to cause diarrhea, malabsorption, decreased productivity, and potential systemic illness in poultry flocks.

8.7.2.2 Risk Factors

- **Host-Related Factors**
  Young chicks (1–6 weeks) are most susceptible due to immature immune systems. Birds affected by viral infections (e.g., infectious bursal disease, Marek's disease, Newcastle disease) or nutritional deficiencies are at higher risk. Rapidly growing broilers may be more vulnerable due to metabolic stress and high feed intake.

- **Nutritional and Dietary Factors**
  Protein-rich diets can favor intestinal *E. coli* proliferation. Poor-quality food or sudden dietary changes can disturb gut microbiota. Vitamin or mineral deficiencies (e.g., vitamin A, E, selenium, and zinc) impair mucosal immunity and increase susceptibility.
- **Environmental and Management Factors**
  Overcrowding and high stocking density stress increase susceptibility and bacterial spread. Poor hygiene and sanitation contaminated litter, feeders, and water sources increase exposure. High humidity and wet litter promote bacterial survival and growth. Inadequate ventilation increases ammonia levels, irritating the mucosa and impairing local defenses. Stress factors such as transport, handling, temperature fluctuations, and co-infections predispose birds to disease.
- **Pathogen-Related Factors**
  Presence of virulent APEC strains with adhesins, fimbriae, and enterotoxins. High environmental contamination from previous flocks or neighboring farms. Concurrent intestinal disease, particularly coccidiosis, which disrupts the mucosal barrier and facilitates colonization.

8.7.2.3 Clinical Signs and Pathology

- **External Findings**
  Enteric colibacillosis in chickens ranges from subclinical infections to acute enteritis with systemic disease, depending on age, bacterial load, and predisposing factors.

  Acute Enteric Form

  Diarrhea, ruffled feathers, depression, lethargy, reduced feed and water intake, dehydration, emaciation, and sudden deaths.

  Chronic or Subclinical Form

  Poor weight gain and uneven flock growth. Reduced feed conversion efficiency. Mild diarrhea or pasty droppings intermittently. Birds often remain alert but underperforming.
- **Necropsy Findings**
  The small and large intestines are distended with fluid and gas; the mucosa may be congested or mildly necrotic. Intestinal content is watery or pasty, sometimes foul-smelling. Mesenteric vessels are engorged in severe infections.

8.7.2.4 Diagnostic Testing

- **Culture**
  Isolation of APEC strains on MacConkey agar or blood agar under aerobic conditions. Serotyping (O1, O2, O78) may be performed for epidemiologic purposes.
- **PCR Assays**
  Detect virulence genes such as fimbriae (fimH), toxins, and siderophores.
- **ELISA**
  Less commonly used but can detect specific antibodies against APEC.

8.7.2.5 Treatment and Therapeutic Interventions

- **Supportive Care**
  Fluid therapy for dehydrated birds. Electrolyte supplementation to correct imbalances caused by diarrhea. Nutritional support, high-quality, easily digestible feed to promote recovery. Maintain optimal temperature, ventilation, and minimal handling.

- **Medications**
  Treatment is primarily antibiotic-based, ideally guided by culture and sensitivity testing due to the risk of resistance.
  Amoxicillin/Clavulanate 125–250 mg/kg by mouth every 8–12 hours for 5–7 days.
  Amoxicillin sodium 50–250 mg/kg intramuscular every 8–12 hours for 5–7 days.
  Amoxicillin trihydrate 55–200 mg/kg by mouth, subcutaneous, or intramuscularly every 4–12 hours for 5–7 days.
  Trimethoprim-sulfamethoxazole 100 mg/kg by mouth every 12 hours for 5 days.
  Follow withdrawal periods for meat and eggs. Avoid indiscriminate use to reduce antimicrobial resistance.

8.7.2.6 Prevention and Control

- **Biosecurity and Management**
  Quarantine new birds and monitor for signs of disease before flock integration. Segregate age groups to prevent spread from older carriers to susceptible chicks. Maintain proper stocking density to reduce stress and fecal contamination. Ensure optimal ventilation to reduce ammonia accumulation and respiratory stress. Litter management keeps bedding dry, clean, and free from caked feces.
- **Nutrition and Feeding**
  Provide high-quality, digestible feed balanced in protein and energy. Avoid sudden diet changes to prevent gut dysbiosis. Include prebiotics and probiotics to promote healthy intestinal microbiome. Ensure adequate vitamin and mineral supplementation, particularly vitamins A and E and selenium.
- **Control of Predisposing Factors**
  Coccidiosis control via vaccination or anticoccidial feed additives. Stress reduction minimizes handling, abrupt environmental changes, and overcrowding. Water quality management to prevent contamination with bacteria or fecal material.
- **Environmental Sanitation**
  Frequent cleaning and disinfection of housing, feeders, and drinkers. Control of vectors, flies and rodents that may mechanically transmit bacteria. Rotational or all-in/all-out flock management to reduce environmental contamination.

8.7.2.7 Nursing Considerations

Nursing care for chickens affected by colibacillosis focuses on supportive management, maintaining hydration and nutrition, and preventing secondary infections. Affected birds should be closely monitored for diarrhea, depression, lethargy, reduced feed intake, weight loss, ruffled feathers, and signs of systemic infection, as early detection improves treatment outcomes. Providing clean, fresh water and easily digestible, high-quality food supports hydration, nutrient absorption, and recovery while minimizing GI stress. Environmental management is essential: maintain clean litter, reduce overcrowding, provide proper ventilation, and implement strict biosecurity measures to limit exposure to pathogenic *E. coli* and other opportunistic bacteria. Nursing care may also involve isolating severely affected birds, reducing stress, and administering supportive veterinary care, including antibiotics or probiotics as prescribed. Overall, nursing considerations for colibacillosis emphasize monitoring clinical signs, ensuring proper hydration and nutrition, maintaining environmental hygiene, and minimizing stress to support recovery, prevent complications, and maintain flock health and productivity.

8.7.3 Avian Intestinal Spirochetosis

8.7.3.1 Overview and Pathogenesis

Avian intestinal spirochetosis (AIS) is a bacterial disease of poultry caused primarily by *Brachyspira* spp., Gram-negative, anaerobic spirochetes that colonize the large intestine of chickens, particularly the cecum and rectum. The disease predominantly affects adult layers and breeders, and is of economic importance due to reduced egg production, poor feed conversion, decreased body weight, and diarrhea, which can compromise flock performance. Transmission occurs via the fecal-oral route, often facilitated by contaminated litter, feed, water, or equipment, and poor biosecurity. Clinically, affected birds may present with mucoid or watery diarrhea, pasty vents, decreased egg production, reduced weight gain, and general lethargy, although subclinical infections are common.

The pathogenesis of AIS begins with ingestion of the spirochetes, which colonize the mucosal surface of the ceca and large intestine, adhering to epithelial cells. The bacteria produce toxins and induce local inflammation, leading to mucosal thickening, hyperplasia, and infiltration by heterophils and lymphocytes, which disrupt normal nutrient absorption and intestinal motility. The resulting intestinal dysfunction manifests as diarrhea, reduced feed efficiency, and poor egg production. Opportunistic bacterial proliferation may exacerbate mucosal damage in chronic or severe infections. Overall, AIS is a bacterial enteric disease in which colonization of the large intestine, toxin production, and host inflammatory responses converge to cause intestinal pathology, diarrhea, and decreased productivity in adult laying and breeding chickens.

8.7.3.2 Risk Factors

- **Host-Related Factors**
  Most cases occur in adult laying hens and meat breeds; younger birds are less commonly affected. Birds stressed by viral infections (e.g., IBD, Marek's disease) or nutritional deficiencies are more susceptible to infections. High metabolic demand and rapid egg production may increase susceptibility.
- **Nutritional and Dietary Factors**
  High-energy diets or diets rich in indigestible carbohydrates may alter gut flora, facilitating spirochete overgrowth. Poor feed quality or sudden dietary changes disrupt normal microbiota and intestinal function. Vitamin and mineral deficiencies (e.g., vitamin E, selenium) may impair mucosal immunity.
- **Environmental and Management Factors**
  Overcrowding increases stress and facilitates fecal–oral transmission. Poor litter management, wet, caked, or contaminated litter serves as a reservoir for *Brachyspira*. Inadequate ventilation increases ammonia levels and respiratory stress, indirectly affecting gut health. Shared waterers or feeders allow rapid spread of spirochetes among birds.
- **Pathogen-Related Factors**
  Presence of virulent *Brachyspira* strains, capable of adhering to and colonizing the cecal epithelium. High environmental contamination from previous flocks increases exposure risk. Concurrent infections, particularly coccidiosis or *E. coli*, exacerbate mucosal damage and promote colonization.

8.7.3.3 Clinical Signs and Pathology

- **External Findings**

  The clinical presentation of AIS is often subtle or chronic, making early detection challenging. Severity depends on bird age, flock density, and presence of concurrent infections.

  Subclinical Form

  Mild diarrhea, poor weight gain, and small reductions in egg production without obvious illness.

  Clinical Form

  Diarrhea, depression, ruffled feathers, lethargy, dehydration, reduced food intake, and drop in egg production.

  Severe or Chronic Form

  Persistent diarrhea leads to weight loss and uneven flock growth. Secondary infections may exacerbate clinical signs. Mortality is rare, but production losses can be significant.
- **Necropsy Findings**

  Ceca are hyperemic, thickened, and sometimes filled with mucoid or watery content. Mucosal surface may have a thin layer of mucus, occasionally mild hemorrhage. Other intestinal segments are usually unremarkable, although mild congestion may be observed. Secondary lesions, in chronic cases, mild hepatomegaly or enteric inflammation may be noted if concurrent infections exist.

8.7.3.4 Diagnostic Testing

- **Wet Mount**

  Detects actively motile spirochetes (spiral-shaped, corkscrew motility). Rapid but not species-specific and may miss low-level infections.
- **Stained Smears**

  Tissue impression smears or cecal scrapings can be stained with Warthin–Starry stain or Giemsa stain. Shows spiral-shaped bacteria attached to mucosa. Confirms the presence but not the species of spirochete.
- **Culture**

  Anaerobic or microaerophilic conditions are required. Cultured from cecal content using selective media (e.g., trypticase soy agar with blood and antibiotics). Culture is time-consuming (3–7 days) but allows for antimicrobial sensitivity testing and species confirmation.

8.7.3.5 Treatment and Therapeutic Interventions

- **Supportive Care**

  Fluid and electrolyte support especially for severely diarrheic or dehydrated birds. Highly digestible feed to compensate for malabsorption and weight loss. Probiotics help restore normal gut microbiota. Vitamin/mineral supplementation particularly vitamins A, D, and B-complex to support mucosal healing and immunity.
- **Medication**

  Tylosin 50 mg/kg by mouth once daily for 5–7 days or 15–30 mg/kg intramuscularly every 6–12 hours for 5–7 days.

  Oxytetracycline 5 mg/kg subcutaneous or intramuscularly every 12–24 hours for 5–7 days or 2500 mg/L of drinking water, 2500mg/kg of feed.

8.7.3.6 Prevention and Control

- **Biosecurity and Management**
  Maintain a closed flock where possible. Quarantine new additions for at least 30 days and monitor for diarrhea or poor growth. Rodent, wild birds, and insect control as these can act as mechanical vectors for *Brachyspira*.
- **Sanitation and Environmental Control**
  Thorough cleaning and disinfection between flocks, remove all organic matter before disinfection. Use effective disinfectants (e.g., oxidizing agents, glutaraldehyde, quaternary ammonium compounds). Keep litter dry and clean to minimize bacterial survival and spread.
- **Nutritional and Flock Health Support**
  Balanced diets to maintain strong intestinal mucosa and immunity. Avoid overcrowding, maintain ventilation, and control temperature to reduce susceptibility. Co-infections can predispose or worsen spirochetosis (e.g., coccidiosis, NE).

8.7.3.7 Nursing Considerations

Nursing care for chickens affected by AIS focuses on supportive management, maintaining hydration and nutrition, and preventing secondary infections. Affected birds should be closely monitored for diarrhea, poor growth, reduced feed intake, lethargy, and signs of systemic illness, as early recognition can help minimize complications and productivity losses. Providing clean, fresh water and easily digestible, nutrient-rich feed supports hydration and nutrient absorption while reducing GI stress. Environmental management is essential: maintain clean litter, implement strict biosecurity, and control vectors such as contaminated feed, water, and rodents that may harbor *Brachyspira* spp. Nursing may also involve isolating severely affected birds, reducing stress, and consulting a veterinarian for appropriate antimicrobial therapy. Overall, nursing considerations for AIS emphasize monitoring clinical signs, supporting hydration and nutrition, maintaining hygiene, controlling environmental contamination, and minimizing stress to promote recovery, reduce morbidity, and maintain flock productivity.

8.8 Noninfectious GI Disorders

1) **Nutritional Enteritis**: Occurs due to sudden diet changes, spoiled feed, or mycotoxins. Signs include diarrhea, poor growth, and uneven flock performance. Treatment involves correcting feed and providing supportive care.
2) **Foreign Body Ingestion**: Birds may ingest plastic, string, or metal leading to crop or intestinal obstruction. Surgery or endoscopy may be required. In cases of metal ingestion, chelation therapy is recommended. Calcium EDTA is administered parenterally (IM, IV) to avoid enhanced GI absorption. This therapy can initially worsen a patient's neurological condition but will resolve with time (Figure 8.11).
3) **Toxin-Related Enteropathies**: Mycotoxins, salt toxicity, and chemical exposure can all damage the GI tract. Nursing care includes supportive fluids and removal of contaminated feed.

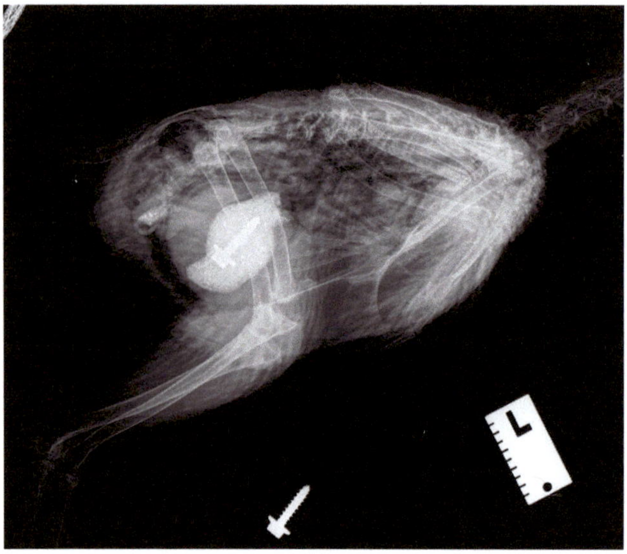

Figure 8.11 Radiograph of hen who consumed a large screw. Courtesy of Unusual Pet Vets.

Further Reading

Coccidiosis in Poultry - Poultry [Internet]. [cited 2025 Nov 29]. Available from: https://www.merckvetmanual.com/poultry/coccidiosis-in-poultry/coccidiosis-in-poultry

Hauck R. Helminthiasis in Poultry [Internet]. Merck Veterinary Manual. 2024. Available from: https://www.merckvetmanual.com/poultry/helminthiasis/helminthiasis-in-poultry

Internal Parasites in Chickens [Internet]. Available from: https://extension.unh.edu/sites/default/files/migrated_unmanaged_files/Resource007786_Rep11398.pdf

Intestinal Health and Necrotic Enteritis in Broilers | Mississippi State University Extension Service [Internet]. Msstate.edu. 2019 [cited 2025 Dec 12]. Available from: https://extension.msstate.edu/publications/intestinal-health-and-necrotic-enteritis-broilers

Tabler T. Department of Animal Science INTERNAL PARASITES OF POULTRY [Internet]. 2022 [cited 2025 Dec 8]. Available from: https://utia.tennessee.edu/publications/wp-content/uploads/sites/269/2023/10/D184.pdf

Yegani M, Korver DR. Factors affecting intestinal health in poultry. *Poultry Science*. 2008 Oct;87(10):2052–2063.

9

Cardiovascular and Respiratory Diseases

9.1 Cardiovascular Disease in Chickens—Risk Factors and Clinical Context

Cardiovascular disease in chickens represents a multifactorial clinical challenge, arising at the intersection of genetics, management practices, environmental stressors, nutrition, and infectious agents. In veterinary care, understanding these risk elements is crucial for effective prevention, early detection, and comprehensive patient support. Often, in the clinical setting, meat-breed birds rescued from production farms are encountered. At 6–7 weeks of age, these birds are slaughtered for consumption; too young to develop cardiovascular disease. However, the rescuer will need explicit education about nutrition to avoid obesity-induced maladies, predominantly circulatory diseases.

9.1.1 Genetic and Breed Predispositions

- **Heavy breeds**, particularly rapidly growing meat birds, are genetically more susceptible to cardiovascular disease due to selective breeding for fast growth and high mass. This predisposition arises because cardiovascular and pulmonary systems often cannot develop fast enough to meet increasing metabolic demands, creating a mismatch that precipitates disease.
- **Meat breed-specific vulnerabilities** include pulmonary hypertension and ascites syndrome (right-sided heart failure), linked to inadequate pulmonary vasculature development and functional capacity in fast-growing breeds.

9.1.2 Metabolic Stress and Rapid Growth

- **Rapid growth pressure** places significant stress on cardiovascular systems, most notably in meat breeds where explosive weight gain outpaces heart-pulmonary adaptation. This can result in arrhythmias, cardiac failure, syncope, and death.
- **Pulmonary hypertension syndrome (ascites)** is triggered specifically by this imbalance between tissue oxygen demand and cardiac-pulmonary supply, often intensified by environmental stress such as hypoxia, particularly at high altitudes and extreme temperatures.

9.1.3 Nutritional and Dietary Influences

- **Improper feeding strategies**, such as unrestricted access to grower feed, predispose meat birds to dilated cardiomyopathy (DCM). This effect is compounded by metabolic overload and rapid musculoskeletal growth.

- **High-fat or high-cholesterol diets**, especially when low in polyunsaturated fats, increase risk for atherosclerosis in adult chickens. Critical factors include dietary balance, cholesterol content, and fatty acid composition.
- **Marek's disease virus (MDV)**, beyond its oncogenic effects, promotes vascular lesions and atherosclerosis-like changes, compounding risk.

9.1.4 Environmental Stressors and Housing Conditions

- **Environmental extremes**—heat, cold, or altitude-induced hypoxia—can exacerbate cardiac stress in predisposed birds. Meat breeds particularly struggle with right ventricular dilation when housed in high-altitude or cold environments.
- **Overcrowding and poor ventilation** increase respiratory effort and systemic inflammation, which indirectly burdens cardiac output. Though not strictly cardiovascular, these conditions facilitate disease progression.

9.1.5 Infectious and Inflammatory Contributors

- **Infectious agents**, especially Marek's disease virus, can directly contribute to cardiac pathology, including arterial thickening and atherosclerosis.
- **Chronic systemic inflammation** stemming from poor hygiene, overcrowding, or subclinical disease mirrors human "dirty chicken" hypotheses, where low-grade inflammation can elevate cardiovascular risk by promoting vascular changes and metabolic disruption.

9.1.6 Other Contributory Factors

- **Age and obesity** add cumulative risk, especially in heavier or high-production layers that may suffer hypocalcemia, fatty infiltration, or stress on the circulatory system.

9.2 Clinical Context for Technicians

Recognizing these risk factors enables early intervention and disease prevention:

- **Assessment should include** breed, age, diet, housing, and husbandry practices.
- **Early identification** of vulnerable birds—especially fast-growing broilers (meat breeds) or high-producing layers—can guide targeted monitoring, dietary adjustment, and environmental mitigation.
- **Client education** about feed selection, growth rates, housing conditions, and vaccination when available, especially for hatchery-purchased chicks (e.g., Marek's), empowers proactive flock health decisions.

9.3 Dilated Cardiomyopathy

9.3.1 Clinical Signs

DCM in chickens is a progressive cardiac muscle disorder, leading to diminished pumping ability and often resulting in congestive heart failure, arrhythmias, syncope, or sudden death. The veterinary team must be alert for these hallmark signs:

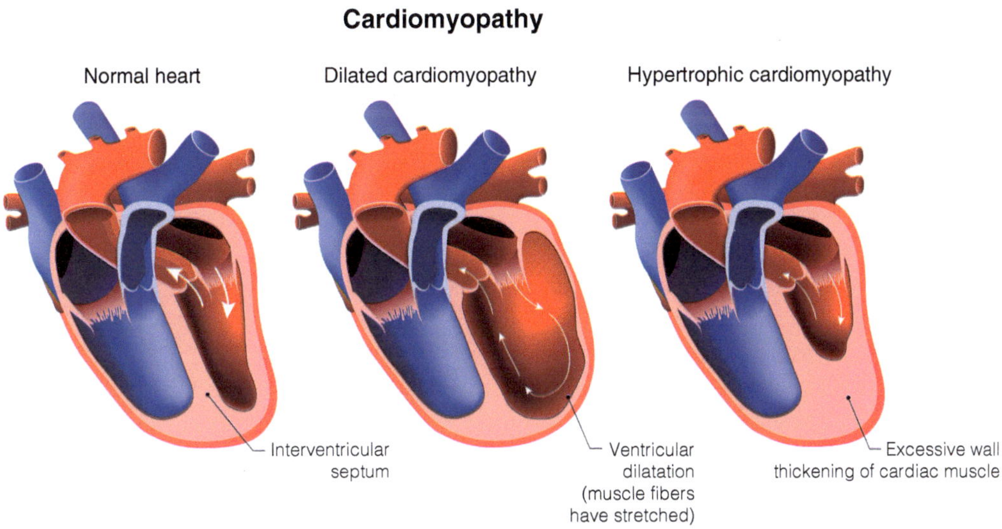

Figure 9.1 Comparative pathology of the heart. designua / Adobe Stock Photos.

- **Exercise intolerance**, lethargy, general weakness, and collapse
- **Increased respiratory rate and effort**; sometimes coughing—indicative of pulmonary congestion, cyanosis of the oral cavity and comb, wattles
- **Abdominal (coelom) distension** from ascites
- **Additional observations**: listlessness, unkempt/ruffled feathers, and possible sudden death (Figure 9.1)

9.3.2 Diagnostic Testing

An accurate diagnosis relies upon a combination of:

- **History and clinical signs**, including noting breed predispositions like heavy meat breeds
- **Physical exam**, focusing on respiratory effort, abdominal (coelom) palpation for fluid accumulation; comb and wattle color
- **Thoracic radiography** for evaluating heart size and pulmonary fluid
- **Echocardiography (echocardiogram)** to visualize cardiac chamber dilation and function
- **Electrocardiogram (ECG/EKG)** for detecting arrhythmias such as atrial fibrillation, supraventricular tachycardia, and ventricular premature complexes

9.3.3 Treatment

Treatment of DCM is multifaceted and focused on supportive care, pharmacologic therapy, and correction of fluid imbalances:

1) **Supportive Care**
   - Isolate the bird in a quiet, warm, draft-free, low-stress environment with easy access to feed and water.
2) **Therapeutic Interventions**
   - **Coelomocentesis:** remove excess coelomic (abdominal) fluid, when present; avoid removing excessive amounts at one time to avoid electrolyte and fluid imbalances

- **Furosemide**: loop diuretic, 0.5–1 mg/kg orally
- **Enalapril**: ACE inhibitor, 1–5 mg/kg to reduce afterload and blunt fluid retention
- **Pimobendan**: inodilator (PDE III inhibitor), 0.25–0.5 mg/kg to increase systolic function
- **Digoxin**: digitalis glycoside, 0.004–0.02 mg/kg, for inotropic support, particularly helpful in arrhythmias
- **Spironolactone**: aldosterone antagonist, dosage extrapolated from dogs, supports fluid balance.

3) **Nutrition and Prevention**
   - **Vitamin D Supplementation**: 25-hydroxycholecalciferol (25OHD$_3$) at 69 mg/kg in feed has shown benefits in reducing cardiac inflammation and sudden death—especially in meat-breed hens.
   - Avoid feeding chickens "grower" feed, especially meat breeds; restrict feed intake to reduce metabolic and cardiac stress.

9.3.4 Nursing Considerations

Effective care involves enabling cardiac function while minimizing stress and supporting recovery:

- **Environment**: Provide a quiet, warm, and safe enclosure, with bedding changed regularly to encourage rest. Monitor fecal/urate output, note coelom distension or increased respiratory effort.
- **Handling**: Be gentle—minimize handling stress and abrupt movements. Transport should be smooth and brief. Avoid restricting the coelom from movement.
- **Monitoring**: Record respiratory rate, effort, heart rate (if possible), posture, and overall demeanor at least twice daily. Note the comb and wattle color for cyanosis.
- **Fluid Management**: Monitor hydration status; ensure that medications are administered accurately by weight. For diuretics, observe for dehydration or electrolyte imbalance.
- **Nutrition and Medication Delivery**: Offer easily accessible feed and water. Administer medications accurately in doses adjusted per weight; observe for adverse reactions—especially the narrow therapeutic window for digoxin.
- **Communication**: Keep clear notes for veterinarians about responses to diuretics, presence or reduction of ascites, and any arrhythmic episodes (syncope, collapse).
- **Education and Record-Keeping**: Inform caregivers about husbandry factors influencing cardiac disease (e.g., rapid growth, overfeeding) and maintain detailed medical records of treatment course and patient responses.

9.4 Ascites Syndrome (Pulmonary Hypertension Syndrome)

9.4.1 Overview and Pathogenesis

Ascites syndrome, also called “water belly” or pulmonary hypertension syndrome, is characterized by right-sided congestive heart failure resulting from elevated pulmonary arterial pressure (pulmonary hypertension). In meat-breed chickens, rapid growth and limited cardiopulmonary development contribute to insufficient oxygen delivery, triggering right ventricular dilation, ascites, hydropericardium, and liver congestion.

Right ventricular overload occurs because the rigid, non-expansile avian lung cannot accommodate increased blood volume, so pulmonary pressure rises to maintain flow—eventually leading to heart failure.

9.4.2 Risk Factors

9.4.2.1 Genetic and Metabolic Predisposition

- Selective breeding for rapid growth and high feed efficiency in meat birds has inadvertently increased their susceptibility to ascites.
- Heritability studies show moderate to high genetic susceptibility, varying across strains; some breeding programs are now selecting against ascites susceptibility directly.

9.4.2.2 Environmental Triggers

- **High altitude (hypoxia)** is a well-recognized trigger due to reduced oxygen availability, increasing pulmonary arterial pressure.
- **Cold stress**, especially early in life (first 3 weeks), markedly increases ascites risk by elevating metabolic demand for thermoregulation, raising cardiac workload.
- **Poor ventilation, overcrowding, temperature extremes, dust, or respiratory disease** further impair oxygen exchange, exacerbating the imbalance between oxygen demand and supply.

9.4.2.3 Nutritional and Management Factors

- Overly dense, unrestricted feed supports super rapid growth and high metabolic demand—key drivers of ascites.
- Early feed or nutrient restriction and lighting management can slow growth rate, helping prevent ascites without compromising final body weight significantly.
- Supplemental arginine has been shown to improve pulmonary vascular dilation, reducing resistance and lowering ascites incidence in colder temperatures.

9.4.3 Clinical Signs and Pathology

Affected birds, older than 5 weeks:

- Abdominal distension ("water belly"), cyanosis, dyspnea or panting, and diminished exercise tolerance.
- Some birds may collapse or die suddenly, even before fluid accumulates visibly.

Necropsy findings:

- Accumulation of noninflammatory fluid in abdominal and pericardial spaces, dilated right ventricle and atrium, hydropericardium, ascites with fibrin clots, congested lungs, and liver.

9.4.4 Diagnostic Testing

- Gross pathology at necropsy is often diagnostic for ascites syndrome.
- Imaging and cardiac diagnostics:
  - Abdominal fluid analysis typically reveals clear or fibrin-containing fluid.
  - Radiographs may show an enlarged cardio-hepatic silhouette and abdominal opacity.

- Electrocardiography (ECG) may demonstrate decreased heart rate, elevated S-wave amplitude, ventricular fibrillation, and electrical axis shift due to right-heart dilation.
- Echocardiography reveals dilated cardiac chambers, atrioventricular valve regurgitation, reduced ventricular fractional shortening, and possible pericardial effusion.

9.4.5 Prevention and Control

Because treatment is limited, prevention is the cornerstone:

- Implement early feed restriction and avoid lighting manipulation to allow neonatal or young bird growth rate.
- Maintain thermoneutral temperatures; ensure proper ventilation; avoid cold stress and overcrowding.
- Consider arginine supplementation to promote pulmonary vascular dilation and mitigate pressure overload.

9.4.6 Nursing Considerations

- **Observation and Monitoring**: Watch for early signs of respiratory distress, coelom swelling, cyanosis, or lethargy in fast-growing meat breeds.
- **Environmental Management**: Maintain stable, appropriate temperatures and ensure adequate ventilation; minimize stress, especially in the neonatal period.
- **Growth Management**: Collaborate on implementing feed and lighting protocols to avoid too rapid growth.
- **Euthanasia Decisions**: In severe cases where welfare is compromised, humane euthanasia may be the most ethical option, given the poor prognosis of established ascites syndrome.

9.5 Atherosclerosis: Chronic Arterial Disease

9.5.1 Overview and Pathogenesis

Atherosclerosis in chickens involves the formation of fibrous, lipid-rich arterial lesions like those in humans—consisting of intimal thickening and lipid deposition within arterial walls. Notably, infection with MDV has been shown to induce atherosclerosis, even in chickens on low-cholesterol diets. This suggests a synergistic role of viral impairment and lipid metabolism in disease development.

MDV appears to disrupt arterial cholesterol processing, enhancing cholesteryl ester synthesis and reducing catabolic activity—leading to lipid accumulation in the aorta. In birds infected with MDV and fed high-cholesterol diets, atherosclerotic plaques develop in major arteries, including the aorta and coronaries—mimicking human pathology. This is why chicken models are used in atherosclerosis research studies.

9.5.2 Risk Factors

- **Marek's Disease Virus (MDV)**: MDV infection is a primary driver of atherogenesis, with viral presence significantly altering cholesterol metabolism.
- **Dietary Cholesterol**: High dietary cholesterol exacerbates MDV-related artery damage, although the virus alone is sufficient to initiate lesions.
- **Viral–Diet Synergy**: Fatty lesions are more pronounced in MDV-infected chickens fed high cholesterol diets, compared to infected birds with normal cholesterol levels.

9.5.3 Clinical Signs and Pathology

- **External Signs**: Atherosclerosis in chickens typically shows no overt clinical signs until it is advanced. In practice, these lesions are more commonly detected during necropsy rather than through clinical observation.
- **Necropsy Findings**: Gross examination reveals plaques in the aorta and major arterial branches, sometimes occlusive. Histologically, lesions show intimal fibromuscular thickening with fibrous caps over lipid cores—paralleling human atherosclerosis.

9.5.4 Diagnostic Testing

- **Definitive Diagnosis**: Relies on necropsy and histopathology. Gross and microscopic arterial examinations are currently the gold standard for detecting plaque formation.
- **Experimental Model Insights**: Research involving MDV infection and cholesterol diets illustrates the pathological progression but does not translate into routine in-field diagnostics.

9.5.5 Treatment and Therapeutic Interventions

While atherosclerosis in chickens typically carries a poor prognosis, it outlines several supportive and off-label treatments:

- **Supportive Care**
  Isolate the bird into a warm, low-stress environment.
- **Dietary Modification and Supplementation**
  Stop feeding table scraps and feed a lower-protein, low-fat, low-cholesterol diet. Supplement EPA/DHA-rich omega-3 (0.22 mL/kg feed) and vitamin E (160 mg/kg). Lower cholesterol with niacin. Vitamin C (600 mg/kg).
- **Medication and Herbal Support**
  Isoxsuprine 5–10 mg/kg PO as a vasodilator
  Propolis 0.25 g/kg as an anti-inflammatory and antioxidative
  Sotalol 1 mg/kg PO BID as an antiarrhythmic
  Diltiazem 3–30 mg/kg PO twice daily as a calcium channel blocker
  Nifedipine 3–30 mg/kg PO twice daily as a calcium channel blocker
  Verapamil 2–20 mg/kg PO twice daily as a calcium channel blocker
  Atorvastatin 10 mg/kg PO BID for reduction in cholesterol plaques

9.5.6 Prevention and Control

- Reduce cholesterol intake and feed low-fat, low-cholesterol diets rich in omega-3s. No table scraps. Fresh, green vegetables and small amounts of fruits in daily feeding.
- Vaccinate chicks against Marek's disease to prevent viral-induced arterial lesions.
- Encourage physical activity daily to decrease lipid accumulation.

9.5.7 Nursing Considerations

- **Monitoring and Prevention**: While clinical detection is rare, veterinary technicians should incorporate prevention into routine flock care—immunization (dependent on availability), balanced nutrition, and controlled feeding.

- **Medication Administration**: For affected individuals, ensure proper dosing, especially when using agents like statins or niacin.
- **Environmental Management**: Maintain low-stress, well-balanced nutritional and enrichment environments, even in the absence of signs.

9.6 Amyloidosis (AA Amyloidosis and Amyloid Arthropathy)

9.6.1 Overview and Pathogenesis

Amyloidosis in chickens manifests primarily as AA (amyloid A) amyloidosis, characterized by extracellular deposition of amyloid—an insoluble, misfolded protein often associated with chronic inflammation. In avian species like waterfowl, amyloidosis commonly follows chronic infections or inflammatory conditions such as pododermatitis (bumblefoot) or tuberculosis.

Chickens typically develop a condition termed amyloid arthropathy, marked by amyloid accumulation in joints—particularly the hock—frequently following infections with *Enterococcus faecalis* or *Mycoplasma synoviae*, and even occasionally linked to contaminated vaccine diluents.

Additionally, systemic AA amyloidosis can be experimentally induced in chickens via repeated inflammatory stimuli, such as oil-emulsified bacterin vaccinations, especially when multiple inoculations are administered. Backyard chicken guardians and veterinary technicians are not likely to see amyloidosis in birds unless they originated from broiler houses.

9.6.2 Risk Factors

- **Chronic Inflammation and Infection**: Conditions such as tuberculosis, bumblefoot (*Staphylococcus* infections in waterfowl), and persistent infections can trigger amyloid deposition in birds.
- **Amyloid Arthropathy—Pathogenic Agents**: Amyloid-associated joint disease is most frequently seen in brown egg layers, meat breeds, turkeys, and guinea fowl. *E. faecalis* is often implicated, detectable in joint tissues, with genetic strains matching outbreaks.
- **Vaccination and Inflammatory Stimuli**: Repeated inoculations using oil-adjuvanted vaccines (e.g., against salmonellosis, infectious coryza) have been strongly associated with amyloidosis—amyloid deposits appear at injection sites, in the liver, spleen, and intestines.
- **Age and Breed Predisposition**: Adult birds, especially egg-laying breeds of hens (e.g., white Leghorn/Lohmann), show a higher incidence.

9.6.3 Clinical Signs and Pathology

- **Amyloid Arthropathy (Joint Form)**: Clinically evident as swollen, often painful hock joints filled with yellow–orange material. Affected birds may exhibit lameness or reluctance to move.
- **Systemic Amyloidosis**: Signs are often vague or absent until advanced. Necropsy may reveal visceral involvement. Common findings include enlarged, pale, or friable liver and spleen with capsule stretching, rounded margins, and liver failure or hemorrhage in severe cases.
- **Post-Vaccination Amyloidosis**: Experimental studies report hepatomegaly, discoloration, hemorrhage, splenomegaly, edema at injection sites, granulomas, and amyloid deposits confirmed by Congo red staining and immunohistochemistry.

9.6.4 Diagnostic Testing

- **Gross and Histopathological Evaluation**: Necropsy revealing enlarged, pale viscera and swollen joints should prompt microscopic confirmation. Congo red staining (apple-green birefringence under polarized light) remains the diagnostic standard, along with histology and immunohistochemistry for AA protein.
- **Injection Sites as Indicator**: Detection of amyloid at prior vaccine administration sites can help trace induction sources.

9.6.5 Treatment and Therapeutic Interventions

Unfortunately, no definitive treatment exists for amyloidosis in chickens; care is largely supportive:

- **Supportive Management**: Provide analgesia via anti-inflammatory and opioid agents and isolate birds. Maintain warm, low-stress environments to preserve welfare. Soft bedding.
- **No Disease-Modifying Therapies Available**: Due to the progressive and systemic nature of amyloidosis, curative treatment is rarely feasible.
- **Preventive Emphasis**: Focus remains on management strategies to prevent development rather than attempt reversal.
- **Humane Management**: Given the lack of treatment and progressive nature, recognize when euthanasia may be more ethical for animal welfare (Figure 9.2).

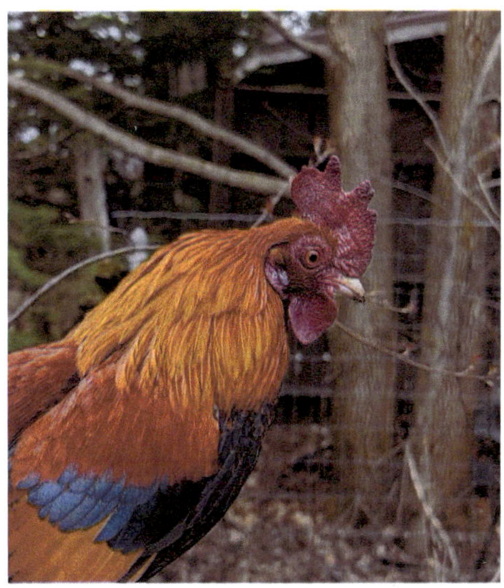

Figure 9.2 Bantam Old English Game rooster with cardiovascular disease. Note the comb and wattle color. Courtesy of Sheila Meharrie.

Further Reading

Greenacre CB, Morishita TY. *Backyard Poultry Medicine and Surgery: A Guide for Veterinary Practitioners*. Hoboken, NJ, John Wiley & Sons, Inc; 2021.

Julian R. The Avian Cardiovascular System Slide Study Set # 25 [Internet]. [cited 2025 Dec 8]. Available from: https://aaap.memberclicks.net/assets/Slides/cardiovascular.pdf

Olkowski AA. Pathophysiology of heart failure in broiler chickens: structural, biochemical, and molecular characteristics. *Poultry Science*. 2007 May;86(5):999–1005.

10

Reproductive Diseases

The reproductive system of the hen is central to the productivity and longevity of the backyard flock. Healthy reproduction directly influences egg production, fertility, hatchability, and the general well-being of the bird. Disorders of the reproductive tract are common in chickens, particularly in high-producing laying hens (specific breed predilection) and older backyard birds that continue to ovulate long past their peak commercial age.

Reproductive diseases may be noninfectious (structural abnormalities that can be malignant or benign, metabolic conditions, or mechanical disorders like egg binding) or infectious (bacterial, viral, or parasitic infections affecting the oviduct and ovary). Both categories can compromise health, reduce egg production, and in severe cases, result in mortality.

For veterinary technicians, early recognition of reproductive disorders is critical. Owners may first notice decreased egg production, abnormal eggs, unusual posture, or hens that appear depressed, strained, or with distended coeloms. Veterinary technicians play a vital role in triage, diagnostics (radiography, cloacal swabs, fecal sampling), continuous nursing support, and client counseling.

This chapter reviews the major reproductive diseases of chickens, emphasizing clinical signs, diagnostic methods, treatment, including medications where applicable—and nursing considerations.

10.1 Anatomy and Physiology of the Reproductive System

10.1.1 Female Reproductive Anatomy

Unlike mammals, the hen has a single functional left ovary and oviduct. The right ovary and oviduct are typically vestigial. The ovary contains thousands of follicles in varying stages of development.

The oviduct is divided into distinct regions:

- **Infundibulum**: captures the ovulated yolk; site of fertilization if sperm is present.
- **Magnum**: secretes albumen (egg white).
- **Isthmus**: adds shell membranes.
- **Uterus (Shell Gland)**: deposits calcium carbonate shell.
- **Vagina**: facilitates egg expulsion.

Normal oviposition occurs approximately every 24–26 hours in peak laying hens (Figures 10.1 and 10.2).

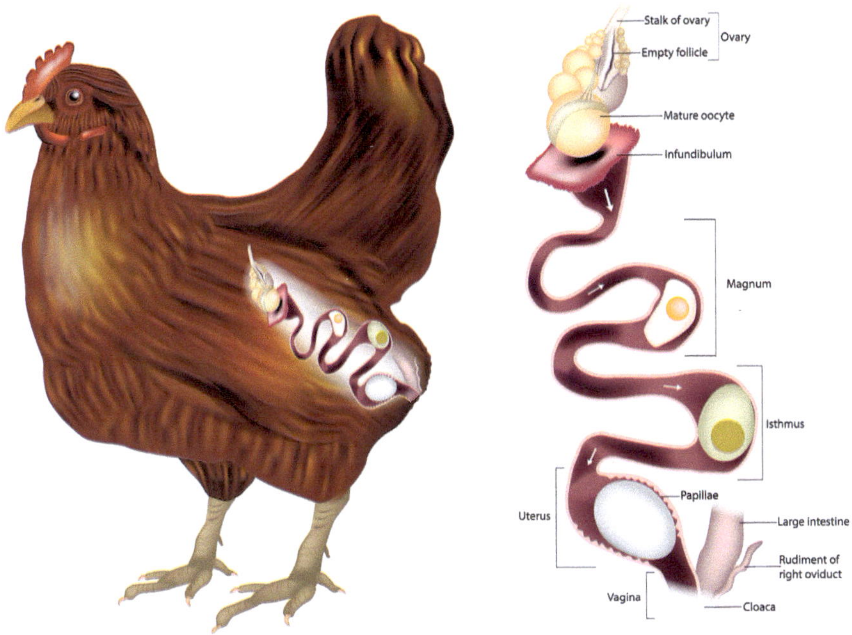

Figure 10.1 Egg formation pathway. sakurra / Adobe Stock Photos.

10.1.2 Endocrine Control

The hypothalamus and anterior pituitary regulate ovulation via gonadotropin-releasing hormone (GnRH), follicle-stimulating hormone (FSH), and luteinizing hormone (LH). Disturbances in photoperiod, nutrition, or disease can disrupt this balance and impair egg laying. Implantation of hormone pellet is controversial and may be prohibited in some states. Deslorelin is a long-acting implant placed every 4–6 months to prevent further development and release of ovarian follicles, thereby reducing future episodes of reproductive disorders.

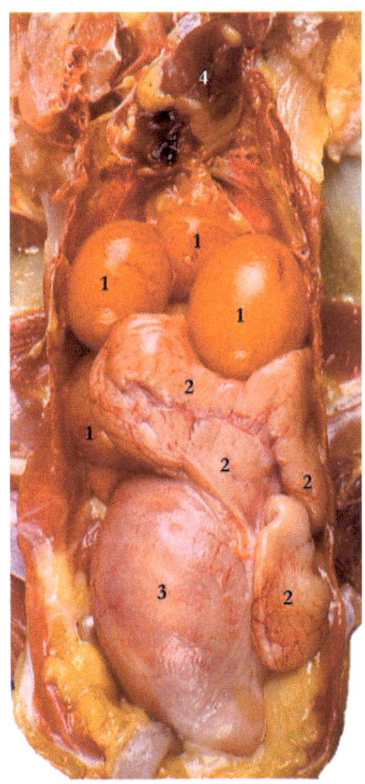

Figure 10.2 Hen reproductive organs. 1. Ovarian follicles, 2. Oviduct, 3. Uterus with egg inside, 4. Heart. Uwe Gille / Wikimedia Commons / CC BY-SA 3.0.

10.2 General Clinical Signs of Reproductive Disease

Because many reproductive diseases manifest nonspecific symptoms, technicians should be vigilant for:

- Reduced or halted egg production
- Abnormal eggs (misshapen, thin-shelled, soft-shelled, shell-less, or with internal deposits)
- Distended abdomen/coelom (suggesting egg peritonitis, internal laying, or tumors)
- Straining, lethargy, abnormal posture, or anorexia

- Cloacal discharge (foul-smelling in cases of infection)
- Feather loss around the vent from persistent straining
- Sudden death in severe or acute conditions

Early intervention is crucial, as reproductive disease often progresses rapidly once clinical signs are evident.

10.3 Noninfectious Reproductive Disorders

Quick reference chart

Disorder	Overview/cause	Key clinical signs	Pathology/lesions	Diagnostic tests
Egg binding (dystocia)	Failure to expel an egg due to oversized egg, dehydration, hypocalcemia, obesity, or stress	Straining, tail pumping, lethargy, swollen vent, wide stance	Egg lodged in lower oviduct or cloaca; edema, congestion	Palpation, radiography, cloacal exam
Prolapse of the oviduct (cloacal prolapse)	Oviduct protrudes through vent due to straining, large eggs, or poor muscle tone	Red, swollen tissue protruding from vent, bleeding, picking by flock mates	Everted oviduct, edema, necrosis if untreated	Visual exam
Internal laying/egg yolk peritonitis	Retrograde movement of egg yolk into abdomen→ inflammation, often due to oviductal dysfunction	Distended abdomen, depression, decreased laying, dyspnea	Yellow fluid and yolk in coelom, inflamed peritoneum, adhesions	Abdominal palpation, ultrasound, postmortem
Soft-shelled or shell-less eggs	Inadequate calcium or vitamin D, poor nutrition, stress, or oviductal dysfunction	Thin, wrinkled, or missing shell; may break internally	Thin-shelled eggs in oviduct, shell gland hypocalcification	Diet evaluation, history
Ovarian cysts/tumors (neoplasia)	Age-related degenerative or neoplastic changes	Progressive weight loss, distension, cessation of laying	Enlarged ovary with cysts or nodules	Radiograph, ultrasound, necropsy
Double yolk/ malformed eggs	Hormonal or ovulatory timing error	Large or irregular eggs, occasional vent trauma	Two yolks in one shell, stretched oviduct	Observation
Vent pecking/ trauma	Secondary to stress, crowding, or lighting imbalance	Bleeding vent, prolapse, tissue damage	Lacerations or peck injuries at vent	Visual exam
Testicular tumors	Neoplastic growths (commonly *Sertoli*, *Leydig*, or seminomas) in roosters, often age-related	Unilateral leg weakness, ataxia, reduced fertility, abdominal swelling, feminization (enlarged comb, plumage changes)	Enlarged testis, pale or nodular mass, compression of kidneys/nerves	Radiograph, ultrasound, necropsy, histopathology

Chart courtesy of Stephanie Freeman.

10.3.1 Testicular Tumors

10.3.1.1 Overview and Pathogenesis

Testicular tumors in chickens are uncommon neoplasms arising from the testicular tissue, which may include germ cells, Sertoli cells, or interstitial (Leydig) cells. These tumors can be benign or malignant, with seminomas representing germ cell neoplasms and Leydig or Sertoli cell tumors arising from the supporting interstitial cells.

Pathogenesis involves uncontrolled proliferation of the respective cell type, leading to enlargement of the testes and potential disruption of normal spermatogenesis and hormone production. Etiology is poorly understood, but age, genetic predisposition, and chronic testicular stimulation may contribute to tumor development. Clinically, affected birds may show testicular enlargement on radiographs or ultrasound, coelomic distention, reduced fertility, or behavioral changes related to hormonal imbalances. Histologically, seminomas are characterized by sheets of uniform germ cells, whereas Leydig and Sertoli cell tumors exhibit proliferation of interstitial or supporting cells with variable degrees of cellular atypia, mitotic activity, and occasional local invasion.

10.3.1.2 Risk Factors

- **Host-Related Factors**
  Older males are at higher risk, reflecting cumulative genetic mutations and prolonged exposure to environmental or metabolic stressors. Certain breeding lines may have an increased incidence due to heritable predisposition. Inbreeding may increase the likelihood of neoplastic transformation in gonadal tissue.
- **Hormonal and Physiological Factors**
  Chronic hormonal stimulation, such as prolonged exposure to androgens or other endocrine imbalances, may promote abnormal proliferation of testicular cells.
- **Environmental and Management Factors**
  Carcinogen exposure (e.g., feed mycotoxins like aflatoxin and chemical contaminants). Chronic stress or poor husbandry that suppresses immunity.

10.3.1.3 Clinical Signs and Pathology

- **External Findings**
  Often asymptomatic in early stages. Reduced fertility or infertility in breeder males. Coelomic distension due to a large intra-abdominal mass. Weight loss and reduced feed intake. Lameness or difficulty perching/walking, if the mass compresses nerves or pelvis. Dyspnea (respiratory distress) if the tumor compresses air sacs or lungs. Altered feathering patterns due to hormonal imbalance.
- **Necropsy Findings**
  Unilateral or bilateral testicular enlargement, often markedly asymmetric. Testis may appear firm, pale, and lobulated, which is common in seminomas or Sertoli cell tumors. They may also appear as yellow-tan, friable, and vascular, which is typical of interstitial/Leydig cell tumors. Large masses may cause compression of adjacent organs (kidneys, intestines, lungs, air sacs). Metastasis is uncommon but may occur with malignant types (especially Sertoli cell tumors or mixed tumors).

10.3.1.4 Diagnostic Testing

- **Imaging**
  Ultrasonography can detect enlarged testes and distinguish between solid masses and cystic structures. Radiographs may reveal a large intra-abdominal mass causing organ displacement.
- **Hormone Assays**
  Elevated estrogen with Sertoli cell tumors. Altered androgen levels with Leydig cell tumors.

10.3.1.5 Treatment and Therapeutic Interventions

- **Surgical Management**
  Orchiectomy may be attempted; it requires advanced avian surgical expertise due to the proximity of the testes to the kidneys, major vessels, and air sacs.
- **Supportive and Palliative Care**
  Analgesics to reduce discomfort in birds with large coelomic masses. Fluid therapy and nutritional support in weakened birds.

10.3.1.6 Prevention and Control

- **Genetic and Breeding Management**
  Avoid inbreeding, which may increase susceptibility to tumors and other reproductive abnormalities.

10.3.1.7 Nursing Considerations

Nursing care of roosters with testicular tumors focuses on monitoring, supportive care, and maintaining overall health, as surgical or medical treatment options are limited. Birds should be observed for signs of discomfort, coelomic distention, reduced fertility, or behavioral changes associated with hormonal imbalance. Gentle handling is recommended to avoid trauma to the vascular enlarged testes. Maintaining optimal nutrition, clean housing, analgesia, and reduced stress supports general well-being. In cases where the tumor compromises quality of life or leads to systemic illness, humane euthanasia should be considered. Breeders should also monitor affected males for reproductive performance, as fertility may be significantly impacted by testicular neoplasia.

10.3.2 Internal Laying

10.3.2.1 Overview and Pathogenesis

Internal laying, also known as egg retention within the abdominal cavity, is a reproductive disorder in laying hens characterized by the release of yolk or eggs into the coelomic cavity rather than the oviduct, which can lead to secondary complications such as egg yolk peritonitis (EYP). This condition primarily affects older hens, high-producing layers, or birds with reproductive tract dysfunction, and is of importance due to reduced egg production, increased risk of infection, and potential mortality. Predisposing factors include ovarian or oviductal abnormalities, oviductal obstruction, hormonal imbalances, nutritional deficiencies (especially calcium and protein), stress, and trauma during oviposition. Clinically, affected hens may show coelomic distension, lethargy, decreased egg production, anorexia, and signs of systemic illness if secondary infection occurs.

The pathogenesis of internal laying begins with the disruption of normal ovulation and oviductal passage, resulting in yolk or eggs being released into the coelomic cavity instead of entering the functional oviduct. Free yolk in the coelomic cavity serves as an excellent medium for opportunistic bacterial growth, predisposing birds to secondary infections such as EYP. The presence of yolk and subsequent bacterial proliferation triggers inflammatory responses, including infiltration by

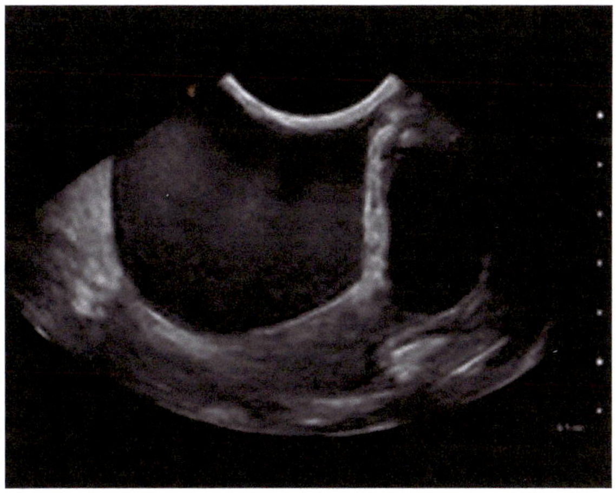

Figure 10.3 Egg yolk peritonitis diagnosed during ultrasonography. Courtesy of Unusual Pet Vets.

heterophils and lymphocytes, fibrin deposition, and accumulation of purulent material, which can compromise organ function and overall health. Chronic or recurrent internal laying can lead to adhesion formation, oviductal fibrosis, and long-term reproductive dysfunction, further reducing egg production. Overall, internal laying is a reproductive and secondary inflammatory disorder in which misplacement of yolk, reproductive tract dysfunction, and opportunistic bacterial infection converge to impair egg production, cause abdominal pathology, and threaten hen health (Figure 10.3).

10.3.2.2 Risk Factors

- **Hen-Specific Factors**
  Common in middle-aged to older laying hens, especially after peak production when oviduct tone declines. Commercial or hybrid layers (e.g., Leghorn-type hens) are more prone due to intense, continuous ovulation. Altered estrogen/progesterone regulation can disrupt oviduct motility and timing, increasing the chance of misdirected ova. Excess fat in the coelomic cavity can physically impede oviductal function or increase ovary fragility.
- **Pathologic and Disease-Associated Factors**
  Prior or ongoing infections (e.g., salpingitis) can damage the oviduct, allowing yolks to miss entry. Egg binding, oviductal prolapse, or rupture may cause scarring or malalignment of the infundibulum. Any illness that disrupts normal ovulation rhythm (e.g., chronic infections, hepatic disease) may increase risk.
- **Environmental and Management Factors**
  Long photoperiods (>14–16 h/day) promote continuous laying with little rest for the reproductive tract. Hens denied a break in laying cycles are more susceptible to reproductive tract fatigue. Social stress, overcrowding, or abrupt environmental changes may disrupt ovulation timing and oviductal coordination.

10.3.2.3 Clinical Signs and Pathology

- **External Signs**
  Internal laying in chickens typically shows recurrent reduction in egg production, coelom distension, penguin-like stance (standing upright with tail tucked), lethargy, weight loss, and intermittent anorexia. May also progress to secondary bacterial peritonitis.

- **Necropsy Findings**
  Free yolk material in the coelomic cavity appears as yellow to orange, oily or pasty material floating in the abdominal cavity. May be present as clumps, strands, or diffuse film coating viscera. Fibrinous strands between intestines, oviduct, ovary, liver, and body wall. Thickened, opaque peritoneum. Active, large follicles along with collapsed or ruptured follicles. Oviduct lumen may contain inspissated (dried) yolk-like material. Purulent or caseous exudate in the coelomic cavity, malodorous fluid, and signs of septicemia (liver enlargement, splenomegaly, congestion) if secondary bacterial infection is present.

10.3.2.4 Diagnostic Testing

- **Imaging**
  Radiographs may reveal soft tissue opacity or silhouettes of yolk material in the coelomic cavity. It can rule out egg binding or other reproductive tract disorders. Ultrasonography shows hyperechoic fluid pockets, fibrin strands, or free yolk-like material. It can help distinguish between ascites and neoplasia.
- **Coelomic Fluid Analysis (If Ascites Present)**
  Coelomic centesis may retrieve yellow, viscous, protein-rich fluid consistent with yolk material. Cytology may show lipid droplets, macrophages, and heterophils.

10.3.2.5 Treatment and Therapeutic Interventions

- **Supportive Therapy**
  Oral or subcutaneous fluid therapy +/− electrolytes to address dehydration. High-quality, easily digestible food to maintain nutritional status. Vitamin and probiotic supplementation to support general health and gut flora.
- **Medications**
  Trimethoprim-sulfamethoxazole 100 mg/kg by mouth every 12 hours for 5–7 days.
  Amoxicillin-Clavulanate 125–250 mg/kg by mouth every 8–12 hours for 7–10 days.
  Meloxicam 0.5 mg/kg by mouth or intramuscularly every 12–24 hours.
  Carprofen 5–10 mg/kg by mouth or intramuscularly once daily.
  Deslorelin is a long-acting implant placed every 4–6 months to prevent further development and release of ovarian follicles, thereby reducing future episodes of internal laying. This intervention is controversial and may be prohibited in some states.
- **Surgical Intervention**
  Salpingohysterectomy (oviduct removal) is considered the only definitive treatment, especially for recurrent or severe cases.

10.3.2.6 Prevention and Control

- **Lighting Control**
  Avoid sudden changes in light duration or intensity. Follow recommended lighting programs for layers to prevent premature or multiple ovulations. Maintain 14–16 hours of consistent light during peak production; avoid overstimulation with continuous lighting. Natural lighting is best practice for a healthy hen, allowing her reproductive system to "rest" during the fall and winter.
- **Stress Reduction**
  Minimize overcrowding, rough handling, and predator threats. Provide adequate perches, dust baths, puzzle toys, and nesting boxes to reduce stress-induced ovulation misplacements. Assess for comorbidities and treat accordingly if present.

- **Weight Management**
  Prevent obesity by balancing diet and avoiding excessive high-energy feeds. Monitor body condition and body weight score regularly.
- **Balanced Diet**
  Ensure adequate calcium, phosphorus, and vitamin D3 to maintain eggshell and reproductive health.
- **Selective Breeding**
  Choose breeds or breed mixes with lower susceptibility to reproductive disorders where possible. Avoid breeding hens with chronic internal laying or reproductive dysfunction.

10.3.2.7 Nursing Considerations

Nursing care for chickens affected by internal laying focuses on supportive management, monitoring reproductive health, and preventing secondary complications. Affected birds should be closely observed for signs of coelomic distension, reduced egg production during normal laying season, lethargy, anorexia, and changes in behavior or posture, as early detection can help prevent more severe reproductive disorders such as egg peritonitis. Providing easy access to clean water and a balanced, nutrient-rich diet supports overall health and helps maintain body condition. Environmental management is essential: maintain clean housing, reduce overcrowding, and provide appropriate perches and nesting areas to minimize stress and facilitate normal egg-laying behavior. Nursing care may also involve reducing stress, isolating affected birds if necessary, and consulting a veterinarian for reproductive assessment and management, including interventions to prevent or treat secondary infections. Overall, nursing considerations for internal laying emphasize monitoring clinical signs, supporting nutrition and hydration, maintaining optimal environmental conditions, and timely veterinary intervention to promote reproductive health and prevent complications. Human euthanasia is an option to alleviate suffering.

10.3.3 Egg Binding (Dystocia)

10.3.3.1 Overview and Pathogenesis

Egg binding, also known as dystocia, is a reproductive disorder in laying hens characterized by the inability to pass an egg through the oviduct and cloaca within the normal timeframe. This condition primarily affects high-producing layers, older hens, obese birds, or hens with underlying reproductive tract abnormalities, and is significant due to reduced egg production, potential reproductive tract injury, and mortality in severe cases. Predisposing factors include large or misshapen eggs, oviductal malformations, inadequate calcium or protein intake, obesity, stress, environmental temperature extremes, and previous reproductive tract trauma. Clinically, affected hens may exhibit straining, lethargy, coelomic distension, ruffled feathers, anorexia, and in severe cases, depression or sudden death. It must be said that "sudden" death is somewhat of a misnomer. Oftentimes, inexperienced caregivers miss initial, subtle clinical signs in an egg-bound hen. Therefore, the hen's death may seem sudden, but the symptoms were misunderstood or ignored.

The pathogenesis of egg binding begins with mechanical or physiological impediments to egg passage in the oviduct. These may arise from egg size exceeding the oviductal lumen, misshapen eggs, or oviductal spasms due to calcium deficiency affecting smooth muscle contraction. Retained eggs exert pressure on the oviductal and coelomic tissues, leading to local inflammation, edema, and potential necrosis. Prolonged retention may compromise blood supply, predisposing the oviduct to secondary bacterial infection, which can progress to EYP or systemic septicemia. In addition, repeated occurrences of egg binding can cause fibrosis, adhesions, and permanent reproductive tract dysfunction, further reducing productivity. Overall, egg binding is a mechanical and secondary inflammatory reproductive disorder in which retained eggs, oviductal dysfunction, and secondary infections converge to impair egg-laying performance and compromise the health of laying hens.

10.3.3.2 Risk Factors

- **Hen-Specific Factors**
  Immature oviduct musculature and poor coordination can predispose dystocia. Advanced age, weakened oviductal tone, and chronic reproductive tract changes may slow egg passage. Excess coelomic fat can impede normal oviduct contractions and constrict the pelvic canal. Bantam or small-framed hens are at higher risk of obstruction when laying large eggs.
- **Reproductive and Physiologic Factors**
  Double-yolked, elongated, or misshapen eggs are more difficult to pass. Thin or soft-shelled eggs are more prone to deforming and lodging in the oviduct. Conditions like salpingitis, scarring from prior trauma, or congenital oviduct malformations narrow the lumen and increase resistance. Hypocalcemia +/− vitamin D deficiency causes poor shell formation and weak smooth muscle contractions. Hormonal imbalance can disrupt oviduct motility and the timing of ovulation.
- **Environmental and Management Factors**
  Cold stress or abrupt environmental changes can delay laying and increase the risk of retention. Inadequate nesting sites or space increases stress and suppresses normal laying behavior. Continuous lighting schedules (>16 h/day) overstimulate ovulation and reduce reproductive rest periods. Deficiency in calcium, phosphorus, or other essential nutrients for reproductive health.

10.3.3.3 Clinical Signs and Pathology

- **External Findings**
  Straining or repeated unproductive attempts to lay, "penguin stance," lethargy, weakness, anorexia, decreased water intake, labored or open mouth breathing, distended or firm coelom or cloacal bulge, and absent or greatly reduced fecal output.
- **Necropsy Findings**
  Impacted egg in the distal oviduct or uterus (shell gland). Oviduct congestion, edema, and hemorrhage. Ischemic necrosis of the oviductal wall. Oviduct rupture and secondary EYP. Compression of cloaca, intestines, ureters, and blood vessels, leading to constipation, decreased urate production, or circulatory shock.

10.3.3.4 Diagnostic Testing

- **Physical Palpation**
  Gentle coelom or cloacal palpation may reveal a firm, ovoid mass corresponding to the retained egg. Care must be taken to avoid rupturing the egg or injuring the oviduct.
- **Imaging**
  Radiology confirms the presence, size, and position of the egg. Can detect multiple retained eggs or concurrent skeletal/soft tissue abnormalities. Ultrasound visualizes the egg within the oviduct and assesses surrounding soft tissue. Can detect coelomic fluid, fibrin, or early peritonitis (Figure 10.4).

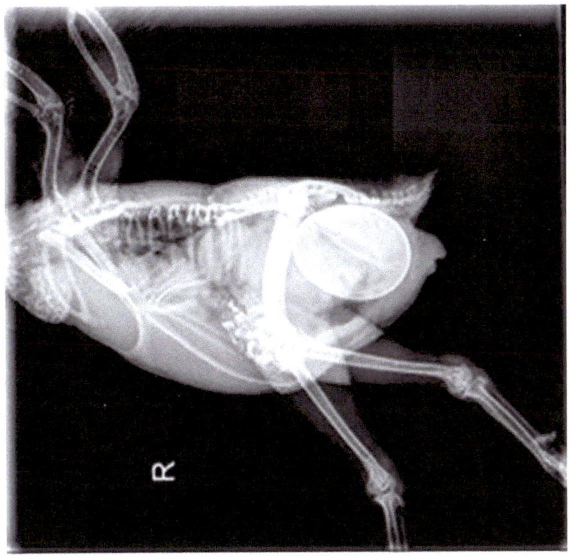

Figure 10.4 Egg-bound hen radiographic image. Adobe Stock.

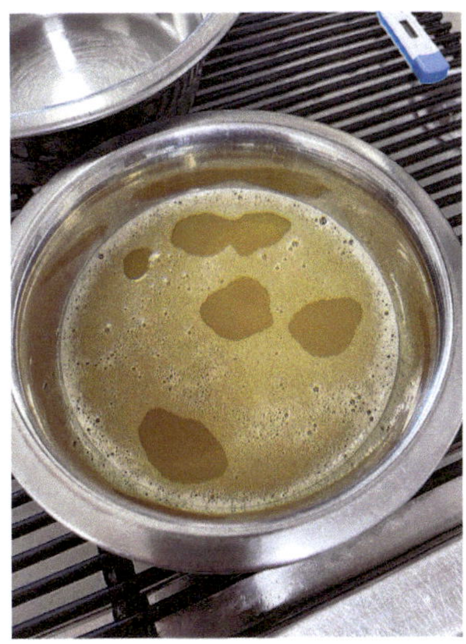

Figure 10.5 Collection of coelomic fluid from an egg-bound hen. Courtesy of Sarah Meyer.

- **Coelomic fluid analysis** (if egg rupture or peritonitis is suspected)
  Reveals protein-rich fluid with yolk material. Cytology may show heterophils, macrophages, or bacteria if secondary infection is present (Figure 10.5).

10.3.3.5 Treatment and Therapeutic Interventions

- **Supportive Care**
  Isolate the bird in a warm, quiet environment. Intravenous or subcutaneous fluid +/− electrolytes administration can be helpful as well. Warm water soak with magnesium sulfate granules soaking of the vent helps to relax the hen, allowing natural release of the egg. Lubrication (water-based jelly with lidocaine 2%) and gentle digital manipulation if the egg is near the cloaca. Ovocentesis and gentle digital extraction in refractory cases (Figure 10.6). Analgesics and benzodiazepines can further provide relief and relax the distressed bird.

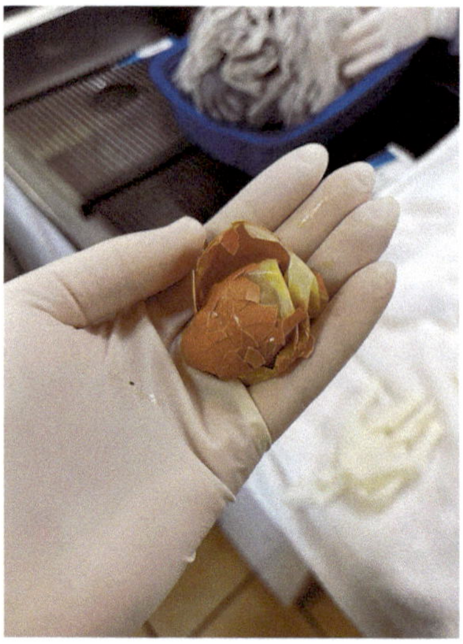

Figure 10.6 Egg after centesis for ease of manual extraction from cloaca of an egg-bound hen. Courtesy of Sarah Meyer.

- **Supplementation**
  Subcutaneous or oral calcium gluconate to enhance smooth muscle contractions, particularly if hypocalcemia is suspected.
- **Surgical Intervention**
  Oviductotomy is indicated if nonsurgical methods fail or the egg is lodged deep in the oviduct. The procedure involves ventral coeliotomy, incision of the oviduct, and removal of the egg. Salpingohysterectomy (rare, for recurrent cases), complete removal of the oviduct +/− ovary can prevent future egg binding in valuable or pet hens. Avian surgical expertise and general anesthesia are essential.
- **Management of Secondary Complications**
  EYP initiates antimicrobial therapy guided by culture and sensitivity. Commonly used antibiotics include enrofloxacin, trimethoprim-sulfamethoxazole, or amoxicillin-clavulanate.

10.3.3.6 Prevention and Control

- **Nutritional Management**
  Adequate calcium provided daily, vitamin D3 supplementation that allows calcium absorption, balanced phosphorus, and an overall balanced diet.
- **Husbandry and Environmental Practices**
  Nest box management to reduce stress, mental stimulation, temperature regulation avoiding extremes, natural lighting programs to ensure appropriate stimulation, and stress reduction.
- **Health Monitoring and Disease Prevention**
  Routine individual bird health checks, vaccination (if available), and biosecurity against infectious bronchitis and Marek's disease, and parasite control.
- **Genetic and Breeding Considerations**
  Selective breeding to avoid hens with chronic reproductive issues and breed awareness to recognize that ornamental breeds and very high-production hybrid breeds may need closer monitoring.

10.3.3.7 Nursing Considerations

Nursing care for chickens affected by egg binding focuses on prompt recognition, supportive care and management, and minimizing stress to facilitate egg passage and prevent complications. Birds should be closely monitored for signs such as straining, frequent sitting, lethargy, fluffed feathers, anorexia, and distended coeloms or cloacal prolapse, as early intervention is critical to prevent rupture or secondary infections. Providing a warm, quiet, and stress-free environment can help relax the hen and support natural egg expulsion. Ensuring easy access to clean water and calcium-rich, well-balanced nutrition supports proper muscle contractions and reproductive health. Gentle supportive care may include warm soaking baths or external cloacal lubrication under veterinary guidance to aid egg passage. Analgesia is advised. Nursing management also involves isolating the affected bird to prevent bullying, monitoring for signs of shock or distress,

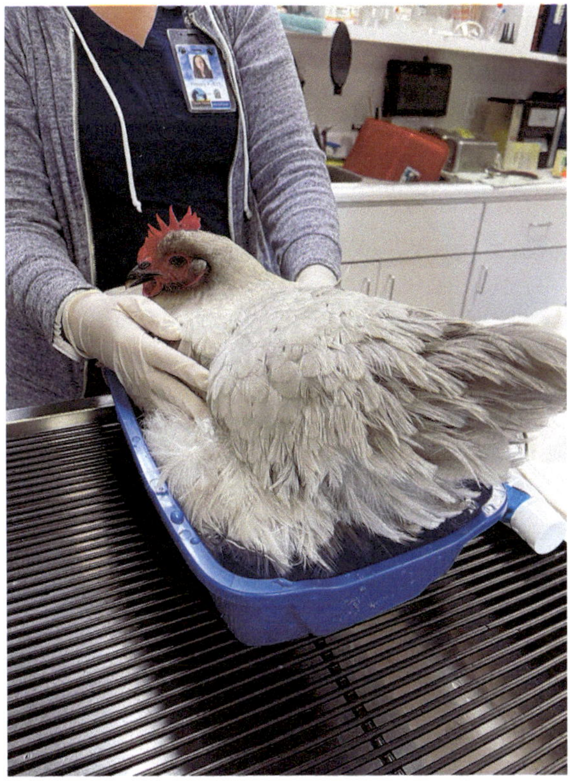

Figure 10.7 Warm magnesium (Epsom salt) soak for an egg-bound Lavender Orpington hen. Courtesy of Sarah Meyer.

and seeking timely veterinary assistance for manual egg removal or medical intervention if needed. Overall, nursing considerations emphasize early detection, supportive care, stress reduction, and timely veterinary involvement to optimize recovery and prevent recurrence or severe complications (Figure 10.7).

10.3.4 Prolapse of the Oviduct

10.3.4.1 Overview and Pathogenesis

Prolapse of the oviduct is a reproductive disorder in laying hens characterized by the eversion and protrusion of the oviduct through the cloaca, often accompanied by exposure of mucosal tissues to the external environment. The condition primarily affects high-producing layers, particularly older hens or birds under stress, and it is significant due to reduced egg production, risk of secondary infection, trauma, and potential mortality. Predisposing factors include obesity, large egg size, poor body condition, nutritional deficiencies (particularly calcium and protein), forced molting, high environmental temperature, and previous reproductive tract injuries. Clinically affected birds present with visible oviductal tissue protruding from the vent, discomfort, straining, decreased egg production, and increased susceptibility to bacterial infection.

The pathogenesis of oviductal prolapse begins with mechanical or physiological stressors that increase intra-abdominal pressure during oviposition, forcing the distal oviduct to evert through the cloaca. Weakening of the pelvic muscles, ligaments, and vent musculature, often associated with nutritional deficiencies or poor body condition, exacerbates the risk of prolapse. Once everted, the exposed mucosa is prone to trauma (self or flock mates), desiccation, and secondary bacterial contamination, frequently leading to bacterial infection, necrosis, or gangrenous changes, which can compromise hen survival. Chronic or recurrent prolapse may result in scarring, adhesion, and permanent reproductive impairment, reducing egg production. Overall, oviductal prolapse is a mechanical and secondary inflammatory reproductive disorder in which structural weakness, reproductive stress, and secondary infections converge to impair reproductive performance and compromise health.

10.3.4.2 Risk Factors

- **Reproductive and Developmental Factors**
  Early sexual maturity before the body frame is fully developed. Premature photo stimulation (light programs started too early). Inadequate pelvic and cloacal muscle tone in young pullets. High-producing commercial egg-laying breeds. Large, elongated, or double-yolked eggs. Misshapen eggs require extra straining during laying. Inherited body conformation issues (narrow pelvis, rapid growth rates).
- **Nutritional Factors**
  Calcium, phosphorus, or vitamin D deficiencies. Imbalanced protein-energy diet. Overfeeding leads to obesity and excessive coelomic fat.
- **Management and Environmental Factors**
  Overcrowding and lack of adequate nest boxes. Poor ventilation or stressful housing conditions. Rough or inappropriate flooring increases straining and vent trauma in chickens primarily by leading to poor hygiene, which causes vent infections, and by causing physical injuries that attract pecking behavior.
- **Health-Related Factors**
  Straining from cloacitis, enteritis, or parasitic irritation. Secondary infections weakening cloacal/oviductal tissue.

10.3.4.3 Clinical Signs and Pathology

- **External Findings**
  Visible protrusion of red, moist oviductal/cloacal tissue through the vent. Straining and frequent visits to the nest box without successful laying. Soiling or trauma of the protruding tissue. Blood-stained feathers or vent region. Reduced egg production.
- **Necropsy Findings**
  Everted, edematous, and congested oviductal mucosa. Hemorrhages, necrosis, or ulceration of exposed tissue. Retained or impacted eggs within the oviduct. Secondary peritonitis in severe or chronic cases.

10.3.4.4 Diagnostic Testing

- **Cytology**
  Assess secondary bacterial or fungal infections of prolapsed tissue.
- **Fecal Flotation**
  Rule out parasitic irritation (e.g., *Capillaria* spp.) causing excessive straining.
- **Bloodwork**
  Evaluate calcium levels and general metabolic status.

10.3.4.5 Treatment and Therapeutic Interventions

- **Supportive Care**
  Isolate the affected hen from the flock to prevent pecking and cannibalism. Place in a clean, quiet, dimly lit area to reduce stress and suppress laying drive. Administration of analgesics is advised.

Cleanse the tissue with warm sterile saline or dilute antiseptic (e.g., chlorhexidine or iodine). With veterinarian supervision, reduce swelling with hyperosmotic agents (sugar, manuka honey, or hypertonic saline applied topically). Administer analgesics with sedation. Lubricate (water-based jelly and lidocaine 2% jelly) thoroughly before attempting manual replacement of the oviduct. If replacement is not possible immediately, keep tissue moist with sterile water-soluble lubricant to prevent desiccation and necrosis. Apply topical antibiotic ointment to reduce the risk of secondary infection by direction of veterinarian. Systemic antibiotics and anti-inflammatory/analgesic therapy may be prescribed by a veterinarian in cases with infection risk. Prevent self-trauma, injury.

10.3.4.6 Prevention and Control

- **Flock Management**
  Do not expose pullets to extended light programs to prevent early stimulation of egg production. Natural lighting is advised. Provide one nest per four to five hens to reduce straining and mislaid eggs. Prevent overcrowding, which increases stress and vent pecking.
- **Nutrition**
  Provide appropriate calcium, phosphorus, and vitamin D to support eggshell quality and muscle function. Prevent obesity by controlling feed intake in meat and egg breeds as pullets. Ensure diets are formulated to support gradual, healthy reproductive development.
- **Egg Production Control**
  Avoid breeds prone to producing excessively large or misshapen eggs. Manage light duration and intensity to regulate egg production rate. Natural lighting is ideal to allow the hen's reproductive organs to "rest."
- **Health and Biosecurity**
  Prevent *Capillaria* spp. and other internal parasites that cause straining. Monitor for infections that predispose to prolapse. Good ventilation, appropriate temperature, and low-stress handling reduce prolapse risk.

10.3.4.7 Nursing Considerations

Nursing care for chickens affected by prolapse of the oviduct focuses on prompt intervention, supportive care/management, and preventing secondary injury or infection. Affected birds should be closely observed for signs of protruding tissue from the vent, straining, lethargy, decreased appetite, and distress, as rapid response can prevent further tissue damage and complications. Immediate nursing actions include isolating the bird in a clean, quiet, and low-stress environment to prevent pecking by flock mates and reduce contamination risk. The exposed tissue should be kept clean, moist, and protected from trauma using sterile saline-moistened gauze until veterinary care is available. Providing easy access to fresh water and a well-balanced diet rich in calcium supports muscle tone and healing, while minimizing stress aids recovery. Nursing staff should monitor for signs of infection, pain, necrosis, or recurrence and ensure veterinary assessment for reduction of the prolapse, possible suturing, and treatment of underlying reproductive issues. Overall, nursing considerations emphasize early detection, gentle supportive care, strict hygiene, stress reduction, and timely veterinary intervention to promote healing and reduce the risk of recurrence or further complications.

10.3.5 Cystic Right Oviduct

10.3.5.1 Overview and Pathogenesis

Cystic right oviduct, also known as cystic remnants of the right oviduct, is a congenital or developmental reproductive abnormality observed in female chickens, most commonly in layer breeds or breeding birds. Normally, the right oviduct regresses during embryonic development, leaving only the left oviduct functional. In cystic right oviduct, incomplete regression leads to the formation of fluid-filled cysts, which can vary in size and may occasionally interfere with the function of the left oviduct. Although often asymptomatic, larger cysts may cause coelomic distension, discomfort, reduced egg production, or predisposition to secondary infections.

The pathogenesis of cystic right oviduct arises during embryogenesis, when hormonal and genetic signals that normally induce regression of the right oviduct are disrupted. The persistent right oviduct may form cystic structures lined with epithelium, capable of secreting fluid and expanding within the abdominal cavity. These cysts can compress adjacent organs or the functional left oviduct, potentially interfering with oviposition and predisposing to internal laying or secondary bacterial infection. The fluid-filled cysts themselves are typically sterile unless secondarily infected. Overall, cystic right oviduct is a developmental reproductive abnormality in which incomplete embryonic regression results in cyst formation, which may impact abdominal organ function, reproductive efficiency, and predispose to secondary complications in affected hens.

10.3.5.2 Risk Factors

- **Developmental and Embryological Factors**
  In female chicks, the right oviduct normally regresses during embryonic development, if regression is incomplete, remnants of the right oviduct can persist and later form cystic structures.
- **Genetic Factors**
  Certain genetic lines or breeding stock may have a higher predisposition. Selection for high egg production may increase the likelihood of reproductive tract anomalies.

10.3.5.3 Clinical Signs and Pathology

- **External Findings**
  Progressive abdominal distension. Decreased egg production, but often otherwise clinically normal until cyst becomes large. In advanced cases: respiratory compromise from coelomic compression.
- **Necropsy Findings**
  Thin-walled, fluid-filled cyst(s) on the right side of the coelomic cavity. Size ranges from small incidental nodules to large cysts occupying a significant portion of the coelom. Cyst contents are usually clear, straw-colored fluid, occasionally thickened or cloudy if secondary infection occurs. Secondary findings are compression of intestines, air sacs, or left oviduct.

10.3.5.4 Diagnostic Testing

- **Diagnostic Imaging**
  Ultrasound confirms a thin-walled, fluid-filled cyst versus a solid mass. Helpful in differentiating from tumors or ascites. Radiographs show a soft-tissue mass in the right coelom cavity, distinct from the egg in the left oviduct.
- **Abdominocentesis**
  May recover clear or straw-colored cystic fluid, ruling out infectious peritonitis (which usually produces fibrinous, turbid exudate).
- **Cytology of Aspirated Fluid**
  Typically, acellular or low cellularity; inflammatory cells only if secondarily infected.

10.3.5.5 Treatment and Therapeutic Interventions

- **Surgery**
  Surgical removal may be considered. Cystectomy or excision of the persistent right oviduct tissue. Postoperative care includes antibiotics, analgesics, and restricted activity.

10.3.5.6 Prevention and Control

- **Understanding the Condition**
  Cystic right oviduct is a congenital anomaly. Because it is developmental, true prevention at the individual bird level is not possible once the defect exists.
- **Preventive Strategies (Flock-Level)**
  Selective breeding, avoid breeding birds with known cystic right oviduct. Select for lines with a lower incidence of reproductive tract malformations. Incubation management maintains correct temperature, humidity, and ventilation during hatching to reduce embryonic stress that could influence abnormal duct development.

10.3.5.7 Nursing Considerations

Nursing care for chickens is affected by a cystic right oviduct center on monitoring reproductive health, providing supportive care, and preventing secondary complications. Since this condition is often chronic and may go unnoticed until advanced, birds should be closely observed for signs of abdominal distension, reduced activity, weight loss, decreased egg production, or respiratory difficulty from pressure on internal organs. Housing should be clean, quiet, and low stress, minimizing environmental challenges that can exacerbate reproductive disorders. Providing a balanced diet rich in essential nutrients and vitamins, especially calcium and protein, supports general health and helps maintain body condition. Affected birds may benefit from isolation to prevent flock aggression or bullying and to allow close observation of their eating, drinking, and droppings. Nursing care also includes prompt veterinary consultation to evaluate the extent of the cystic changes and to manage pain or secondary infections, which may involve anti-inflammatories, antibiotics, or in some cases surgical intervention. Overall, nursing considerations emphasize supportive husbandry, close observation, minimizing stress, and ensuring timely veterinary involvement to maintain quality of life and reduce the risk of complications.

10.3.6 Ovarian and Oviductal Neoplasia

Figure 10.8 is consistent with mass effect in coelom. The cranial pole of the kidney as well as the region of oviduct may be involved. Impacted oviduct (can be related to colibacillosis), neoplasia (including ovarian carcinoma and lymphosarcoma), and coelomic fluid, among others are differentials. Image courtesy of Katherine Gaskill CVT, VTS-ECC. Image interpretation by Jennifer Graham DVM, DABVP, DACZM.

10.3.6.1 Overview and Pathogenesis

Ovarian and oviductal neoplasia in chickens refers to benign or malignant tumors arising from the ovarian or oviductal tissues, most commonly affecting older laying hens. The condition is important due to reduced egg production, abnormal eggs, coelomic distension, decreased body condition, and potential mortality. Tumor development is multifactorial, with genetic predisposition, prolonged reproductive activity, hormonal imbalances, and chronic inflammation serving as predisposing factors. Clinical signs vary depending on tumor location, size, and malignancy, and may include coelomic swelling, lethargy, anorexia, decreased egg production, abnormal egg morphology, and cachexia in advanced cases.

The pathogenesis of ovarian and oviductal neoplasia involves aberrant cellular proliferation within the ovarian or oviductal epithelium, potentially triggered by chronic hormonal stimulation,

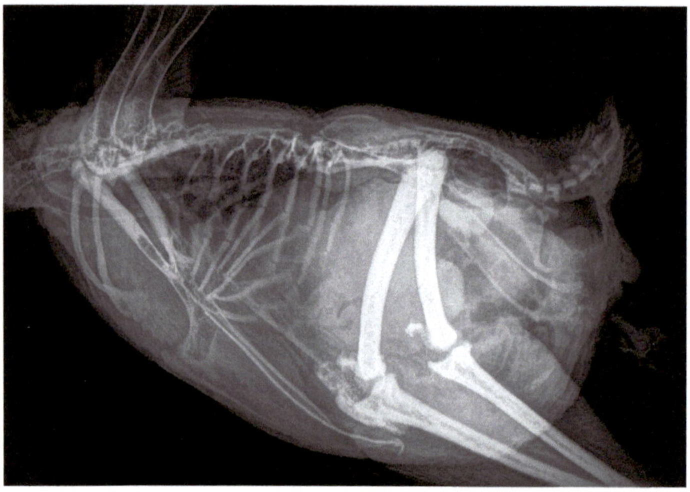

Figure 10.8 Ovarian neoplasia. Image courtesy of Katherine Gaskill CVT, VTS-ECC. Image interpretation by Jennifer Graham DVM, DABVP, DACZM.

inflammatory stimuli, or genetic mutations affecting tumor suppressor genes and oncogenes. In malignant cases, neoplastic cells invade surrounding tissues, including the coelomic cavity, leading to ascites, secondary bacterial infections, and systemic illness. Tumor growth may obstruct normal ovulation and oviduct function, causing internal laying, EYP, or salpingitis. Some neoplasms, particularly adenocarcinomas of the ovary or oviduct, can metastasize to the liver, kidneys, and abdominal serosa, further impairing organ function. Overall, ovarian and oviductal neoplasia is a reproductive tract neoplastic disease in which dysregulated cellular proliferation, local tissue invasion, and secondary complications disrupt normal egg production and compromise health and productivity in laying hens.

10.3.6.2 Risk Factors

- **Age and Reproductive History**
  Advanced age, prolonged egg production, and reproductive fatigue can predispose them to neoplastic transformation.
- **Genetic and Breed Predisposition**
  Commercial egg breeds selected for continuous laying, increasing lifetime exposure to risk factors. Hereditary susceptibility, some lines demonstrate a higher incidence of ovarian carcinomas, suggesting a genetic component.
- **Infectious and Viral Factors**
  Certain avian retroviruses can promote tumor formation. Marek's disease is known for causing lymphoid tumors but can also affect the reproductive tract indirectly.
- **Environmental and Management Factors**
  Artificial lighting that extends the laying period increases ovulation frequency, contributing to neoplastic risk. Chronic exposure to mycotoxins, pesticides, or endocrine-disrupting agents may also play a role. Chronic inflammation, such as recurrent salpingitis, EYP, or trauma to the reproductive tract, can predispose to neoplasia through long-term irritation and repair cycles.

10.3.6.3 Clinical Signs and Pathology

- **External Findings**
  Abdominal distension decreased or irregular egg production, lethargy, weakness, dyspnea, anorexia, coelomic fluid accumulation, and occasional palpable masses.
- **Necropsy Findings**
  Enlarged ovary with nodular or lobulated masses may be unilateral or bilateral. Thickened oviductal wall, often forming polypoid or irregular masses. Accumulation of clear or straw-colored fluid in the coelomic cavity. Malignant tumors may implant on serosal surfaces or other abdominal organs.

10.3.6.4 Diagnostic Testing

- **Diagnostic Imaging**
  Radiographs aid visualization of soft tissue masses and coelomic fluid. Ultrasound detects solid or cystic ovarian/oviductal masses, coelomic fluid, and organ displacement.
- **Cytology of Coelomic Fluid**
  May reveal neoplastic cells, inflammatory cells, or secondary infection.
- **Bloodwork**
  Can identify anemia, electrolyte imbalances, or signs of systemic illness in chronic cases.

10.3.6.5 Treatment and Therapeutic Interventions

- **Supportive Care**
  Provide comfort, nutrition, and safe housing for affected hens. Monitor for ascites; coelomic fluid may occasionally need drainage under veterinary supervision. Pain management is recommended.
- **Surgical Excision**
  Laparotomy or oophorectomy may be attempted. Reserved for benign or localized tumors. Requires intensive postoperative care. Avian surgeon expertise is required.

10.3.6.6 Prevention and Control

- **Flock Management**
  Neoplasia is primarily age-related, so risk increases in older hens. Maintain good overall flock health to reduce secondary complications. Monitor older layers closely for coelomic distension or changes in egg production.
- **Genetic Selection**
  Avoid breeding birds with known predisposition to reproductive tract tumors.
- **Nutrition**
  Provide a balanced diet with adequate vitamins, minerals, and protein to support reproductive tract health. Avoid overfeeding or underfeeding that may compromise general health or reproductive function.
- **Environmental and Health Management**
  Minimize stressors, provide proper ventilation, reduce overcrowding, and provide adequate nesting space. Regular parasite control and biosecurity help maintain reproductive tract health, indirectly reducing secondary complications.

10.3.6.7 Nursing Considerations

Nursing care for chickens affected by ovarian and oviductal neoplasia focuses on providing supportive management, maintaining comfort, and preventing secondary complications, as these tumors are typically progressive and often detected late. Birds should be monitored closely for clinical signs such as coelomic distension, reduced egg production, lethargy, weight loss, respiratory difficulty, or changes in droppings, as these may indicate tumor growth or associated fluid accumulation. Housing should be kept clean, quiet, and stress-free, with easy access to food and water at an appropriate height to encourage intake despite reduced mobility or appetite. Boredom must be mitigated. Providing a nutrient-dense, balanced diet rich in protein, vitamins, and minerals supports general health and helps maintain body condition. Isolating the affected bird can prevent bullying and allow for careful observation of feeding behavior and droppings. Nursing care also involves prompt veterinary evaluation for diagnostic imaging, fluid drainage (if ascites is present), and palliative medical management, including analgesics or anti-inflammatories to improve comfort. Overall, nursing considerations emphasize supportive care, stress reduction, analgesia, close monitoring, and timely veterinary involvement to enhance the bird's quality of life and reduce/prevent suffering associated with neoplastic disease.

10.3.7 Double Yolk/Malformed Eggs

10.3.7.1 Overview and Pathogenesis

Double-yolk and malformed eggs in chickens are noninfectious reproductive abnormalities that occur due to disruptions in the normal ovulation and egg formation processes. These conditions are most often seen in young pullets at the onset of lay, when the hormonal system is still maturing, or in older hens with irregular ovulatory cycles. While these eggs are typically benign from a health perspective, they can indicate temporary reproductive imbalance or environmental or nutritional influences affecting the hen's physiology.

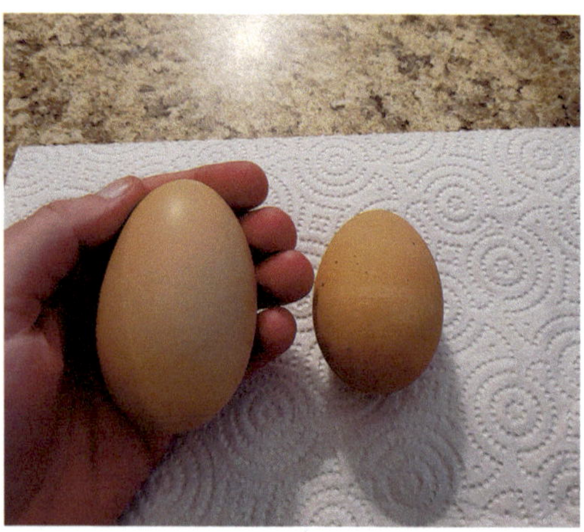

Figure 10.9 Abnormally large egg from the same hen on different days. the egg on the left contained a double yolk. Courtesy of Sarah Meyer.

Double-yolk eggs form when two yolks are released from the ovary into the oviduct within a short time, usually within a few hours. Under normal conditions, the ovary releases a single mature ovum (yolk) at a time. However, hormonal irregularities, particularly excessive or uncoordinated LH surges, can trigger the release of multiple follicles simultaneously. Both yolks then enter the infundibulum together and become enclosed within a single albumen and shell. Young hens with immature hypothalamic-pituitary-ovarian axis regulation are especially prone to this, as their reproductive hormones have not yet stabilized. Genetic predisposition and high-protein diets may also contribute (Figure 10.9).

Malformed eggs result from disturbances in the oviduct's function, especially within the magnum (albumen-secreting region) and shell gland (uterus). These disturbances can arise from stress, nutritional imbalances (notably calcium or vitamin D3 deficiency), mechanical strain from oversized eggs, or transient oviductal inflammation. The result is eggs that are misshapen, soft-shelled, rough-surfaced, or otherwise irregular in appearance. In some cases, premature expulsion of the egg before complete shell deposition, often due to stress or excessive uterine contractions, produces thin-shelled or shell-less eggs.

Overall, the pathogenesis of both double-yolk and malformed eggs reflects temporary physiological or hormonal dysregulation rather than infectious or structural disease. Most hens recover normal laying patterns once reproductive hormone levels stabilize and environmental or nutritional conditions are optimized (Figure 10.10).

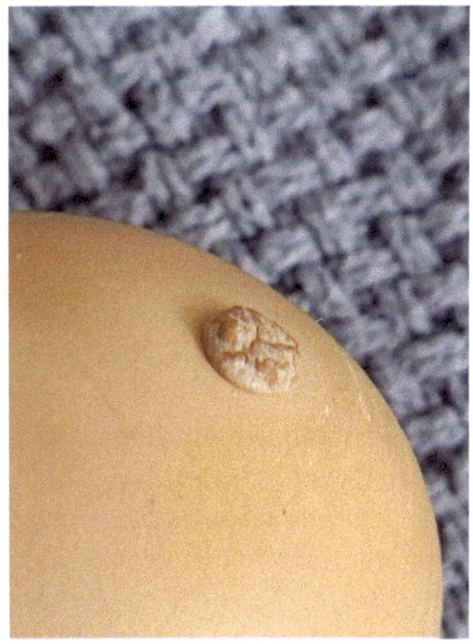

Figure 10.10 Eggshell abnormality; excess calcium deposit. Courtesy of Sarah Meyer.

10.3.7.2 Risk Factors

- **Nutritional Deficiencies**
  Calcium deficiency causes poor eggshell formation, thin shells. Vitamin D3 deficiency causes impaired calcium absorption. Protein or amino acid imbalance causes inadequate yolk formation. Trace mineral deficiencies cause structural shell defects.
- **Environmental Stress**
  Heat stress causes decreased laying. Cold stress leads to reduced appetite and delayed ovulation. High ammonia levels or poor ventilation leads to respiratory discomfort affecting laying. Sudden changes in lighting disrupt hormonal control of ovulation.
- **Management Practices**
  Overcrowding increases stress, pecking, and reduced food access. Frequent handling or transport causes stress-induced drop in production. Inconsistent photoperiod affects hypothalamic-pituitary-ovarian axis. Molting induced improperly may result in a temporary drop in egg production.
- **Reproductive Stress**
  Overproduction and prolonged laying cycles lead to fatigue of the reproductive system. Early sexual maturity causes immature oviduct or shell-gland function.
- **Disease-Associated Factors (Secondary, Noninfectious Contribution)**
  Subclinical reproductive disorders (e.g., salpingitis, ovarian cysts) without infection can predispose to production drops. Previous nutritional or metabolic stress may reduce egg quality or frequency.

10.3.7.3 Clinical Signs and Pathology

- **External Findings**
  Sudden drop in egg numbers (may decline 10–50% in affected flock). Thin-shelled, soft, or malformed eggs; misshapen or wrinkled shells; sometimes pale or brittle shells. Birds may appear otherwise healthy; feeding intake is usually normal; mild lethargy may occur in some cases. Delayed oviposition; occasionally abnormal yolk coloration; no systemic illness or fever. Often affects a subset of laying hens; pattern may be flock-wide if due to environmental or nutritional stress.

- **Necropsy Findings**
  Typically, no overt systemic lesions. Shell gland (uterus) may appear pale, underdeveloped, or flaccid in affected birds. Ovaries are usually normal, unless concurrent reproductive disorders are present. Occasionally, soft or thin-shelled eggs are retained in the oviduct.

10.3.7.4 Diagnostic Testing

- **Rule Out Infectious Causes**
  Viral Egg Drop Syndrome (EDS-76 virus), Newcastle disease, or infectious bronchitis virus (IBV) via serology (ELISA, HI test) or PCR. No viral particles should be detected in noninfectious cases.

10.3.7.5 Treatment and Therapeutic Interventions

- **Nutritional Support**
  Provide layer feed with adequate calcium (3–4% for adult layers). Offer oyster shell or crushed limestone as a free choice for shell formation. Vitamin D3 supports calcium absorption and eggshell quality. Ensure diet meets recommended daily allowance or provide supplemental vitamin D3 in feed or water. Ensure adequate high-quality protein in the diet (16–18% for layers). Manganese, zinc, and selenium are critical for shell quality and reproductive health. Refer to Chapter 4, Nutrition.

10.3.7.6 Prevention and Control

- **Age-Appropriate Bird Management**
  Young pullets are the most frequent producers of double yolks and malformed eggs as their ovulation and shell gland cycles are not yet synchronized. Delay onset of lay until birds reach appropriate physiological maturity by avoiding unnatural lighting stimulation in immature birds. Gradually increase day length in a controlled manner rather than making abrupt lighting changes. Premature light stimulation may trigger multiple ovulations, increasing the incidence of double yolks and irregular shell formation.
- **Environmental Management and Stress Reduction**
  Stress is a significant contributing factor to egg malformations, including slab-sided, shell-less, or misshapen eggs. Maintain consistent temperature, natural lighting, and ventilation. Sudden temperature spikes or drops can disturb oviposition timing. Avoid prolonged heat stress, which can reduce shell quality and increase malformation rates. Limit unnecessary catching, chasing, or disturbances during the laying cycle. Secure housing to prevent predator intrusion, which can induce sudden fright and interrupt egg formation. Avoid overcrowding, which increases stress and disrupts laying patterns. Provide sufficient nest boxes (minimum 1 nest per 4–5 hens) to reduce competition and accidental breakage.
- **Disease Prevention and Reproductive Health**
  Certain reproductive tract infections or inflammatory conditions can lead to misshapen, shell-less, or thin-shelled eggs. Internal and external parasites cause stress and nutrient diversion, indirectly affecting egg formation. Implement regular deworming and mite control as indicated. Conditions such as salpingitis, oviductal cysts, or neoplasia can cause persistent malformations.

10.3.7.7 Nursing Considerations

Nursing care for hens producing double-yolk or malformed eggs centers on supportive care, stress reduction, and optimization of nutrition and environmental conditions to restore normal ovulatory rhythm and shell formation. Birds should be maintained in a calm, stable environment with

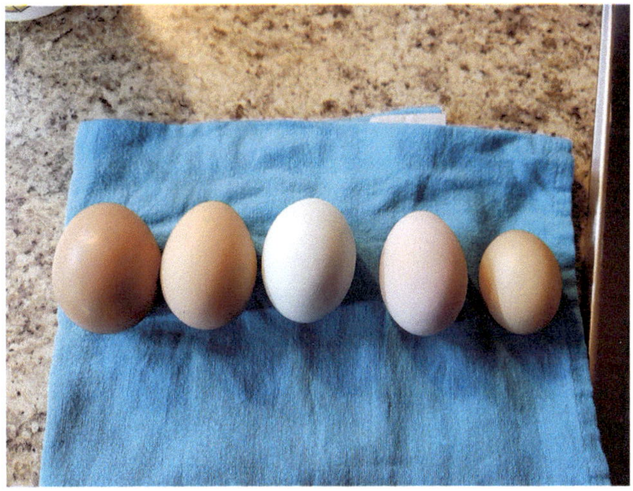

Figure 10.11 Normal eggs, shells from a healthy mixed breed flock. Photo by Sarah Meyer.

minimal handling and noise to prevent stress-induced hormonal fluctuations that can disrupt ovulation and egg passage. Consistent lighting schedules are particularly important; abrupt changes in photoperiod can cause multiple ovulations or premature egg expulsion. History taking from the chicken guardian and documentation are key nursing responsibilities. Record any changes in egg size, shell texture, or laying frequency to help identify patterns or potential contributing factors. Birds straining to lay an oversized or double-yolk egg should be monitored closely for signs of egg binding, such as lethargy, tail pumping, or cloacal protrusion. If egg binding occurs, prompt veterinary attention is required. Education of chicken guardians plays an important preventive role, highlighting the need for gradual light increases during the onset of lay, balanced nutrition, and stress minimization. With appropriate care and environmental stability, most hens experiencing double-yolk or malformed eggs return to normal laying patterns without long-term reproductive issues (Figure 10.11).

10.3.8 Soft-Shelled or Shell-Less Eggs

10.3.8.1 Overview and Pathogenesis

Soft-shelled and shell-less eggs in chickens are noninfectious reproductive abnormalities characterized by eggs laid with thin, pliable shells or no calcified shell layer at all, often enclosed only by the inner membranes. These eggs are common in young pullets starting their laying cycle, older hens nearing the end of production, or birds experiencing nutritional deficiencies or environmental stress. While occasional soft-shell eggs are usually benign, persistent production indicates an underlying physiological or nutritional disturbance affecting shell formation in the oviduct's shell gland (uterus).

Pathogenesis primarily involves disruption of calcium metabolism or interference with the normal timing and function of shell deposition. Calcium carbonate, the main component of the eggshell, is derived from dietary calcium absorbed through the intestine and mobilized from medullary bone under the influence of vitamin D3 and parathyroid hormone. Inadequate calcium, phosphorus, or vitamin D3 intake impairs mineral availability, preventing proper shell calcification. Additionally, disturbances in the shell gland's ability to retain the egg long enough for mineral deposition, often caused by stress, disease, or hormonal imbalances, result in premature egg expulsion before shell formation is complete. Other contributing factors include excessive dietary salt, exposure to mycotoxins, or consumption of high-energy, low-calcium feed formulations. Heat stress and sudden environmental changes can alter circulating corticosterone and prostaglandin levels, affect uterine contractions, and reduce the time available for shell mineralization. Infectious or inflammatory conditions of the reproductive tract, such as salpingitis, can also impair shell gland function, although these represent secondary complications rather than primary noninfectious causes.

10.3.8.2 Risk Factors

- **Physiological and Age-Related Factors**
  Immature reproductive systems may ovulate before the shell gland is fully synchronized, resulting in thin or missing shells. Double ovulations or rapid successive ovulations may shorten time in the shell gland, producing soft shells. Shell gland function declines with age, resulting in reduced calcium deposition efficiency and more frequent shell defects. Some breeds are more prone to thin-shelled or shell-less eggs due to inherited differences in calcium metabolism or shell gland structure.
- **Nutritional Factors**
  Proper shell formation depends on adequate and balanced mineral and vitamin intake, particularly calcium (Ca), phosphorus (P), and vitamin D3. Inadequate dietary calcium (<3.5–4% for layers) leads to insufficient shell deposition, resulting in soft or shell-less eggs. Birds mobilize calcium from medullary bone to compensate, but prolonged deficits cause depletion and shell defects. Excess phosphorus or insufficient phosphorus relative to calcium interferes with calcium absorption and utilization, weakening shells. Vitamin D3 is essential for calcium metabolism and shell formation; deficiency leads to thin shells, reduced production, and possible egg binding. Spoiled feed, mold contamination, or irregular feeding can disrupt nutrient intake and oviposition timing. Hens without access to oyster shells or limestone grit may not meet daily calcium needs, especially during peak laying season (spring and summer months).
- **Environmental and Management Factors**
  Environmental conditions and husbandry practices have major impacts on shell gland function and ovulation timing. Loud noises, mishandling, predator attacks, or abrupt environmental changes can interrupt the calcification phase, resulting in soft or shell-less eggs. Inconsistent or inappropriately timed lighting can trigger premature ovulation before shell formation is complete. Abrupt changes in photoperiod may disrupt hormonal regulation of ovulation. Natural lighting is advised, and unnatural lighting should be avoided. Heat stress (84–86°F) reduces feed intake, calcium absorption, and shell quality. Prolonged heat exposure leads to thinner shells and higher rates of shell-less eggs. Lack of comfortable nest boxes may cause hens to retain or pass eggs abnormally, sometimes prematurely.
- **Infectious Disease Factors**
  Several infectious agents, particularly those affecting the oviduct and shell gland, can cause persistent soft-shelled or shell-less egg production. One of the most significant causes. IBV can damage the shell gland permanently, resulting in misshapen, thin, or shell-less eggs even after recovery. Some strains specifically target reproductive tissues. Newcastle disease and avian influenza are severe systemic diseases that can disrupt ovulation and shell formation, often alongside other reproductive and respiratory signs. Infection and inflammation of the oviduct can alter shell-gland secretions, resulting in defective shells.

10.3.8.3 Clinical Signs and Pathology

- **External Findings**

  Thin-shelled eggs have a soft, pliable shell that may collapse easily during handling. The surface may appear wrinkled, translucent, or irregular. Shell-less eggs are passed surrounded only by the shell membranes, without any calcified layer. These are often fragile, misshapen, and prone to rupture in the cloaca or nest. Intermittent production of normal and soft-shelled eggs may occur, especially with stress-induced or hormonal causes. Due to the fragile membrane breaking as the egg is laid, releasing albumen and yolk that soil feathers around the vent. If the soft or shell-less egg fails to pass normally, hens may exhibit tenesmus, tail pumping, or prolonged nest sitting. Fewer eggs, out-of-sequence laying, or changes in laying time may signal oviductal dysfunction or disease.

- **Necropsy Findings**

  Shell Gland (Uterus)

  Thinning or pallor of the mucosa may be seen with chronic calcium deficiency. Atrophy or scarring of the shell gland wall may occur in birds with previous IBV infection, indicating permanent loss of shell-secreting function.

  Oviduct

  May be inflamed (salpingitis) in bacterial infections (*E. coli, Mycoplasma, Pasteurella*), with thickened walls, caseous exudate, or fibrinous deposits. Tears, adhesions, or deformities may be present in hens with chronic internal laying or trauma.

10.3.8.4 Diagnostic Testing

- **Infectious Disease Testing**

  Confirm or rule out viral and bacterial pathogens that damage the shell gland and oviduct.

- **Diagnostic Imaging**

  Radiography is useful for visualizing retained eggs, oviduct dilation, or abnormal shell deposition. Soft-shelled or shell-less eggs may appear as soft tissue density masses in the caudal coelom. Ultrasound detects oviductal dilation, fluid accumulation, internal egg material, or shell-gland abnormalities.

10.3.8.5 Treatment and Therapeutic Interventions

- **Supportive and Immediate Individual Care**

  This is indicated for hens that are actively passing soft-shelled or shell-less eggs, or showing signs of straining, retention, or secondary complications. If a soft-shelled egg becomes retained, it may not stimulate the same expulsion reflex as a hard-shelled egg. Analgesic administration is advised. Lubrication (water-based jelly +/− lidocaine 2% topical jelly) of the cloaca and gentle massage may assist passage of the egg in calm, restrained birds. Avoid aggressive manipulation, as shell membranes are fragile and can rupture, causing contamination or trauma. Place the bird in a warm, quiet, low-stress environment to reduce straining and allow natural expulsion. If the bird is dehydrated, oral or subcutaneous fluids (e.g., lactated Ringer's solution, warm) help restore hydration and support muscular function during egg passage. NSAIDs (e.g., meloxicam, carprofen) may be used to reduce inflammation and discomfort, especially if salpingitis or irritation is suspected. Corticosteroids are avoided, as they can interfere with calcium metabolism and ovulation cycles. If shell-less eggs rupture internally or in the cloaca, bacterial contamination can lead to vent soiling or ascending salpingitis.

- **Calcium Correction**
  Calcium Supplementation
  - **Immediate Supplementation**: 50–100 mg/kg by mouth or subcutaneously.
  - **Long-term Supplementation**: Ensure layer diets with 3.5–4% calcium. Offer supplemental oyster shell in separate feeders to allow voluntary intake, especially during peak lay. Never force calcium unless a known deficiency exists.

10.3.8.6 Prevention and Control

- **Nutritional Management**
  Proper nutrition is the cornerstone of shell quality. Preventing deficiencies or imbalances in calcium, phosphorus, and vitamin D3 is essential for consistent shell formation. Provide layer feed containing 3.5–4.0% calcium (35–40 g/kg) during the laying period. Use large particle calcium sources (e.g., oyster shell, coarse limestone >2 mm) to ensure prolonged retention in the gizzard and steady release during nighttime shell formation. Offer free-choice oyster shell or limestone grit in a separate feeder so birds can self-regulate intake. Maintain Ca:P ratio around 10:1 for layers; avoid excess phosphorus, which impairs calcium uptake. Ensure feed contains adequate vitamin D3 (not D2), critical for calcium absorption and shell gland function. Supplementation through water-soluble premixes may be useful in backyard flocks with inconsistent sunlight exposure or during high production periods (spring through early summer). Provide cool water to help hens with heat. Store feed in dry, cool, rodent-proof areas to prevent mold and nutrient degradation.
- **Environmental and Management Practices**
  Stress, excessive lighting, and temperature extremes are major noninfectious triggers of soft-shelled or shell-less eggs. Preventive management aims to minimize disturbances and support physiological laying rhythms. Protect flocks from sudden loud noises, predators, and abrupt environmental changes. Provide adequate nesting boxes (one box per four to five hens minimum), lined with comfortable material to encourage normal, relaxed laying behavior.

10.3.8.7 Nursing Considerations

Nursing care for hens producing soft-shelled or shell-less eggs focuses on restoring calcium metabolism, minimizing stress, and ensuring optimal reproductive health. The priority is to evaluate and correct the bird's nutritional intake. A balanced layer ration containing adequate calcium (3–4%), phosphorus, and vitamin D3 is essential for proper shell formation. Free-choice calcium supplements such as crushed oyster shell, limestone grit, or soluble calcium sources should always be available, particularly during peak laying periods. Vitamin D3 supplementation may be recommended under veterinary supervision to enhance calcium absorption and utilization. Observation and documentation are vital nursing responsibilities. Monitor for recurrence of soft-shelled eggs, changes in shell quality, or signs of reproductive distress such as straining or reduced laying frequency. If multiple hens are affected, review flock nutrition, feed storage (to prevent mold and mycotoxin exposure), and water quality. In some cases, soft-shelled eggs may precede or follow reproductive tract inflammation; therefore, veterinary technicians should monitor for abnormal discharge from the vent, vent swelling, or lethargy and report findings promptly for veterinarian evaluation. Education of chicken guardians is key for prevention, emphasizing proper nutrition, enrichment, and stress reduction. With early intervention and supportive care, most hens recover normal egg quality within several laying cycles once calcium metabolism and environmental conditions are corrected.

10.3.9 Vent Pecking/Trauma

10.3.9.1 Overview and Pathogenesis

Vent pecking, also known as cloacal or posterior pecking, is a behavioral and traumatic condition in chickens characterized by pecking, pulling, or tearing of the skin and tissues around the vent (cloaca). This behavior often begins as mild curiosity or social dominance but can escalate into severe cannibalism, resulting in open wounds, prolapse, hemorrhage, and even death if not promptly managed. It is primarily a management- and environment-related disorder rather than an infectious disease.

The pathogenesis of vent pecking is multifactorial and closely linked to social, nutritional, and environmental stressors. It frequently occurs in high-density flocks or under conditions of boredom, poor lighting, or limited foraging opportunities. Bright lighting, especially directly over nest boxes, can make the reddened, moist vent of a hen (freshly laid egg) more conspicuous and trigger pecking by nearby birds. Once pecking starts, the sight of blood or exposed tissue reinforces the behavior within the flock, leading to rapid spread.

10.3.9.2 Risk Factors

- **Environmental and Management Factors**
  Overcrowding increases competition, stress, and physical contact between birds, facilitating pecking. Overcrowded conditions often also lead to ventilation issues, heat buildup, and increased aggressive interactions. High light intensity or prolonged photoperiods can overstimulate birds and make the vent region more conspicuous. Bright, direct lighting at vent level (e.g., from uncovered bulbs) increases pecking frequency. Sudden changes in light schedule or intensity can disrupt normal behavior and trigger aggression. Boredom and lack of foraging opportunities increase the likelihood of redirected pecking at flock mates. Bare housing systems with no litter, pecking substrates, or perches are at higher risk. High temperatures and inadequate airflow cause discomfort and agitation, leading to aggressive pecking behaviors. Abrupt changes in feeding schedules and unnatural lighting programs can precipitate vent-pecking episodes, particularly in large groups.
- **Nutritional Factors**
  Dietary deficiencies and imbalances can alter normal behavior, increase irritability, or make vents more attractive to flock mates. Diets deficient in protein or essential amino acids (especially methionine) have been associated with increased injurious pecking. Conversely, excess protein or imbalances can cause wetter droppings and increased cloacal soiling, making vents more noticeable. Sodium deficiency is a recognized risk factor for feather and vent pecking, as birds seek alternative sources (including skin). Imbalances in calcium and phosphorus can also affect behavior indirectly through effects on laying and cloacal appearance. Low dietary fiber leads to insufficient satiety and foraging activity, increasing the incidence of redirected pecking behaviors.
- **Bird-Related/Physiological Factors**
  The cloaca enlarges and becomes moist during egg laying, drawing attention from other birds, especially in young pullets starting to lay. Erratic oviposition or soft-shelled eggs can lead to temporary prolapse or vent eversion, increasing vulnerability. Birds with cloacal or oviductal prolapse expose bright mucosal tissue, which triggers pecking reflexes in flock mates. Some birds exhibit increased aggressiveness and bullying behaviors, acting as initiators of pecking behavior.

10.3.9.3 Clinical Signs and Pathology

- **External Findings**

  Early Stage

  Feather loss and bare skin surrounding the vent. Mild erythema, edema, or small scabs on the pericloacal skin. Increased restlessness or irritation of the vent area. Repeated preening, tail lifting, or turning to peck at the affected site. Mild decreases in feed intake or activity if pain is present.

  Moderate Stage

  Visible wounds or ulcerations around the cloaca with scabbing or bloody feathers. Fresh blood on the feathers surrounding the vent, tail, or undercarriage, a common early sign noticed during flock inspection. Pecking attracts additional birds, leading to escalating trauma and increased aggression. Reduced egg production or intermittent laying. Signs of pain, such as reluctance to perch or move. Increased vocalization or isolation from the flock. Affected birds may strain during defecation or laying, especially if swelling is significant.

  Advanced Stage

  Large, deep lacerations around or into the vent and surrounding tissues. Prolapse of the cloaca or oviduct is common; protruding bright red tissue becomes the primary target for pecking. Severe hemorrhage, sometimes life-threatening, may occur rapidly if pecking damages blood vessels. Pale combs and wattles, tachypnea, or weakness secondary to blood loss. Sudden death in severe group outbreaks, especially if pecking occurs overnight without monitoring.

- **Necropsy Findings**

  Pericloacal skin lesions ranging from superficial abrasions to deep lacerations penetrating subcutaneous tissue or musculature. Cloacal prolapse is frequently present in advanced cases; prolapsed tissue is often edematous, congested, and covered in necrotic debris from repeated pecking. Hemorrhage may be focal or extensive. Secondary cellulitis, vent gleet, or cloacitis may be evident due to bacterial contamination.

10.3.9.4 Diagnostic Testing

The diagnosis of vent pecking and related trauma relies on a combination of flock behavioral observation, individual bird examination, necropsy findings, and selective laboratory testing to rule out infectious or reproductive conditions that may mimic or contribute to the lesions. Timely and accurate diagnosis is essential for intervening before the behavior escalates and causes flock-wide morbidity or mortality.

10.3.9.5 Treatment and Therapeutic Interventions

- **Isolation and Triage of Affected Birds**

  Promptly isolate injured birds to prevent further pecking and blood loss. Place in a clean, quiet, dimly lit hospital ward or recovery pen with easy access to food and water. Provide soft, clean bedding (do not use shredded paper or wood shavings) to reduce contamination of wounds. Blankets and towels with disposable potty pads are preferable. Stabilize first; assess viability. Birds with irreversible prolapse, severe hemorrhage, or necrotic cloacal tissue may require humane euthanasia for welfare reasons.

- **Wound Management**

  Pre-emptive analgesia administration is advised. Wearing exam or sterile gloves, gently clean wounds with warm sterile saline or dilute antiseptic solutions (e.g., chlorhexidine 0.05% or povidone-iodine as a "weak tea" color). Remove debris, blood clots, and necrotic tissue carefully. Local anesthetic jelly, e.g., lidocaine 2%, can be applied with a gloved hand to decrease painful manipulation. A paste of jelly and sugar or manuka honey can be used to osmotically reduce the edematous tissue prior to attempted replacement. Avoid caustic agents that may damage mucosa (e.g., alcohol). Apply broad-spectrum topical antiseptics (e.g., povidone-iodine) or antimicrobial sprays labeled for poultry. Flystrike prevention may be necessary in warm climates; use appropriate insect repellents or protectants on intact skin around the cloaca (never use toxic fly sprays directly on wounds). Use nonirritant, non-bright-colored wound dressings; bright red or pink ointments can trigger further pecking. Semipermeable dressings, wet-to-dry bandaging, and frequent bandage changes are helpful for wound healing and comfort. Human-grade menstrual pads are useful. Control bleeding with gentle pressure, styptic powder, or silver nitrate sticks if needed; local anesthetic jelly is advisable prior to the application of any hemostatic agents. Birds with significant hemorrhages should be warmed and hydrated to counteract hypovolemia.

- **Cloacal Prolapse Management**
  Prolapse is a frequent complication of vent pecking or laying disorders. Clean prolapsed tissue gently with saline. Apply a water-based lubricant or osmotic agent (e.g., granulated sugar or hypertonic saline; adding povidone-iodine to either agent will mitigate bacterial infections) to reduce edema. Administer analgesics +/− sedation to manually replace the prolapsed tissue into the vent with a gloved, lubricated finger. Purse-string sutures may be placed in birds to prevent recurrence, leaving enough room for defecation and egg passage. Prevent self-trauma, injury.

10.3.9.6 Prevention and Control

- **Environmental Management**
  Allow natural light to avoid stress-induced pecking. Avoid sudden light interruptions or flashes, which can trigger aggression. Provide additional feeders, drinkers, and nesting areas to minimize competition and reduce flock stress. Maintain optimal barn temperature, 68–75°F for layers; avoid heat stress. Ensure adequate ventilation to reduce humidity, ammonia buildup, and discomfort/stresses that can trigger pecking.
- **Behavioral and Environmental Enrichment**
  Introduce pecking blocks, hanging food objects, or attractive, colored items to divert attention from the vent region. Scatter small amounts of scratch grains or seeds in litter to encourage foraging. Allow supervised free range. Provide perches at multiple heights to allow birds to escape potential aggressors and reduce stress. Maintain a dynamic environment, rotating enrichment objects to sustain interest. Avoid large barren floor areas where birds have no stimulation.
- **Health and Hygiene Practices**
  Regular parasite control (lice, mites, helminths) to prevent irritation that attracts pecking. Keep vent areas clean and dry, particularly during molting or peak production. Monitor for reproductive tract disorders, which can increase vent exposure and vulnerability. Clean vent feathers of stool buildup, which can lead to skin irritation.
- **Monitoring and Early Intervention**
  Conduct daily inspections for blood-stained feathers, early feather loss, or vent irritation, redness. Observe flock behavior during feeding, laying, and perching periods. Rapid action prevents escalation into widespread cannibalism.

10.3.9.7 Nursing Considerations

Nursing care for vent pecking and trauma focuses on immediate wound care, prevention of further injury, stress reduction, and correction of environmental or nutritional triggers. Affected birds should be immediately isolated in a quiet, clean area to allow healing and prevent continued aggression from flock mates. Wounds should be gently cleaned with sterile saline or an antiseptic solution, and topical antimicrobials or protective dressings can be applied to prevent infection and discourage pecking. In severe cases, temporary physical barriers or devices such as vent covers or collars may be used under veterinarian guidance. Close observation is necessary to monitor wound healing, detect signs of secondary infection (swelling, discharge, foul odor), and ensure that the bird maintains appetite and normal behavior. Diligent observation and recordkeeping of affected birds and flock behavior help identify patterns and evaluate the effectiveness of interventions. Education of caretakers is important to maintain proactive management and reduce recurrence. Early intervention typically results in full recovery and prevents severe injury or flock-wide outbreaks.

10.4 Infectious Reproductive Diseases

Infectious reproductive diseases in chickens are caused by bacteria, viruses, and occasionally fungi that infect the ovary, oviduct, or peritoneum. These pathogens can directly damage reproductive tissues or indirectly impair egg production through systemic illness.

10.4.1 Salpingitis (Infectious)

Figure 10.12.

10.4.1.1 Overview and Pathogenesis

Salpingitis is an inflammation of the oviduct in laying hens, commonly associated with bacterial infection, particularly *Escherichia coli*, *Mycoplasma gallisepticum*, *Staphylococcus*

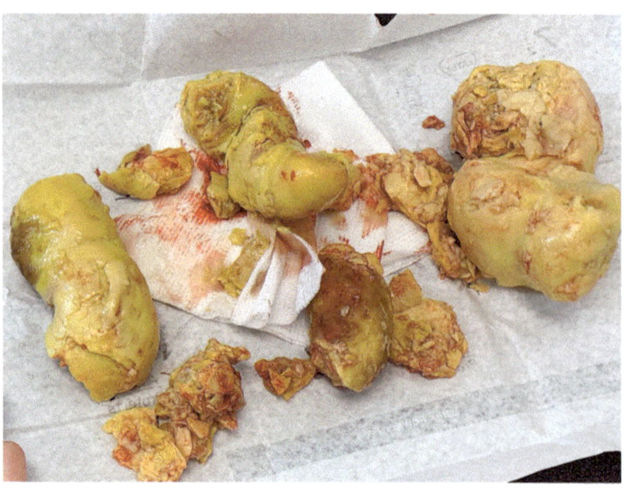

Figure 10.12 Coelomic contents removed during necropsy of hen suffering from salpingitis. Courtesy of Stephanie Freeman.

spp., and *Salmonella* spp. The disease primarily affects adult layers, especially high-producing or older hens, and is of importance due to reduced egg production, poor egg quality, reproductive tract lesions, and occasional mortality. Transmission occurs via ascending infection from the cloaca, contamination of the reproductive tract, or systemic spread through bacteremia, often facilitated by reproductive tract trauma, egg-binding, immunosuppression, or co-infections. Clinically, affected hens may exhibit decreased egg production, lethargy, anorexia, abdominal distension, abnormal eggs (soft-shelled, misshapen, or bloody), and sometimes sudden death.

The pathogenesis of salpingitis begins with bacterial colonization of the oviduct, often entering through the vent or cloaca following ascending infection, or via hematogenous spread in systemic infections. The bacteria adhere to and invade the oviductal epithelium, triggering local inflammation, edema, and infiltration of heterophils and lymphocytes. In severe or chronic cases, fibrinous exudates, mucosal necrosis, and adhesion formation may occur, impairing oviduct function and egg passage. Opportunistic bacteria proliferate in the presence of retained eggs, egg yolk, or damaged epithelium, exacerbating inflammation and predisposing to secondary infection, such as EYP. Overall, salpingitis is a bacterial reproductive tract disease in which colonization, local inflammation, and opportunistic secondary infections lead to impaired egg production, reproductive tract pathology, and decreased flock performance.

10.4.1.2 Risk Factors

- **Infectious Agents**
  Bacterial pathogens are the most common cause. Viral infections such as IBV damage the oviduct lining, predispose to secondary bacterial infection. Fungal causes are rare but may occasionally spread to the reproductive tract.
- **Reproductive and Physiological Factors**
  Continuous laying increases fatigue on the oviduct. Retained eggs create a nidus for infection. Internal laying and EYP provide a medium for bacterial growth. Straining with large, misshapen, or double-yolked eggs can damage mucosa, allowing infection entry.
- **Nutritional Factors**
  Calcium deficiency leads to poor eggshells and soft-shelled eggs, which break in the oviduct and increase infection risk. Vitamin deficiencies (A, E, and Selenium) impair immune defenses and mucosal health. Obesity can also increase the risk of reproductive dysfunction and oviduct infections.
- **Environmental and Husbandry Factors**
  Dirty nesting material and contaminated litter to the cloaca can introduce bacteria into the oviduct. Overcrowding can increase stress and exposure to infectious organisms.

10.4.1.3 Clinical Signs and Pathology

- **External Findings**
  Reduced or ceased egg production, abnormal eggs, distended coelom, depression, lethargy, decreased appetite, dyspnea, and foul-smelling discharge from the cloaca in some cases.
- **Necropsy Findings**
  Thickened, inflamed oviduct walls with congestion and edema. Exudate in the oviduct lumen may be caseous, purulent, or fibrinous depending on chronicity. Retained eggs or yolk material inside the oviduct. Adhesions between the oviduct, intestines, or abdominal wall in chronic cases. Yolk peritonitis is if yolk material escapes into the coelomic cavity. Distended abdomen with serous or fibrinous exudate (Figure 10.13).

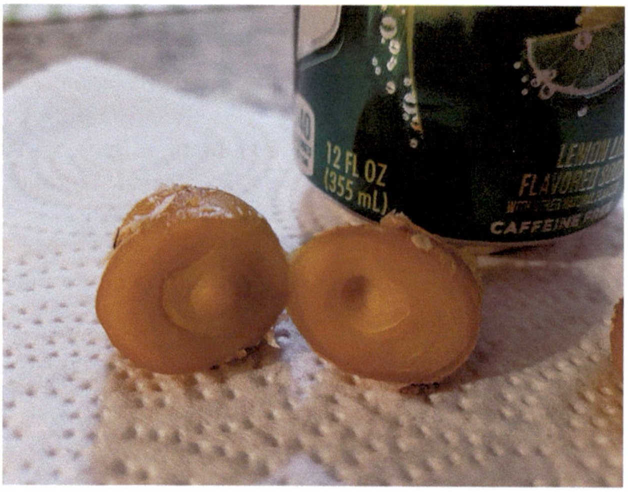

Figure 10.13 "Lash egg" is the common name for salpingitis. This "egg" was naturally passed by a hen who later died from this chronic condition. Courtesy of Sarah Meyer.

10.4.1.4 Diagnostic Testing

- **Palpation**
  Thickened oviduct or coelomic masses.
- **Imaging**
  Ultrasonography can show fluid accumulation, thickened oviduct walls, or retained eggs/yolk. Radiology may reveal abnormal oviduct silhouette, soft tissue masses, or fluid.
- **Culture**
  Swabs from the oviduct, cloaca, or exudate cultured for *E. coli, Salmonella, Mycoplasma,* and other bacteria. Helps confirm causative agents and guide antimicrobial choice.
- **Cytology of Exudate**
  Reveals inflammatory cells (heterophils, macrophages) and bacteria.

10.4.1.5 Treatment and Therapeutic Interventions

- **Supportive Care**
  High-quality feed, vitamins (especially vitamins A and E to support mucosal health), and electrolytes. Reduce stress, provide warmth, isolate from other birds during treatment.
- **Surgical or Manual Intervention**
  In severe, chronic cases where the oviduct is filled with concealed exudate or eggs, manual evacuation of caseous material under general anesthesia or salpingectomy may be attempted though it carries a risk and is not commonly performed. Requires advanced avian surgical expertise.
- **Medications**
  Broad-spectrum antibiotics (enrofloxacin, amoxicillin, or tetracyclines) and anti-inflammatories (meloxicam).
- **Hormonal Therapy**
  To suppress further ovulation during recovery, deslorelin acetate hormone implants can cease ovulation and allow the oviduct to rest and heal. This can help prevent recurrence while underlying infection is treated. This intervention is controversial and may be prohibited in some states and countries since the chicken is classified as a food animal.

10.4.1.6 Prevention and Control

- **Flock Management and Husbandry**
  Sanitation of enclosures, vent protection, and stress reduction can help prevent.

- **Nutritional Support**
  Adequate calcium, phosphorus, and vitamin D3 to reduce soft-shelled eggs. Vitamin A for mucosal integrity, vitamin E and selenium for immune defense, and balanced protein for tissue repair.
- **Disease Prevention and Biosecurity**
  Vaccination against IBV is available. Control human traffic, disinfect footwear/equipment, and 30-day quarantine new birds before introduction. Manage internal and external parasites to reduce overall immune suppression.
- **Breeding and Genetic Strategies**
  Choose breeds less prone to reproductive tract infections and abnormalities.
- **Monitoring and Early Intervention**
  Watch for reduced egg production, abnormal eggs (thin shells, misshapen), coelomic swelling, or signs of depression. Address egg binding, prolapse, or internal laying quickly before secondary infection occurs.

10.4.1.7 Nursing Considerations

Nursing care for chickens affected by salpingitis centers on prompt intervention, supportive therapy, and prevention of complications associated with this painful reproductive tract infection. Birds should be closely monitored for signs such as lethargy, decreased appetite, reduced egg production, abnormal or retained eggs, straining, and coelom distension, as these may indicate worsening inflammation or infection. Affected hens should be immediately isolated in a clean, dry, and quiet environment to reduce stress, prevent bullying, and allow close observation of food and water intake as well as droppings. Providing a balanced, nutrient-dense diet rich in calcium, protein, and vitamins supports recovery and immune function, while ensuring constant access to clean, fresh water helps maintain hydration. Nursing care also involves maintaining good hygiene to prevent secondary infections and assisting with gentle handling to avoid exacerbating pain or rupturing infected tissue. Collaboration with the veterinarian is essential for appropriate antimicrobial therapy, anti-inflammatory treatment, and drainage or surgical removal of retained egg material if needed or elected. Overall, nursing considerations emphasize supportive care, stress reduction, infection control, and close monitoring to improve outcomes and support recovery from salpingitis.

10.4.2 Egg Yolk Peritonitis

10.4.2.1 Overview and Pathogenesis

EYP is a common reproductive disorder in laying hens characterized by the accumulation of yolk material in the coelom cavity, often associated with secondary bacterial infection. This disorder is subsequent to internal laying. The condition primarily affects older hens and high-producing layers, with economic significance due to reduced egg production, decreased feed efficiency, poor body condition, and increased mortality in severe cases. EYP is not directly infectious but is frequently associated with opportunistic bacteria, such as *E. coli*, *Staphylococcus* spp., and *Streptococcus* spp., which exacerbate inflammation and systemic illness. Predisposing factors include ovarian or oviductal dysfunction, reproductive organ trauma, delayed oviposition, endocrine (hormone) imbalances, nutritional deficiencies, and immunosuppression, often in combination with poor husbandry or environmental stressors. Clinically, affected hens may exhibit coelomic distension, lethargy, anorexia, ruffled feathers, decreased egg production, and sometimes sudden death. It must be noted that sudden death is a misnomer; death occurs due to missed clinical signs.

The pathogenesis of EYP begins when yolk is released into the abdominal cavity instead of entering the oviduct, a phenomenon known as internal laying. Free yolk acts as an excellent medium for bacterial proliferation, facilitating secondary infection by opportunistic pathogens that enter via the cloaca, reproductive system, or bloodstream. The presence of yolk and bacterial invasion triggers inflammatory responses, leading to fibrinous exudation, adhesion formation, and accumulation of purulent fluid in the coelomic cavity. Chronic or recurrent cases result in peritoneal fibrosis, organ adhesion, and systemic illness, which impair nutrient absorption, reproductive performance, and overall health. Overall, EYP is a secondary, opportunistic inflammatory condition in which misplaced yolk, bacterial infection, and host inflammatory responses converge to produce abdominal inflammation, decreased productivity, and potential mortality in affected hens.

10.4.2.2 Risk Factors

- **Reproductive and Physiological Factors**
  Modern high-production breeds (especially commercial layers) are predisposed due to frequent ovulations. Malformations, scarring, or adhesions in the oviduct can prevent normal yolk capture. Yolk misses the oviduct and ends up in the coelom, triggering inflammatory response. Older hens have cumulative reproductive organ fatigue and higher incidence of oviductal disease.
- **Infectious Predispositions**
  E. coli (most common), *Salmonella* spp., *Mycoplasma* spp., *Staphylococcus* spp. ascend from the cloaca or spread systemically. IBV damages the oviduct, predisposing to egg misplacement and secondary bacterial infection.
- **Nutritional Factors**
  Calcium, vitamin D3, vitamin A, and vitamin E deficiency.
- **Environmental and Husbandry Factors**
  Fecal contamination introduces bacteria that can ascend the cloaca. Stress and competition for nest boxes lead to rushed or abnormal laying. Heat stress, transport, or predator threats lower immune function.

10.4.2.3 Clinical Signs and Pathology

- **External Findings**
  Lethargy, depression, reluctance to move, pain elicited from handling, ruffled feathers, unkempt appearance, anorexia, weight loss, dehydration, and pale or shrunken comb and wattles. Reduced or cessation of egg production, soft-shelled, shell-less, or misshapen eggs. Distended, firm, or fluctuant coelomic cavity. Penguin-like stance or waddling gait due to abdominal distention and discomfort. Open-mouth breathing, tail-bobbing, increased respiratory effort (due to pressure on air sacs from coelomic fluid accumulation). Collapse and death (in acute peritonitis with sepsis).
- **Necropsy Findings**
  Yellow to orange, pasty or liquid, often mixed with fibrin and cellular debris. Fibrinous or caseous exudate covering serosal surfaces (liver, intestines, oviduct, peritoneum). Thickened, inflamed peritoneum and serosal tissues. Yolk adhered to organs, forming adhesions between intestines, ovary, and abdominal wall. Ovary and oviduct may show active follicular regression, rupture, or hemorrhage.

10.4.2.4 Diagnostic Testing

- **Diagnostic Imaging**
  Ultrasonography is more sensitive than radiographs for coelomic fluid and soft tissue changes. Echogenic coelomic fluid with suspended particles, echogenic strands, and adherent masses or yolk clumps. Useful for guiding coelomic fluid aspiration (abdominocentesis).

Radiographs may reveal soft tissue opacity in coelomic cavity, loss of normal organ detail from fluid or inflammatory exudate. Can help rule out other causes (eggs bound in oviduct, neoplasia, ascites from cardiac and/or liver disease).

- **Coelomic Fluid Analysis (Abdominocentesis)**
  Gross appearance: yellow-orange, viscous, opaque. Cytology reveals high protein content, yolk globules, cholesterol clefts, degenerate heterophils, macrophages, and possible intracellular bacteria.
- **Bloodwork**
  Nonspecific inflammatory pattern leukocytosis, hyperglobulinemia, and anemia of chronic disease. Elevated liver enzymes if hepatic involvement.

10.4.2.5 Treatment and Therapeutic Interventions

- **Supportive Care**
  Fluid therapy (oral, subcutaneous, or IV) to correct dehydration and support circulation. Thermal support keeps patients warm and in a quiet, stress-free environment. Probiotics to help maintain gut flora during antibiotic use. Pain management alleviates discomfort.
- **Surgical Interventions**
  Salpingohysterectomy. Definitive but invasive option in valuable birds or chronic recurrent cases. Requires advanced avian surgical expertise and general anesthesia. The ovary is usually left in place (difficult to remove), so hormonal implant therapy is often still needed post-operatively.
- **Abdominocentesis**
  Can provide temporary relief if significant coelomic fluid is present. Always combined with antibiotics fluid reaccumulates without addressing the underlying cause.
- **Medications**
  Meloxicam 0.5 mg/kg by mouth or intramuscularly every 12–24 hours.
  Carprofen 5–10 mg/kg by mouth or intramuscularly once daily.
  Trimethoprim-sulfamethoxazole 100 mg/kg by mouth every 12 hours for 5–7 days.
  Oxytetracycline 5 mg/kg subcutaneously or intramuscularly every 12–24 hours. 2500 mg/L drinking water and 2500 mg/kg feed.
  Deslorelin Acetate Implants
  Suppresses ovulation to prevent further yolk release and allow inflammation to resolve.

10.4.2.6 Prevention and Control

- **Husbandry and Environmental Management**
  Provide clean, dry, and well-ventilated housing to reduce bacterial load and stress. Prevent overcrowding (avoid competition, pecking injuries, stress-induced ovulation problems). Avoid sudden changes in lighting, feed, or environment. Reduce stress by handling birds gently and reducing predator threats or loud disturbances. Chickens like routine and familiarity.
- **Nutritional Management**
  Balanced layer diet with correct levels of protein, energy, and essential fatty acids. Calcium, phosphorus, and vitamin D3 for shell quality. Vitamins A and E for epithelial and immune health. Preventing obesity, overweight hens have a higher rate of reproductive tract disorders. Ensure constant access to clean water; dehydration predisposes hens to reproductive problems.
- **Reproductive Management**
  Avoid excessive reproductive cycling; use hormonal implants in chronic internal layers or birds not intended for breeding. Selectively breed for reproductive health; avoid breeding from hens with a history of internal laying or reproductive tract disease.

- **Infectious Disease Control and Biosecurity**
  Prevent the introduction of pathogenic bacteria (notably *E. coli*, *Salmonella*). Quarantine new birds for 30 days.

10.4.2.7 Nursing Considerations

Nursing care for chickens with EYP focuses on supportive management, infection control, and comfort care, as this condition can rapidly become life-threatening if not addressed promptly. Affected birds should be monitored closely for signs such as lethargy, fluffed feathers, decreased appetite, reduced egg production, coelomic distension, and labored breathing caused by fluid and inflammation within the coelomic cavity. They should be housed in a clean, warm, quiet, and stress-free environment to promote rest and reduce metabolic demands, while being isolated from the flock to prevent bullying and allow diligent observation of food and water intake as well as droppings. Providing a high-quality, easily digestible diet with balanced protein, vitamins, and minerals supports overall health and immune function, and ensuring constant access to clean, fresh water helps maintain hydration. Gentle handling is important to prevent rupture of fragile tissues or worsening internal inflammation. Nursing care also involves prompt veterinary involvement for diagnostic evaluation, fluid drainage if ascites is present, and administration of systemic antibiotics, anti-inflammatory agents, and supportive therapy as prescribed. Overall, nursing considerations emphasize close observation, stress reduction, hygiene, supportive nutrition, and timely veterinary collaboration to improve comfort and recovery potential in birds with EYP.

10.4.3 Pullorum Disease

10.4.3.1 Overview and Pathogenesis

Pullorum disease is a highly contagious systemic bacterial infection of poultry caused by Salmonella enterica subsp. Enterica serovar *Pullorum*, a Gram-negative, nonmotile bacterium closely related to *S. gallinarum*. The disease predominantly affects young chicks under 3 weeks of age, although older birds may act as asymptomatic carriers, making it a significant concern for poultry production. Pullorum disease is important due to high mortality in young chicks, poor growth, decreased hatchability, reduced flock productivity, and the risk of persistent environmental contamination. Transmission occurs mainly via vertical infection through contaminated eggs, but horizontal spread through feces, litter, feed, water, and contaminated equipment is also possible. Clinically, affected chicks often present with weakness, depression, huddling, pasty vent, anorexia, dehydration, and sudden death, whereas older carrier birds may appear clinically normal yet perpetuate the infection.

The pathogenesis of pullorum disease begins with oral ingestion of the bacteria, which colonizes the intestinal mucosa and invades M cells of the gut-associated lymphoid tissue (GALT). After breaching the intestinal barrier, *S. pullorum* enters the bloodstream, causing systemic bacteremia and dissemination to organs such as the liver, spleen, lungs, and yolk sac in young chicks. Virulence factors, including invasins, endotoxins, and intracellular survival mechanisms, allow the bacterium to evade host defenses and persist within macrophages and reticuloendothelial tissues. The resulting inflammation, organ necrosis, and tissue damage contribute to clinical signs and high mortality. Older birds that recover or remain subclinical carriers may intermittently shed the bacteria via feces or eggs, facilitating environmental persistence and new infections. Overall, pullorum disease is a systemic septicemic bacterial disease in which intestinal invasion, bacteremia, and organ colonization lead to severe mortality in young chicks, chronic carrier states in adults, and substantial economic losses in poultry operations.

10.4.3.2 Risk Factors

- **Host-Related Factors**
  Pullorum disease primarily affects young chicks (high mortality within the first 2–3 weeks). Fowl typhoid can affect all ages, but more severe in young growing birds and adults. Chicks with poor maternal antibody transfer (from unvaccinated or infected hens) are at higher risk. No strong breed predisposition, but commercial meat or egg breeds with high-density production are more affected.
- **Environmental and Management Factors**
  Eggs laid by carrier hens may contain bacteria, and infected chicks hatch already infected. Fecal-oral spread via contaminated litter, feed, water, or equipment. Inadequate cleaning and disinfection of housing and equipment increases bacterial load. Older carrier birds can transmit bacteria to susceptible chicks. Transport, handling, temperature fluctuations, and nutritional deficiencies can predispose birds to infection.
- **Epidemiological Factors**
  Bringing new or untested birds into the flock increases risk. Poorly sanitized incubators and egg-handling equipment serve as reservoirs. Backyard flocks in regions with a history of Pullorum Disease have higher risk if biosecurity is lax.

10.4.3.3 Clinical Signs

- **External Findings**
  Sudden death without premonitory signs. Weakness, depression, and lethargy. White, pasty diarrhea ("white diarrhea"). Poor growth or stunted development.
- **Necropsy Findings**
  The liver is enlarged, pale, or mottled with necrotic foci. The spleen is enlarged and congested. The heart has pericardial congestion and edema. The lungs are congested and edematous. The kidneys are enlarged and pale. Joints have swelling, inflammation, and sometimes fibrinous exudate in chronic cases. The gastrointestinal tract is enlarged and congested with fibrinous exudate and Peyer's patches may show necrosis.

10.4.3.4 Diagnostic Testing

- **Culture**
  Liver, spleen, heart, yolk sac, cecal tonsils (from necropsy). Cloacal swabs (from live birds, especially young chicks).
- **PCR**
  Detect *S. pullorum* DNA from tissues or swabs. Faster and more sensitive than culture.

10.4.3.5 Treatment and Therapeutic Interventions

- **No Effective Treatment:** eradication and depopulation are recommended. Supportive antibiotics may temporarily reduce signs but do not eliminate infection.

10.4.3.6 Prevention and Control

- **Biosecurity Measures**
  Limit visitors and enforce footbaths, protective clothing, and hand hygiene. Quarantine new birds for 30–45 days and test for S. pullorum before introduction if possible. Disinfect equipment, feeders, drinkers, and housing regularly. Rodent and wild bird control as these animals can harbor and spread *Salmonella*.
- **Flock Monitoring and Testing**
  Cloacal swabs or tissue sampling in suspect birds.

10.4.3.7 Nursing Considerations

Nursing care for chickens affected by Pullorum disease focuses on strict biosecurity, supportive care, and regulatory compliance, as this condition, caused by *Salmonella pullorum*, is highly contagious and vertically transmitted. Affected birds, especially young chicks, should be immediately isolated from the rest of the flock to prevent further spread, and caretakers must implement rigorous hygiene measures, including disinfecting equipment, washing hands, wearing dedicated footwear and clothing, and preventing cross-contamination between sick and healthy birds. The environment should be kept warm, clean, and dry, as chicks are vulnerable to chilling and stress, which can worsen clinical signs. Birds should be closely monitored for lethargy, white pasty diarrhea, drooping wings, and poor growth, and supportive care should include readily accessible clean water, electrolyte supplementation, and easily digestible, nutrient-rich feed to help maintain strength and hydration. Nursing responsibilities also involve prompt notification of veterinarian or state agricultural authorities, as Pullorum Disease is a reportable disease, and assisting with testing or flock eradication programs if required. Because survivors may become lifelong carriers, culling of infected birds is often recommended, and veterinary technicians should provide compassionate handling to minimize stress and suffering. Overall, nursing considerations center on infection control, supportive management, environmental hygiene, careful monitoring, and compliance with control regulations to protect both the affected birds and the rest of the flock.

10.4.4 Fowl Typhoid

10.4.4.1 Overview and Pathogenesis

Fowl typhoid is a systemic bacterial disease of poultry caused by *Salmonella enterica* subspecies enterica serovar *Gallinarum*, a Gram-negative, nonmotile, facultatively anaerobic bacterium. The disease primarily affects adult chickens and layers, though birds of all ages can be susceptible, and is significant due to high mortality, decreased egg production, and inhibited growth. Transmission occurs via the fecal-oral route, through contaminated feed, water, litter, equipment, and by vertical transmission from infected parent birds to progeny via eggs. Clinically, affected birds may exhibit depression, ruffled feathers, anorexia, diarrhea, dehydration, anemia, and sudden death, with chronic cases showing poor growth and reduced egg production.

The pathogenesis of fowl typhoid begins with ingestion of the bacterium, which colonizes the intestinal epithelium and invades M cells of the GALT. Following translocation across the intestinal barrier, *S. Gallinarum* enters the bloodstream, leading to bacteremia and systemic dissemination of the liver, spleen, bone marrow, and other organs. Virulence factors, including invasins, endotoxins, and survival mechanisms within macrophages, enable the bacterium to evade host defenses and persist in reticuloendothelial tissues. The resulting inflammatory response and tissue damage contribute to clinical signs such as organomegaly, necrosis, and hemorrhages in visceral organs. Chronic carriers may shed the bacterium intermittently, perpetuating environmental contamination and transmission. Overall, fowl typhoid is a systemic septicemic bacterial disease in which intestinal invasion, bacteremia, and organ colonization lead to high morbidity, mortality, and production losses in large flocks.

10.4.4.2 Risk Factors

- **Host-Related Factors**
  Older chicks, juveniles, and adult chickens are susceptible; disease is uncommon in neonates. Birds stressed by disease, poor nutrition, or immunosuppression are at higher risk.

- **Environmental and Management Factors**
  Contaminated litter, feeders, drinkers, and housing increase bacterial exposure. Transport, mishandling, temperature fluctuations, and nutritional deficiencies predispose birds to infection.
- **Epidemiological and External Factors**
  Bringing new, untested birds into a flock can introduce Fowl typhoid. Feed or water contaminated with *S. gallinarum* is a major source of infection. Flocks in regions with a history of fowl typhoid are at increased risk if biosecurity is lax. Wild birds and rodents can act as mechanical vectors for bacteria.

10.4.4.3 Clinical Signs and Pathology

- **External Findings**
  Sudden onset of depression, weakness, and lethargy. Reduced feed and water intake. Pale combs and wattles; sometimes cyanosis is noted.
- **Necropsy Findings**
  The liver is enlarged, friable, dark bronze or greenish, with necrotic foci. The spleen is enlarged and congested. Kidneys are swollen, pale, with urate deposition in chronic cases. Pericardial congestion and occasional fibrinous exudate. Ovarian and oviductal congestion, follicular atresia, or oviduct inflammation. The gallbladder is distended and thickened in some birds.

10.4.4.4 Diagnostic Testing

- **Culture**
  Liver, spleen, heart, kidney, gallbladder, and cecal tonsils (from necropsy). Cloacal swabs from live birds. Plating on XLD (Xylose Lysine Deoxycholate) or Brilliant Green Sulfa (BGS) agar.
- **PCR**
  Detects *S. gallinarum* DNA in tissues, swabs, or environmental samples. Highly sensitive and rapid, useful for carrier detection and outbreak confirmation.

10.4.4.5 Treatment and Therapeutic Interventions

- **Supportive Care**
  Easily digestible, energy-dense feed; small frequent meals if birds are weak. Assisted feeding if indicated. Maintain warm, dry, and low-stress housing.
- **Medication**
  Reduce bacterial load, treat septicemia, and prevent secondary infections. Tetracyclines, sulfonamides, and amoxicillin are commonly used.

10.4.4.6 Prevention and Control

- **Biosecurity Measures**
  Limit visitors; enforce footbaths, personal protection equipment, and hand hygiene. Quarantine new birds for 30 days; test before introduction if possible. Regularly clean and disinfect housing, feeders, drinkers, and equipment.

10.4.4.7 Nursing Considerations

Nursing care for chickens affected by fowl typhoid, caused by *S. gallinarum,* centers on strict biosecurity, supportive management, and adherence to regulatory control measures, as the disease is highly contagious and can cause high mortality, especially in adult birds. Affected chickens should be promptly isolated from the flock to prevent transmission, and all caretakers should practice meticulous hygiene and disinfection protocols, including cleaning and sanitizing housing, feeders, and waterers, as well as using dedicated clothing and footwear to avoid cross-contamination. The birds should be kept in a clean, warm, and stress-free environment to support their immune system, with easy access to clean water and highly palatable, nutrient-rich food to prevent dehydration and weight loss. Veterinary nursing staff must observe birds closely for signs of lethargy, anorexia, diarrhea, pale combs, and sudden deaths, and provide supportive measures such as electrolytes and vitamin-enriched nutritional support to improve resilience during illness. Because fowl typhoid is a reportable disease, veterinary technicians also play a vital role in reporting suspected cases to the veterinarian or state agricultural authorities and assisting with diagnostic testing or flock eradication programs. Survivors often become chronic carriers, so nursing duties may include assisting in humane euthanasia procedures as recommended by veterinarians to prevent further spread of disease. Overall, nursing considerations emphasize infection control, supportive care, vigilant monitoring, stress reduction, and regulatory compliance to protect the health of both affected and at-risk birds.

10.5 Prevention and Client Education

Reproductive diseases in chickens represent a major source of morbidity, mortality, and decreased productivity in backyard flocks. Disorders range from noninfectious conditions such as egg binding and internal laying to infectious diseases like salpingitis, egg peritonitis, and viral infections. If vaccines are available, veterinarians can administer or recommend them to backyard flock guardians.

Ultimately, success in managing reproductive disease depends on a combination of early detection, appropriate veterinary medical or surgical interventional therapy, proper nutrition, and strong preventive husbandry practices. The education of clients about early signs of reproductive disease, zoonotic risks, and the importance of veterinary consultation completes the collaborative effort to maintain healthy chickens.

Further Reading

AnimalDVM LLC. Signs of Reproductive Disease in Hens Infographic [Internet]. PoultryDVM. Signs of Reproductive Disease in Hens Infographic; 2024 [cited 2025 Dec 8]. Available from: https://www.poultrydvm.com/featured-infographic/signs-of-reproductive-disease-in-chickens

Greenacre CB. Reproductive diseases of the backyard hen. *Journal of Exotic Pet Medicine*. 2015 Apr;24(2):164–171.

Most Prevalent Reproductive Diseases in Chickens [Internet]. Dvm360.com. dvm360; 2018 [cited 2025 Dec 8]. Available from: https://www.dvm360.com/view/most-prevalent-reproductive-diseases-in-chickens

Reproductive Tract Disease in Chickens – Bird Vet Melbourne [Internet]. Bird-vet.com. 2025. Available from: https://www.bird-vet.com/ReproductiveTractDiseaseinChickens.aspx

Reproductive Diseases of Pet Birds – Exotic and Laboratory Animals [Internet]. MSD Veterinary Manual. Available from: https://www.msdvetmanual.com/exotic-and-laboratory-animals/pet-birds/reproductive-diseases-of-pet-birds

11

Viral, Bacterial, and Fungal Diseases

11.1 Infectious Diseases of Chickens: Viral, Bacterial, and Fungal Etiologies

Chickens (*Gallus gallus domesticus*) are susceptible to a wide range of infectious diseases caused by viruses, bacteria, and fungi. These pathogens affect not only the health and welfare of individual birds but also flock productivity, food safety, and public health. Backyard flocks are increasingly common, which expands the role of veterinary professionals in diagnosing, treating, and preventing disease in small-scale settings.

For chickens, infectious diseases are often present in clusters, with overlapping respiratory, gastrointestinal, reproductive, and systemic clinical signs. Because many pathogens are highly contagious and some are reportable (e.g., Newcastle disease [ND], highly pathogenic avian influenza [HPAI]), prompt recognition and appropriate response are critical.

This chapter reviews viral, bacterial, and fungal diseases in chickens, emphasizing

- **Clinical signs** recognizable to veterinary technicians and guardians
- **Diagnostic testing** methods accessible in practice
- **Treatment**, including medications where feasible
- **Nursing considerations**, such as supportive care and client education

Frequently, vaccination as a preventive measure is mentioned throughout this chapter. Again, it must be noted that vaccines are not readily available to backyard flocks unless the guardian acquired chicks from a commercial hatchery or National Poultry Improvement Plan (NPIP)-certified breeder. Guardians are encouraged to purchase vaccinated birds or hatching eggs from NPIP-certified providers. This is discussed further in Chapter 1. By the end of this chapter, veterinary technicians should be able to support veterinarians in triaging cases, implementing biosecurity, administering treatments, and providing flock guardians with clear guidance. Education regarding the zoonotic potential of some of the viral, bacterial, and fungal diseases discussed in this text must occur as the veterinary professional's duty to public health. Veterinary professionals consult the National List of Reportable Animal Disease, which is updated annually. https://www.aphis.usda.gov/livestock-poultry-disease/surveillance/reportable-diseases?page=1

There are currently 65 National Animal Health Laboratory Network-approved laboratories in the United States. This network provides diagnostics for disease surveillance, disease event response, and communication with veterinarians regarding diagnostic outcomes for veterinarians (https://www.aphis.usda.gov/labs/nahln/approved-labs/all-labs).

Veterinary reference laboratories offer poultry disease testing as well. Examples include

IDEXX Poultry Diagnostics https://www.idexx.com/en/livestock/livestock-tests/poultry-tests/

Each state's department of agriculture provides testing resources or can guide veterinary healthcare teams in specimen collection, testing procedures, and shipping details.

11.2 Viral Diseases of Chickens

Viral diseases remain the most impactful category in poultry medicine, as most lack curative treatments and are best managed through preventive measures and strict biosecurity (Table 11.1).

11.3 Newcastle Disease (Avian Paramyxovirus-1)

11.3.1 Overview and Pathogenesis

Newcastle disease (ND) is a highly contagious viral disease of poultry caused by avian paramyxovirus type 1 (APMV-1), a single-stranded, negative-sense RNA virus of the family *Paramyxoviridae*. The disease affects chickens of all ages and other avian species, with considerable economic importance due to high mortality, decreased egg production, poor growth, and trade restrictions. ND viruses are classified based on virulence into velogenic (highly pathogenic), mesogenic (moderately pathogenic), and lentogenic (low pathogenic) strains. Transmission occurs via direct contact with infected birds, respiratory secretions, feces, contaminated equipment, feed, water, and fomites, and virus spread is facilitated by wild birds. Clinically, ND may present as respiratory signs (coughing, sneezing, nasal discharge), neurological signs (tremors, paralysis, torticollis), gastrointestinal signs (diarrhea), decreased egg production, and sudden death, depending on the virulence of the strain.

The pathogenesis of ND begins with infection of the respiratory or gastrointestinal epithelium following exposure to the virus. Velogenic strains replicate rapidly in epithelial cells and subsequently spread systemically via the bloodstream and lymphoid tissues, causing widespread infection. Virulence is largely determined by the cleavage site of the viral fusion (F) protein, which dictates the ability of the virus to infect multiple tissues. Viral replication induces cellular necrosis, vascular damage, and inflammatory responses, leading to edema, hemorrhages, and organ dysfunction. In velogenic neurotropic forms, the virus invades the central nervous system, producing neurological signs such as ataxia, paralysis, and torticollis. The host immune response contributes to tissue damage through cytokine release and inflammatory cell infiltration. Overall, ND is a systemic, multiorgan viral disease in which viral replication, tissue tropism, and host immune responses converge to produce respiratory, neurological, gastrointestinal, and reproductive pathology, often resulting in high mortality and severe economic losses in poultry flocks.

11.3.2 Risk Factors

- **Host-Related Factors**
  All ages are susceptible, but young birds often suffer more. Immunocompromised or stressed birds are more susceptible. Poor maternal antibody transfer in chicks increases vulnerability. High-production commercial egg layers and meat birds are at increased risk due to intense production cycles. Unvaccinated or improperly vaccinated birds are highly susceptible.

Table 11.1

Quick reference chart				Disease	Causative agent
Transmission	**Key clinical signs**	**Diagnostic testing**	**Treatment**	**Newcastle disease (NDV)**	**Avian paramyxovirus-1**
Aerosol, direct contact, fomites, wild birds	Respiratory distress, nasal discharge, coughing, neurologic signs (torticollis, paralysis), ↓ egg production	Virus isolation, RT-PCR, HI test, ELISA, AGID	No specific; supportive care	Infectious bronchitis (IB)	Coronavirus
Aerosol, direct contact, fomites, contaminated equipment	Sneezing, coughing, rales, watery eyes, ↓ egg production, misshapen eggs	Virus isolation in embryos, RT-PCR, ELISA serology	No specific; supportive care, warmth, reduce stress	Infectious bursal disease (IBD/Gumboro)	Birnavirus (serotype 1)
Fecal–oral, contaminated litter, fomites	Depression, ruffled feathers, trembling, high morbidity, mortality in young chicks (3–6 wks)	Histopathology of bursa, AGID, ELISA, RT-PCR	No specific; supportive care, reduce stress	Marek's disease	Gallid herpesvirus-2
Inhalation of feather dander, long environmental persistence	Progressive paralysis, wing/leg paresis, wasting, grey eye (ocular form), tumors	Histopathology, PCR, immunohistochemistry	No treatment	Avian leukosis	Avian leukosis virus (ALV)
Vertical (egg), horizontal (fecal–oral, contact)	Wasting, anemia, decreased egg production, tumors (liver, spleen, kidneys)	ELISA, virus isolation, PCR, histopathology	No treatment	Fowl pox	Avipoxvirus
Mosquito vectors, skin abrasions, aerosols (wet form)	Cutaneous scabs on comb/wattles (dry form); diphtheritic lesions in mouth/trachea (wet form); ↓ production	Histopathology (Bollinger bodies), PCR, virus isolation	No specific; supportive care, reduce secondary infection	Avian influenza (AI)	Influenza A virus
Aerosols, feces, fomites, wild waterfowl	Respiratory distress, cyanosis, edema, ↓ production, sudden death (HPAI)	RT-PCR, virus isolation, serology (HI, AGID), sequencing	No treatment; depopulation for HPAI	Chicken infectious anemia (CIA)	Gyrovirus
Vertical, horizontal (fecal–oral, contaminated surfaces)	Anemia, pallor, depression, immunosuppression, growth retardation	PCR, histopathology, virus isolation	No treatment; supportive	Laryngotracheitis (ILT)	Gallid herpesvirus-1
Aerosol, contaminated equipment, carrier birds	Coughing, gasping, bloody mucus, nasal discharge, reduced productivity	Histopathology (intranuclear inclusions), PCR, virus isolation	No specific; supportive, reduce stress	Swollen head syndrome	Avian metapneumovirus + secondary bacteria (e.g., *E. coli*)
Aerosol, direct contact	Periorbital swelling, sinusitis, torticollis, ↓ egg production	Virus isolation, PCR, ELISA	No specific antiviral; supportive + antibiotics for secondary infection		

Courtesy of Stephanie Freeman.

- **Management and Environmental Factors**
  Poor ventilation and housing conditions. Older birds may act as reservoirs, exposing younger susceptible birds. Mixed species farms such as turkeys, pigeons, and wild birds may harbor and transmit NDV.
- **Epidemiological and External Factors**
  Movement of birds without quarantine. Shared equipment, vehicles, feed sacks, footwear, and clothing from infected sites. Migratory waterfowls, feral pigeons, and other wild birds can carry APMV-1. High traffic and mixing of birds from different sources increase exposure risk.

11.3.3 Clinical Signs

- **External Findings**
  Coughing, sneezing, dyspnea, rales, nasal and ocular discharge. Tremors, torticollis, opisthotonus, paralysis, ataxia, and circling behavior. Greenish, watery diarrhea, sudden drop in feed and water consumption, severe depression, lethargy, cyanosis, and edema of combs and wattles. Sharp drop in egg production, production of thin-shelled, soft-shelled, or misshapen eggs, and poor internal egg quality (watery albumen, mottled yolks).
- **Necropsy Findings**
  Congested, edematous trachea and lungs. Mucus or hemorrhage in the trachea. Cloudy, thickened air sacs, often with caseous or fibrinous exudate (especially if complicated by bacteria). Hemorrhages in the proventriculus are one of the most characteristic lesions of ND. Hemorrhages may also be present in the intestinal tract, especially at the ileocecal junction, cecal tonsils, and Peyer's patches.

11.3.4 Diagnostic Testing – Reference Laboratory

- **RT-PCR (Reverse Transcription Polymerase Chain Reaction)**
  Detects NDV RNA from tracheal/cloacal swabs, tissues (trachea, lungs, brain, spleen, cecal tonsils). Rapid, sensitive, and highly specific. Can differentiate virulent versus avirulent strains using pathotyping assays.
- **Real-Time Quantitative RT-PCR (qRT-PCR)**
  Provides viral load quantification. Used during outbreaks for rapid screening.
- **LAMP (Loop-Mediated Isothermal Amplification)**
  Field-adaptable rapid molecular test for NDV detection.
- Reportable disease

11.3.5 Treatment and Therapeutic Interventions

Because ND is caused by avian avulavirus 1 (APMV-1), there is no specific antiviral treatment available. Management therefore focuses on supportive care, controlling secondary infections, and preventing further spread within and between flocks.

- **Supportive Care**
  On the farm/in the backyard, offer easily accessible clean water and oral electrolytes to counter dehydration from diarrhea and reduced intake. Ensure palatable, high-quality feed is offered to maintain energy intake in sick birds. Reduce stress by keeping birds warm, dry, and well-ventilated. Clinical treatment includes intravenous fluids, antibiotics for secondary bacterial infections, nutritional supplementation, a clean/warm/quiet environment, and a strict quarantine protocol. Minimize handling and disturbances.

11.3.6 Prevention and Control

- **Biosecurity Measures**
  Because NDV spreads rapidly through secretions, feces, equipment, and even windborne particles, biosecurity is the most critical defense.
- **Vaccination Programs**
  Vaccination (often occurs in commercial flocks) is the cornerstone of ND control but must be properly managed. Vaccine failures often result from poor administration, stress, maternal antibody interference, or mismatch with circulating strains. Vaccination is often not available for backyard flocks, so strict biosecurity must be practiced.
- **Management Practices**
  Proper ventilation, a reasonable number of birds in an enclosure, and temperature control. Dry, clean litter reduces viral persistence and bacterial co-infections. Avoid raising chickens alongside other bird species, i.e., turkeys, ducks, or pigeons.

11.3.7 Nursing Considerations

Nursing care for chickens affected by ND focuses on strict biosecurity, supportive management, and comfort care, as this viral infection is highly contagious and can cause severe respiratory, digestive, and neurological signs. Affected birds should be immediately isolated from the flock to prevent disease spread, and all caretakers should follow rigorous hygiene and disinfection protocols, including handwashing, use of dedicated clothing, and proper cleaning of equipment and housing. Birds should be kept in a warm, quiet, and stress-free environment to reduce metabolic demands and prevent exacerbation of clinical signs. Close monitoring is essential to monitor for progression of respiratory distress, diarrhea, or neurological symptoms such as tremors, paralysis, or torticollis, and to ensure birds are still able to access to and the ability to consume food and water. Offering easily accessible, palatable, and nutrient-rich feed and clean water can help maintain strength, though handfeeding or assisted hydration may be needed if neurological impairment is severe. Prompt reporting to veterinary authorities, as ND is a notifiable disease, and assisting veterinarians with diagnostic sampling and supportive treatments as necessary. Clinical treatment will require intensive nursing care and a strict isolation protocol. Because affected birds often deteriorate quickly, humane euthanasia may be recommended in severe cases to prevent suffering. Overall, nursing considerations emphasize infection control, intensive supportive care, stress reduction, careful monitoring, and regulatory compliance when managing chickens with ND.

11.4 Avian Influenza (AI)

11.4.1 Overview and Pathogenesis

Avian influenza (AI) is a highly contagious viral disease of poultry caused by avian influenza virus (AIV), an enveloped, single-stranded RNA virus of the family *Orthomyxoviridae*. The virus is classified into low pathogenicity (LPAI) and high pathogenicity (HPAI) strains based on the severity of clinical disease and mortality. AI affects chickens, turkeys, ducks, and other avian species, with major economic importance due to rapid flock mortality, production losses, trade restrictions, and zoonotic potential. Transmission occurs via direct contact with infected birds, contaminated fomites, feed, water, and aerosols, with wild waterfowl as natural reservoirs. Clinically, LPAI infections may be subclinical or mild, causing respiratory signs, decreased egg production, and mild diarrhea, whereas HPAI infections can lead to sudden death, severe respiratory distress, edema, cyanosis of combs and wattles, and hemorrhages in multiple organs.

The pathogenesis of AI begins with inhalation or ingestion of the virus, which initially infects respiratory and gastrointestinal epithelial cells. Viral replication in epithelial tissues leads to cellular damage, inflammation, and impaired barrier function, facilitating secondary infections. HPAI strains possess a multi-basic cleavage site in the hemagglutinin protein, allowing systemic viral spreading via the bloodstream and resulting in multiorgan hemorrhages, edema, and necrosis. Host immune responses, including cytokine release and infiltration of heterophils and lymphocytes, contribute to tissue pathology. The severity and clinical outcome depend on viral strain virulence, host age and immunity, and environmental stressors. Overall, AI is a highly pathogenic viral disease in which epithelial cell destruction, systemic viral dissemination, and immune-mediated damage lead to respiratory, gastrointestinal, and systemic lesions, rapid mortality, and significant economic impact in poultry flocks.

11.4.2 Risk Factors

- **Host-Related Factors**
  Young birds tend to show more severe clinical disease and higher mortality. Chickens and turkeys are highly susceptible, especially to highly pathogenic AI (HPAI). Incomplete or poor vaccination response (for LPAI in endemic areas).
- **Environmental Factors**
  Presence of wild birds (especially migratory waterfowl) as natural reservoirs and primary introducers of the AI virus. Virus survives longer in cool, moist environments.
- **Management and Biosecurity Factors**
  Poor housing and ventilation increase respiratory stress and susceptibility. Contaminated equipment, incubation egg trays, and clothing/footwear without disinfection can cause spread.

11.4.3 Clinical Signs and Pathology

- **External Findings**
  - *Low Pathogenic Avian Influenza (LPAI)*
    Often mild, sometimes subclinical. Respiratory signs are seen, such as coughing, sneezing, nasal discharge, and mild conjunctivitis. Drop in egg production or thin-shelled, soft-shelled, or misshapen eggs. Mortality is usually low, unless complicated by secondary infections.
  - *High Pathogenic Avian Influenza (HPAI)*
    Peracute Form
    Sudden death without prior clinical signs. Mortality can reach 80–100% within days.
    Acute Form
    Severe depression, huddling, and ruffled feathers. Cyanosis of comb, wattles, and legs. Edema of the head, face, and neck.
    Chronic Form
    Lower mortality but poor growth, persistent respiratory and egg production problems.
- **Necropsy Findings**
  - *Low Pathogenic Avian Influenza (LPAI)*
    Congestion of trachea, sinuses, and lungs. Mild airsacculitis (if complicated by bacteria). Catarrhal enteritis in some cases.

– *High Pathogenic Avian Influenza (HPAI)*
  Edema, congestion, and hemorrhages in multiple organs. Petechiae on serosal and mucosal surfaces. Cyanosis of combs, wattles, and shanks. Subcutaneous hemorrhages and edema, especially around head and neck. Congestion, edema, and hemorrhages in trachea and lungs. Hemorrhages in proventriculus and gizzard. Petechiae in the intestines and cecal tonsils. Enlarged, congested, and mottled spleen. Hepatomegaly with hemorrhages or necrotic foci. Renal adenopathy with paleness and urate deposits. Hemorrhagic and regressing ovaries. In some cases, encephalitis and congestion in the brain.

11.4.4 Diagnostic Testing—Reference Laboratory

- **Reverse Transcription Polymerase Chain Reaction (RT-PCR)**
  Detect viral RNA in clinical samples, highly sensitive and specific; can subtype (H and N).
- **Real-Time RT-PCR (rRT-PCR)**
  Quantitative version of RT-PCR. Used for rapid diagnosis and surveillance.
- Reportable disease

11.4.5 Treatment and Therapeutic Interventions

Because AI is a highly contagious and notifiable disease, there are no approved curative treatments for affected poultry. Management primarily focuses on eradicating infection, controlling spread, and intensive supportive care (only under strict isolation protocol). Euthanasia is advised.

- **Supportive Care**
  Fluids, electrolytes, warmth, and oxygen therapy (if respiratory signs are present). Isolation of affected birds to prevent spreading. Broad-spectrum antibiotics not to treat the virus, for secondary bacterial infections (e.g., *Escherichia coli or Mycoplasma gallisepticum*).

11.4.6 Prevention and Control

- **Biosecurity (Most Important Defense)**
  Keep chicken flock away from wetlands, wild waterfowl, and backyard birds. Use closed houses or netting to prevent wild bird entry. If AI is reported to be in the area, limit farm/yard access; use footbaths, yard-only boots, and clothing. Disinfect transport crates, egg trays, feeders, and waterers before use or if used with previous flocks. Avoid multi-age or mixed-species flocks.
- **Surveillance and Monitoring**
  Regular flock health checks for sudden mortality, cyanosis, or reduction in egg production. Serological and virological testing via a reference laboratory in endemic regions. AI (especially HPAI) is a notifiable disease; therefore, any suspicion must be reported to veterinary or state authorities.
- **Vaccination**
  Not universally used; depends on the country policy. Recombinant vector vaccines provide better cross-protection but still limited. Backyard flocks do not generally have access to the vaccine.

11.4.7 Nursing Considerations

Nursing considerations for birds with AI should focus on preventing disease spread, protecting human health, and supporting affected birds. Caregivers must implement strict biosecurity measures, including isolating infected birds, restricting movement of birds and equipment, and thoroughly disinfecting all housing areas and tools. Personal protective equipment (PPE) such as gloves, masks, and protective clothing should always be worn to reduce the risk of zoonotic transmission. Birds should be kept in a warm, quiet, and stress-free environment, with easy access to and ability to consume clean water and nutritious food to help maintain their strength. Intensive nursing care if the bird is in a clinical facility. Continuous monitoring for signs of deterioration, such as respiratory distress, neurological signs, or sudden death, is essential, and any suspected cases must be reported to veterinary and regulatory authorities immediately, as AI is a notifiable disease. Accurate documentation, strict adherence to quarantine protocols, and reinforcement of biosecurity practices are vital to control the outbreak and prevent future infections. Human euthanasia is always an option.

11.5 Avian Chlamydiosis

11.5.1 Overview and Pathogenesis

Avian chlamydiosis, caused by *Chlamydia psittaci*, is an important zoonotic bacterial infection that can affect a wide range of avian species, including chickens. The organism is an obligate intracellular bacterium with a biphasic life cycle consisting of infectious, environmentally resistant elementary bodies (EBs) and metabolically active reticulate bodies (RBs) that replicate within host cells. Transmission typically occurs through inhalation or ingestion of contaminated feces, feather dust, or respiratory secretions. Once inhaled, EBs are phagocytosed by epithelial cells and macrophages in the respiratory tract, where they transform into RBs and replicate within intracellular inclusions. The bacteria spread through the bloodstream, resulting in a systemic infection that can affect multiple organs, including the liver, spleen, lungs, and air sacs.

Pathogenesis is primarily due to intracellular replication, cellular lysis, and the associated inflammatory response, which leads to tissue damage, necrosis, and dissemination. In chickens, clinical expression can vary widely depending on strain virulence and host factors. Some birds remain asymptomatic carriers, intermittently shedding organisms, while others develop conjunctivitis, nasal discharge, dyspnea, diarrhea, lethargy, weight loss, and decreased egg production. Lesions often include airsacculitis, pericarditis, perihepatitis, and splenomegaly, reflecting systemic spread. Stressors such as overcrowding, concurrent infections, or transport can trigger recrudescence and increased shedding, contributing to flock outbreaks and zoonotic risk.

11.5.2 Risk Factors

- **Host-Related Factors**
  Young birds are more prone to clinical disease due to immature immunity. Older birds may carry subclinical infections and shed intermittently. Birds under stress, malnourished, or immunocompromised are at a higher risk of severe disease.
- **Environmental Factors**
  Accumulation of feces, dust, and feathers contaminated with *Chlamydia* increases transmission. Dense housing facilitates aerosol transmission and increases stress. Poorly ventilated cages or houses allow pathogen accumulation in dust and droppings. Chlamydia can survive longer in cool, damp environments, promoting environmental contamination.

- **Management Factors**
  Transport, handling, breeding, molt, or concurrent disease increases shedding and susceptibility. Bringing in infected or subclinical carriers without quarantine increases flock risk. Housing different bird species together can facilitate cross-species transmission. Shared feeders, waterers, or contaminated surfaces can serve as indirect sources of infection (Figure 11.1).

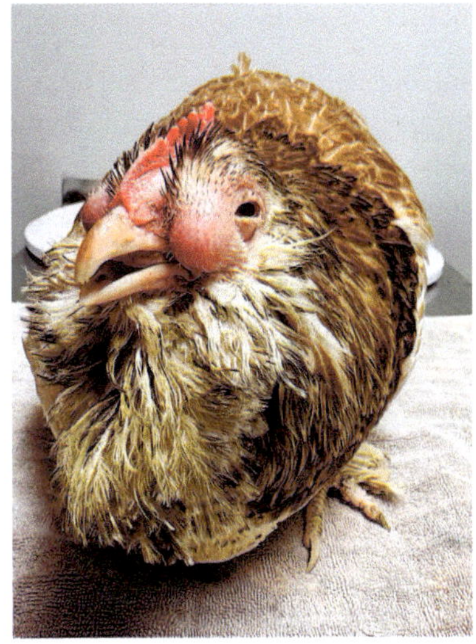

Figure 11.1 Severe sinus infection swelling. Courtesy of Funky Chicken Rescue.

11.5.3 Clinical Signs and Pathology

- **External Findings**
  Sneezing, nasal discharge, conjunctivitis, and dyspnea. Diarrhea, green or watery droppings. Lethargy, anorexia, weight loss, ruffled feathers, and dehydration. Severe cases may progress to hepatosplenomegaly, jaundice, and sudden death.
- **Necropsy Findings**
  Hepatomegaly, splenomegaly, pneumonia, air sacculitis, conjunctivitis, and sinusitis.

11.5.4 Diagnostic Testing—Reference Laboratory

- **ELISA**
  Detects antibodies, useful for flock screenings but cannot always differentiate active versus past infection.
- **PCR**
  Cloacal or choanal swabs, highly sensitive and specific. Detects organism even in subclinical carriers.
- Reportable disease

11.5.5 Treatment and Therapeutic Interventions

- **Supportive Care**
  Maintain hydration and nutrition. Reduce stress and overcrowding during treatment.
- **Medication**
  Oxytetracycline
  5 mg/kg subcutaneous or intramuscular every 12–24 hours. 2500 mg/L drinking water and 2500 mg/kg feed.

11.5.6 Prevention and Control

- **Environmental Management**
  Regular cleaning and disinfection of cages, perches, feeders, and waterers. Good ventilation to reduce aerosolized bacteria. Avoid damp conditions; remove wet litter or bedding promptly.
- **Flock Management**
  Quarantine new birds for at least 30 days with testing. Avoid mixing species prone to chlamydiosis with others. Reduce stress from transport, handling, or environmental changes.

11.5.7 Nursing Considerations

Nursing care for birds affected by avian chlamydiosis focuses on supporting the patient, preventing disease spread, and protecting human health, since *Chlamydia psittaci* is a significant zoonotic pathogen. Veterinary technicians should follow strict biosecurity and PPE protocols, including gloves, masks or respirators, and protective clothing when handling affected birds or contaminated materials. Infected or suspected birds should be isolated in a well-ventilated, low-stress environment, ideally with separate air handling if available. Enclosures and equipment must be thoroughly cleaned and disinfected with agents effective against *Chlamydia*, such as quaternary ammonium compounds, and litter should be carefully removed and disposed of to minimize aerosolization. Humane euthanasia is always an option.

11.6 Avian Leukosis

11.6.1 Overview and Pathogenesis

Avian leukosis is a group of neoplastic diseases in chickens caused by avian leukosis virus (ALV), a retrovirus in the *Alpharetrovirus* genus. These viruses are classified into several subgroups (A–J), with subgroups A, B, and J being most associated with disease in commercial poultry. Transmission occurs both vertically (from hen to chick via the egg) and horizontally (through close contact, contaminated equipment, or secretions). Vertical transmission, especially through infected hens shedding virus into the egg, is the most important route and results in congenitally infected chicks that may become persistent carriers. Horizontally infected birds usually develop transient viremia, often clearing the virus if exposure occurs after the development of immune competence. The likelihood of observing and diagnosing this virus in clinical practice is rare unless the bird originates from a commercial hatchery or production farm.

Pathogenesis depends on the age at infection, viral subgroup, and host immune status. In congenitally infected birds, the virus integrates into the host genome, leading to immune tolerance and persistent viremia, which allows the virus to replicate without immune clearance. Over time, viral insertion near host oncogenes can activate uncontrolled cell division, leading to neoplastic transformation, most commonly in the bursa of Fabricius, liver, spleen, and other lymphoid or parenchymal organs. The classic presentation is lymphoid leukosis, characterized by the development of discrete or diffuse lymphoid tumors in affected organs. Birds typically show progressive weight loss, loss of pallor, depression, reduced egg production, and sometimes sudden death. Gross lesions often include enlarged, pale livers with smooth nodules, splenomegaly, and tumor masses in various organs, without the bursal distortion typical of Marek's disease (MD).

11.6.2 Risk Factors

- **Host-Related Factors**
  Certain chicken lines and breeds are more susceptible to ALV. Congenital infection occurs when infected hens transmit the virus to embryos. Young chicks, especially those infected vertically (in ovo), are more likely to develop tumors later in life. Immunocompromised birds or those co-infected with other viruses (e.g., MD) have higher expressions for disease.
- **Environmental Factors**
  Crowded housing facilitates horizontal virus transmission via feces, respiratory secretions, and contaminated feed/water. ALV is shed in feces and secretions; dirty litter and equipment increase

exposure risk. Extreme temperatures, poor ventilation, or handling stress can exacerbate susceptibility and viral shedding.

- **Management Factors**
  Infected breeders can pass ALV directly to embryos, which is a primary route of infection in commercial flocks. Spread via direct contact, shared feeders, waterers, and contaminated equipment. The presence of older infected birds increases the exposure risk to susceptible chicks.

11.6.3 Clinical Signs and Pathology

- **External Findings**
  Most common presentations are lymphoid or myeloid tumors in various organs. Tumors may affect the spleen, liver, kidneys, bone marrow, heart, and intestines. Poor growth in affected birds. Chronic disease often leads to gradual death, sometimes with sudden mortality if tumors cause organ failure.
- **Necropsy Findings**
  Enlarged spleen, liver, kidneys, or heart. Multiple nodular masses in visceral organs; may be white, pale, or firm. Bone marrow involvement leads to pale bones and anemia in some birds. Lymphoid infiltration, prominent in bursa, spleen, and thymus in lymphoid leukosis.

11.6.4 Diagnostic Testing—Reference Laboratory

- **ELISA**
  Detects group- or subgroup-specific viral antigens in serum or egg yolk. Cannot distinguish between active infection and past exposure.
- **PCR**
  Detects viral DNA in blood, tissue, or embryos. Highly sensitive and specific, and can identify subgroups of ALV (A, B, C, D, J). Detects subclinical carriers before clinical signs or tumors appear.

11.6.5 Treatment and Therapeutic Interventions

No specific antiviral treatment exists for ALV. Disease is chronic and often progressive, so management focuses on prevention, intensive supportive care, and flock-level control. Birds with tumors or immunosuppression generally cannot be cured, and infected birds are often humanely euthanized to prevent spread and suffering.

- **Supportive Care**
  Provide a high-quality, balanced diet to maintain body condition. Ensure adequate water intake, particularly in birds with diarrhea or anorexia. Minimize handling and environmental stressors to support immune function. Treat concurrent bacterial or viral infections as needed (antibiotics for bacterial infections). Intravenous fluids and other therapies if the bird is in a clinical facility.

11.6.6 Prevention and Control

- **Biosecurity Measures**
  Isolate for at least 30 days and test for ALV before introducing them into the main flock. Minimize movement of people, equipment, and supplies between flocks to reduce horizontal transmission. Regularly clean and disinfect housing, feeders, drinkers, and equipment using approved virucidal agents.

11.6.7 Nursing Considerations

Nursing care for chickens affected by avian leukosis centers on supportive management, biosecurity, and flock-level control, as there is no effective treatment for the viral infection or associated tumors. Veterinary technicians should monitor affected birds for progressive weight loss, weakness, and signs of organ failure, ensuring they have easy access to feed and water and are housed in a low-stress, comfortable environment to maintain quality of life for as long as possible. Severely affected birds should be isolated to prevent bullying and allow closer monitoring, though horizontal transmission is relatively inefficient compared to vertical spread. Intensive veterinary therapies and nursing care increase the likelihood of positive outcomes. Humane euthanasia is recommended if the condition worsens.

11.7 Avian Tuberculosis

11.7.1 Overview

Avian tuberculosis is a chronic, contagious granulomatous disease caused primarily by *Mycobacterium avium* subsp. *avium*, a slow-growing acid-fast bacterium. The disease is most seen in older or backyard flocks, wild birds, and environments where birds are kept for extended periods, as the organism can persist in the environment for months to years.

11.7.2 Nursing Considerations

Nursing care for chickens with avian tuberculosis focuses primarily on supportive management, infection control, and biosecurity measures, as there is no effective treatment or cure for the disease in poultry. Birds suspected or confirmed to be infected should be immediately isolated from the flock to minimize environmental contamination and prevent transmission. Because *Mycobacterium avium* is zoonotic, particularly posing a risk to immunocompromised individuals, strict hygiene protocols must be observed, including the use of gloves, masks, protective clothing, and thorough handwashing after handling affected birds or contaminated materials. Because treatment is generally not practical or effective, humane euthanasia of clinically affected birds is usually recommended to control the disease within the flock. Veterinary technicians should provide chicken guardians with compassionate education about the chronic nature of avian tuberculosis, its environmental persistence, and the need for thorough depopulation and sanitation before reestablishing a new flock.

11.8 Chicken Infectious Anemia

11.8.1 Overview and Pathogenesis

Chicken Infectious Anemia (CIA) is a highly contagious viral disease of young chickens caused by the Chicken Anemia Virus (CAV), a member of the *Circoviridae* family. The disease is characterized primarily by immunosuppression, anemia, and increased susceptibility to secondary infections. It occurs worldwide and is of particular concern in commercial poultry operations where it can lead to significant economic losses through increased mortality, poor growth rates, and reduced vaccine efficacy. Transmission occurs both vertically (from infected breeder hens to offspring via the egg) and horizontally through the fecal–oral route, contact with contaminated surfaces, or through shedding by infected birds. Chicks infected vertically often develop clinical disease during the first 2 weeks of life, while horizontal infection tends to result in subclinical or delayed disease depending on the age and immune status of the birds. Veterinary professionals are not likely to observe this disease unless birds are from a commercial hatchery or production farm.

The pathogenesis of CIA involves the virus's tropism for hemocytoblasts in the bone marrow and precursor T lymphocytes in the thymus, leading to aplasia of the bone marrow, lymphoid depletion, and profound immunosuppression. Following infection, the virus replicates in lymphoid tissues, causing destruction of hematopoietic progenitor cells and T-cell precursors, which results in anemia, leukopenia, and atrophy of the thymus and other lymphoid organs. Clinically, affected chicks present with pale combs and wattles, depression, anorexia, increased mortality, and poor growth. Subclinical infections in older or immune birds often go unnoticed but can interfere with vaccine responses and flock health. The immunosuppression induced by CAV predisposes birds to secondary bacterial, viral, or fungal infections, exacerbating clinical disease. Maternal antibodies in chicks provide protection during the critical early period; thus, disease is most severe in chicks lacking adequate maternal immunity.

11.8.2 Risk Factors

- **Host-Related Factors**
  Young chicks (≤2 weeks old) are at greatest risk for clinical disease because their immune system is immature, and they lack adequate maternal antibodies. Older birds usually experience subclinical infection but may still shed the virus.
- **Vertical Transmission**
  The most important route of infection in young chicks is vertical transmission through the egg from infected breeder hens. Breeder hens infected just before or during egg production may shed the virus into eggs before seroconversion occurs. This results in uniform infection of entire hatches, leading to outbreaks in day-old chicks.
- **Horizontal Transmission**
  Contaminated equipment, personnel, or dust can spread viruses horizontally. CAV is extremely resistant to disinfectants and environmental degradation, making persistence in hatcheries and poultry houses a key risk factor. Overcrowding, inadequate cleaning, and multi-age flocks facilitate transmission between age groups.
- **Poor Hygiene and Biosecurity**
  Inadequate disinfection between flocks allows virus survival in litter, dander, and dust. Reuse of contaminated houses or equipment without thorough cleaning and downtime increases risk. Lapses in hatchery sanitation (e.g., poor egg handling, inadequate disinfection) contribute to early chick exposure.

11.8.3 Clinical Signs and Pathology

- **External Findings**
  Lethargy and weakness. Pale comb, wattles, and skin due to severe anemia. Anorexia, poor growth, and poor weight gain. Watery, sometimes greenish droppings.
- **Necropsy Findings**
  Bone marrow is typically pale, watery, and gelatinous, instead of normal dark red. This indicates hypoplasia or aplasia of erythroid and myeloid precursors. Thymus and bursa of Fabricius show

marked atrophy. Spleen may be small, with lymphoid depletion and reduced white pulp. Subcutaneous and intramuscular hemorrhages (especially in breast and thigh muscles) may occur due to thrombocytopenia and endothelial damage. Pale, atrophic liver, sometimes with focal necrosis. Kidneys can appear pale and swollen. Proventriculus and intestines are usually unremarkable unless secondary infections are present.

11.8.4 Diagnostic Testing—Reference Laboratory

- **PCR**
  Gold standard for rapid, sensitive detection of CAV DNA in tissues, feces, and environmental samples. It can be performed on fresh, frozen, or formalin-fixed tissues. It is useful for detecting both vertical and horizontal infections, even in subclinical cases.

11.8.5 Treatment and Therapeutic Interventions

- **Supportive Care**
  Provide optimal environmental conditions. Warm, draft-free, and dry housing to reduce additional stress. Clean, dry litter or bedding to prevent secondary bacterial growth. Ensure unrestricted access to clean water and balanced feed, with adequate levels of vitamins and minerals to support hematopoiesis and immune function. Electrolytes can be added to water for dehydrated or weak chicks. Crop feeding is recommended by trained veterinary professionals.

11.8.6 Prevention and Control

- **Biosecurity and Flock Management**
  Strict biosecurity is essential to prevent horizontal spread between flocks. Avoid multi-age systems where older birds can shed virus to younger, unprotected chicks. Use dedicated clothing, footwear, and equipment for each flock. Isolation protocols in the clinical setting.
- **Environmental Sanitation and Disinfection**
  Remove all organic matter (litter, feces, feathers, dust). Wash surfaces with detergents to break down biofilms. Apply disinfectants effective against non-enveloped viruses. Allow complete drying and downtime of at least 2–3 weeks before introducing new birds. Clean and disinfect

11.8.7 Nursing Considerations

Nursing care for chickens affected by CIA focuses on supportive management, prevention of secondary infections, and flock-level biosecurity, as there is no specific antiviral treatment for the disease. Veterinary technicians should monitor young chicks closely for pallor, weakness, anorexia, and delayed growth, providing easily accessible, high-quality feed and clean water to maintain hydration and nutritional support. Intensive nursing care is advised if guardians elect to treat birds. This may include assisted feeding, oxygen therapy, and parenteral fluid therapy. Because CIA causes immunosuppression, affected birds are highly susceptible to secondary bacterial, viral, or fungal infections; therefore, maintaining a clean, stress-free environment and minimizing overcrowding are critical.

11.9 Infectious Bronchitis Virus (IBV), AKA, Avian Infectious Bronchitis

11.9.1 Overview and Pathogenesis

Infectious bronchitis (IB) is an acute, highly contagious viral disease of chickens caused by infectious bronchitis virus (IBV), a single-stranded RNA virus of the genus *Gammacoronavirus*. The disease primarily affects commercially raised young meat birds and production layers, although birds of all ages are susceptible. IB is significant due to respiratory disease, reduced growth, poor feed conversion, decreased egg production, and defective egg quality. Transmission occurs via aerosolized respiratory secretions, contaminated equipment, and personnel, with rapid spread within and between flocks. Clinically, affected birds may exhibit coughing, sneezing, nasal discharge, dyspnea, watery eyes, decreased feed intake, and reduced egg production with poor shell quality.

The pathogenesis of IBV begins with entry through the respiratory tract, where the virus replicates in the nasal turbinates, trachea, and bronchi, causing destruction of ciliated epithelial cells, epithelial sloughing, and mucosal inflammation. The resulting impairment of mucociliary clearance predisposes birds to secondary bacterial infections, exacerbating respiratory disease. In addition to the respiratory system, certain strains of IBV can infect the kidneys, oviducts, and reproductive tissues, leading to nephritis, urate deposition, and reduced egg production or malformed eggs in layers. Viral replication triggers local immune responses, including heterophilic infiltration and cytokine release, which contribute to tissue damage. The severity of disease depends on strain virulence, age, immune status, and environmental stressors. Overall, IBV is a respiratory and systemic viral disease in which epithelial damage, impaired mucociliary function, and organ tropism result in respiratory signs, decreased productivity, and increased susceptibility to secondary infections in poultry flocks.

11.9.2 Risk Factors

- **Host-Related Factors**
  Chicks and young birds are more susceptible due to immature immune systems. Some commercial breeds (especially high-producing layers and meat birds) are more susceptible. Inadequate maternal antibody transfer.
- **Environmental and Management Factors**
  Poor ventilation promotes the accumulation of respiratory irritants (ammonia, dust), which compromise respiratory defenses. Cold stress or heat stress reduces immune competence. Wet or soiled litter encourages persistence of viruses and co-infections. Older birds may serve as reservoirs for younger susceptible birds.
- **Pathogen-Related Factors**
  IBV mutates frequently, leading to many serotypes/variants. Cross-protection between strains is often poor, so vaccinated or previously exposed birds may still get sick. Virus spreads rapidly via respiratory secretions, feces, contaminated equipment, and personnel. Virus can survive for weeks in organic material, dust, and equipment under favorable conditions.
- **Biosecurity and Human Factors**
  Inadequate biosecurity, movement of people, vehicles, and equipment between farms without proper disinfection. Introducing new birds without quarantine. Windborne spread and fomites can transfer the virus between farms or backyard flocks.

- **Nutritional and Stress-Related Factors**
  Deficiencies in protein, vitamins (esp. A, E, C), and minerals weaken immunity. Transport, handling, vaccination, or production stresses (onset of lay, feed restriction) reduce resistance.

11.9.3 Clinical Signs

- **External Findings**
  Coughing, sneezing, nasal discharge, and dropping in egg production. Abnormal eggs such as thin-shelled, misshapen, watery albumen. In chronic cases, false layers.
- **Necropsy Findings**
  Congestion, hyperemia, and edema of mucosa in the trachea. Tracheal rings may be softened, collapsed, or hemorrhagic. Cloudy and thickened air sacs may contain yellow, foamy, or caseous exudate, especially with secondary bacterial infections (E. coli, Mycoplasma). Kidneys enlarged, pale, swollen. Ureters distended with urates. Tubular nephrosis and urate nephritis visible on cut surfaces. Oviduct is regressed, cystic, or atrophied.

11.9.4 Diagnostic Testing—Reference Laboratory

- **Serological Testing**
  Detects antibodies against IBV to assess exposure or immune status. Hemagglutination inhibition (HI) assay is widely used to detect strain-specific antibodies. Enzyme-Linked Immunosorbent Assay (ELISA)-sensitive method for flock-level monitoring. Cannot distinguish active infection from vaccination-induced antibodies; must consider vaccination history.
- **Reverse Transcriptase Polymerase Chain Reaction (RT-PCR)**
  Detects IBV RNA from tracheal, kidney, or oviduct samples. Rapid and highly sensitive. It can be used for genotyping and strain identification. Used to identify variant strains and inform vaccination strategies.
- Reportable disease

11.9.5 Treatment and Therapeutic Interventions

Because IBV is a highly contagious viral disease, there is no specific antiviral therapy available. Management focuses on supportive care, secondary infection control, and flock-level interventions to reduce morbidity and mortality.

- **Supportive Care**
  Ensure warm, dry, well-ventilated housing to reduce stress on the respiratory system. Avoid overcrowding to reduce viral spread. Provide easy access to clean water and high-quality feed to support immune function. Use electrolyte or vitamin supplements (especially vitamins A, D, E, and C) to help mitigate stress and support recovery. Intensive nursing care with hydration and supplemental nutrition.
- **Medications**
  Broad-spectrum antibiotics (under veterinary prescription) may be used to prevent or treat secondary bacterial infections (e.g., *Escherichia coli* colibacillosis and *Mycoplasma gallisepticum*). Commonly used tetracyclines and sulfonamides. Reducing bacterial complications lowers mortality and improves recovery rates.

11.9.6 Prevention and Control

- **Biosecurity Measures**
  Strong biosecurity is the foundation of IBV control because the virus spreads rapidly and survives in the environment. Regularly clean houses, feeders, waterers, and equipment with effective disinfectants (IBV is sensitive to heat and many disinfectants but persists in organic matter). Limit visitors, require clean or pen-specific boots/clothing, and disinfect equipment.
- **Management Practices**
  Prevent buildup of ammonia, dust, and humidity that damage the respiratory tract. Avoid overcrowding to reduce stress and transmission. Prevent extreme temperature changes, which worsen respiratory disease. Keep bedding dry and clean to reduce viral survival.
- **Control of Secondary Infections**
  IBV predisposes chicken to *E. coli, Mycoplasma, Pasteurella*, etc.

11.9.7 Nursing Considerations

Nursing considerations for birds affected by IBV should prioritize supportive care, prevention of secondary infections, and strict biosecurity measures to limit disease spread. Affected birds should be isolated from the healthy flock to reduce transmission, and caregivers should use dedicated clothing, footwear, and equipment when handling sick birds to prevent cross-contamination. Providing a warm, draft-free environment with good ventilation is essential to ease respiratory distress, along with ensuring constant access to clean water and high-quality feed to maintain hydration and nutritional status. Because IBV can predispose birds to bacterial complications, close observation for secondary infections is critical, and veterinary consultation may be needed for antimicrobial therapy if such infections are suspected. Caregivers should monitor egg production and shell quality in laying hens, as IBV can cause long-term reproductive issues. Meticulous cleaning and disinfection of housing, equipment, combined with vaccination programs as advised by a veterinarian, are vital to preventing future outbreaks and maintaining flock health. Vaccines are typically not available for backyard flocks. Intensive nursing care and isolation protocols are advised in a clinical setting.

11.10 Infectious Bursal Disease (IBD, Gumboro Disease)

11.10.1 Overview and Pathogenesis

Infectious bursal disease (IBD), also known as Gumboro disease, is a highly contagious viral disease of poultry caused by Infectious bursal disease virus (IBDV), a double-stranded RNA virus of the family *Birnaviridae*. The disease primarily affects young chickens between 3 and 6 weeks of age, with older birds generally experiencing subclinical infections. IBD is significant due to immunosuppression, increased susceptibility to secondary infections, poor vaccine response, growth retardation, and occasional mortality. Transmission occurs via the fecal-oral route, with the virus persisting in litter, feed, water, and contaminated equipment for weeks to months. Clinically, IBD may be presented as depression, ruffled feathers, diarrhea, dehydration, prostration, and sudden mortality in acute outbreaks.

The pathogenesis of IBD begins with ingestion of the virus, which first replicates in the intestinal epithelium and associated lymphoid tissues before disseminating via the bloodstream to the bursa of Fabricius, the primary lymphoid organ responsible for B-cell maturation. Viral replication within the bursa leads to lymphoid depletion, apoptosis of B lymphocytes, and destruction of follicular architecture, resulting in profound immunosuppression. The immunocompromised state predisposes birds to secondary bacterial and viral infections and reduces the efficacy of vaccinations. In severe cases, systemic spread and high viral loads can cause mortality, while subclinical infections impair long-term flock immunity and productivity. Recovered birds may remain carriers for short periods, contributing to environmental contamination. Overall, IBD is a lymphotropic viral disease in which viral replication in the bursa causes immunosuppression, increased susceptibility to secondary infections, and significant commercial/production farm economic losses in susceptible poultry populations. Veterinary professionals will likely not observe IBD in clinical practice unless birds are from a commercial hatchery or production farm.

11.10.2 Risk Factors

- **Host-Related Factors**
  Very young chicks (<3 weeks) may be subclinical but become immunosuppressed. Chicks 3–6 weeks old are most susceptible because the bursa of Fabricius is well-developed.
- **Virus-Related Factors**
  IBDV is highly resistant to disinfectants and survives for months in poultry houses. A small number of viruses is enough to infect; heavy contamination increases risk.
- **Management and Environmental Factors**
  Poor biosecurity such as movement of people and equipment without proper disinfection. Virus spreads easily via fecal–oral route.
- **Hatchery and Vaccination Factors**
  Chicks hatched from infected or contaminated hatcheries. Incorrect vaccination timing, too early (maternal antibodies neutralize vaccine) or too late (birds already infected). Poor handling of live vaccines (heat inactivation, chlorine in water).

11.10.3 Clinical Signs and Pathology

- **External Findings**
  Sudden onset, rapid spread, depression, and ruffled feathers. Whitish, watery, sometimes bloody diarrhea. Unsteady gait and trembling.
- **Necropsy Findings**
  Enlarged, edematous, and gelatinous bursa. Cream colored or hemorrhagic bursal folds and sometimes streaks of hemorrhage on serosa. Hemorrhages in pelvic limb and breast muscles (especially at proventriculus and gizzard junction). Swollen, pale kidneys with urate deposits (due to dehydration, nephrosis). Congested, edematous liver.

11.10.4 Diagnostic Testing—Reference Laboratory

- **Reverse Transcriptase Polymerase Chain Reaction (RT-PCR)**
  Detects viral RNA, high sensitivity and specificity; widely used.
- **ELISA**
  Detect viral antigen in bursal tissue, rapid and suitable for field samples.
- Reportable disease

11.10.5 Treatment and Therapeutic Interventions

There is no specific antiviral treatment for IBD because it is a viral disease. Management focuses on supportive therapy, reducing secondary infections with antibiotics and a clean enclosure, and flock-level interventions to limit losses and prevent spread.

- **Supportive Care**
  Provide electrolyte-enriched drinking water to counteract dehydration from diarrhea. Especially vitamins A, E, C, and B-complex to support immune function and reduce oxidative stress. Maintain warm, dry, stress-free housing to reduce immunosuppression and mortality. Improve air quality and ventilation to reduce irritation and secondary infections.
- **Control of Secondary Infections**
  IBD-induced immunosuppression predisposes birds to bacterial infections (especially *Escherichia coli*). Broad-spectrum antibiotics (e.g., oxytetracycline, enrofloxacin, or trimethoprim-sulfa) may be administered under veterinary direction to reduce secondary bacterial infections.
- **Restriction and Biosecurity Measures**
  Isolate affected flocks to prevent spread. Strict biosecurity, including limiting human and equipment movement between flocks, using dedicated footwear and clothing, and thorough cleaning and disinfection with effective virucidal agents. Litter management to reduce viral load in the environment. In a clinical setting, frequently changed bedding and isolation protocols.

11.10.6 Prevention and Control

- **Biosecurity and Hygiene**
  Strict biosecurity is the cornerstone of IBD prevention by limiting visitors, personnel, and equipment movement between poultry flocks. Thorough cleaning and disinfection between flocks if mass human euthanasia is performed. Allow adequate downtime (2–3 weeks) to break the cycle.
- **Management Practices**
  Maintain optimal environmental conditions (temperature, humidity, ventilation) to reduce stress. Avoid overcrowding, which can facilitate viral spread. Implement good nutritional support, especially vitamins and trace minerals, to promote strong immune systems.

11.10.7 Nursing Considerations

Nursing considerations for birds affected by (IBD, Gumboro disease) focus on supportive care, immune system protection, and strict biosecurity to control the spread of infection. Affected birds should be promptly isolated from the healthy flock to minimize transmission, and caretakers must practice stringent hygiene, including handwashing, wearing dedicated protective clothing, and disinfecting equipment and housing areas. Because IBD primarily damages the bursa of Fabricius and suppresses the immune system, birds are highly vulnerable to secondary bacterial infections; therefore, they should be closely monitored for signs of concurrent illness, with veterinary evaluation for possible antimicrobial support if secondary infections are suspected. Supportive care includes maintaining a warm, stress-free environment, ensuring constant access to clean water, and providing easily digestible, nutrient-rich feed to support recovery. Caregivers must implement thorough cleaning and disinfection protocols between flocks, as the virus is highly resistant and can persist in the environment for long periods. Intensive nursing care for hospitalized birds under veterinary care.

11.11 Listeriosis

11.11.1 Overview and Pathogenesis

Listeriosis in poultry is a bacterial disease caused by *Listeria monocytogenes*, a gram-positive, facultative intracellular pathogen. While more commonly reported in ruminants, listeriosis can affect chickens, turkeys, and other birds, usually leading to septicemia, encephalitis, or sporadic mortality in flocks. Infection typically occurs via ingestion of contaminated feed, water, or bedding, particularly spoiled silage or decomposed organic matter, though wound contamination can also lead to localized infections. *L. monocytogenes* is ubiquitous in the environment, can survive in a wide range of temperatures, and persists in soil and litter, making environmental management important for control.

Pathogenesis involves the bacteria's ability to invade intestinal epithelial cells and macrophages, enabling dissemination through the bloodstream to multiple organs, including the liver, spleen, heart, and central nervous system. Once inside host cells, *Listeria* escapes the phagosome, replicates in the cytoplasm, and spreads to adjacent cells, evading humoral immune defenses. In the gastrointestinal tract, invasion of mucosal epithelium may lead to enteritis and diarrhea, while systemic spread can cause septicemia, granulomatous hepatitis, splenitis, and occasionally encephalitis. Clinically, affected birds may present with lethargy, inappetence, drooping wings, diarrhea, torticollis, or sudden death, depending on the organs involved. Chronic infections often produce granulomatous lesions in the liver, spleen, and intestines, reflecting the host's cell-mediated immune response to the intracellular pathogen.

11.11.2 Risk Factors

- **Age and Immune Status**
  Young chicks and immunocompromised birds are more susceptible to severe disease. Older or immunologically stressed birds may develop subclinical infections that act as carriers. Concurrent immunosuppression (e.g., due to IBDV and CAV) increases susceptibility.
- **Environmental Factors**
  Contaminated feed and water are the main sources of infection. *Listeria* thrives in silage, spoiled grains, moldy feed, or wet feed. Poor sanitation and damp housing favor bacterial survival. Soil contamination with feces or decaying organic matter can harbor Listeria. Cold, wet conditions may increase environmental persistence, as *Listeria* is psychotropic (can thrive at low temperatures).
- **Management and Husbandry Practices**
  Poor hygiene in housing, feeders, waterers, and litter. High stocking density or overcrowding, leading to stress and increased exposure. Multi-age flocks increase the risk of horizontal transmission. Improper feed storage (moldy silage, wet feed) is a significant predisposing factor.

11.11.3 Clinical Signs and Pathology

- **External Findings**
  Septicemia Form
  Depression, lethargy, anorexia, poor weight gain, huddling, reluctance to move, pale comb and wattles, and diarrhea.

Neurologic Form (Encephalitis/Circling Disease)
Head tilt, circling, or torticollis. Ataxia and incoordination. Tremors or convulsions in severe cases. Loss of appetite and depression.

Localized Form (Arthritis/Synovitis)
Swelling of joints (hock, stifle). Lameness or reluctance to move.

- **Necropsy Findings**
  Small, pale foci of necrosis or diffuse mottling on liver. Spleen enlargement, congestion, or focal necrosis. Brain may appear congested or edematous in neurologic cases. Joints may have swelling and synovial inflammation in localized infections. Kidneys and intestines may show congestion or necrotic foci.

11.11.4 Diagnostic Testing – Reference Laboratory

- **Culture**
  Gold standard for diagnosis. *L. monocytogenes* can be isolated from liver, spleen, brain, or joint tissue. Cloacal or fecal swabs can be taken for surveillance.
- **PCR**
  PCR assays detect *L. monocytogenes* DNA in tissue, feed, water, or environmental samples. Highly sensitive and rapid; useful for subclinical infections or outbreak investigations. Can identify serotype or strain, aiding epidemiologic tracking.
- Reportable disease in some states

11.11.5 Treatment and Therapeutic Interventions

- **Medication**
  Listeria monocytogenes is generally susceptible to several antibiotics, but antimicrobial treatment is most effective in early stages, particularly the septicemic form.
  Penicillin G 0.5–3 mL by mouth for 3–5 days.
  Oxytetracycline 5 mg/kg subcutaneous or intramuscular every 12–24 hours. 2500 mg/L drinking water and 2500 mg/kg feed.
  Trimethoprim-Sulfamethoxazole 100 mg/kg by mouth every 12 hours for 5–7 days.
  Tylosin 50 mg/kg by mouth once daily for 5–7 days or 15–30 mg/kg intramuscularly every 6–12 hours for 5–7 days.
- **Supportive Care**
  Isolation of clinically affected birds to reduce transmission. Fluid therapy (oral electrolytes or supportive fluids) to counter dehydration in septicemic cases. Nutritional support, including easily digestible feed and vitamin supplementation (especially vitamin E and selenium to support immune function). Temperature control and reduce stress to improve recovery chances. If hospitalized, birds undergo intensive nursing care such as fluid therapy, nutritional supplementation, antibiotic therapy, analgesics, and warm, clean bedding with frequent changes. Though not zoonotic, appropriate PPE should be considered during handling and sanitation of enclosure.

11.11.6 Prevention and Control

Because *Listeria monocytogenes* is a hardy environmental organism capable of persisting in soil, water, litter, and feed, prevention focuses on biosecurity, feed management, environmental sanitation, and flock health. Unlike many viral diseases, there is no vaccine for listeriosis in poultry, making management and hygiene the primary control measures.

- **Feed and Water Management**
  Contaminated feed is one of the most important sources of infection in chickens. *Listeria* grows well in wet, moldy, or poorly stored feed, including spoiled silage. Provide birds with fresh, clean feed; discard any moldy, wet, or spoiled feed immediately. Store feed in dry, sealed containers, protected from moisture, rodents, and wild birds. Avoid feeding improperly fermented silage or feed with visible mold. Clean and disinfect feeders regularly to prevent buildup of biofilms and bacterial growth. Ensure a clean, chlorinated water supply; clean drinkers daily to remove organic matter and biofilm or algae.
- **Environmental Sanitation**
  Listeria is persistent and resistant to many environmental stresses. Effective environmental control measures are crucial. Thoroughly clean and disinfect hen houses, equipment, and surfaces. Effective disinfectants include properly diluted hypochlorite (bleach), peracetic acid, and iodine-based products. Quaternary ammonium compounds are less effective against *Listeria*. Remove organic matter (manure, litter, spilled feed) before disinfection, as it can protect bacteria from chemicals. Maintain dry litter and good drainage to minimize bacterial survival. Implement regular cleaning schedules for feeders, drinkers, nest boxes, and perches. Dispose of dead birds promptly and properly (incineration, composting, or rendering); do not leave carcasses accessible to scavengers.
- **Biosecurity Measures**
  Strict biosecurity is essential to prevent the introduction and spread of *Listeria*. Restrict access to the flock. Clean and disinfect equipment used in the house/coop and pen. Control rodents, wild birds, and insects, which can mechanically carry *Listeria* into houses or pens or contaminate feed and water. Prevent cross-contamination between different age groups or species through dedicated equipment.
- **Flock Health and Immunity**
  Maintaining a healthy, immunocompetent flock reduces susceptibility and severity of disease. Reduce stressors such as overcrowding, poor ventilation, temperature extremes, or abrupt management changes. Provide balanced nutrition, including adequate vitamin E and selenium, to support immune function. Control concurrent infections (e.g., IBD and CIA) that may predispose birds to *Listeria* infection. Avoid unnecessary handling or transport.

11.11.7 Nursing Considerations

Nursing care for chickens affected by listeriosis focuses on supportive care, preventing secondary infections, and environmental management, as antibiotic treatment may be limited and often requires veterinary guidance. Veterinary technicians should monitor affected birds for lethargy, inappetence, diarrhea, neurological signs, and weight loss, providing easily accessible feed and clean water to maintain hydration and nutritional support. Birds showing severe neurological signs or systemic illness require isolation to reduce stress and facilitate monitoring. Strict biosecurity and hygiene are essential because *Listeria monocytogenes* is widespread in the environment. Contaminated feed, bedding, or water sources should be removed and properly disposed of, and housing should be cleaned, disinfected, and well-ventilated to reduce bacterial load. Veterinary technicians should ensure that all equipment follows strict sanitation protocols. Record-keeping of clinical signs, morbidity, and mortality helps identify outbreak patterns and supports veterinary interventions. Educating caretakers on proper feed storage, prevention of spoiled or contaminated feed, and minimizing stressors are crucial to reduce incidence and limit spread. Supportive nursing combined with early detection and veterinary oversight improves survival rates and reduces flock-level losses. If a bird is hospitalized, intensive nursing care includes hydration, supplemental nutrition, antibiotic therapy, and analgesics and anti-inflammatory agents as needed.

11.12 Marek's Disease

11.12.1 Overview and Pathogenesis

MD is a highly contagious, neoplastic, and immunosuppressive disease of chickens caused by Marek's disease virus (MDV), an alphaherpesvirus of the family *Herpesviridae*. The disease primarily affects chickens between 8 and 30 weeks of age, though all ages are susceptible. It is significant due to lymphoid tumors, paralysis, immunosuppression, decreased egg production, and mortality. Transmission occurs via inhalation of virus-laden dust or dander from infected birds, with environmental persistence facilitated by virus shedding from feather follicles. Clinically, MD may present as asymmetric paralysis of wings or legs, atrophy of the breast muscles, weight loss, vision impairment, immunosuppression, and death in severe cases.

The pathogenesis of MD begins when the virus is inhaled and infects the respiratory epithelium, where it undergoes primary replication in B and T lymphocytes. Following systemic spread, MDV establishes a latent infection in $CD4^+$ T lymphocytes, which can persist for the bird's lifetime. During the latent phase, the virus can reactivate and induce clonal proliferation of transformed T lymphocytes, leading to lymphoid tumors in nerves, visceral organs, and skin. Infiltration of nerves, particularly the sciatic and brachial nerves, causes neurological signs such as paralysis and ataxia. Concurrent immunosuppression occurs due to the destruction and functional impairment of lymphoid tissues, predisposing birds to secondary infections. The disease may progress to visceral tumors, nerve enlargement, and systemic immunodeficiency, resulting in decreased growth and production. Overall, MD is a lymphoproliferative viral disease in which viral latency, T-cell transformation, and immunosuppression collectively produce tumors, paralysis, and significant economic losses in commercial and production poultry flocks. Commercial hatcheries will vaccinate all production chicks, but will only vaccinate chicks if requested by the ordering customer.

11.12.2 Risk Factors

- **Host-Related Factors**
  Chicks are highly susceptible from hatch until 6 weeks of age. Clinical disease usually appears at 8–24 weeks but can occur later. Birds without proper vaccination at hatch are at the highest risk.
- **Virus-Related Factors**
  More virulent strains can cause disease even in vaccinated flocks. Virus is shed in feather dander for life, making infected birds permanent carriers.
- **Environmental and Management Factors**
  Overcrowding causes a faster spread of feather dander. Poor ventilation and dusty houses due to the virus spread more easily in the air. Poor litter management causes virus to build up in the environment.
- **Vaccination-Related Factors**
  Lack of vaccinations or improper administration at hatch. If chicks are exposed before immunity develops, vaccination fails.

11.12.3 Clinical Signs and Pathology

- **External Findings**
  - *Classical Tumor Form (Lymphomatous Marek's Disease)*
    Age affected is usually 8–24 weeks, but can occur earlier in highly susceptible flocks. Asymmetric paralysis of wings, legs, or neck. Torticollis and ataxia. Drooping wings, inability to stand, and progressive lameness. Birds may be thin and depressed. Nodules or enlargement of feather follicles in wings, neck, or body. Gray-white iris tumors, irregular pupil shape (rare). Pallor of comb and wattles.
  - *Acute Form*
    Sudden death with few premonitory signs, high mortality, and birds may show severe depression or diarrhea just before death.
- **Necropsy Findings**
  Enlarged, grayish, or pale nerves (sciatic, brachial, vagus). Nodular lymphomas in liver, spleen, kidneys, gonads, proventriculus, heart, lungs, gut, and skin. Nodules in the feather pulp, especially wings and neck. Enlargement of sciatic or brachial nerves with asymmetric paralysis. Iris tumors are grayish-white, often unilateral or bilateral. The iris tumors can cause irregular pupil shape or blindness. Spleen and liver are swollen, grayish-white nodules. Kidneys are enlarged with lymphoid infiltration.

11.12.4 Diagnostic Testing—Reference Laboratory

- **PCR**
  Detects MDV DNA from tissues (tumors, nerves, feather pulp, buffy coat). Allows differentiation between virulent field strains and vaccine strains.
- **Histopathology**
  Confirms lymphoid infiltration, differentiates from Lymphoid Leukosis.

11.12.5 Treatment and Therapeutic Interventions

MD is caused by an oncogenic *Gallid herpesvirus* 2 (serotype 1), and once clinical signs or tumors develop, there is no curative treatment. Management therefore focuses on supportive care of affected birds (when feasible), immediate flock-level interventions to limit further spread, and long-term prevention through vaccination and biosecurity.

- **Supportive/Palliative Care**
  Isolation of affected birds prevents pecking injuries and reduces viral shedding to flock. Assisted feeding and hydration if the bird can still consume food and water. Soft, easily digestible feed is placed at the beak level for paralyzed birds. Keep warm, dry, and stress-free environment to reduce immunosuppression. Intensive nursing care for hospitalized birds may increase survivability. Humane euthanasia is recommended for severely paralyzed or emaciated birds with a poor prognosis. MD-affected birds remain lifelong carriers and shedders, even if they survive.

11.12.6 Prevention and Control

- **Vaccination**
  Vaccination is essential. Rispens (CVI-988) vaccine is more protective, especially against very virulent strains. Administered at hatch via subcutaneous infection. Vaccine is sensitive to light,

heat, and disinfectants. Vaccinated birds may carry the virus and do not prevent infection entirely. Vaccines prevent tumor formation and clinical disease but do not prevent infection or viral shedding. If Marek's vaccine is offered by the hatchery, it is highly recommended for chicks to receive this preventive measure.

- **Biosecurity Measures**
  MDV is shed in feather dander and can survive for months, remove litter and thoroughly clean surfaces, and use effective disinfectants. Restrict visitors.

11.12.7 Nursing Considerations

Nursing considerations for birds affected by MD focus on supportive care, prevention of secondary infections, and minimizing stress to enhance quality of life, as there is no curative treatment for this viral disease. Affected birds should be monitored closely for neurological signs such as paralysis, ataxia, or wing droop, as well as for tumors, weight loss, and lethargy, with careful handling to avoid injury. Housing must be clean, warm, well-ventilated, and low-stress, and affected birds may need isolation from healthy flock mates to prevent bullying and allow focused care. Providing easy access to clean water and nutrient-dense, easily digestible feed supports hydration and maintains body condition despite reduced mobility or appetite. If the bird cannot self-feed, crop feeding under a veterinarian's direction is preferable. Nursing care also involves vigilant observation for secondary bacterial or fungal infections due to immune compromise, and consultation with a veterinarian for palliative care, including analgesics or anti-inflammatories if appropriate. Overall, nursing considerations emphasize supportive management, stress reduction, careful monitoring, and maintenance of environmental hygiene to optimize welfare and quality of life in birds affected by MD. Humane euthanasia is always a reasonable option.

11.13 Swollen Head Syndrome

11.13.1 Overview and Pathogenesis

Swollen Head Syndrome (SHS) is a multifactorial respiratory and sinus disease of chickens and turkeys characterized by periorbital and infraorbital sinus swelling, respiratory distress, and reduced productivity. The condition is most associated with infection by Avian Metapneumovirus (aMPV), often complicated by secondary bacterial pathogens such as *Escherichia coli*, *Staphylococcus spp.*, or *Mycoplasma gallisepticum*. SHS typically affects broiler breeders, commercial layers, and broilers, and is most severe in young or immunologically naïve flocks. Transmission occurs mainly through aerosols, direct bird-to-bird contact, and contaminated equipment or personnel, with rapid flock spread once introduced. It is unlikely that veterinary professionals will observe SHS in clinical practice.

The pathogenesis begins with inhalation or contact with the virus, which targets and replicates in the epithelial cells of the upper respiratory tract, including the nasal turbinates and infraorbital sinuses. Viral replication damages the ciliated epithelium, impairing mucociliary clearance and predisposing the bird to opportunistic bacterial invasion. The subsequent inflammatory response in the sinus tissues leads to the accumulation of serous to mucopurulent exudate, causing the characteristic swelling around the eyes and head. In severe cases, extension of infection into the middle ear or cranial bones can lead to neurological signs, such as torticollis or incoordination.

Clinical signs vary with the severity of infection and include nasal discharge, sneezing, conjunctivitis, facial edema, open-mouth breathing, and decreased feed intake. In complicated cases, morbidity is high, though mortality is usually low unless secondary infections become systemic.

11.13.2 Risk Factors

- **Pathogen-Related Factors**
  Secondary *E. coli* infection is the major cause of the characteristic periorbital swelling and cellulitis of SHS. Other opportunists (e.g., *Ornithobacterium rhinotracheale (ORT), Mycoplasma gallisepticum, and Pasteurella multocida*) may exacerbate disease. Poor biosecurity or high bacterial loads in the environment increase the likelihood of secondary infection.
- **Host-Related Factors**
  Young meat birds (3–6 weeks) and pullets are commonly affected. Birds without prior exposure or vaccination against aMPV are more susceptible. Immunosuppression from other diseases (e.g., IBD, CIA) or stress increases risk.
- **Environmental and Management Factors**
  Poor ventilation, high ammonia levels, and dust irritate the respiratory mucosa, making birds more vulnerable to aMPV infection and bacterial invasion. Inadequate air exchange increases the concentration of airborne pathogens. Sudden drops in ambient temperature, chilling, or drafts are common triggers for SHS outbreaks, especially in poorly insulated houses. Thermal stress impairs mucociliary clearance and suppresses immune function. Overcrowding, wet litter, and inadequate cleaning between large commercial flocks contribute to increased bacterial load and stress. Poorly sanitized water lines and feeders can serve as reservoirs for opportunistic bacteria.

11.13.3 Clinical Signs and Pathology

- **External Findings**
  Affected birds typically show signs 2–5 days after exposure to aMPV, with bacterial complications developing shortly after. The onset in a flock is rapid, often affecting a large proportion of birds within a short period.
  Early Phase
  Clear to mucoid nasal discharge. Sneezing, coughing, and rales (tracheal or nasal). Conjunctivitis with watery or foamy ocular discharge. Swollen infraorbital sinuses cause mild periorbital swelling in early stages. Head shaking due to irritation and mucus accumulation.

  Progressive Phase
  Unilateral or bilateral periorbital and supraorbital swelling, sometimes extending to the submandibular region, giving birds a puffy, distorted facial appearance. Swelling of eyelids leads to partial or complete closure of the eyes. Edema and cellulitis of the periorbital and cranial subcutaneous tissues. Crepitus may be palpable in severe cases due to gas-forming bacteria (less common).
- **Necropsy Findings**
  Serous to mucopurulent exudate in the nasal passages and infraorbital sinuses. Edema and cellulitis of the periorbital and cranial subcutaneous tissues; sometimes gelatinous or caseous material on dissection. Conjunctival hyperemia, sinus distension, and turbid sinus contents. Mucosal thickening of the upper respiratory tract. In severe cases, exudate may extend into the

middle ear or cranial bones. Tracheas are usually clear or with mild catarrhal inflammation, as the disease is primarily localized to the upper respiratory tract.

11.13.4 Diagnostic Testing—Reference Laboratory

- **Reverse Transcriptase PCR (RT-PCR)**
  Gold standard for rapid detection of avian metapneumovirus RNA in choanal/tracheal swabs or tissue samples. It can distinguish subtypes A, B, C, and D of aMPV. High sensitivity and specificity; detects virus before seroconversion.
- **ELISA**
  Widely used for flock screening and monitoring vaccine responses. Detects antibodies to aMPV; a rising titer in paired samples confirms recent infection. Useful for retrospective diagnosis in later stages of outbreaks.
- **Culture**
  Aerobic culture and sensitivity from sinus aspirates, nasal swabs, or subcutaneous lesions. Isolation of heavy pure or mixed growth of *E. coli* supports the diagnosis. Antimicrobial sensitivity testing (AST) is essential to guide treatment, as *E. coli* resistance patterns vary widely between flocks and regions.
- Reportable disease

11.13.5 Treatment and Therapeutic Interventions

- **Medication**
  Early initiation is critical, ideally within the first 24–48 hours of clinical onset, to limit the severity of cellulitis and sinusitis. Choice of antibiotics should be based on culture and sensitivity testing.
- **Supportive and Nursing Care**
  Provide clean, easily accessible water and palatable feed to counteract reduced intake due to facial swelling and impaired vision. Electrolytes and vitamins (especially vitamins A, E, and C) can support the immune response and help birds tolerate infection. Remove crusts and discharge from the eyes and nares gently to maintain airway patency. Separate severely affected birds to reduce competition and allow for targeted treatment. Supplemental nutrition, oxygen therapy, nebulization, fluid therapy, and anti-inflammatory agents are advised for severely compromised birds.

11.13.6 Prevention and Control

- **Biosecurity Measures**
  Strict biosecurity is the cornerstone of SHS control. Avian metapneumovirus spreads rapidly through flocks via aerosol, direct contact, and contaminated equipment or personnel. The virus can also persist in the environment for short periods, especially under cool, damp conditions. Restrict movement between flocks of different ages to minimize viral spread. Remove all organic matter before applying effective virucidal disinfectants. Prevent contact with wild birds, which can serve as reservoirs of aMPV. Control rodents, flies, and insects, which can mechanically transmit pathogens.
- **Environmental and Management Practices**
  Maintain optimal ventilation to reduce viral and bacterial loads and prevent humidity elevation. Control dust and ammonia to protect respiratory mucosa and enhance vaccine effectiveness. Ensure good litter quality, with low moisture levels, to reduce bacterial proliferation.

11.13.7 Nursing Considerations

Nursing care for chickens affected by SHS focuses on supportive respiratory management, controlling secondary infections, and strengthening biosecurity to limit disease spread. Technicians should monitor flocks closely for nasal discharge, periorbital swelling, conjunctivitis, sneezing, or neurological signs, and isolate clinically affected birds to reduce transmission and allow targeted care. Providing warm, well-ventilated, and dust-free housing helps ease respiratory distress and supports mucociliary clearance. Clean, easily accessible water and high-quality feed should always be available, as facial swelling and sinus congestion may impair feeding and drinking. If the bird is unable to self-feed, assisted feeding is advised. Parenteral fluid and oxygen therapies, if indicated. Strict biosecurity and hygiene are essential, as avian metapneumovirus spreads rapidly through aerosols and contaminated equipment. Environmental cleaning to reduce dust and ammonia, along with effective ventilation, helps decrease viral persistence and bacterial overgrowth. Veterinary technicians should keep detailed records of clinical signs and treatments to assist veterinarians in management.

11.14 Fowl Pox

11.14.1 Overview and Pathogenesis

Fowl pox is a viral disease of poultry caused by Fowl Pox virus, a double-stranded DNA virus of the family *Poxviridae*. The disease affects chickens, turkeys, and other avian species and is of economic significance due to morbidity, decreased egg production, growth retardation, and occasional mortality, especially in naive flocks. Transmission occurs via direct contact with infected birds, contaminated equipment, or biting insects (mechanical vectors), with aerosol spread being less common. Fowl pox manifests in two primary forms: cutaneous ("dry") form, characterized by nodular lesions on unfeathered skin and combs, and diphtheritic ("wet") form, affecting mucous membranes of the oral cavity, pharynx, larynx, and upper respiratory tract (Figure 11.2).

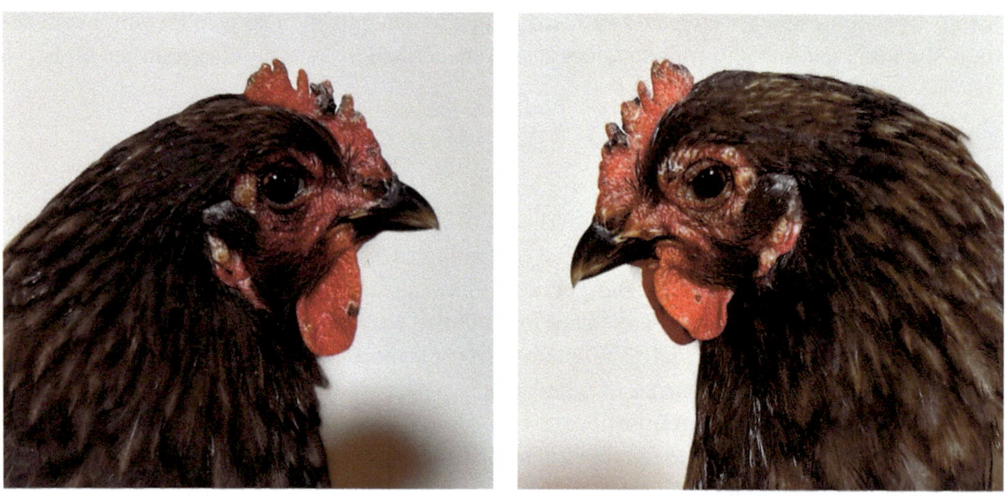

Figure 11.2 Cochin hen with dry fowl pox lesions. Photo courtesy of Stephanie Freeman.

The pathogenesis of fowl pox begins when the virus enters through skin abrasions or mucosal surfaces. In the cutaneous form, viral replication occurs in epithelial cells, leading to cell hypertrophy, cytoplasmic inclusion bodies, and necrosis, which manifests as raised, wart-like lesions. In the diphtheritic form, infection of the respiratory or oral epithelium causes necrotic lesions, fibrin deposition, and obstruction of the upper airways, potentially leading to respiratory distress and asphyxiation. Viral replication elicits localized inflammatory responses with infiltration of heterophils and lymphocytes, which contribute to lesion formation. Although mortality is generally low in the cutaneous form, the diphtheritic form can be more severe, particularly in young or immunocompromised birds. Recovered birds develop long-lasting immunity, and the virus persists in the environment or in scabs, facilitating further outbreaks. Overall, fowl pox is a viral epithelial disease in which viral replication, lesion formation, and localized inflammation result in cutaneous nodules or mucosal diphtheritic lesions, leading to morbidity and production losses in poultry.

11.14.2 Risk Factors

- **Host-Related Factors**
  All ages are susceptible, but young chickens (2–12 weeks) often show more severe disease. Some commercial breeds may have partial resistance; backyard or indigenous breeds are often more affected. Vitamin A and other micronutrient deficiencies increase severity.
- **Virus-Related Factors**
  Fowl pox virus exists in different strains; some are more pathogenic, causing high morbidity. Virus can survive for months in scabs, dust, and contaminated equipment.
- **Environmental Factors**
  Crowded, poorly ventilated, or unsanitary conditions increase transmission. Mosquitoes (*Culex spp., Aedes spp.*) are the main vectors for cutaneous/wet pox. Mosquito abundance in warm, wet seasons increases outbreaks.
- **Management and Biosecurity Factors**
  Sharing of equipment, feeders, and waterers without disinfection. Chickens recently introduced to the flock without the recommended 30-day quarantine.
- **Vaccination-Related Factors**
  Unvaccinated flocks are highly susceptible. Incorrect method or poor storage/handling reduces the efficacy of the vaccine. Younger birds in endemic areas may be exposed before immunity develops. Vaccines are not typically available for backyard flocks unless immunized at a commercial hatchery.

11.14.3 Clinical Signs and Pathology

- **External Findings**
  - *Cutaneous Form*
    Lesions on comb, wattles, eyelids, beak, legs, and feet. Small, raised papules develop into vesicles, then turn to scabs within 1–2 weeks. Lesions may coalesce into larger crusts. Low mortality, mainly due to secondary infections or severe cases in young chicks.
  - *Diphtheritic Form*
    Lesions in mouth, pharynx, larynx, trachea, and esophagus. Yellowish or grayish plaques/membranes on mucous membranes. Respiratory distress seen by coughing, sneezing, open-mouth breathing, and dyspnea.

- **Necropsy Findings**
  - *Cutaneous Form*

    Papules, vesicles, and scabs on comb, wattles, eyelids, legs, and feet. Nodular or thickened lesions in severe cases. Mild edema; usually no deep organ involvement.
  - *Diphtheritic Form*

    Thick, yellowish, or gray pseudomembranes in oral cavities, larynx, trachea, and esophagus. Plaques may cause airway obstruction. Congestion and mild inflammation of trachea and lungs due to secondary bacterial infections. Usually minimal systemic involvement; occasionally dehydration-related changes in liver and kidney.

11.14.4 Diagnostic Testing—Reference Laboratory

- **Histopathology**

  Skin or mucosal lesion biopsy reveals hyperplasia, ballooning degeneration, and intracytoplasmic Bollinger bodies in epithelial cells; confirms viral etiology.
- **PCR**

  Detects viral DNA; differentiates field strains from vaccine strains (Figure 11.3).

11.14.5 Treatment and Therapeutic Interventions

Fowl pox is a viral disease with no specific antiviral treatment, so management focuses on supportive care, prevention of secondary infections, and minimizing stress. Clinical outcomes depend on the form of the disease and the overall health and immune status of the flock.

- **Supportive Care**

  Ensure clean, fresh water is always available. Provide high-quality food; for birds with oral lesions, they offer soft or moistened food to facilitate eating. If the bird is reluctant to self-feed,

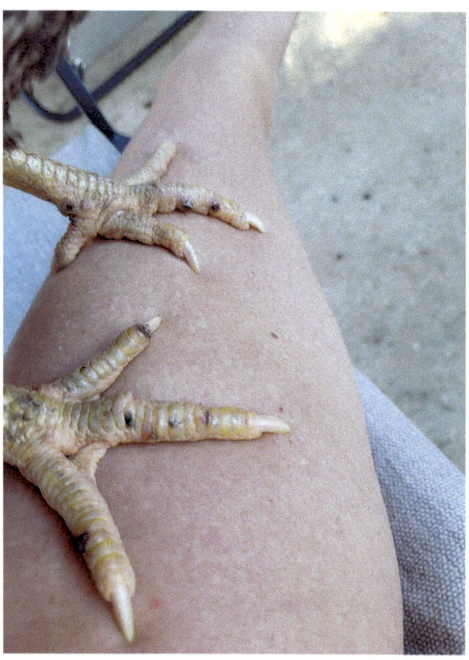

Figure 11.3 Fowl pox lesions on the feet. Courtesy of Sarah Meyer.

crop-feeding is advised. Reduce crowding, dust, and ammonia levels to minimize stress and secondary infections. Limit stress from handling, transport, or mixing with other birds, which can exacerbate disease. Anti-inflammatory agents can be administered for comfort.

- **Control of Secondary Infections**
  Bacterial infection may complicate skin or diphtheritic lesions. Antibiotics prescribed by the veterinarian if secondary bacterial infections are evident. Keep lesions clean and dry to reduce bacterial colonization.
- **Lesion Management**
  Topical antiseptics may be applied to cutaneous lesions if practical to prevent secondary infection. Avoid attempting to remove scabs manually, as this can worsen viral spread and cause discomfort for the bird.

11.14.6 Prevention and Control

- **Vaccination**
  Fowl pox vaccines are highly effective and widely used. The wing-web stab method is the most common administration method. It can also be given via intradermal or feather follicle routes in some protocols. Typically administered at 8–12 weeks of age for layers and breeders in commercial flocks. For backyard chicks in endemic areas, may vaccinate as early as 6 weeks if offered by hatcheries.
- **Biosecurity Measures**
  Remove scabs in the environment from previous outbreaks, clean and disinfect housing and equipment. Virus can survive for months in scabs and dust. Control the movement of people and equipment to prevent mechanical spread. Quarantine for a minimum of 30 days before introducing new birds to the flock.
- **Vector Control**
  Mosquito control is critical, especially for cutaneous to diphtheritic transmission. Eliminate standing water on property and near hen houses. Use insect screens, repellents, or larvicides.
- **Management Practices**
  Avoid overcrowding, sudden environmental changes, and rough handling. A balanced diet and adequate vitamins (A, E, and selenium) support immunity.

11.14.7 Nursing Considerations

Nursing considerations for birds affected by Fowl Pox focus on supportive care, prevention of secondary infections, and minimizing stress to aid recovery, as there is no specific antiviral treatment for this disease. Affected birds should be monitored closely for the presence of cutaneous or diphtheritic lesions, reduced food intake, lethargy, and difficulty swallowing or breathing, depending on the form of the disease. Housing should be clean, dry, well-ventilated, and low-stress, and affected birds may benefit from isolation from healthy flock members to reduce pecking injuries and allow careful observation. Providing easy access to clean water and nutrient-rich, easily digestible feed supports hydration and maintains body condition, while softening feed may help birds with oral or pharyngeal lesions. Assisted feeding or crop-feeding for anorexic birds. Nursing care also involves maintaining good hygiene of lesions to prevent secondary bacterial infections, reducing environmental stressors, and consulting a veterinarian if lesions are severe or complicating feeding and breathing. Overall, nursing considerations emphasize supportive management, environmental hygiene, stress reduction, and careful monitoring to promote recovery and minimize complications from Fowl Pox.

11.15 Avian Encephalomyelitis (AE)

11.15.1 Overview and Pathogenesis

Avian encephalomyelitis (AE) is a viral disease of poultry caused by Avian encephalomyelitis virus (AEV), a small, single-stranded RNA virus belonging to the *Picornaviridae* family. The disease primarily affects young chickens under 3 weeks of age, although older birds and other avian species can serve as reservoirs. AE is significant due to morbidity, growth retardation, and reduced egg production in commercial breeder flocks. Transmission occurs vertically from infected hens to progeny via eggs and horizontally through fecal-oral exposure to contaminated litter, feed, or water. Clinically, AE may present as tremors, ataxia, incoordination, leg paralysis, and stunted growth, with older birds often showing subclinical infections.

The pathogenesis of AE begins with ingestion or hatching from infected eggs, allowing the virus to replicate initially in the intestinal epithelium and lymphoid tissues. The virus then disseminates via the bloodstream to the central nervous system, where it preferentially infects neurons in the brainstem, cerebellum, and spinal cord. Viral replication in neurons causes neuronal degeneration, inflammation, and gliosis, leading to characteristic tremors, incoordination, and paralysis. Concurrently, the virus may replicate in pancreatic and hepatic tissues, contributing to reduced growth and production performance. Infection in adult birds is often subclinical but can result in a temporary reduction in egg production. Recovered birds develop immunity, but infected chicks may suffer permanent neurological deficits depending on the severity and timing of infection. Overall, AE is a neurotropic viral disease in which viral replication in neurons and lymphoid tissues leads to neurological signs, growth retardation, and decreased productivity in susceptible poultry. Veterinary professionals in clinical practice are not likely to observe this disease unless the bird originates from a commercial flock.

11.15.2 Risk Factors

- **Host-Related Factors**
  Chicks 1–3 weeks old are most susceptible to clinical disease. Older birds may become infected but usually remain subclinical. Maternal antibodies protect chicks for the first 1–2 weeks. Chicks from unvaccinated or poorly vaccinated breeders are at higher risk.
- **Virus-Related Factors**
  Some AE virus strains are more pathogenic, causing severe neurological disease. AE can survive in contaminated litter, feces, feed, and water, though it is less hardy than some other poultry viruses.
- **Transmission and Environmental Factors**
  Virus can be transmitted from infected breeder hens to eggs, resulting in infected chicks at hatch. Fecal–oral spread among young chicks in contaminated litter, feeders, or waterers. Cold or fluctuating temperatures may worsen disease severity in young chicks.
- **Management and Biosecurity Factors**
  Introduction of infected chicks from unvaccinated or contaminated sources. Older birds can act as carriers, exposing naïve chicks. Virus persists in feces and dust.
- **Vaccination-Related Factors**
  Unvaccinated breeders cause chicks to lack protective maternal antibodies. Improper breeder vaccination timing causes insufficient immunity to be passed to progeny. Vaccine handling errors because live AE vaccines are sensitive to temperature and light. Vaccines are not typically available for backyard flocks.

11.16 Clinical Signs and Pathology

- **External Findings**
  - *In Young Chicks (1–3 weeks, most susceptible)*
    Neurologic signs are the classic signs such as ataxia, fine tremors of head and neck, weakness, progressive paralysis of legs and wings, sitting on hocks, reluctance to move, loss of balance, and falling backward. Other signs that are seen are depression, failure to thrive, and cataracts may develop in some survivors. Survivors are also often stunted and unthrifty.
  - *In Adult Chickens (layers/breeders)*
    Usually subclinical infection. The main effect is a drop in egg production. Some birds may develop cataracts weeks to months after infection.
- **Necropsy Findings**
  Often absent or non-specific, especially in young chicks. In some cases, pale and emaciated birds. Proventriculus and gizzard may show mild catarrhal inflammation. Cataracts or cloudy lenses in some affected birds. Lymphocytic infiltration in gizzard and proventriculus in some cases. Lymphocytic perivascular cuffing in brain and spinal cord. Neuronal degeneration and gliosis in cerebellum.

11.16.1 Diagnostics Testing—Reference Laboratory

- **Reverse Transcriptase PCR (RT-PCR)**
  Detects AEV RNA; highly sensitive and specific.
- **Histopathology**
  Shows neuronal degeneration, necrosis, and perivascular cuffing; confirms neurotropic viral infection.

11.16.2 Treatment and Therapeutic Interventions

AE is a viral disease with no specific antiviral treatment.

- **Supportive Care**
  Ensure clean, fresh water is always available. Provide high-quality feed; chicks with neurological impairment may require soft or easily accessible feed. Maintain warm, dry, well-ventilated housing. Reduce stressors such as overcrowding, sudden noise, or handling. Isolation of severely affected chicks to minimize pecking or injury. Intensive nursing care includes fluid therapy, analgesics, and supplemental nutrition.
- **Control of Secondary Infections**
  AE-induced weakness and immobility predispose chicks to bacterial infections, especially in the skin or gastrointestinal tract. Antibiotics may be used under veterinary guidance to control secondary bacterial infections, but they do not affect the virus itself.

11.16.3 Prevention and Control

- **Vaccination (Main Preventive Measure)**
  Breeder vaccination is the cornerstone of control. Breeder pullets should be vaccinated at 10–15 weeks of age, well before the onset of lay. This ensures they develop strong immunity and pass protective maternal antibodies to chicks. Maternal antibodies protect chicks for the first

2–3 weeks of life, which is the critical period when they are most susceptible. Vaccines are not typically available for backyard flocks.

- **Biosecurity Measures**
  Prevent the introduction of virus into clean flocks by restricting visitors. Eggs should be sourced only from vaccinated and/or NPIP-certified breeder flocks. Proper disinfection and handling in hatcheries to minimize fecal contamination. Restrict movement of personnel, equipment, and vehicles between poultry houses. Use dedicated clothing, boots, and footbaths for each flock. Limit contamination by rodents, wild birds, or insects that may carry the virus.

11.16.4 Nursing Considerations

Nursing considerations for birds affected by AE focus on supportive care, prevention of secondary infections, and minimizing stress, particularly in young chicks, as there is no specific antiviral treatment. Affected birds should be closely monitored for neurological signs such as tremors, ataxia, weakness, or paralysis, as well as for decreased feed and water intake and lethargy, with gentle handling to avoid injury. Housing should be warm, draft-free, quiet, and low-stress, and affected birds may require isolation from healthy flock members to prevent bullying and allow targeted care. Providing easy access to clean water and nutrient-rich, easily digestible feed supports hydration, maintains body condition, and aids recovery in weakened birds. Nursing care also involves monitoring for secondary bacterial infections, particularly in birds with compromised mobility, and supportive interventions such as fluid therapy or supplemental feeding if necessary. Analgesia should be considered. Overall, nursing considerations emphasize supportive care, environmental management, stress reduction, careful observation, and maintenance of hydration and nutrition to optimize recovery and minimize complications in birds affected by AE. Euthanasia is always a humane treatment option.

11.17 Infectious Laryngotracheitis (ILT)

11.17.1 Overview and Pathogenesis

Infectious Laryngotracheitis (ILT) is an acute, highly contagious respiratory disease of chickens caused by *Gallid alphaherpesvirus* 1, a DNA virus belonging to the family *Herpesviridae*. The disease primarily affects older chickens and layers, although all ages are susceptible. ILT is of economic importance due to respiratory morbidity, decreased egg production, and occasional mortality. Transmission occurs mainly via aerosolized respiratory secretions, contaminated equipment, or personnel, and the virus can persist in recovered birds as a latent infection. Clinically, ILT may manifest as gasping, coughing, nasal discharge, expectoration of bloody mucus, conjunctivitis, and reduced egg production, with severe cases resulting in death.

The pathogenesis of ILT begins with inhalation of the virus, which infects the respiratory epithelium of the trachea and larynx. Viral replication causes destruction of ciliated epithelial cells, syncytia formation, and intranuclear inclusion bodies, leading to tracheal inflammation, edema, and hemorrhage. The loss of mucociliary clearance results in the accumulation of exudates and secondary bacterial infections, exacerbating respiratory distress. In severe cases, tracheal obstruction from fibrinous casts or mucus plugs can cause suffocation and death. Following recovery, the virus establishes latency in the trigeminal ganglia, with potential reactivation under stress or immunosuppression, enabling persistence and transmission within flocks. Overall, ILT is a viral respiratory disease characterized by epithelial destruction, airway inflammation, and latent infection, leading to acute respiratory signs and production losses in poultry. Veterinary professionals in clinical practice will likely not see this disease unless the bird originates from a commercial flock.

11.17.2 Risk Factors

- **Host-Related Factors**
  Most severe in chickens over 3 weeks old (broilers, layers, breeders). Rare in very young chicks. Immunosuppressed birds (due to MD, IBD, and stress) are more susceptible. No strong breed predisposition, but high-producing commercial layers and broilers are at greatest risk due to density.
- **Virus-Related Factors**
  Field strains range from mild (conjunctivitis, nasal discharge) to severe (dyspnea, high mortality). Inadequately attenuated live vaccines can revert to virulence and spread between birds. Recovered or vaccinated birds may become lifelong carriers and shed virus under stress.
- **Environmental and Management Factors**
  Overcrowding facilitates rapid respiratory spread. Poor ventilation and dusty housing worsen respiratory irritation, making birds more vulnerable. Older carrier birds can transmit viruses to younger birds. Mixing vaccinated and unvaccinated birds can perpetuate circulation.
- **Transmission-Related Factors**
  Direct transmission by coughing, sneezing, or respiratory secretions. Indirect transmission by contaminated equipment, litter, water, and clothing. Recovered or latently infected birds are the main reservoir.

11.17.3 Clinical Signs and Pathology

- **External Findings**
  Severe dyspnea, coughing and expectoration of bloody mucus, nasal discharge, conjunctivitis, watery eyes, laryngeal rales, and gurgling sounds. Depression, lethargy, and decreased appetite.
- **Necropsy Findings**
  Hemorrhage, congestion, and edema of the larynx and trachea. Fibrinous or diphtheritic membranes lining the trachea and larynx. Blood-stained mucus is often present in the trachea. Lungs are usually congested, occasionally with secondary bacterial pneumonia. Necrosis and sloughing of tracheal and laryngeal epithelium.

11.17.4 Diagnostic Testing—Reference Laboratory

- **PCR**
  Detects ILTV DNA from tracheal or conjunctival swabs, or tissue samples. Can differentiate vaccine strains from field strains using strain-specific primers (differential PCR or sequencing). Useful in early infection and carrier detection.
- Reportable disease in many states

11.17.5 Treatment and Therapeutic Interventions

Because *Gallid alphaherpesvirus* 1 is a herpesvirus, ILT infections cannot be cured once birds are infected. Management focuses on supportive care, outbreak control, and prevention of secondary infections.

- **Supportive Care**
  Reduce stressors (handling, overcrowding, heat/cold stress) to limit disease severity. Improve air quality and ventilation to reduce irritation and secondary infections. Ensure easy access to feed and clean water, sick birds often stop eating/drinking. Provide electrolytes and vitamins (especially vitamins A and C) in drinking water to support mucosal healing and immunity. Provide intensive nursing care to include fluid therapy, antibiotic, analgesics, and clean enclosure. Isolate clinically affected birds to limit virus spread.
- **Control of Secondary Bacterial Infections**
  Broad-spectrum antibiotics are used to reduce the risk of secondary infections, i.e., *Escherichia coli* or *Mycoplasma gallisepticum*. Common classes are tetracyclines, macrolides, or sulfonamide-trimethoprim combinations.

11.17.6 Prevention and Control

- **Vaccination (Main Preventive Tool)**
  Vaccination should be based on local disease prevalence and risk assessment. Avoid overuse of live vaccines in ILT-fee regions to prevent vaccine-virus cycling. Vaccines are not typically available for backyard flocks.
- **Biosecurity Measures**
  Quarantine new or returning birds for at least 30 days. Avoid mixing vaccinated and unvaccinated birds. Limit visitors to the property, access to birds.
- **Management During Outbreaks**
  Immediate isolation of affected birds if virus is suspected to prevent spread. Restrict movement of birds, eggs, and equipment off the premises. Emergency vaccination applies live attenuated vaccine to birds in the outbreak zone to reduce spread. This is not typically an option for backyard flocks.

11.17.7 Nursing Considerations

Nursing considerations for birds affected by Infectious Laryngotracheitis focus on supportive care, prevention of secondary infections, and reducing stress to aid respiratory recovery. Affected birds should be closely monitored for signs of respiratory distress, including coughing, sneezing, nasal discharge, and labored breathing, as well as for reduced feed and water intake, lethargy, and ruffled feathers. Housing should be clean, well-ventilated, draft-free, and low-stress, with affected birds isolated from the healthy flock to reduce disease spread and prevent pecking injuries. Providing easy access to clean water and soft, easily digestible food helps maintain hydration and nutrition, while supplemental electrolytes or vitamins may support recovery. Intensive nursing care includes fluid therapy if indicated, oxygen therapy, supplemental nutrition, antibiotic(s) for prevention of secondary bacterial infection(s), and anti-inflammatory/analgesic agents. Further nursing care also involves reducing environmental irritants such as dust and ammonia. Overall, nursing considerations emphasize supportive management, respiratory care, stress reduction, environmental hygiene, and careful observation to optimize recovery and maintain flock health in birds affected by ILT. To alleviate suffering, humane euthanasia is considered.

11.18 Bacterial Diseases of Chickens

Bacterial diseases play a significant role in poultry morbidity and mortality. Unlike viral diseases, many bacterial infections are treatable with antimicrobials if diagnosed early, though antimicrobial resistance and residue concerns limit indiscriminate use. Veterinary technicians are often involved in sample collection, administering and monitoring therapeutic responses, and client education about biosecurity and husbandry (Table 11.2).

11.19 Fowl Cholera

11.19.1 Overview and Pathogenesis

Fowl Cholera is an acute, subacute, or chronic bacterial disease of poultry caused by *Pasteurella multocida*, a Gram-negative, non-motile, encapsulated bacterium. The disease affects chickens, turkeys, and other avian species. Transmission occurs via direct contact with infected birds, contaminated water, feed, equipment, and fomites, and chronic carriers play a major role in maintaining infection within flocks. Clinically, fowl cholera may manifest as sudden death in acute outbreaks, respiratory signs, diarrhea, swollen wattles, joint inflammation, and decreased egg production in subacute or chronic cases. The disease is particularly common in California, Texas, Nebraska, and the Lower Missouri River Basin. It also occurs in other countries, though outbreaks in wild birds appear less frequent outside North America. Fowl cholera can occur throughout the year, but is most prevalent in late summer and fall, and winter months.

The pathogenesis of fowl cholera begins with colonization of the upper respiratory tract or mucous membranes following exposure to *P. multocida*. The bacterium then invades the bloodstream, leading to bacteremia and septicemia. Virulence factors such as the capsule, adhesins, lipopolysaccharide (LPS), and exotoxins facilitate evasion of host immunity, adherence to tissues, and tissue damage. Septicemia results in systemic lesions, including hemorrhages, fibrinous exudates on serosal surfaces, hepatomegaly, splenomegaly, and joint inflammation. Acute cases often result in rapid death without prior clinical signs, while subacute or chronic infections may produce localized lesions, decreased performance, and persistent environmental contamination. Environmental persistence of *P. multocida* and the presence of asymptomatic carriers contribute to repeated outbreaks. In summary, fowl cholera is a systemic, septicemic disease in which bacterial invasion, virulence factors, and host susceptibility combine to produce rapid mortality or chronic infection in poultry.

11.19.2 Risk Factors

- **Host-Related Factors**
  More common in mature and older birds (layers, breeders, turkeys). Rare in chicks under 16 weeks of age. Turkeys are highly susceptible, chickens somewhat less so.
- **Pathogen-Related Factors**
  Birds that recover may harbor *P. multocida* in the respiratory tract, tonsils, or sinuses, shedding bacteria intermittently. Some strains cause peracute outbreaks with sudden death, while others cause chronic localized infections.

Table 11.2

Quick reference chart

Disease	Causative agent	Transmission	Key clinical signs	Diagnostic testing	Treatment
Mycoplasmosis (CRD, infectious synovitis)	*Mycoplasma gallisepticum*, *M. synoviae*	Aerosols, direct contact, vertical (eggs), fomites	Chronic respiratory signs: coughing, rales, nasal discharge; swollen joints/synovitis with *M. synoviae*	PCR, culture, ELISA, HI	Tylosin, tiamulin, tetracyclines (reduce signs, not eliminate)
Colibacillosis	*Escherichia coli* (pathogenic strains)	Fecal–oral, inhalation of contaminated dust, secondary to viral infections	Respiratory distress, septicemia, peritonitis, omphalitis in chicks	Culture, PCR, serotyping	Broad-spectrum antibiotics (based on sensitivity), supportive
Fowl cholera	*Pasteurella multocida*	Ingestion, inhalation, contaminated equipment, carrier birds	Acute: sudden death; Chronic: localized swellings (wattles, joints), respiratory distress	Culture, PCR, Gram stain	Sulfonamides, tetracyclines, penicillin (based on sensitivity)
Paratyphoid	*Salmonella enterica* (non-host adapted serovars)	Fecal–oral, contaminated feed/water, rodents, wild birds	Often subclinical; sometimes diarrhea, decreased growth, septicemia	Culture, serotyping, PCR	Antibiotics based on sensitivity (care: carrier risk)
Erysipelas	*Erysipelothrix rhusiopathiae*	Skin wounds, ingestion, contaminated soil, carriers	Sudden death, swollen snood/face (turkeys), lameness, cutaneous lesions	Culture, Gram stain, PCR	Penicillin (effective), supportive care
Staphylococcosis	*Staphylococcus aureus*	Skin wounds, contaminated environment, secondary to trauma	Lameness, bumblefoot, arthritis, septicemia, osteomyelitis	Culture, Gram stain, sensitivity testing	Antibiotics based on culture, wound care
Avian chlamydiosis	*Chlamydia psittaci*	Inhalation of dried droppings, secretions; zoonotic	Lethargy, ruffled feathers, green droppings, nasal discharge, conjunctivitis	PCR, culture (specialized labs), ELISA, histopathology	Tetracyclines (e.g., doxycycline), prolonged courses
Necrotic enteritis	*Clostridium perfringens* (Type A/C)	Overgrowth in gut (predisposed by coccidiosis, diet), fecal-oral	Depression, ruffled feathers, diarrhea, sudden death	Histopathology, anaerobic culture, PCR for toxins	Bacitracin, penicillin, supportive
Botulism	*Clostridium botulinum* toxin	Ingestion of preformed toxin in carcasses, spoiled feed, wet litter	Flaccid paralysis, limp neck ("limberneck"), death from respiratory failure	Mouse bioassay, ELISA, PCR	Antitoxin (early), supportive, remove source
Gangrenous dermatitis	*Clostridium septicum*, *C. perfringens*, *Staph. aureus* (mixed)	Skin trauma, immunosuppression (IBD, CAV), contaminated litter	Rapid mortality, skin discoloration, moist lesions, subcutaneous emphysema	Impression smears, culture, histopathology	Penicillin, bacitracin, improve environment

Table courtesy of Stephanie Freeman.

- **Environmental and Management Factors**
  High stocking density and overcrowding facilitate spread. Poor ventilation and wet litter cause stressed birds and support bacterial survival. Older carriers can infect younger birds.
- **Transmission-Related Factors**
  Wild birds, rodents, and other animals (cats, dogs) can carry and introduce *P. multocida*. Bacteria can survive for weeks in moist environments. Dead birds not promptly removed can be a major source.

11.19.3 Clinical Signs and Pathology

- **External Findings**
  - *Peracute Form (Sudden Outbreaks)*
    Sudden death without prior clinical signs.
  - *Acute Form*
    Depression, lethargy, ruffled feathers, high fever, anorexia, increased thirst, nasal and oral discharge, dyspnea, cyanosis, greenish diarrhea, and a drop in egg production.
  - *Chronic Form*
    Localized infections due to survival of bacteria in tissues, swollen wattles, swollen joints, and footpads. Abscesses in sinus, ear, or conjunctiva. Chronic wasting and reduced productivity.
- **Necropsy Findings**
  - *Peracute/Acute Cases*
    Septicemia is the hallmark sign. Petechial and ecchymotic hemorrhages on heart, liver, and gizzard mucosa. Enlarged, congested liver and spleen (often with small necrotic foci). Congested lungs with possible pneumonia. Fibrinous exudates on serous membranes (pericarditis, perihepatitis, peritonitis). Congested intestines; enteritis with mucus or blood.
  - *Chronic Cases*
    Caseous exudates in wattles, sinuses, joints, and tendon sheaths. Swollen wattles filled with pus. Chronic pneumonia and air sacculitis.

11.19.4 Diagnostic Testing—Reference Laboratory

- **Culture**
  Collect samples aseptically from heart blood, liver, spleen, and bone marrow (acute cases). Swabs from lesions or exudates in chronic cases. Culture on blood agar or chocolate agar under aerobic conditions. Identify small Gram-negative coccobacilli with characteristic morphology and biochemical profile.
- **PCR**
  Detects Pasteurella multocida DNA directly from tissues or swabs. Highly sensitive and specific. Useful when birds have received antibiotics or when rapid confirmation is needed.
- **Impression Smears**
  Impression smears from liver or heart blood (acute deaths). Stain with Gram, Giemsa, or Wright stain. Observe bipolar-staining Gram-negative coccobacilli, which is a characteristic of *P. multocida*.
- Reportable disease in some states

11.19.5 Treatment and Therapeutic Interventions

- **Antibiotic Therapy**
  Pasteurella multocida is usually sensitive to many antibiotics, but treatment reduces mortality rather than eliminating carrier states. Usually given in drinking water or feed for flock treatment. Individual treatment (e.g., injections) may be feasible in small flocks or valuable birds.

- **Supportive Therapy**
  Provide good nutrition and clean water. Add vitamins (A, C, E, and K) and electrolytes to support recovery and reduce stress. Reduce overcrowding and environmental stressors.
- **Therapeutic Interventions in Flock Settings**
  Implement immediate antibiotic treatment to reduce losses, but follow with long-term prevention strategies (vaccination, biosecurity). Remove and properly dispose of dead birds quickly to reduce environmental contamination.

11.19.6 Prevention and Control

- **Biosecurity (Most Important Measure)**
  Prevent introduction of *P. multocida*. Quarantine new or replacement birds for at least 30 days. Limit access to visitors. Disinfect feeders, drinkers, and housing regularly. Remove and properly dispose of carcasses quickly (burning, composting, or deep burial). Rodents and wild birds are major reservoirs of *P. multocida*. Seal feed bins, eliminate standing water, and reduce vegetation around enclosures.
- **Vaccination**
  Protection is often strain-specific therefore vaccines may not protect against all field isolates. Vaccination should be combined with biosecurity, not used alone. Vaccines are typically not available to backyard flocks.
- **Environmental Management**
  P. multocida survives for weeks in moist soil, litter, and water. Thorough cleaning, drying, and disinfection are critical. Rotate pasture for free-range birds to prevent build-up in soil.

11.19.7 Nursing Considerations

Nursing considerations for birds affected by Fowl Cholera focus on supportive care, prevention of secondary infections, and strict biosecurity, as this bacterial disease can cause rapid morbidity and mortality. Affected birds should be closely monitored for signs such as lethargy, ruffled feathers, reduced feed and water intake, diarrhea, swollen wattles or joints, and sudden deaths, with early detection improving recovery outcomes. Housing should be clean, dry, well-ventilated, and stress-free, and affected birds should be isolated from the healthy flock to reduce disease spread. Providing readily accessible, high-quality feed and clean water supports hydration and nutrition, while environmental management, including disinfection of feeders, waterers, and housing, helps limit pathogen exposure. Nursing care also involves monitoring hydration, supplemental nutrition as needed, antibiotic(s) for secondary infections when indicated, and reducing flock stress. Overall, nursing considerations emphasize supportive care, husbandry, stress reduction, careful monitoring, and biosecurity to improve recovery and protect flock health in cases of Fowl Cholera. Euthanasia is always a humane treatment option to alleviate suffering.

11.20 Colibacillosis (*E. coli*)

11.20.1 Overview and Pathogenesis

Colibacillosis is a common bacterial disease of poultry caused by *Escherichia coli*, a Gram-negative, facultatively anaerobic bacterium. It primarily affects chickens of all ages but is especially significant in commercial-raised meat birds, layers, and immunocompromised birds. The disease is opportunistic, often arising secondary to stress, viral infections, or poor management, and is a major cause of respiratory disease, septicemia, and mortality in affected flocks. Transmission occurs via direct contact, contaminated feed, water, equipment, and the environment, with vertical transmission possible in some cases. Clinically, colibacillosis may present as air sacculitis, pericarditis, perihepatitis, septicemia, cellulitis, and swollen joints, leading to poor growth, decreased egg production, and increased mortality. Veterinary professionals in clinical practice may see affected birds formerly living in squalid conditions.

The pathogenesis of colibacillosis involves the colonization of mucosal surfaces, primarily the respiratory and gastrointestinal tracts, by pathogenic strains of *E. coli*. Predisposing factors such as viral infections (e.g., IB and ND), environmental stress, high stocking density, poor ventilation, and immunosuppression facilitate bacterial invasion. Once the bacterium breaches mucosal barriers, it enters the bloodstream, causing septicemia and systemic infection. Pathogenic *E. coli* strains produce a variety of virulence factors, including adhesins, fimbriae, hemolysins, endotoxins, and capsules, which enhance attachment, immune evasion, and tissue damage. The result is widespread inflammation, fibrinous exudation, and necrosis in affected organs such as the liver, heart, air sacs, and joints. Clinical severity depends on host immunity, bacterial virulence, and environmental conditions. Recovered or subclinical infected birds may become carriers, shed bacteria, and maintain environmental contamination. Overall, colibacillosis is an opportunistic, systemic bacterial disease in which stress, co-infections, and virulence factors converge to produce localized lesions, septicemia, and production losses in poultry.

11.20.2 Risk Factors

- **Environmental and Management Factors**
  Poor ventilation, buildup of ammonia, and dust irritate the respiratory tract, allowing bacterial invasion. Overcrowding increases stress, competition, and contamination load. High humidity and wet litter promote bacterial growth and contamination of feathers, feet, and equipment. Inadequate sanitation and disinfection of housing, feeders, and drinkers. Poor quality feed or contaminated water sources.
- **Host-Related Factors**
  Young birds with immature immune systems are less able to fight infection. Immunosuppression from other diseases (e.g., IBD, MD, and CAV) or stress. Nutritional deficiencies, especially vitamins A, E, and selenium, impair immune function. Concurrent respiratory infections (e.g., IB, Mycoplasmosis, and ND) damage the respiratory epithelium and allow secondary *E. coli* invasion. Breaches in skin or mucous membranes, such as wounds, pecking injuries, or navels in newly hatched chicks.
- **Pathogen-Related Factors**
  Presence of virulent APEC (Avian Pathogenic *Escherichia coli*) strains with fimbriae, toxins, and iron-acquisition systems that enhance colonization and immune evasion. High environmental contamination levels for feces of infected or carrier birds.

11.20.3 Clinical Signs and Pathology

- **External Findings**
  Depression, ruffled feathers, loss of appetite, and poor growth. Sneezing, coughing, rales, nasal discharge, dyspnea, and swollen sinuses. Infected leg and/or foot lesions. Sudden death, cyanosis of comb and wattles, and fever, followed by weakness and dehydration.

- **Necropsy Findings**
  - *Acute Colibacillosis (Septicemia)*
    Enlarged, congested liver (hepatomegaly), sometimes with small necrotic foci. Splenomegaly and congestion. Petechial hemorrhages of heart, liver, and generalized musculature. Septicemia may occur without obvious localized lesions.
  - *Subacute/Chronic Colibacillosis*
    Thickened, cloudy, fibrinous exudate in air sacs (hallmark lesion). Pericarditis, perihepatitis, peritonitis, salpingitis/oophoritis, arthritis/osteomyelitis, and omphalitis in chicks.

11.20.4 Diagnostic Testing—Reference Laboratory

- **Culture**
  Gold standard for confirming colibacillosis. Collect samples from internal organs showing lesions (heart, liver, spleen, air sacs, joints, yolk sac) using aseptic technique. Culture on MacConkey agar or blood agar colonies are lactose-fermenting, Gram-negative rods. Confirm identity using biochemical tests or automated systems (e.g., API and VITEK).
- **PCR**
  Detects *E. coli*-specific or APEC virulence genes (e.g., iss, tsh, iroN, iutA). It is useful for confirming pathogenic strains and differentiating from commensal isolates.

11.20.5 Treatment and Therapeutic Interventions

Escherichia coli infections require prompt and targeted therapy because the disease can progress rapidly to septicemia and death. Effective treatment includes antimicrobial therapy, supportive care, and flock-level management measures.

- **Supportive Care**
  Improve hydration and electrolyte balance (especially during septicemia) orally, subcutaneously, or intravenously. Vitamin supplementation (especially vitamins A, E, and selenium) to support immunity. Reduce stress (optimize temperature, reduce handling, avoid overcrowding).
- **Medications**
  Antibiotics are the primary treatment, but therapy must be guided by AST due to widespread resistance among avian *E. coli* strains.
  Amoxicillin/Clavulanate: 125–250 mg/kg by mouth every 8–12 hours for 5–7 days.
  Amoxicillin Sodium: 50–250 mg/kg intramuscular every 8–12 hours for 5–7 days.
  Amoxicillin Trihydrate 55–200 mg/kg by mouth, subcutaneous, or intramuscularly every 4–12 hours for 5–7 days.
  Oxytetracycline 5 mg/kg subcutaneous or intramuscular every 12–24 hours. 2500 mg/L drinking water and 2500 mg/kg feed.

11.21 Prevention and Control

- **Biosecurity and Management**
  Quarantine. Control rodents, wild birds, and insects (mechanical carriers of *E. coli*). Restrict visitor access and disinfect equipment/footwear.

- **Environmental Control**
  Maintain good airflow, reduce ammonia and dust, which protects the respiratory tract. Fresh, clean water. Keep feeders clean and avoid moldy feed. Clean pen and house regularly. Disinfect perches, nest boxes, houses, and pens after cleaning.
- **Control of Predisposing Factors**
  Vaccination against primary respiratory pathogens IBV, NDV, and *Mycoplasma gallisepticum*. Hatcheries offer vaccinations; backyard flocks typically do not have vaccines available. Control of coccidiosis prevents gut damage and secondary *E. coli* infection. Reduce stress.
- **Vaccination and Probiotics**
  Autogenous or commercial vaccines are available in some regions (e.g., live attenuated aroA mutant strains). Mainly used in breeder or layer flocks in endemic farms. Probiotics, prebiotics, and competitive exclusion products help maintain healthy gut flora and reduce colonization by pathogenic *E. coli*.
- **Therapeutic Control**
  Antibiotics (based on culture and sensitivity) tetracyclines, sulfonamides, enrofloxacin (where permitted). Supportive therapy such as enteral or parental fluids for hydration; vitamins A, E, C, selenium, and electrolytes to boost immunity.

11.21.1 Nursing Considerations

Nursing considerations for birds affected by Colibacillosis focus on supportive care, maintaining hydration and nutrition, and preventing secondary infections. Affected birds should be closely monitored for signs such as depression, lethargy, reduced feed and water intake, ruffled feathers, diarrhea, and evidence of systemic infection, with early recognition improving outcomes. Housing should be clean, dry, well-ventilated, and stress-free, and affected birds may need to be isolated from healthy flock members to prevent further spread and reduce competition at feeders and waterers. Providing easy access to fresh water and high-quality, easily digestible feed supports hydration and nutritional status, while reducing gastrointestinal stress. Nursing care also involves monitoring for secondary bacterial infections, minimizing stressors, veterinarian-prescribed appropriate antimicrobial therapy, and/or supportive treatments. Open wounds require frequent cleaning and dressing. When handling affected birds, appropriate PPE should be worn. Overall, nursing considerations emphasize supportive management, environmental hygiene, careful observation, stress reduction, and veterinarian collaboration to optimize recovery and maintain flock health. Humane euthanasia is an option to alleviate bird suffering.

11.22 Mycoplasmosis

11.22.1 Overview and Pathogenesis

Mycoplasmosis in poultry is a chronic, significant respiratory and systemic disease caused primarily by *Mycoplasma gallisepticum* (MG) and, to a lesser extent, *Mycoplasma synoviae* (MS). The disease affects chickens and turkeys of all ages, although young and immunocompromised birds are particularly susceptible. It is highly contagious and spreads via direct contact, aerosols, or contaminated equipment, with vertical transmission from infected breeders to offspring also possible. Clinically, Mycoplasmosis may manifest as respiratory signs, reduced growth, decreased egg production, lameness, and, in severe cases, increased mortality. The disease often predisposes flocks to secondary bacterial infections, compounding economic losses. MS is very common in backyard flocks, likely due to a lack of biosecurity.

The pathogenesis of Mycoplasmosis begins with colonization of the respiratory epithelium or, in the case of MS, synovial membranes. *Mycoplasma* species lack a cell wall, allowing them to adhere tightly to epithelial cells using specialized attachment organelles. Once attached, they evade the host immune response through antigenic variation and suppression of local immunity, leading to chronic infection. The bacteria induce ciliary damage, epithelial sloughing, and mucosal inflammation, resulting in impaired mucociliary clearance and respiratory distress. In the case of *M. synoviae*, joint colonization triggers synovitis, lameness, and reduced mobility. Immunosuppressive factors, stress, and concurrent infections exacerbate disease severity. Chronic carriers may harbor *Mycoplasma* in the respiratory tract or reproductive organs, facilitating long-term transmission within and between flocks. Overall, Mycoplasmosis is a chronic, opportunistic infection in which bacterial adhesion, immune evasion, and tissue damage lead to respiratory, articular, and systemic manifestations.

11.22.2 Risk Factors

- **Host-Related Factors**
  All ages are susceptible, but chronic respiratory disease (CRD) is more severe in older birds. Commercial broilers and layers are more susceptible than native breeds.
- **Environmental and Management Factors**
  Poor ventilation causes ammonia and dust damage to respiratory mucosa. Overcrowding causes stress and rapid disease spread.
- **Transmission-Related Factors**
  Infected breeder hens transmit *Mycoplasma* via eggs. Aerosol droplets, contaminated equipment, feed, water, or people can also transmit disease.
- **Co-Infections**
- Viral infections (IBV, NDV, AI) damage the respiratory tract and increase severity. ORT co-infection worsens disease.

11.22.3 Clinical Signs and Pathology

- **External Findings**
  - *Respiratory Form (Mycoplasma gallisepticum or CRD)*
    Coughing, sneezing, nasal discharge, rales, conjunctivitis, watery eyes, swollen infraorbital sinuses.
  - *Reproductive Form*
    Drop in egg production and hatchability. Reduced fertility in breeders. Misshapen, thin-shelled, or rough eggs in layer.
  - *Joint Form (Mycoplasma synoviae or Infectious Synovitis)*
    Lameness, reluctance to move, swollen hock joints and footpads, and tendon sheath swelling (especially gastrocnemius).
- **Necropsy Findings**
  - *Respiratory Form (Mycoplasma gallisepticum or CRD)*
    Thickened, cloudy, or caseous exudate in air sacs (often fibrinous). Mucous or caseous plugs in trachea, cloudy exudate in sinuses. Swollen eyelids and frothy exudate.

- *Reproductive Form*
  Oophoritis, salpingitis, and peritonitis in severe or chronic infections.
- *Joint Form (Mycoplasma synoviae or Infectious Synovitis)*
  Yellow, turbid exudate in hock joints, footpads, and tendon sheaths. Chronic cases thickened synovial membranes, caseous exudate, and lameness. Deformities or ankylosis (fusion) of joints in long-term cases.

11.22.4 Diagnostic Testing—Reference Laboratory

- **Serology (for Screening Flocks)**
  Rapid Plate Agglutination (RPA): Quick but prone to false positives.
  ELISA: More reliable for flock-level monitoring.
- **Culture**
  Requires specialized media; slow but confirms viable organisms.
- **PCR**
  Highly sensitive and specific; detects MG/MS DNA from swabs or tissues.

11.22.5 Treatment and Therapeutic Interventions

- **Medication**
  Tylosin 50 mg/kg orally once daily for 5–7 days or 15–30 mg/kg intramuscularly every 6–12 hours for 5–7 days.
  Tiamulin 25–50 mg/kg orally every 24 hours for 3–5 days.
  Oxytetracycline 5 mg/kg subcutaneous or intramuscular every 12–24 hours. 2500 mg/L drinking water and 2500 mg/kg feed.
- **Supportive Care**
  Treat concurrent *E. coli* or viral infections to reduce mortality. Anti-inflammatories for discomfort.

11.22.6 Prevention and Control

- **Biosecurity and Management**
  Acquire *Mycoplasma*-free chicks or hatching eggs from certified sources. Quarantine new birds for at least 3–4 weeks before introduction. Rodent and wild bird control (important reservoirs and vectors). Restrict visitor access and enforce footwear/clothing disinfection.
- **Environmental Management**
  Good ventilation prevents buildup of ammonia and dust that damages the respiratory tract. Avoids overcrowding to minimize stress and spread.
- **Hatchery and Breeder Flock Management**
  Keep breeder flocks *Mycoplasma*-free (testing, culling positives). Use SPF (specific-pathogen-free) eggs where possible. Maintain strict hatchery hygiene (egg fumigation/sanitization, clean hatchers).
- **Vaccination**
  Vaccination (when available) is recommended in endemic areas.
- **Control of Predisposing Factors**
  Vaccinate (when available) against respiratory viruses (NDV, IBV, ILT, AI) to prevent co-infections. Control *E. coli* and coccidiosis to reduce secondary infections. Provide balanced

nutrition (adequate vitamins A, E, selenium, zinc) for mucosal immunity. Minimize stress from handling, vaccination, or transport.

- **Medication/Therapeutic Control**
  Antibiotics do not eliminate *Mycoplasma* but can reduce signs and transmission. Should be combined with biosecurity and vaccination.

11.22.7 Nursing Considerations

Nursing care for birds affected by Mycoplasmosis focuses on supportive management, minimizing stress, and preventing secondary infections. Affected flocks should be housed in clean, well-ventilated environments with optimal temperature and humidity to reduce respiratory strain. Isolate infected birds to prevent transmission and monitor them closely for signs of respiratory distress, lethargy, reduced feed intake, or a drop in egg production. Provide easily digestible, high-quality food and fresh water to maintain hydration and nutritional status. Intensive nursing interventions can potentially improve outcomes: fluid therapy, oxygen therapy, and supplemental nutrition. Stressful handling should be minimized, as stress exacerbates clinical signs and bacterial proliferation. Implement strict biosecurity measures, including disinfection of equipment, proper waste disposal, and limiting visitors to the flock. Administer approved, prescribed antibiotics, ensuring correct dosage and duration to avoid resistance.

11.23 Paratyphoid

11.23.1 Overview and Pathogenesis

Paratyphoid in poultry refers to infections caused by non-host-adapted *Salmonella* spp., most commonly *Salmonella enterica* serovars such as *S. Typhimurium*, *S. Enteritidis*, *S. Heidelberg*, and others. Unlike *Salmonella pullorum* and *S. Gallinarum*, which cause host-specific diseases (Pullorum Disease and fowl typhoid), paratyphoid infections affect a broad range of avian species and are important zoonotic pathogens, posing food safety concerns. The disease can occur in birds of all ages but is particularly severe in young chicks and poults, often leading to septicemia and high mortality, whereas older birds may become asymptomatic carriers. Transmission occurs both vertically (through eggs from infected breeders) and horizontally through contaminated feed, water, litter, fomites, rodents, wild birds, and humans, making biosecurity critical to prevention.

Pathogenesis begins with the ingestion of *Salmonella* organisms, which colonize the intestinal mucosa, particularly in the ceca, and then invade enterocytes and macrophages. The bacteria are capable of intracellular survival and replication, allowing them to bypass host defenses and disseminate systemically via the bloodstream. In young or immunocompromised birds, this results in bacteremia and septicemia, with localization in the liver, spleen, yolk sac, joints, and other organs. Lesions typically include focal necrosis and white pinpoint foci in the liver and spleen, catarrhal enteritis, and omphalitis in chicks. Clinical signs vary depending on the age and immune status of the flock but commonly include depression, ruffled feathers, watery diarrhea, dehydration, anorexia, huddling, and increased mortality in young birds. Older or carrier birds may not show obvious signs, but shed bacteria intermittently, contributing to environmental contamination and perpetuating infection cycles.

11.23.2 Risk Factors

- **Host-Related Factors**
  Young chicks and turkey poults are highly vulnerable; infections are often more severe in the first few weeks of life. Older birds may act as carriers, shedding bacteria without obvious clinical disease.
- **Environmental Factors**
  Poor sanitation in housing, hatcheries, or equipment (incubators, drinkers, feeders). Contaminated hatcheries (eggs, incubators, trays, and transport boxes). Wet, dirty litter that supports bacterial survival and multiplication.
- **Management Factors**
  Overcrowding increases stress and contamination load. Inadequate biosecurity (movement of people, equipment, and vehicles between flocks). Poor ventilation and hygiene weaken bird immunity and promote bacterial spread. Mixing different age groups of birds, allowing carriers to infect younger, more susceptible chicks.
- **Nutritional and Health Factors**
  Poor nutrition or contaminated feedstuffs (fish meal, meat meal, or poorly stored grains). Stress factors (transport, handling, temperature extremes). Concurrent immunosuppressive diseases (e.g., IBD, MD) reduce resistance.

11.23.3 Clinical Signs and Pathology

- **External Findings**
  Sudden death without warning. Lethargy, huddling, and drooping wings. Anorexia and poor growth. Watery, whitish or greenish diarrhea, causing pasted vents. Dehydration, ruffled feathers, and weakness. Swollen, painful joints in some cases (arthritis).
- **Necropsy Findings**
  Enlarged, congested liver and spleen. Small gray-white necrotic foci ("paratyphoid nodules") on liver. Inflamed, catarrhal to hemorrhagic small intestine with watery contents. Yolk sacculitis with cheesy, caseous material. Congested lungs, sometimes with fibrinous pneumonia.

11.23.4 Diagnostic Testing—Reference Laboratory

- **PCR**
  PCR provides rapid and sensitive detection of Salmonella DNA in tissues, feces, or environmental samples. Targets include the invA gene, present in all Salmonella species. PCR is especially useful in detecting low-level or intermittent shedders that may be missed by culture.
- **Culture**
  Sample Types
  Living birds: Cloacal swabs, feces, or guardian boot swabs.
  Deceased birds: Liver, spleen, ceca, intestinal contents, and yolk sac in chicks.
  Environmental: Litter, hatchery fluff, feed, water, and dust samples.
  Culture is the definitive test for regulatory and surveillance programs.
- Reportable disease in many states

11.23.5 Treatment and Therapeutic Interventions

- **Supportive Care**
  Young chicks and stressed adults are most susceptible to systemic disease. Supportive therapy should be initiated immediately upon suspicion, even before laboratory confirmation. Provide oral rehydration solutions (ORS) with electrolytes and glucose via drinking water to counteract dehydration from enteritis. In severely ill, subcutaneous fluids (e.g., Lactated Ringer's solution at 20–30 mL/kg, warmed) may be indicated. Maintain optimal brooding temperatures in chicks to reduce stress. Avoid chilling or overheating, which can exacerbate disease progression. Offer easily digestible feeds, free of contaminants. Vitamin supplementation, especially vitamins A, D3, E, and B-complex, may aid recovery. Crop feeding when indicated. Use prebiotics and probiotics to restore normal intestinal microbiota and reduce *Salmonella* colonization.
- **Medication**
  Amoxicillin/Clavulanate 125–250 mg/kg by mouth every 8–12 hours for 5–7 days.
  Trimethoprim-Sulfamethoxazole 100 mg/kg by mouth every 12 hours for 5–7 days.
  Oxytetracycline 5 mg/kg subcutaneous or intramuscular every 12–24 hours. 2500 mg/L drinking water and 2500 mg/kg feed.

11.23.6 Prevention and Control

- **Biosecurity Measures**
  Biosecurity is the cornerstone of paratyphoid prevention, aimed at preventing introduction and spreading *Salmonella* into flocks. Restrict flock access. Disinfect equipment (waterers and feeders) and tools entering flock areas. Establish rodent, wild bird, and insect control programs, as these vectors play a major role in *Salmonella* spread. Avoid introducing birds of unknown health status; purchase chicks or pullets from NPIP-approved or *Salmonella*-monitored sources.
- **Feed and Water Control**
  Contaminated feed is a major source of infection. *Salmonella* can survive for months in feed ingredients and multiply if moisture is present. Source feed from reputable, *Salmonella*-monitored suppliers. Use heat-treated or pelleted feed, as pelleting temperatures kill *Salmonella*. Store feeds in clean, dry bins that protect them from moisture, rodents, and wild birds. Clean feeders regularly and removing old or spilled feed. Wash and disinfect feeders and waterers. Avoid standing water, which can harbor *Salmonella* and other pathogens. *Salmonella* can persist in biofilms.
- **Environmental Sanitation**
  Because paratyphoid salmonellae survive for months in damp litter and dust, between-flock cleaning and downtime are crucial. Remove all organic matter (manure, litter, dust) before applying disinfectants. Use effective disinfectants such as phenolics, oxidizing agents, or quaternary ammonium compounds. Thoroughly dry the house after disinfection; dry conditions significantly reduce *Salmonella* survival. Allow a downtime period of at least 2 weeks, ideally longer, between flocks. Clean and disinfect all equipment, nest boxes, feeders, and waterers. Proper sanitation is often the most effective and economical control step for *Salmonella*.

11.23.7 Nursing Considerations

Nursing care for chickens affected by paratyphoid focuses on supportive management, strict biosecurity, and prevention of spread, as *Salmonella* infections pose both animal health and public health (zoonotic) concerns. Veterinary technicians should monitor birds, especially young chicks, closely for depression, diarrhea, dehydration, poor growth, and increased mortality, providing clean, easily accessible water and nutritionally balanced feed to support hydration and recovery. Crop feeding and fluid therapy are recommended for critically ill birds. Severely affected birds should be isolated promptly to limit environmental contamination and to facilitate individualized care. Brooding temperatures and environmental conditions should be optimal and stress-free, as chilling or overcrowding exacerbates disease severity. Rodent and wild bird control is critical, as these are common reservoirs and vectors. Education of caretakers about zoonotic risk, emphasizing hand hygiene and safe handling of eggs and raw poultry products, is essential. Vaccination (when available) may be part of a comprehensive prevention plan. Humane euthanasia of suffering birds is always a reasonable clinical option.

11.24 Necrotic Enteritis

11.24.1 Overview and Pathogenesis

Necrotic Enteritis (NE) is an economically important enteric disease of poultry caused primarily by *Clostridium perfringens*, a Gram-positive, spore-forming, anaerobic bacterium. The disease predominantly affects commercial facility chickens aged 2–6 weeks but can also occur in older birds under predisposing conditions. NE may present as an acute clinical form with sudden mortality or as a subclinical form characterized by poor weight gain, decreased feed conversion, and reduced overall performance. Although *C. perfringens* is a normal component of the intestinal microbiota, disease occurs when intestinal homeostasis is disrupted, allowing pathogenic strains to proliferate. Predisposing factors include high-protein diets, non-starch polysaccharides, coccidial infections that damage intestinal mucosa, immunosuppression, and environmental stressors. The pathogenesis of necrotic enteritis begins with overgrowth of pathogenic *C. perfringens* in the small intestine, especially the jejunum and ileum, under favorable conditions created by predisposing factors. The bacteria produce potent toxins, primarily alpha-toxin and, in some strains, NetB toxins, which damage enterocytes, disrupt the mucosal barrier, and trigger an inflammatory response. This results in necrosis intestinal epithelium, fibrin deposition, and heterophilic infiltration, producing the characteristic fibrin necrotic lesions observed on necropsy. Clinically, acute NE manifests as depression, ruffled feathers, diarrhea with foul odor, and sudden death, whereas subclinical NE leads to impaired nutrient absorption and poor flock performance. Recovered or subclinical affected birds may continue to shed pathogenic clostridia, contributing to environmental contamination and recurrent outbreaks. Overall, necrotic enteritis is a toxin-mediated enteric disease in which intestinal mucosal damage, bacterial overgrowth, and predisposing factors converge to produce either acute mortality or chronic production losses.

11.24.2 Risk Factors

- **Host-Related Factors**
  Most common in 2–6-week-old commercial facility broilers but can occur in older birds under stress. Fast-growing broilers due to higher nutrient demand and gut stress predispose to NE.
- **Pathogen-Related Factors**
  Clostridium perfringens overgrowth triggered by high-protein diets. Non-starch polysaccharides increase gut viscosity and undigested nutrients. NetB toxin-producing strains are most pathogenic.

- **Environmental and Management Factors**
  Wet litter supports *Clostridium* growth and spore survival. Suddenly cold or heat waves compromise gut integrity.
- **Dietary Risk Factors**
  Diets rich in animal protein (fishmeal, meat, and bone meal). High-energy diets with poorly digestible fats. Mycotoxin-contaminated feed damages gut lining.
- **Co-Infections**
  Coccidiosis is a major predisposing factor because it damages intestinal epithelium, providing a niche for *C. perfringens*. Other gut pathogens also disrupt gut balance.

11.24.3 Clinical Signs and Pathology

- **External Findings**
  Depression, ruffled feathers, reduced feed and water intake, diarrhea, dehydration, drooping wings, huddling, poor growth, and a drop in egg production in layers/breeders.
- **Necropsy Findings**
  Jejunum and ileum were most affected. Ballooning and distension of intestines with foul-smelling brown fluid. The intestinal wall is thickened and fragile. Necrotic mucosa covered by a yellow to brown diphtheritic membrane. Sloughed mucosa may form a cast inside the intestine. Focal or extensive hemorrhages in the intestinal wall. Liver may be enlarged and congested (secondary septicemia). Carcasses may be dehydrated and emaciated in chronic cases.

11.24.4 Diagnostic Testing–Reference Laboratory

- **Culture**
  Collect samples from the small intestine shortly after death (autolysis occurs quickly). Culture under anaerobic conditions on blood agar. *C. perfringens* colonies are large, opaque, and hemolytic. Confirmation by Gram stain (Gram-positive rods without spores in clinical cases).
- **PCR**
  Detects toxin genes (alpha-toxin *cpa*, NetB toxin *netB*) to confirm pathogenic strains. Useful for distinguishing pathogenic versus commensal strains.

11.24.5 Treatment and Therapeutic Interventions

- **Medications**
  - *First-Line Antibiotics*
    Amoxicillin/Clavulanate: 125–250 mg/kg by mouth every 8–12 hours for 5–7 days.
    Amoxicillin Sodium: 50–250 mg/kg intramuscular every 8–12 hours for 5–7 days.
    Amoxicillin Trihydrate: 55–200 mg/kg by mouth, subcutaneous, or intramuscularly every 4–12 hours for 5–7 days.
  - *Alternative Antibiotics*
    Tylosin 50 mg/kg by mouth once daily for 5–7 days or 15–30 mg/kg intramuscularly every 6–12 hours for 5–7 days.
    Lincomycin 25–50 mg/kg by mouth every 12 hours.
- **Supportive Therapy**
  Since coccidiosis is a major predisposing factor, treat concurrent *Eimeria* spp. infections (e.g., with Amprolium or toltrazuril). Remove high-protein, poorly digestible ingredients (fishmeal,

wheat, barley); provide easily digestible balanced rations. Intensive nursing care, including fluid therapy and nutritional supplementation; crop feeding if indicated. Prebiotics and probiotics.

11.24.6 Prevention and Control

- **Biosecurity and Management**
  Good litter management by keeping the bedding clean and dry. Remove wet patches around drinking water. Reduce humidity and ammonia that weaken gut and respiratory health. Prompt removal and disposal of dead birds to limit bacterial spread.
- **Control of Predisposing Diseases**
  Coccidiosis control is the single most important step. Manage other intestinal parasites or infections that damage the gut lining.
- **Dietary and Nutritional Management**
  Avoid diets with excess animal proteins (fishmeal, meat meal) that favor *Clostridium* growth. Minimize wheat, rye, and barley to reduce intestinal viscosity. Use enzymes (xylanases, β-glucanases) to improve digestion and reduce undigested feed in intestines. Ensure balanced vitamins (A, E) and trace minerals (selenium, zinc) to support gut immunity. Avoid sudden diet changes. Prevent mycotoxin contamination in feed.
- **Probiotics, Prebiotics, and Feed Additives**
  Probiotics/direct fed microbials (e.g., *Bacillus subtilis*, *Lactobacillus*) to compete with *Clostridium*. Prebiotics to improve gut health. Organic acids (formic, butyric, propionic acid) reduce pH, inhibit *Clostridium* growth.
- **Integrated Approach**
  Combine biosecurity, coccidiosis control, feed/nutrition management, and probiotics. Reserve antibiotics for outbreaks and only under veterinary guidance. Regular monitoring of flock health and feed quality.

11.24.7 Nursing Considerations

Nursing care for birds affected by Necrotic Enteritis emphasizes supportive management, environmental control, and prevention of secondary complications. Birds should be housed in clean, dry, and well-ventilated facilities to reduce stress and environmental contamination, which can exacerbate *Clostridium perfringens* proliferation. Isolate severely affected birds when possible and monitor the flock closely for signs of depression, diarrhea, decreased feed and water intake, and sudden mortality. Ensure access to high-quality, easily digestible feed and fresh water to maintain hydration and nutritional status, as affected birds are often weak and dehydrated. Intensive nursing care, including fluid therapy, antibiotics, nutritional supplementation, and analgesics. If hospitalized in a clinical setting, isolation protocol and PPE are of utmost importance. Minimize stressful handling and sudden changes in diet, as abrupt feed transitions can worsen intestinal pathology. Strict biosecurity practices, including routine litter management, disinfection of feeders and waterers, and limiting movement between flocks, are essential to prevent spread. Administer medications such as prescribed antibiotics or other therapeutics under veterinary guidance, monitoring response to treatment and adjusting care as necessary. Additionally, educate farm staff on recognizing early clinical signs, maintaining optimal flock management, and implementing preventive measures, including coccidiosis control, which can significantly reduce the risk and severity of Necrotic Enteritis. Veterinary-assisted euthanasia is always a humane option for critically ill birds.

11.25 Avian Botulism

11.25.1 Overview and Pathogenesis

Avian botulism is an acute neuroparalytic disease of poultry caused by botulinum neurotoxins (BoNTs) produced by *Clostridium botulinum*, a Gram-positive, spore-forming, obligatory anaerobic bacterium. The disease affects chickens, turkeys, waterfowl, and wild birds, and is of major concern due to rapid onset, high mortality, and economic losses. Birds are exposed primarily through ingestion of preformed toxin in contaminated feed, water, or decomposing carcasses, though wound contamination and, rarely, intestinal colonization can also occur. Among poultry, toxin types C and E are most implicated. The disease manifests as neurotoxicosis rather than a conventional bacterial infection, meaning the bacterium does not need to colonize tissues to cause clinical disease.

The pathogenesis of avian botulism begins with ingestion of preformed BoNT, which survives passage through the gastrointestinal tract and is absorbed into the bloodstream. Once systemic, the neurotoxin targets presynaptic motor nerve terminals at neuromuscular junctions, where it binds to receptors and cleaves SNARE proteins essential for acetylcholine release. This results in flaccid paralysis of voluntary muscles, starting with the neck and eyelid muscles ("limberneck"), progressing to wings, legs, and ultimately respiratory muscles, which can lead to death. Clinical severity depends on toxin dose, type, and bird susceptibility. Environmental factors, such as decaying organic matter, stagnant water, and anaerobic conditions, facilitate spore germination and toxin production, perpetuating outbreaks. Birds that survive sublethal exposure may recover but can contribute to environmental contamination, maintaining risk for further cases. In summary, avian botulism is a toxin-mediated neuromuscular disease in which rapid neuroparalysis and high mortality occur following ingestion of preformed toxin, with environmental management being critical for prevention.

11.25.2 Risk Factors

- **Host-Related Factors**
  All ages can be affected, but young chicks may show milder signs, while adult birds can die rapidly. Chickens with weakened immunity (due to stress, concurrent infections, or malnutrition) are more susceptible. Chickens, turkeys, and waterfowl are all susceptible, with waterfowl often more prone to outbreaks.
- **Environmental and Management Factors**
  Exposure to rotting carcasses, spoiled feed, or decomposing vegetation are ideal for *C. botulinum* growth.
- **Transmission-Related Factors**
  Ingestion of preformed toxin (the most common route in chickens). Wound botulism is rare, but spores entering injuries may produce toxin locally. Vectors such as maggots, insects, and rodents can carry toxins.

11.25.3 Clinical Signs and Pathology

- **External Findings**
  Progressive flaccid paralysis is a hallmark sign. Early signs can be seen such as weakness in legs and wings, difficulty standing, walking, or perching. Advanced signs include lateral or dorsal

recumbency, unable to right themselves, inability to swallow, watery drooling, and respiratory distress due to paralysis of intercostal muscles. Onset is usually sudden within hours to a few days after ingesting toxin.

- **Necropsy Findings**
  Typically, there are no specific gross lesions in organs. Minimal lesions in tissues. Most diagnoses are clinical and epidemiological, rather than based on gross pathology.

11.25.4 Diagnostic Testing—Reference Laboratory

- **ELISA**
  Detect botulinum toxins directly.
- **PCR**
  Detects *C. botulinum* genes in feed, litter, or carcass samples. Confirms bacterial presence but does not prove toxin activity.
- **Culture**
  Isolation of *C. botulinum* from intestines or environment under anaerobic conditions. Must be paired with toxin testing, since non-toxigenic strains also exist.

11.25.5 Treatment and Therapeutic Interventions

- **Botulinum Antitoxin**
  Administered subcutaneously or intravenously in valuable birds (individual pet chickens, rare breeds). Dose: varies by product, usually 1000–10,000 IU per bird. Most practical in small flocks or individual cases, not commercial facility birds. Neutralizes circulating toxins but cannot reverse damage already done to nerve endings.
- **Supportive Care**
  Oral, subcutaneous, or intravenous fluids (lactated Ringer's or 0.9% sodium chloride) for dehydrated birds. Oral activated charcoal or bentonite clay may help bind residual toxin if administered early. Provide easy-to-eat feed and fresh water within easy reach (paralyzed birds cannot reach feeders). Tube feeding may be necessary for weak or recumbent birds. Supportive slings or wheelchairs help birds stand and avoid pressure sores if recumbent. Passive range of motion for all joints. Clean and soft bedding.
- **Antibiotic Therapy**
  It is not directly effective against toxin but may help control secondary bacterial infections.

11.25.6 Prevention and Control

- **Feed Hygiene**
  Avoid spoiled or decaying feed. Discard moldy, rancid, or wet feed. Prevent contamination with deceased animals (dead rodents, birds, or insects). Keep feed dry and cool in sealed containers. Rotate feed to prevent prolonged storage and spoilage. Avoid high-risk feed ingredients such as fishmeal, meat meal, or poultry byproducts unless properly processed.
- **Environmental and Farm Management**
  Dead birds or animals must be removed immediately to prevent toxin production. Use clean, fresh water. Avoid stagnant water, ponds, or puddles where spores may proliferate. Control decaying vegetation in pens or free-range areas. Maintain dry litter and bedding to reduce anaerobic conditions.

- **Rodent and Insect Control**
  Rodents, maggots, and flies can carry botulinum toxins. It is necessary to implement pest control programs. Prevent access to wild birds or animals to food and water sources.
- **Stress Reduction and Husbandry**
  Avoid overcrowding and temperature extremes. Minimize handling stress. Provide balanced nutrition to maintain immunity.
- **Vaccination**
  Botulinum toxoid vaccines are available in some regions for prevention in endemic areas or high-risk flocks. Vaccination is primarily used in hatchery breeder or layer flocks, not typically in commercial birds.
- **Therapeutic Measures**
  Antitoxin administration can neutralize circulating toxins if available. Antibiotics are not effective, since the disease is caused by preformed toxin, not active bacterial infection in tissues.

11.25.7 Nursing Considerations

Nursing care for birds affected by Avian Botulism centers on supportive management, environmental control, and prevention of further toxin exposure. Immediately remove affected birds from contaminated water or feed sources and isolate them to prevent cross-contamination. Provide supportive care, including easily accessible fresh water and high-quality, easily digestible feed, as affected birds often have difficulty swallowing and reduced feed intake. Intensive nursing care, including fluid therapy, antibiotics for secondary infections, supplemental nutrition, and analgesics if indicated. Handle birds gently to minimize stress and avoid injury, since flaccid paralysis increases the risk of trauma. Maintain optimal temperature and ventilation to reduce additional metabolic stress. Monitor flocks closely for early signs such as weakness, drooping wings, limber neck, or respiratory distress, and promptly report cases to a veterinarian for potential antitoxin therapy where available. Implement strict biosecurity measures, including removal of decaying carcasses, control of maggots and other vectors, and disinfection of contaminated areas, to prevent further infection. Educate guardians on early recognition, environmental management, and the importance of rapid intervention to reduce mortality and support recovery in affected birds. Veterinarians may alleviate bird suffering with humane euthanasia.

11.26 Gangrenous Dermatitis

11.26.1 Overview and Pathogenesis

Gangrenous dermatitis (GD) is an acute, rapidly progressive necrotizing skin disease of poultry, primarily caused by *Clostridium septicum*, often in association with *Clostridium perfringens* and *Staphylococcus aureus*. The disease predominantly affects commercial flocks aged 3–12 weeks, though older birds can also be affected under predisposing conditions. GD is of major economic concern due to high mortality in acute outbreaks and rapid flock spread. Transmission is opportunistic, typically occurring through skin abrasions, feather follicles, or minor wounds, with environmental contamination and poor husbandry contributing to disease occurrence.

The pathogenesis of gangrenous dermatitis begins with predisposing factors that compromise skin integrity or immunity, such as trauma, pecking, overcrowding, wet litter, elevated ammonia levels, or immunosuppressive viral infections like MD or IBD. Once the skin barrier is breached, *C. septicum* colonizes damaged tissues and produces potent alpha-toxins that cause rapid necrosis, edema, and hemorrhage. Secondary infections by *C. perfringens* or *S. aureus* can exacerbate tissue destruction. Lesions commonly develop in ventral areas such as the breast, abdomen, and under the wings. Clinically, acute GD may result in sudden death with minimal prior signs, whereas subacute or chronic cases present with swelling, erythema, and necrotic skin patches that may progress to systemic toxemia. Environmental persistence of clostridial spores and colonization of recovered birds contribute to recurring outbreaks, making GD a significant management challenge in poultry production.

11.26.2 Risk Factors

- **Host-Related Factors**
  Usually affects commercial chickens 2–6 weeks old, but layers and breeders can also be affected. Fast-growing commercial broilers are more prone than backyard breeds.
- **Environmental and Management Factors**
  Wet, damp, or caked litter favors bacterial proliferation. High humidity increases skin maceration. Scratches, pecking, or trauma allow bacteria to enter skin.
- **Pathogen-Related Factors**
  Clostridium septicum, *Clostridium perfringens*, and *Staphylococcus aureus* are opportunistic pathogens that invade damaged skin. Overgrowth of clostridia in litter or gut increases risk. Co-infections, especially coccidiosis, increase bacterial load and skin vulnerability.
- **Dietary and Nutritional Risk Factors**
  Diets high in fishmeal, animal proteins, or poorly digestible feed increase gut clostridial proliferation.

11.26.3 Clinical Signs and Pathology

- **External Findings**
  - *Acute Form*
    Sudden onset with rapid progression. Birds are depressed, reluctant to move, and often prostrate. Ruffled feathers, pale comb, and wattles. Rapid mortality, birds may die within hours.
  - *Skin Lesions (Hallmark Sign)*
    Dark red to black, necrotic patches on the skin. Lesions commonly on breast, vent, abdomen, and thighs. Skin may appear edematous and tense, with a foul odor. Sometimes gas formation under skin causes swelling or crepitation.
- **Necropsy Findings**
  - *Skin and Subcutaneous Tissue*
    Necrosis of skin and subcutaneous tissue with black discoloration. Fibrinous exudate and hemorrhage may be present. Skin may slough off in severe cases. Gas bubbles under skin due to clostridial fermentation.
  - *Muscle Involvement*
    Necrosis may extend into underlying muscles (pectoralis, thigh muscles). Muscles may appear dark, soft, and friable.
  - *Visceral Lesions*
    Usually minimal unless secondary infections occur. Occasionally fibrinous pericarditis or perihepatitis if *Clostridium perfringens* spreads systemically.

11.26.4 Diagnostic Testing—Reference Laboratory

- **Bacterial Culture (Definitive Diagnosis)**
  Culture on anaerobic media (blood agar under anaerobic conditions) to isolate Clostridium spp. Identification via biochemical testing or MALDI-TOF for species confirmation.
- **PCR**
  Detects toxigenic genes of *C. septicum* or *C. perfringens*. Useful for epidemiological studies or outbreak confirmation.

11.26.5 Treatment and Therapeutic Interventions

- **Medication**
  Amoxicillin/Clavulanate: 125–250 mg/kg by mouth every 8–12 hours for 5–7 days.
  Amoxicillin Sodium: 50–250 mg/kg intramuscular every 8–12 hours for 5–7 days.
  Amoxicillin Trihydrate: 55–200 mg/kg by mouth, subcutaneous, or intramuscularly every 4–12 hours for 5–7 days.
  Oxytetracycline 5 mg/kg subcutaneous or intramuscular every 12–24 hours. 2500 mg/L drinking water and 2500 mg/kg feed.
  – *Alternative Antibiotics*
  Lincomycin 25–50 mg/kg by mouth every 12 hours.
- **Supportive Care**
  Move affected birds to dry, clean, well-ventilated housing. Remove wet, contaminated litter that supports bacterial growth. Consider adding vitamin and mineral supplements (especially Vitamin E and selenium) to boost immunity. Clean and disinfect wounds with properly diluted iodine or chlorhexidine 0.5–1%. Apply topical antibiotics to reduce secondary infection. Fluid therapy and supplemental nutrition if prescribed by the veterinarian.

11.26.6 Prevention and Control

- **Environmental and Litter Management**
  Keep litter dry and clean remove wet, caked, or damp areas promptly. Good ventilation reduces humidity, ammonia, and skin maceration. Avoid overcrowding minimizes stress and skin injuries. Prompt removal of dead birds prevents proliferation of clostridial spores.
- **Biosecurity and Farm Management**
  Disinfection of houses, equipment, and tools. Rodent, insect, and wild bird control reduces bacterial and mechanical vectors. 30-day quarantine of new birds before introducing them to the flock.
- **Feed and Water Management**
  Avoid spoiled or wet feed that can harbor clostridia. Use well-balanced diets and avoid sudden nutritional changes. Clean waterers regularly prevent stagnant water accumulation. Limit high-risk feed ingredients (fishmeal, meat meal) unless properly processed.
- **Disease Control/Predisposing Factors**
  Control coccidiosis because damaged gut increases clostridial proliferation. Minimize other infections that compromise immunity.
- **Therapeutic Measures**
  Antibiotics may be used during outbreaks. Intensive supportive care for affected birds. Mortality is often rapid; prevention is far more effective than treatment.

11.26.7 Nursing Considerations

Nursing care for birds affected by Gangrenous Dermatitis focuses on supportive management, environmental control, and rapid intervention to prevent spread and secondary complications. Affected birds should be immediately isolated to reduce transmission, as the disease progresses rapidly and has high mortality. Maintain clean, dry, and well-ventilated housing, as wet litter and high humidity exacerbate skin lesions and bacterial proliferation. Minimize stress through gentle handling and stable flock routines, since stress can worsen disease progression. Monitor birds closely for early signs, including skin discoloration, swelling, or necrotic lesions, and provide access to clean water and easily digestible feed to support hydration and nutrition. Intensive nursing therapeutics, including fluids for hydration, analgesics, and nutritional supplementation. Implement strict biosecurity measures, including thorough disinfection of housing, equipment, and footwear, and promptly remove and properly dispose of deceased birds. Administer antibiotics or other veterinary-prescribed treatments by observing dosage and duration to improve outcomes. Educate caregivers on early recognition of lesions, environmental management, and preventive strategies to reduce incidence and severity of Gangrenous Dermatitis in chicken flocks.

11.27 Staphylococcosis

11.27.1 Overview and Pathogenesis

Staphylococcosis is a bacterial disease of poultry caused primarily by *Staphylococcus aureus*, a Gram-positive, facultatively anaerobic coccus. It is an opportunistic pathogen that affects chickens of all ages, though growing broilers and layers are most affected. The disease is significant because it can lead to localized infections such as subcutaneous abscesses, dermatitis, arthritis, and osteomyelitis, as well as systemic conditions like septicemia and endocarditis, resulting in reduced growth, poor egg production, and increased mortality. Transmission occurs through direct contact with infected birds, contaminated equipment, or via mechanical vectors (insects, rodents), with entry typically through skin wounds, mucous membranes, or areas of trauma.

The pathogenesis of staphylococcosis begins with colonization of compromised skin, feather follicles, or injured tissues by *S. aureus*. The bacteria adhere to host tissues using surface proteins and produce a variety of virulent factors, including coagulase, hyaluronidase, and proteases, which facilitate tissue invasion and immune evasion. Localized infections manifest as abscesses, swelling, or necrosis in subcutaneous tissue, joints, and bones, while systemic spread can result in septicemia and organ involvement, including endocarditis of the heart. Opportunistic infections are often exacerbated by predisposing factors such as immunosuppressive viral infections, poor environmental conditions, trauma, or concurrent diseases. Recovered birds may become carriers, harboring *S. aureus* on skin or in the respiratory tract and perpetuating environmental contamination. Overall, staphylococcosis in chickens is a multifactorial opportunistic disease in which host susceptibility, bacterial virulence, and environmental stressors collectively determine disease severity and clinical outcome.

11.27.2 Risk Factors

- **Host-Related Factors**
  All ages can be affected, but young chicks and broilers are more susceptible to omphalitis and septicemia. Fast-growing commercial meat breeds and layers are more prone than backyard breeds.

- **Environmental and Management Factors**
  Poor sanitation such as contaminated litter, feeders, and waterers. Ventilation issues, elevated ammonia damages skin and respiratory tract. Skin injuries, scratches, pecking, or abrasions allow bacterial entry. Overcrowding leads to pecking and bullying wounds.
- **Feed-Related Factors**
  Spoiled or contaminated feed can harbor *Staphylococcus aureus*. High-protein or animal-based feed may favor bacterial overgrowth if hygiene is poor.

11.27.3 Clinical Signs and Pathology

- **External Findings**
  - *Omphalitis ("Mushy Chick Disease")*
    Affects day-old chicks, especially from contaminated hatcheries. Swollen, unhealed navel, yolk sac may appear cloudy or foul smelling, weak, depressed, and reluctant to move.
  - *Acute Form (Septicemia)*
    Sudden death in young or immunocompromised birds. Weakness, depression, ruffled feathers, pale comb, and wattles.
  - *Arthritis (Tenosynovitis)*
    Lame and reluctance to move. Swollen hock joints, footpads, or tendon sheaths. Reduced growth and feed conversion in broilers. Chronic cases, joint deformities, or ankylosis.
  - *Skin and Subcutaneous Infections*
    Abscesses under the skin, often on breast, back, or wings. Swelling, redness, heat, and occasionally pus formation. Slow-growing abscesses that may rupture in chronic cases.
- **Necropsy Findings**
  - **Omphalitis:** Inflamed, sometimes necrotic navel. Enlarged, cloudy, or fibrinous yolk sac. Foul odor common.
  - **Arthritis (Tenosynovitis):** Swollen joints filled with yellowish or greenish caseous exudate. Thickened joint capsules or tendon sheaths. Sometimes necrosis of cartilage.
  - **Skin and Subcutaneous Infections:** Abscesses, localized necrosis, pus accumulation, and sometimes gas formation. Often blackened or discolored necrotic tissue.
  - Visceral Lesions: Occasionally mild fibrinous pericarditis, perihepatitis, or liver congestion in septicemic cases. Typically, minimal unless secondary infections occur.

11.27.4 Diagnostic Testing—Reference Laboratory

- **Bacterial Culture (Definitive Diagnosis)**
  Culture on blood agar, colonies are usually golden-yellow, smooth, and hemolytic.
- **PCR**
  Detects specific *Staphylococcus* genes, particularly virulence or antibiotic resistance genes. Useful for epidemiological studies or outbreaks in valuable flocks.
- **Antibiotic Susceptibility Testing**
  Essential for selecting appropriate treatment, especially given widespread resistance in *S. aureus* strains.

11.27.5 Treatment and Therapeutic Interventions

- **Medication**
  Oxytetracycline 5 mg/kg subcutaneous or intramuscular every 12–24 hours. 2500 mg/L drinking water and 2500 mg/kg feed.

- **Surgical or Physical Management**
  Using local, regional, or general anesthesia, the veterinarian or credentialed veterinary technician lances and drains localized abscesses, followed by warm flushes of a diluted antiseptic. Ensure strict aseptic technique to prevent secondary infection. Chronic cases may require long-term systemic antibiotics; prognosis is guarded.
- **Supportive Care**
  Provide clean water ad libitum; consider electrolyte supplementation for weak birds. High-quality, easily digestible food to support immune function. Minimize stress and provide clean, dry housing to aid recovery. If indicated, fluid therapy and supplemental nutrition. Analgesia.

11.27.6 Prevention and Control

- **Hatchery and Chick Management**
  Disinfect incubators and brooders thoroughly. Use NPIP-certified eggs and chicks from healthy breeders (discussed in Chapter 1). Prevent omphalitis, proper navel care and handling of day-old chicks. Quarantine new chicks before introduction to the flock.
- **Environmental and Housing Management**
  Maintain dry, clean litter to reduce skin trauma and bacterial proliferation. Good ventilation reduces humidity and ammonia, which weaken skin and respiratory tract. Prompt removal of dead birds to limit environmental contamination. Control rodents, insects, and wild birds that can carry bacteria. Prevent overcrowding. Eliminate sharp edging of enclosures.
- **Feed and Water Management**
  Provide clean, dry feed; avoid moldy or spoiled feed. Ensure clean water.
- **Therapeutic Measures**
  Antibiotics may be used for acute outbreaks or lameness cases.

11.27.7 Nursing Considerations

Nursing care for birds affected by Staphylococcosis emphasizes supportive management, wound care, and environmental hygiene to prevent secondary infections. Affected birds should be housed in clean, dry, and well-ventilated environments, with careful attention to litter quality and perches to reduce trauma that can serve as entry points for *Staphylococcus* spp. Isolate birds showing clinical signs such as swollen joints, abscesses, lameness, or dermatitis to prevent cross-contamination. Provide easy access to fresh water and high-quality, easily digestible feed to maintain hydration and nutritional status, especially in debilitated birds. Intensive nursing care that includes fluid therapy, analgesia, surgical debridement, and supplemental nutrition. Handle birds gently to minimize stress and further injury. Clean and dress any visible lesions under veterinary guidance and administer prescribed antibiotics following correct dosages and treatment durations. Implement strict biosecurity, including disinfection of equipment and prompt removal of dead birds or other animals, to limit environmental contamination. Educate caregivers on early recognition of clinical signs, proper wound management, and environmental control measures to reduce the incidence and severity of Staphylococcosis in backyard flocks.

11.28 Erysipelas

11.28.1 Overview and Pathogenesis

Erysipelas is a systemic bacterial disease of poultry caused by *Erysipelothrix rhusiopathiae*, a Gram-positive, slender rod-shaped organism. It primarily affects adult birds but can also occur in younger birds. The disease is significant due to sudden mortality in acute outbreaks and chronic manifestations such as arthritis, endocarditis, and reduced egg production. Transmission occurs through direct contact with infected birds, contaminated feed, water, litter, or via mechanical vectors such as equipment and insects.

The pathogenesis of erysipelas involves the entry of *E. rhusiopathiae* either orally, through contaminated feed or water, or via skin abrasions. Upon entering the host, the bacterium colonizes blood vessels and internal organs such as the liver, spleen, and joints, evading host defenses through its capsule and enzymatic virulence factors like neuraminidase. Rapid multiplication in the bloodstream results in septicemia and endotoxemia, leading to widespread tissue damage. Vascular endothelial injury triggers hemorrhages, fibrin deposition, and inflammatory infiltration, which manifest as clinical signs including lethargy, ruffled feathers, anorexia, swollen joints, and sudden death in acute cases. Chronic infections may result in arthritis, endocarditis, and decreased egg production.

Environmental persistence plays a critical role in disease recurrence, as *E. rhusiopathiae* can survive in soil, litter, and water for extended periods. Carrier birds further contribute to the maintenance of infection within the flock, creating ongoing risk for new outbreaks. In summary, erysipelas in chickens is a vascular and systemic disease in which septicemia, toxin-mediated tissue injury, and immune evasion collectively lead to high mortality in acute cases and productivity losses in chronic infections.

11.28.2 Risk Factors

- **Host-Related Factors**
  All ages are susceptible, but adult chickens and breeders are more commonly affected. Commercial broilers, layers, and breeders may be more at risk than hardy backyard breeds.
- **Environmental and Management Factors**
  Contaminated litter, soil, and water harbor bacteria. Contaminated litter, soil, and water harbor bacteria. Rodent and wild bird presence are potential carriers of *E. rhusiopathiae.*
- **Feed and Water Factors**
  Contaminated feed or water sources can serve as a route of infection. Poor feed hygiene or storage can promote bacterial proliferation.
- **Stress and Predisposing Factors**
  Transportation, handling, or vaccination stress increases susceptibility. Concurrent infections (IBD, coccidiosis, other bacterial infections) compromise immunity. Nutritional deficiencies (vitamins A, E, selenium) reduce resistance.
- **Transmission Factors**
  Erysipelas is transmitted directly via contact with infected birds or indirectly via contaminated environment, feed, water, or fomites. Skin wounds or abrasions facilitate bacterial entry. Chronic carriers may shed bacteria intermittently.

11.28.3 Clinical Signs and Pathology

- **External Findings**
  - *Acute Form*
    Sudden onset, often in adult birds. Depression, ruffled feathers, reluctance to move. Fever and anorexia. Cyanosis or purple discoloration of combs, wattles, and legs. Lameness due to arthritis. Rapid mortality may occur in severe outbreaks.

- *Subacute/Chronic Form*
  Swollen joints, particularly hocks and stifles. Arthritis or tenosynovitis. Skin lesions, red or purple blotches, sometimes necrotic. Reduced egg production in layers or breeders. Weight loss and poor growth in chronic cases.
- **Necropsy Findings**
  - *Skin and Subcutaneous Tissue*
    Hemorrhages and dark purple-red areas on legs, feet, and ventrum. Occasionally necrotic skin lesions or vesicles.
  - *Joints and Muscles*
    Swollen joints with fibrinous or serous exudate. In chronic cases, thickened joint capsules and fibrous adhesions. Muscles may appear pale or edematous.
  - *Visceral Lesions*
    Splenomegaly and hepatomegaly. Congestion of kidneys and liver. Fibrinous pericarditis or perihepatitis in septicemic cases.

11.28.4 Diagnostic Testing—Reference Laboratory

- **Bacterial Culture (Definitive Diagnosis)**
  Culture on blood agar: smooth, translucent, small colonies with alpha-hemolysis. Identification: Gram-positive, slender rods, non-spore forming, catalase negative.
- **PCR**
  Detects *E. rhusiopathiae* DNA from tissue or blood. Useful in acute cases or when culture is difficult.
- **Serology**
  ELISA or agglutination tests can detect antibodies, indicating prior exposure or vaccination. It is useful for flock-level surveillance but cannot differentiate active infection from past exposure.

11.28.5 Treatment and Therapeutic Interventions

- **Medication**
  Short-acting penicillin or amoxicillin. Oral or intravenous route for 10–14 days.
- **Supportive Care**
  Provide electrolytes for dehydrated or weak birds. Offer high-quality, easily digestible feed to support immune recovery. Avoid feed changes that could stress the flock further. Intensive nursing care including fluid therapy, nutritional supplementation, analgesics, and clean bedding. Maintain optimal ambient temperature and ventilation. Fluid therapy, analgesics, and nutritional supplementation.

11.28.6 Prevention and Control

- **Biosecurity and Husbandry**
  Quarantine new birds for at least 30 days before introducing them. Disinfection of houses, equipment, feeders, and waterers. Rodent, wild birds, and insect control, since they can carry pathogenic bacteria. Prompt removal of dead birds to reduce environmental contamination.
- **Environmental and Housing Management**
  Maintain dry litter and prevent damp or caked bedding. Ensure good ventilation to reduce humidity and ammonia accumulation. Avoid overcrowding to minimize stress and bacterial spread. Clean waterers and provide clean, fresh water.

- **Vaccination**
  Inactivated (killed) or live-attenuated vaccines are available in endemic areas, but typically for commercial breeder and layer flocks only.
- **Therapeutic Measures**
  Antibiotics can be used in acute outbreaks.

11.28.7 Nursing Considerations

Nursing care for birds affected by Erysipelas focuses on supportive management, rapid isolation, and strict biosecurity to limit disease spread and support recovery. Affected birds should be housed in clean, well-ventilated facilities with dry litter or clean bedding to reduce environmental stress and prevent secondary infections. Immediately isolate birds showing signs such as sudden death, depression, lameness, swollen joints, or skin lesions, and monitor the flock closely for additional cases. Provide easy access to fresh water and high-quality, easily digestible food to maintain hydration and nutritional status, particularly for weakened or immobile birds. Provide fluid therapy and tube feeding if indicated by the veterinarian. Minimize handling and other stressors, as stress can exacerbate disease progression. Administer antibiotics or other veterinary-prescribed treatments ensuring correct dosage and duration to optimize therapeutic outcomes. Implement rigorous biosecurity measures, including disinfection of housing, equipment, and footwear, and proper disposal of dead birds or other animals, to reduce environmental contamination and prevent further outbreaks. Educate guardians on early recognition of clinical signs, the importance of vaccination where available, and effective preventive strategies to control Erysipelas in free-range backyard flocks. If bird's condition worsens, humane euthanasia is a reasonable option.

11.29 Fungal Diseases of Chickens

Although less common than viral and bacterial infections, fungal diseases significantly impact flock health, particularly under conditions of poor ventilation, damp litter, or immunosuppression. Veterinary technicians are frequently involved in identifying risk factors, monitoring clinical signs, and implementing husbandry changes that prevent recurrence (Table 11.3).

11.30 Aspergillosis

11.30.1 Overview and Pathogenesis

Aspergillosis is a fungal disease of chickens caused primarily by ubiquitous, opportunistic *Aspergillus fumigatus*, and less commonly by *A. flavus* or *A. niger*. It primarily affects the respiratory system, although systemic infections occur typically in immunocompromised or young birds. Infection usually occurs via inhalation of fungal spores from contaminated litter, feed, or bedding, which then colonize the respiratory tract, particularly the air sacs and lungs.

The pathogenesis involves spore germination in the respiratory mucosa, followed by tissue invasion, inflammation, and formation of granulomatous lesions. These lesions impair respiratory function and can cause dyspnea, gasping, and cyanosis, while systemic spread may lead to organ involvement and mortality. Predisposing factors include poor ventilation, high humidity, dusty or moldy litter, overcrowding, and immunosuppression, all of which facilitate spore proliferation and

Table 11.3

Quick reference chart				
Disease	**Causative agent**	**Transmission/source**	**Key clinical signs**	**Diagnostic testing**
Aspergillosis (brooder pneumonia)	*Aspergillus fumigatus* (most common), *A. flavus*, *A. niger*	Inhalation of spores from contaminated litter, feed, hatchery air; not contagious bird-to-bird	Respiratory distress, open-mouth breathing, gasping, lethargy, weight loss; high chick mortality in outbreaks	Direct microscopy (wet mounts), histopathology (fungal hyphae), culture (Sabouraud agar), PCR
Candidiasis (thrush, mycosis of crop)	*Candida albicans* (yeast)	Overgrowth of normal flora after antibiotics, contaminated water/feeders; opportunistic	Inappetence, delayed crop emptying, white plaques in mouth/crop, regurgitation	Wet mounts (budding yeast, pseudohyphae), culture, histopathology
Mycotoxicosis (aflatoxicosis, ochratoxicosis, T-2 toxicosis, etc.)	Mycotoxins produced by *Aspergillus*, *Fusarium*, *Penicillium* spp.	Ingestion of contaminated/moldy feed or litter; not infectious	Reduced growth, poor feed conversion, immunosuppression, ruffled feathers, sometimes nervous signs; aflatoxins → liver damage	Feed testing (HPLC, ELISA), clinical signs, necropsy findings
Mucormycosis (zygomycosis)	*Mucor*, *Rhizopus*, *Absidia* spp.	Inhalation of spores from contaminated litter or feed, opportunistic	Similar to aspergillosis but less common; respiratory distress, weight loss, poor growth	Histopathology (broad, non-septate hyphae), culture
Cryptococcosis (rare)	*Cryptococcus neoformans*	Inhalation; contaminated soil/pigeon droppings	Respiratory signs, CNS signs in advanced cases	Culture, histopathology (encapsulated yeast), PCR

Table courtesy of Stephanie Freeman.

increase susceptibility. The disease can present acutely, with sudden deaths in young chicks, or chronically, with gradual weight loss, lethargy, respiratory distress, and reduced productivity in adult birds. Overall, aspergillosis is a fungal opportunistic infection whose severity depends on the infectious dose, host immunity, and environmental conditions.

11.30.2 Risk Factors

- **Host-Related Factors**
  Young chicks (1–3 weeks old) are highly susceptible; older birds can be affected but usually less severely. Commercial broilers and layers are often more susceptible due to intensive production systems.
- **Environmental and Housing Factors**
  Accumulation of dust and spores. High humidity favors mold growth. Moldy straw, wood shavings, or hay are common sources. Moldy grains or feed promote fungal growth. Inhalation of spores into the respiratory system is the main route of infection.

- **Feed and Water Factors**
  Moldy feed or improperly stored grains are major sources of spores. Contaminated food with mycotoxins may worsen immune suppression. Moist feed encourages fungal growth.
- **Transmission Factors**
  Inhalation of spores (conidia) is the primary route. Rarely, ingestion of heavily contaminated feed or bedding can lead to visceral infection. Spores are ubiquitous in the environment, making hygiene and litter/feed management critical.

11.30.3 Clinical Signs

- **External Findings**
  - *Acute Form (Young Chicks)*
    Sudden onset of respiratory distress, gasping, open-mouth breathing, and audible wheezing. Depression, ruffled feathers, and reluctance to move. Cyanosis of comb and wattles in severe cases. Mortality can be high. Reduced feed intake and stunted growth in surviving chicks.
  - *Chronic Form (Adults)*
    Respiratory signs chronic coughing, dyspnea, nasal discharge, and wheezing. Reduced egg production in layers. Weight loss and poor growth in meat bird breeds. Often subclinical until secondary infections or stress occur.
- **Necropsy Findings**
  Air sacs thickened, cloudy, or caseous exudate; often "cheesy" or gray-white plaques. Lungs nodular, firm, or yellowish-gray lesions. Trachea occasionally shows fibrinous exudate or plaques. Sinuses and nares may have thick exudate. Liver and kidneys occasionally have nodular granulomas. Less common infections in the eyes, brain, skin, viscera, and joints.

11.30.4 Diagnostic Testing—Reference Laboratory

- **Fungal Culture**
  Culture samples on Sabouraud dextrose agar at 25–37°C. Colonies are cottony, white to green, turning yellow or brown with age, depending on species. Culture confirms species and allows antifungal susceptibility testing in research or severe cases.
- **Direct Microscopy**
  Samples of tracheal swabs, air sac exudate, or lung tissue. Stains used are lactophenol cotton blue or PAS (Periodic Acid-Schiff). Look for septate hyphae with dichotomous branching at ~45° angles, characteristic of *Aspergillus*.
- **Radiographs**
  Detects pulmonary nodules, air sac opacities, or granulomas. Useful in chronic or subclinical cases.
- **Endoscopy**
  Visualization of air sac lesions or fungal plaques in research, valuable, or birds of dedicated caregivers.

11.30.5 Treatment and Therapeutic Interventions

- **Systemic Antifungals**
  Itraconazole is a referred antifungal in poultry, effective against *Aspergillus*. Dose is 5–10 mg/kg orally for 5–7 days.

- **Supportive Care**
  Move affected birds to clean, well-ventilated housing. Reduce dust and mold exposure in bedding and feed. Provide high-quality, easily digestible feed to support immune function. Isolation and intensive nursing therapies, including fluids, supplemental nutrition, and a warm enclosure with soft, clean bedding. Avoid overcrowding and handling to minimize immunosuppressive stress. Immunosuppressed birds are susceptible to bacterial pneumonia; antibiotics may be used only for confirmed secondary infections.

11.30.6 Prevention and Control

- **Environmental and Housing Management**
  Maintain dry, clean litter to prevent fungal growth. Ensure good ventilation to reduce humidity and dust accumulation. Avoid overcrowding, which increases stress and respiratory exposure to spores. Regularly clean and disinfect housing, feeders, and waterers.
- **Feed and Bedding Management**
  Store feed properly to prevent mold growth. Discard moldy feed immediately. Use dry, uncontaminated bedding; avoid moldy hay, straw, or wood shavings. Minimize dust in feed and bedding, as spores are easily airborne.

Nursing care for birds affected by *Candidiasis* focuses on supportive management, hygiene, and prevention of further fungal overgrowth. Affected birds should be housed in isolated clean, dry, and well-ventilated facilities, and litter and feeding equipment should be regularly cleaned and disinfected to reduce fungal contamination. Monitor birds for signs such as decreased appetite, crop stasis, regurgitation, or white plaques in the oral cavity and esophagus, and provide easy access to fresh water and easily digestible, palatable feed to maintain hydration and nutritional status. Minimize stress and handling, as stress can exacerbate susceptibility and clinical severity. Where prescribed by a veterinarian, administer antifungal treatments following recommended dosages and duration. Provide fluid therapy and nutritional supplementation if indicated. Implement strict biosecurity and hygiene practices, including rotation and cleaning of feeders and waterers, to prevent recurrence. Educate caregivers on early recognition of clinical signs, proper sanitation, and management of feed and water sources to reduce the risk of *Candidiasis* outbreaks in backyard flocks.

11.31 Mycotoxicosis

11.31.1 Overview and Pathogenesis

Mycotoxicosis in chickens is a toxicological condition caused by ingestion of feed contaminated with mycotoxins, secondary metabolites produced by fungi such as *Aspergillus*, *Fusarium*, and *Penicillium* species. Mycotoxins occur naturally in crops before and after harvest, such as grass hay, oats, peanuts, barley, wheat, and soybeans. The disease primarily affects the liver, kidneys, immune system, and gastrointestinal tract, although systemic effects can occur depending on the type and dose of mycotoxin.

Pathogenesis involves absorption of mycotoxins from the gastrointestinal tract into the bloodstream, followed by cellular and organ-specific toxicity, which can disrupt metabolic pathways, damage epithelial and hepatic cells, and suppress immune function. Clinical signs vary depending on the mycotoxin and exposure level but commonly include reduced feed intake, poor growth, immunosuppression, organ enlargement or degeneration, hemorrhages, and increased susceptibility to secondary infections. Predisposing factors include poor storage of feed, high humidity, temperature fluctuations, and fungal contamination, which favor mycotoxin production. Chronic exposure may lead to reproductive failure, decreased egg production, and poor flock performance, while acute exposure can result in rapid morbidity and mortality. Overall, mycotoxicosis is a toxin-mediated disease that reflects both environmental contamination and host susceptibility, emphasizing the importance of feed quality and storage management in prevention.

11.31.2 Risk Factors

- **Feed-Related Factors**
  Contaminated food or ingredients are the primary source. Use of poor-quality or recycled feed ingredients (e.g., peanut meal, improperly stored oilseed meals). High moisture content in feed (>14%) favors mold growth. Prolonged storage under suboptimal conditions increases mycotoxin concentration.
- **Environmental and Storage Factors**
  Warm, humid climates favor fungal growth. Poor storage facilities with inadequate ventilation or insulation. Use of contaminated feed containers.
- **Host-Related Factors**
  Young chicks and immunosuppressed birds are more sensitive to some mycotoxins (aflatoxin, T-2 toxin). Breed or genetic lines may influence susceptibility to certain mycotoxins. Brown-egg layers were the most sensitive; meat-type birds were intermediate, and white-egg layers were the most resistant. The New Hampshire breed is particularly susceptible to aflatoxin, with detrimental effects at levels that do not seriously affect other breeds.
- **Stress and Predisposing Factors**
  Concurrent infections (IBD, MD, coccidiosis) worsen the effects. Overcrowding, poor nutrition, and handling stress may exacerbate toxicity. Vitamin or mineral deficiencies (e.g., vitamins A, E, selenium, zinc) reduce detoxification and immunity.
- **Feed Processing and Additives**
  Improper feed processing (heating, pelleting) may not destroy mycotoxins. Lack of mycotoxin binders or detoxifying additives in feed increases risk.

11.31.3 Clinical Signs and Pathology

- **External Findings**
  - *General Signs (all mycotoxins)*
    Poor feed intake and weight gain. Drop in egg production and hatchability. Depression, lethargy, ruffled feathers. Poor feed conversion efficiency.
  - *Specific Toxin-Associated Signs*
    - **Aflatoxins**
      Anorexia, listlessness. Pale comb/wattles, anemia. Immunosuppression, reduced egg production.
    - **Ochratoxins**
      Increased thirst and urination. Dehydration and stunted growth.
    - **Trichothecenes (e.g., T-2 toxin)**
      Ulcers and necrotic plaques in mouth and esophagus. Painful swallowing which leads to anorexia.
    - **Fumonisins**
      Poor growth, weakness, and occasionally nervous system clinical signs.

- **Necropsy Findings**
  - *Liver (aflatoxins)*
    Enlarged, pale, friable, fatty. Petechial hemorrhages. Bile duct hyperplasia (chronic).
  - *Kidneys (ochratoxin)*
    Enlarged, pale, swollen kidneys. Uric acid deposits (visceral gout).
  - *Digestive Tract (T-2 toxin)*
    Necrosis/ulcers in mouth, esophagus, and proventriculus. Thickened gut lining.
  - *Immune Organs*
    Atrophy of bursa of Fabricius, thymus, and spleen.

11.31.4 Diagnostic Testing—Reference Laboratory

- **Bloodwork**
  Liver enzymes (AST, ALT, GGT) may indicate hepatic damage from aflatoxins or other hepatotoxins. Immunosuppression markers (lymphocyte counts, antibody response) may be reduced in chronic exposure.
- **Feed Analysis**
  Confirms the presence and quantity of mycotoxins in the feed. Private agriculture testing laboratories and some university extension services also provide this information and resources for testing.

11.31.5 Treatment and Therapeutic Interventions

- **Supportive Care**
  Ensure adequate access to clean water. Provide balanced, high-quality feed rich in protein, vitamins, and minerals to support recovery. Tube feeding and fluid therapy with electrolytes if indicated, i.e., dehydration and diarrhea. Minimize stress and overcrowding to allow the immune system to recover.
- **Stop Exposure**
  Immediately remove contaminated feed from the flock. Provide clean, high-quality feed to prevent ongoing toxin ingestion. Avoid feeding feed from suspect sources until properly tested.
- **Antioxidants and Hepatoprotective Agents**
  Some mycotoxins, especially aflatoxins, cause liver damage. Vitamin E and selenium supplementation may reduce oxidative stress. Silymarin or milk thistle extracts (if approved and available) can support hepatic recovery.
- **Antibiotics**
  Only indicated if secondary bacterial infections occur due to immunosuppression. Should not be used routinely for mycotoxicosis itself.

11.31.6 Prevention and Control

- **Preventative Measures**
  Purchase food from reputable suppliers with low mold contamination. Keep grains and feed dry (moisture <12%). Use well-ventilated, cool, and clean storage facilities. Avoid prolonged storage of feed. Regularly inspect feed for discoloration, odor, or visible mold. Use older feed first to reduce storage time and mold growth risk.

11.31.7 Nursing Considerations

Nursing care for chickens affected by mycotoxicosis focuses on supportive management, prevention of further exposure, and mitigation of secondary complications. Affected birds should be isolated from contaminated feed sources and provided with clean, high-quality, uncontaminated food and fresh water to restore nutrition and hydration. If prescribed by the veterinarian, fluid therapy and supplemental feeding. Housing should be well-ventilated, dry, clean, and stress-free, as environmental stressors can worsen clinical signs and suppress immune function. Birds should be closely monitored for lethargy, reduced feed intake, growth retardation, immunosuppression, and organ dysfunction, with veterinary consultation for supportive therapies such as liver-protective agents, antioxidants, or vitamin supplementation as indicated. Nursing care also includes maintaining strict biosecurity, handling birds gently to reduce stress, and observing secondary infections, which are common due to toxin-induced immunosuppression. Overall, nursing considerations emphasize removing the source of mycotoxins, supportive feeding and hydration, environmental management, close monitoring, and veterinary collaboration to promote recovery, minimize morbidity, and prevent recurrence in affected flocks.

11.32 Mucormycosis (Zygomycosis)

11.32.1 Overview and Pathogenesis

Mucormycosis, also known as zygomycosis, is a fungal disease of chickens caused by opportunistic fungi belonging to the order *Mucorales*, including genera such as *Mucor*, *Rhizopus*, and *Absidia*. These organisms are saprophytic in the environment, commonly found in decaying organic matter, contaminated feed, litter, and soil. Disease typically develops in birds that are immunocompromised, stressed, or have disrupted mucosal barriers, allowing the fungi to invade tissues. In chickens, mucormycosis most frequently affects the gastrointestinal tract and the respiratory system, but systemic or disseminated infections may occur in severe cases. Spores are usually inhaled or ingested, after which they adhere to and invade epithelial surfaces, particularly where mucosal defenses are compromised by concurrent infections, trauma, or poor husbandry. Once inside tissues, the fungi grow as broad, non-septate hyphae that invades blood vessels, leading to thrombosis, tissue necrosis, and granulomatous inflammation.

Pathogenesis involves both mechanical tissue invasion by hyphae and vascular compromise, which causes localized ischemia and enhances fungal spread. Lesions may appear as nodular or ulcerative masses in the proventriculus, gizzard, intestines, air sacs, or lungs, and systemic dissemination can affect organs like the liver and kidneys. Clinical signs are often nonspecific, including weight loss, depression, anorexia, and respiratory distress, and disease is often diagnosed postmortem through histopathology and fungal culture. Mucormycosis is considered opportunistic rather than contagious, with outbreaks usually linked to environmental contamination and poor litter management.

11.32.2 Risk Factors

- **Environmental Conditions**
  Accumulation of wet, moldy, or decomposing litter provides ideal conditions for Zygomycete growth and spore release. High humidity and poor airflow favor fungal proliferation in poultry houses. Spores can be inhaled or ingested from moldy feed, straw, or shavings. Zygomycetes thrive in moist, organic matter typical of poorly controlled housing conditions.

- **Management and Husbandry Factors**
  Overcrowding increases moisture buildup, litter degradation, and environmental contamination. Infrequent litter replacement or turning promotes fungal colonization deep in bedding. Use of contaminated hatchery or brooder equipment, particularly if not thoroughly cleaned and dried between flocks. Poor feed storage practices allowing feed to become damp or moldy supports spore growth.
- **Host-Related Factors**
  Birds under stress, malnourished, or affected by viral immunosuppressive diseases (e.g., CIA, IBD) are more susceptible. Immature immune systems or weakened birds are less able to resist opportunistic fungal invasion. Damage to mucosal defenses by viruses, bacteria, or ammonia exposure increases fungal penetration and colonization.
- **Iatrogenic or Secondary Factors**
  Prolonged or indiscriminate antibiotic use alters normal flora, allowing opportunistic fungi to overgrow. Corticosteroid use can suppress local immunity and increase fungal susceptibility.

11.32.3 Clinical Signs and Pathology

- **External Findings**
  Respiratory Form
  Dyspnea, open beak breathing, gasping, increased respiratory effort with extended neck posture, rales, lethargy, weight loss, poor growth, and reduced food intake.

  Gastrointestinal or Disseminated Form
  Diarrhea, poor weight gain, stunting in young birds, dehydration, pale comb, and generalized weakness. Occasionally, neurological signs may occur if fungal invasion reaches the CNS (central nervous system).
- **Necropsy Findings**
  Respiratory Tract Lesions
  Nodular to plaque-like granulomas in lungs, air sacs, and occasionally trachea and syrinx. Nodules are white to yellow, firm, and irregularly distributed. Air sacs may appear thickened and opaque, sometimes with fuzzy fungal mats. Less distinct margins compared to aspergillosis plaques. Caseous exudate may be present in advanced cases.

  Gastrointestinal Lesions
  Thickened intestinal walls with granulomatous foci. Ulceration or nodules in the proventriculus, gizzard, or intestines. Occasional hepatic granulomas or splenic involvement.

  Disseminated Lesions
  In severe immunocompromised birds, fungi may disseminate hematogenously, causing multifocal granulomas in liver, spleen, kidneys, or CNS. Lesions may mimic tuberculosis or neoplasia grossly.

11.32.4 Diagnostic Testing—Reference Laboratory

- **Cytology**
  Wet mount or impression smears from lesion exudate can reveal typical fungal hyphae. Rapid, inexpensive, and useful for preliminary differentiation from *Aspergillus* spp. (which are septate with acute-angle branching).

- **Histopathology**
  Fixed tissues (e.g., 10% buffered formalin) are stained with HandE, GMS (Gomori methenamine silver), or PAS to highlight fungal elements. Histopathology is considered one of the most reliable methods for definitive diagnosis.
- **Culture**
  Culture from fresh tissue or swabs on Sabouraud dextrose agar or similar fungal media. Colonies are fast-growing, fluffy, and white to grey. Culture confirms viability and allows differentiation from other fungi.

11.32.5 Treatment and Therapeutic Interventions

- **Supportive Care**
  Provide warmth, hydration, and easily digestible food. Reduce stress and optimize ventilation to aid respiratory function. Administer vitamin/mineral supplements to support recovery, particularly vitamins A, D3, and E which aid mucosal immunity and tissue repair. Treat or remove underlying immunosuppressive conditions (e.g., concurrent viral infections, parasitism, or malnutrition).
- **Medication**
  - *Itraconazole*
    5–10 mg/kg by mouth every 12–24 hours
    Nebulization with clotrimazole, amphotericin B, or F10 antiseptic solution (diluted) can deliver drugs directly to the respiratory tract. Requires daily treatments for several days to weeks, specialized equipment, and careful monitoring. May be cost-prohibitive.

11.32.6 Prevention and Control

- **Environmental Management**
  The most critical preventive measure is maintaining a dry, clean, well-ventilated environment to prevent fungal growth. Use dry, clean litter material (e.g., wood shavings, chopped straw) and avoid excessive moisture accumulation. Remove wet spots promptly, especially around waterers and low areas with water accumulation. Turn deep litter regularly to improve aeration and reduce fungal colonization. Ensure adequate airflow to maintain humidity below levels favorable for fungal growth (ideally <70%). Avoid temperature–humidity combinations that create warm, damp microclimates in corners and under equipment. Store feed in dry, cool, well-ventilated areas to prevent mold growth. Discard all feed showing signs of clumping, discoloration, or musty odor; do not sift or pick through. Keep unused bedding materials elevated off the ground and protected from moisture prior to use.
- **Hygiene and Sanitation**
  Thorough and regular cleaning and disinfection of houses, pens, incubators, brooders, feeders, and waterers. Use mechanical cleaning (scraping, washing) before applying disinfectants; fungal spores are resistant to many disinfectants unless organic matter is removed. Allow areas to dry completely, as Zygomycete spores are vulnerable to desiccation.
- **Flock Health and Management**
  Maintain appropriate bird: space ratio to reduce humidity buildup and litter degradation. Overcrowding predisposes birds to stress and environmental contamination. Provide balanced nutrition, adequate space, and stable environmental conditions. Control viral immunosuppressive diseases (e.g., CAV, IBDV) through vaccination (if available) and biosecurity. Avoid

prolonged use of antibiotics or corticosteroids, which predispose birds to fungal overgrowth. Young chicks and immunocompromised birds are most susceptible; extra care with litter and ventilation is warranted in brooders.

- **Source Control and Biosecurity**
  Inspect and test feed and litter sources for fungal contamination, especially after heavy rains or in humid climates. Do not introduce damp or visibly moldy bedding or feed to houses or pens. Implement strict visitor control, equipment disinfection.

11.32.7 Nursing Considerations

Nursing care for chickens affected by mucormycosis focuses on supportive management, environmental control, and strict hygiene, as antifungal treatment is often limited in efficacy for systemic infections. Affected birds should be isolated in a clean, warm, low-stress environment to reduce secondary stressors and prevent exposure to additional pathogens. Veterinary technicians should provide easily accessible feed and water, using high-quality, mold-free feed to avoid further fungal exposure. Assisted feeding, oxygen and fluid therapy if indicated. Careful observation for respiratory distress, weight loss, and changes in droppings is essential, with daily monitoring and documentation to track disease progression. Because mucormycosis is primarily associated with environmental contamination, husbandry protocols should emphasize deep cleaning and disinfection of housing, removal of wet litter and spoiled feed, and improved ventilation to lower humidity and fungal spore load. Any bird with compromised immunity or concurrent illnesses should receive prompt supportive care to minimize susceptibility. In cases where localized lesions are detected (e.g., proventriculus or air sacs), veterinary-directed surgical debridement or localized antifungal therapy may be attempted, though prognosis is often guarded. Veterinary technicians play a key role in educating backyard flock owners on prevention, focusing on proper feed storage, routine litter replacement, and controlling environmental moisture. Necropsy and laboratory testing of deceased birds should be encouraged to confirm diagnosis and guide flock-level interventions. If birds are suffering, humane euthanasia is always a reasonable treatment option.

11.33 Cryptococcosis

11.33.1 Overview and Pathogenesis

Cryptococcosis in poultry is a fungal disease caused primarily by *Cryptococcus neoformans* and *Cryptococcus gattii*. These yeast-like fungi are environmental saprophytes, commonly found in soil contaminated with bird droppings, particularly from pigeons and other wild birds. Chickens are generally less susceptible than mammals, but infections can occur in immunocompromised birds or when there is high environmental exposure to spores. The disease is zoonotic, posing a potential risk to immunocompromised humans handling infected birds or contaminated materials. In chickens, infection occurs through inhalation of airborne spores or, less commonly, via ingestion. Once in the host, the yeast cells colonize the upper respiratory tract, especially the nasal passages, sinuses, and air sacs, and can disseminate systemically in severe cases.

Pathogenesis involves yeast proliferation, capsule formation, and evasion of host immune defenses, leading to localized granulomatous inflammation. The fungus can invade surrounding tissues, causing sinusitis, air sacculitis, and occasionally involvement of internal organs such as the liver and spleen. Lesions are often nodular or caseous granulomas, with minimal necrosis, reflecting the host's cell-mediated immune response. Clinically affected birds may show respiratory distress, nasal discharge, dyspnea, depression, and reduced feed intake, although subclinical infections are common. Environmental contamination with feces and litter contributes to continued exposure and sporadic cases in flocks.

11.33.2 Risk Factors

- **Host-Related Factors**
  Birds with weakened immune systems (due to chronic disease, stress, or concurrent infections) are more susceptible to fungal colonization and invasion. Juvenile or geriatric chickens may have reduced immune defenses. Damage to the respiratory epithelium from ammonia exposure, viral infections, or other irritants facilitate fungal penetration. Conditions such as nutritional deficiencies, or parasitism can predispose birds to opportunistic fungal infections.
- **Environmental Factors**
  Contaminated lofts, coops, or barns near pigeon populations increase exposure risk. Enclosed housing with inadequate air flow and persistent dampness promotes fungal growth and spore aerosolization. Old, moist litter can harbor fungal spores, increase inhalation risk when disturbed. Proximity to large numbers of pigeons or other bird species that serve as environmental reservoirs can increase flock exposure.
- **Management and Husbandry Factors**
  Infrequent cleaning or poor sanitation allows organic material and droppings to accumulate, creating a breeding ground for Cryptococcus. Movement of people, equipment, or wild birds between contaminated and clean areas can introduce the fungus into chicken environments. Overcrowding increases stress and respiratory irritation, predisposing birds to infection.

11.33.3 Clinical Signs and Pathology

- **External Findings**
  Respiratory System (Most Common)
  Nasal discharge (serous to mucoid), sneezing, open beak breathing, dyspnea, head shaking, and frequent scratching at the nares.

  Neurologic Signs
  Infrequent but possible if the fungus disseminates hematogenous to the brain and meninges. Ataxia, head tilt, circling, or depression. In advanced cases, seizures or inability to stand.

  Ocular Signs
  Swelling around the eyes and conjunctivitis if sinus involvement occurs. Occasionally, exophthalmos or ocular opacity with local granuloma formation.
- **Necropsy Findings**
  Upper Respiratory Tract
  Caseous to gelatinous exudate within nasal passages, sinuses, and choanal slit. Thickened mucosa with whitish to cream-colored plaques or mucoid masses adherent to nasal turbinates or sinus walls. In some cases, granulomatous lesions may be found in infraorbital sinuses.

  Lower Respiratory Tract
  Less commonly affected, but may show focal pneumonia with small, gray-white nodules on the lung surface if spores penetrate deeply.

Central Nervous System
If dissemination occurs, gelatinous meningeal exudates, focal granulomas, or softening of brain tissue may be observed. Lesions are typically found in the meninges and brain parenchyma.

Other Organs
In advanced systemic cases, granulomatous foci may occur in the liver, spleen, or kidneys. Lesions are usually firm, pale nodules surrounded by minimal inflammation.

11.33.4 Diagnostic Testing

- **Cytology**
  - **India Ink** reveals encapsulated, budding yeast cells (clear capsule halo around dark cell).
  - **Gram Stain or PAS (Periodic Acid-Schiff)** the yeast appears gram-positive and magenta with PAS.
  - **Grocott's methenamine silver (GMS)** stains fungal cell walls black for clear visualization.
- **Culture**
  Samples from nasal exudate, cerebrospinal fluid, and tissue from affected organs (lungs, sinuses, brain).
- **PCR**
  Confirms Cryptococcus DNA from tissue or culture. Differentiates C. neoformans from C. gattii. Useful in cases with low fungal burden or when culture is inconclusive.

11.33.5 Treatment and Therapeutic Interventions

- **Supportive Care**
  Isolate affected birds to prevent stress and potential environmental contamination. Remove and replace contaminated litter, droppings, and organic material. Disinfect with 1% sodium hypochlorite or formalin (kills fungal spores). Provide balanced diet, vitamin supplementation (especially A and E for immune support). Supplemental nutrition, oxygen therapy, or assisted feeding with/out fluid therapy may be indicated. Maintaining low dust and humidity helps reduce fungal proliferation in the environment. Ensure access to clean water; electrolytes may be added during prolonged illness.
- **Medication**
  Amphotericin B 7 mg/mL for 15 minutes (Nebulized) q12h, 1.5 mg/kg (IV) q8h, 1 mg/kg intratracheal/nasal flush q8–12h diluted to 1 mL with sterile saline.
  Fluconazole 2–5 mg/kg by mouth every 24 hours for 3–6 weeks.
  Itraconazole 5–10 mg/kg by mouth every 12–24 hours.
- **Surgical Intervention**
  Localized lesions (e.g., sinus or subcutaneous nodules) may be surgically debrided or drained to reduce fungal load before systemic antifungal therapy. Local or general anesthesia.

11.33.6 Prevention and Control

- **Environmental Management**
  Remove organic debris, droppings, and damp litter frequently. Disinfect housing and equipment with 1–10% sodium hypochlorite (bleach), then allow it to thoroughly dry. Keep housing dry and well-ventilated to prevent fungal growth. Avoid accumulation of moldy feed or bedding. Replace

litter regularly and avoid reusing contaminated material. Dispose of contaminated litter away from housing. Replace contaminated soil or apply lime in heavily affected outdoor runs to reduce fungal load.

- **Control of Reservoir Hosts**
  Pigeons and wild birds are major carriers of *Cryptococcus neoformans*. Exclude wild birds from chicken houses by sealing openings and using netting. Avoid storing feed or water sources in open areas accessible to pigeons. Remove nesting sites and droppings from roofs, attics, and around coops.
- **Flock Health and Immune Support**
  Maintain good nutrition, adequate vitamins A, E, and selenium support immune function. Minimize stress (avoid overcrowding, ensure proper ventilation and temperature control). Control concurrent diseases (e.g., respiratory or immunosuppressive infections) that can predispose birds to fungal infection.
- **Health Safety**
  Cryptococcus is a zoonotic pathogen. Avoid dry sweeping, moisten droppings before removal to reduce airborne spores. Wash hands thoroughly after contact with birds or litter. Appropriate PPE should be worn while cleaning houses and pens.

11.33.7 Nursing Considerations

Nursing care for chickens affected by cryptococcosis focuses on supportive management, environmental hygiene, and prevention of further exposure, as treatment options for systemic infection are limited and prognosis is often guarded. Veterinary technicians should monitor affected birds for respiratory signs such as nasal discharge, dyspnea, wheezing, and lethargy, ensuring they have easy access to food and water to maintain hydration and nutrition. Cleaning of nares, assisted feeding, oxygen and fluid therapy may be indicated. Housing should be clean, dry, well-ventilated, and free from mold or contaminated droppings, with frequent litter changes to reduce exposure to fungal spores. Isolation of clinically affected birds is recommended to minimize stress and prevent additional exposure, though bird-to-bird transmission is uncommon. Veterinary technicians should employ strict biosecurity measures, including gloves, masks, and protective clothing, due to the zoonotic potential of *Cryptococcus*, particularly for immunocompromised caregivers. Environmental control is critical: removal of contaminated litter, regular disinfection, and limiting access of wild birds or pigeons can significantly reduce risk. Supportive care may include anti-inflammatory therapy or symptomatic treatment for respiratory distress, under veterinary supervision. Technicians should document clinical signs, mortality, and treatment responses, and educate caretakers on zoonotic risks, proper hygiene, and environmental management to prevent future infections.

Infectious (viruses, bacteria, and fungus) diseases of chickens pose significant challenges for flock health. Veterinary technicians play a vital role in early recognition, diagnostic sample collection, supportive care, and client education.

- **Viral Diseases:** largely prevented through vaccination; treatment is supportive.
- **Bacterial Diseases:** treatable with antimicrobials, but resistance and carrier states complicate management.
- **Fungal Diseases:** often environmental in origin; control hinges on husbandry improvements.

Ultimately, successful management requires an integrated approach combining vaccination, biosecurity, husbandry, supportive therapies, judicious antimicrobial use, and vigilant nursing care.

Further Reading

Common Bacterial Diseases in Backyard Chickens [Internet]. Vin.com. 2023. Available from: https://veterinarypartner.vin.com/default.aspx?pid=19239andcatId=254010andid=10048768

Sato Y. Common Infectious Diseases in Backyard Poultry – Exotic and Laboratory Animals [Internet]. Merck Veterinary Manual. 2024. Available from: https://www.merckvetmanual.com/exotic-and-laboratory-animals/backyard-poultry/common-infectious-diseases-in-backyard-poultry

Shamoun K. *Erysipelothrix rhusiopathiae* Infection Associated with Swollen ... [Internet]. Avian Diseases; [cited 2025 Nov 24]. Available from: https://meridian.allenpress.com/avian-diseases/article/67/1/119/491680/Erysipelothrix-rhusiopathiae-Infection-Associated

12

Musculoskeletal Diseases and Disorders

Musculoskeletal diseases in chickens interfere with mobility, feeding, reproduction, and overall health and quality of life. Most commonly seen in rapidly growing meat breeds and in high-producing egg-laying breeds. This can be caused by nutritional imbalances, infectious agents, mechanical stress, traumatic events, or genetic predisposition. Clinical signs noted are lameness, skeletal deformities, joint swelling, and fractures (Table 12.1).

12.1 Arthritis

12.1.1 Overview and Pathogenesis

Arthritis in chickens refers to inflammation of one or more joints, often resulting in swelling, pain, and impaired mobility. It can arise from infectious or noninfectious causes. Infectious arthritis is most associated with bacterial pathogens such as *Staphylococcus aureus*, *Escherichia coli*, or *Mycoplasma synoviae*, which invade joint tissues following systemic infection, penetrating wounds, or extension from surrounding tissues. Viral agents and fungi may also contribute to some cases. Noninfectious arthritis can result from trauma, nutritional imbalances (such as deficiencies of vitamins or minerals affecting cartilage integrity), or degenerative joint disease related to rapid growth or mechanical stress.

Pathogenesis involves inflammation of the synovial membrane, infiltration of leukocytes, and accumulation of exudate within the joint capsule, leading to swelling and pain. Chronic inflammation may cause cartilage erosion, pannus formation, and periarticular fibrosis, ultimately impairing joint function. In severe cases, lameness and reduced productivity are common, and systemic illness may develop with bacterial septic arthritis.

12.1.2 Risk Factors

- **Trauma and Mechanical Factors**
  Leg injuries from rough handling, aggressive birds, or poor flooring. Excessive body weight in meat-bird breeds predisposes them to joint stress and damage.
- **Nutritional and Metabolic Factors**
  Vitamin deficiencies (e.g., vitamin D, vitamin C, and manganese) cause weakened joint integrity. Rapid growth rate in meat bird breeds causes biomechanical stress on joints. An imbalance of calcium and phosphorus weakens bones and cartilage, predisposing to arthropathy.

Table 12.1

Quick reference chart

Condition	Etiology/cause	Key clinical signs	Pathology/lesions	Diagnostic methods	Treatment/therapeutic interventions	Prevention and control
Osteomalacia "Rickets"	Nutritional deficiency—inadequate vitamin D3, calcium, or phosphorus	Lameness, soft or pliable bones, beading of ribs, reluctance to walk, stunted growth	Soft, rubbery bones, bending of long bones, widening of physes (growth plates)	Clinical signs, diet history, radiographs, necropsy	Correct diet (vitamin D3 + Ca:P balance), improve lighting for D3 synthesis	Balanced diet, proper Ca:P ratio (1.8–2:1), sunlight/UVB exposure
Perosis (slipped tendon)	Manganese deficiency, rapid growth, genetic predisposition	Enlargement/swelling of hock, lateral deviation of distal leg, lameness, poor growth	Gastrocnemius tendon slips from condyle, hock swelling	Physical exam, necropsy findings	Dietary manganese supplementation, early correction may help mild cases	Balanced diet, adequate Mn and choline, genetic selection
Splay leg (spraddle leg)	Incubation issues (slippery surfaces), trauma, nutritional factors	Legs splayed outward, inability to stand, often seen in chicks	No bony lesions, ligamentous laxity	Clinical signs (early chick)	Hobbles to bring legs under body, improve footing, supportive care	Proper hatcher floor texture, early intervention, correct nutrition
Curly toe paralysis	Riboflavin (Vit B2) deficiency, especially in young chicks	Flexion of toes, inability to walk properly, leg weakness, decreased weight gain	Peripheral nerve demyelination, esp. sciatic nerve	Clinical signs, necropsy (nerve histopath), dietary history	Riboflavin supplementation; may reverse early cases	Balanced starter diet with adequate B2, good feed storage
Tibial dyschondroplasia (TD)	Rapid growth, genetic predisposition, Ca/P imbalance, metabolic	Swollen joints, reluctance to move, angular leg deformities	Plug of unmineralized cartilage in growth plate (proximal tibiotarsus)	Radiographs, necropsy (growth plate plug), flock history	No specific treatment; dietary correction, reduce growth rate	Genetic selection, dietary management, avoid excessive energy diets
Bacterial (septic) arthritis/ tenosynovitis	Staphylococcus aureus, *E. coli*, others via wounds, hematogenous spread	Hot, swollen joints, lameness, reluctance to bear weight, poor performance	Purulent or caseous exudate in joints/ tendons, synovial hyperplasia	Joint aspirates for culture, necropsy, radiographs	Systemic antibiotics (based on sensitivity), supportive care, culling severe cases	Good biosecurity, prompt wound care, reduce trauma, sanitation

(Continued)

Table 12.1 (Continued)

Quick reference chart

Condition	Etiology/cause	Key clinical signs	Pathology/lesions	Diagnostic methods	Treatment/therapeutic interventions	Prevention and control
Osteomyelitis/bacterial chondronecrosis with osteomyelitis (BCO)	Hematogenous bacterial infection in fast-growing birds	Sudden lameness, birds sitting on hocks, inability to stand, sometimes with no external swelling	Necrosis of femoral head or vertebral bodies, bacterial colonies	Necropsy (typical femoral head lesions), histopathology, culture	No practical flock treatment; cull severely affected birds, reduce stressors	Litter management, ventilation, reducing rapid weight gain, biosecurity
Angular leg deformities (varus/valgus)	Multifactorial—genetic, incubation, nutrition, rapid growth	Abnormal leg angulation (inward/outward), impaired walking, deformities worsen with age	Angular deviation of long bones at joints (often tibiotarsal)	Physical exam, radiographs, necropsy	No effective treatment in advanced cases; mild cases may improve with diet	Genetic selection, balanced diet, manage growth rate, good flooring
Fractures/trauma	Accidents, handling, aggressive flock behavior	Lameness, swelling, abnormal limb position, crepitus	Fracture of long bones or keel	Physical exam, radiographs	Splinting or surgical stabilization (valuable birds), pain control	Safe housing design, gentle handling, reduce aggression
Gout (articular)	High protein diets, dehydration, renal dysfunction, vitamin A deficiency	Swollen joints, chalky white deposits, lameness, reduced mobility	Urate crystal deposits in joints and periarticular tissues	Necropsy, aspirate smears (urate), uric acid tests	Address underlying cause, improve hydration, dietary correction	Balanced protein levels, proper hydration, monitor renal health
Chondrodystrophy/dwarfism	Genetic defects (especially in broilers), sometimes viral (e.g., reovirus)	Shortened long bones, disproportionate body size, stunted growth	Disorganized cartilage columns in growth plates	Necropsy, histopathology, flock history	No treatment; culling affected chicks	Genetic control, breeder flock management

Table courtesy of Stephanie Freeman.

12.1.3 Clinical Signs and Pathology

- **External Findings**
  Reluctance or inability to walk, stand, or perch. Hock, stifle, or foot joints were visibly enlarged. Crepitus, warmth, and pain on palpation. Reduced feed and water intake due to immobility.
- **Necropsy Findings**
  Swollen joints (hock, stifle, intertarsal, or wing joints). Excess synovial fluid is often turbid or caseous in bacterial infections. Thickened synovial membrane with hyperemia. Cartilage erosion in chronic cases, with ankylosis.

12.1.4 Diagnostic Imaging

- **Radiographs**
  May reveal joint effusion, cartilage erosion, or bone involvement.

12.1.5 Treatment and Therapeutic Interventions

- **Medications**
  Meloxicam 0.5 mg/kg by mouth or intramuscularly every 12–24 hours.
  Carprofen 5–10 mg/kg by mouth or intramuscularly once daily.
  Supplemental glucosamine, chondroitin, and omega-3 fatty acids.
  Other options include vitamin E, selenium, turmeric, and avocado/soybean unsaponifiables.
  Polysulfated glycosaminoglycan or PSGAG 1 mg/kg IM once monthly.
- **Adjunctive Therapeutics**
  Low-level laser therapy
  Water treadmill therapy
  Physical therapy, passive range of motion
  Acupuncture

12.1.6 Prevention and Control

- **Environmental and Husbandry Management**
  Soft perches and flooring reduce trauma and pressure on joints. Flat surfaces if unable to hop, climb to a perch. Ensure that feed and water are easily accessible.

12.1.7 Nursing Considerations

Nursing care for chickens with arthritis emphasizes pain relief, infection control, and supportive management to maintain mobility and welfare. Affected birds should be housed on clean, dry, and soft bedding to reduce pressure on swollen joints and minimize secondary trauma. Nutrition must be optimized, with attention to adequate protein, vitamins, and minerals to support joint and immune health. For infectious arthritis, antimicrobial therapy may be prescribed under veterinary supervision, while noninfectious cases may benefit from anti-inflammatory support and careful weight management. Low-level laser therapy. Birds should be monitored closely for lameness, reluctance to move, or reduced access to feed and water, with provisions made to keep food and water easily accessible. Regular observation for progression or systemic illness is important, and humane euthanasia should be considered if birds experience chronic pain or severely reduced mobility that compromises quality of life.

12.2 Curly Toe Paralysis

12.2.1 Overview and Pathogenesis

Curly toe paralysis is a congenital or early-onset musculoskeletal disorder primarily observed in young chicks, characterized by curling of the toes, impaired weight-bearing, and difficulty walking. The condition is most associated with a deficiency of riboflavin (vitamin B2) in the diet, though genetic predisposition, incubation conditions, or secondary nutritional imbalances may contribute.

Pathogenesis involves impaired neuromuscular development, including degeneration of motor neurons in the lumbar and sacral regions of the spinal cord, leading to weakness or paralysis of distal limb muscles. Muscle atrophy and contracture of tendons ensue, producing the characteristic curled toes. Clinically, affected chicks may exhibit lameness, reluctance to move, and abnormal gait, which can compromise access to feed and water, predisposing them to poor growth and secondary health issues. Histologically, lesions include neuronal degeneration, demyelination, and atrophy of affected skeletal muscles.

12.2.2 Risk Factors

- **Nutritional Deficiency**
  Biotin deficiency (vitamin B7) is the primary cause. Low biotin in the diet during the first 2–3 weeks of life. Poorly balanced starter feeds or feed processing errors are contributors. High avidin content in raw egg whites can bind biotin and reduce its availability.
- **Environmental and Management Factors**
  Stressful conditions such as poor temperature control, overcrowding, or rough handling can exacerbate neuromuscular weakness.

12.2.3 Clinical Signs and Pathology

- **External Findings**
  Curled toes, typically the middle and lateral toes bend inward or upward. Impaired gait, chicks may walk on the hock or drag toes. Weak or unsteady legs; may struggle to stand. Difficulty perching or feeding due to impaired mobility.
- **Necropsy Findings**
  No major lesions internally; skeletal structures are normal but appear deformed due to tendon and nerve dysfunction.

12.2.4 Diagnostic Testing

None.

12.2.5 Treatment and Therapeutic Interventions

- **Response to Treatment**
  Rapid improvement after biotin supplementation confirms nutritional etiology. Improved leg strength within 3–5 days, with progressive correction of toe curling.

- **Supportive Care**
  Soft bedding to prevent secondary abrasions or footpad injuries. Reduced activity minimizes stress and prevents further deformity while recovery occurs. Isolation of severely affected chicks may help ensure they can access feed and water. Passive range of motion of pelvic limbs several times daily. May need to prop chick up when drinking, eating to avoid aspiration pneumonia.
- **Nutritional Therapy**
  Biotin supplementation is the treatment of choice. Corrects neuromuscular dysfunction and prevents progression. Early treatment often leads to rapid improvement within 3–5 days.
  Water-Soluble Biotin 0.5–1 mg/L of drinking water for 3–5 days.
  Feed Supplementation: starter feed should contain at least 0.2–0.3 mg/kg biotin.

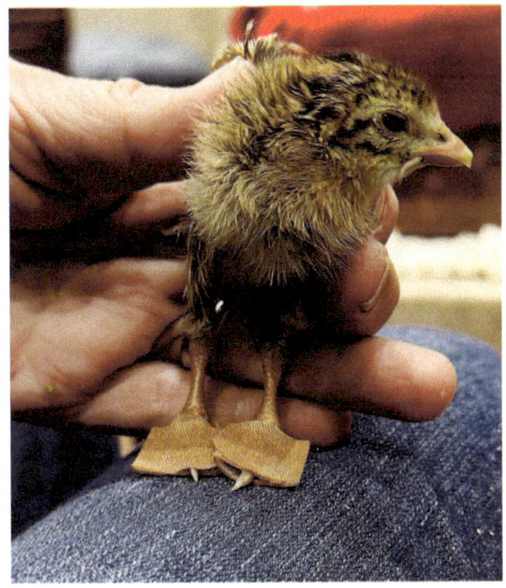

Figure 12.1 Coaptation placement for curly toe paralysis. Courtesy of Funky Chicken Rescue.

12.2.6 Prevention and Control

- **Nutritional Management**
  Ensure adequate biotin in feed. Avoid feeding antagonists; high levels of raw egg whites bind biotin and reduce its availability (Figure 12.1).

12.2.7 Nursing Considerations

Nursing care of curly toe paralysis focuses on correcting underlying nutritional deficiencies, supporting mobility, and preventing secondary complications. Ensuring an adequate supply of riboflavin and a balanced diet during early growth stages is critical to prevent further neuromuscular damage. Affected chicks should be provided with clean, soft, non-slippery bedding to reduce stress on their legs and prevent pododermatitis or injuries. Physical support, such as splints or gentle manipulation, may help maintain toe alignment and improve walking in mild cases. Birds should be closely monitored for feed and water intake, as impaired mobility can lead to dehydration, poor growth, or secondary infections. Early intervention often improves prognosis, but severely affected chicks with compromised mobility or feeding ability may require humane euthanasia to prevent prolonged suffering.

12.3 Gout

12.3.1 Overview and Pathogenesis

Gout in chickens is a metabolic disorder characterized by the deposition of uric acid crystals in tissues, most commonly in joints (articular gout) or on visceral organs such as the kidneys and serous membranes (visceral gout). It is broadly classified into two types: primary (metabolic) and secondary (renal).

Pathogenesis involves either excessive production of uric acid due to high-protein diets or impaired excretion resulting from kidney dysfunction, dehydration, or nephrotoxic injury.

Accumulation of uric acid crystals triggers inflammation, causing joint swelling, pain, and tissue damage in affected organs. Predisposing factors include rapid growth, excessive dietary protein or calcium, vitamin imbalances (particularly vitamin A), and underlying renal disease. Clinically, affected birds may show lameness, reluctance to move, enlarged joints, and in severe cases, sudden death due to systemic urate deposition. Histologically, tissues exhibit tophi (deposits of monosodium urate crystals) accompanied by heterophilic inflammation, fibrosis, and tissue necrosis.

12.3.2 Risk Factors

- **Nutritional Factors**
  Excess dietary protein increases uric acid production. Calcium-phosphorus imbalance causes kidney damage and reduced uric acid clearance. Vitamin A deficiency causes epithelial degeneration in renal tubules, impairing urate excretion. Excessive sodium bicarbonate or salt causes dehydration and kidney stress. Mycotoxins are nephrotoxic, causing renal dysfunction.
- **Environmental and Management Factors**
  Poor water availability, faulty drinkers, or heat stress causes dehydration. High environmental temperatures cause increased water loss, leading to uric acid precipitation. Chronic stress weakens kidney function and general metabolism.
- **Infectious and Toxic Factors**
  Nephropathogenic strains of infectious bronchitis virus (IBV) can cause kidney damage and gout. Heavy metal poisoning leads to nephrotoxicity.

12.3.3 Clinical Signs and Pathology

- **External Findings**
  Reduced feed intake, depression, and lethargy. Weight loss and poor growth in young birds. Increased water intake (polydipsia) in chronic renal damage. High mortality in acute visceral gout outbreaks. Swollen joints (hock, foot, wing joints). Lameness, reluctance to move, or inability to perch.
- **Necropsy Findings**
  Visceral Gout
  White, chalky urate deposits on serosal surfaces of heart, liver, kidneys, air sacs, and peritoneum ("frosted appearance"). Kidneys enlarged, pale, and swollen. Ureters are often distended with urates.

  Articular Gout
  White to yellow chalky masses of urates in joints and tendon sheaths. Joint capsules were thickened and inflamed. Surrounding tissues may be fibrotic.

12.3.4 Diagnostic Testing

- **Bloodwork**
  Elevated uric acid levels in serum (>10 mg/dL typical in gout). Increased creatinine and urea may support the diagnosis of renal failure.

12.3.5 Treatment and Therapeutic Interventions

- **Supportive Care**
  Provide abundant, clean, cool drinking water to help flush uric acid. Electrolytes may improve kidney function and reduce dehydration. Acidification of drinking water (e.g., ammonium

chloride, potassium chloride, or citric acid) helps dissolve urates and reduce precipitation in tissues. Reduce dietary protein (especially nonprotein nitrogen) and balance calcium–phosphorus levels to decrease uric acid production. Clean, soft bedding. Cold laser therapy. Cool packing of joints.

- **Medication**
  Allopurinol
  10–30 mg/kg by mouth every 12 hours.

12.3.6 Prevention and Control

- **Nutritional Management**
  Avoid excessive crude protein and nonprotein nitrogen sources that increase uric acid production. Correct calcium-phosphorus ratio. Adequate vitamin A prevents epithelial damage in kidney tubules. Excess sodium, sulfate, or calcium predisposes to renal overload and gout. Use binders or high-quality feed to reduce the risk of nephrotoxic aflatoxins, ochratoxin, and citrinin.
- **Water Quality and Availability**
  Provide constant access to clean, fresh water to promote uric acid excretion. Monitor for salt contamination, hardness, and heavy metals. Prevent dehydration from heat stress, crowding, or waterer failure.
- **Environmental and Management Practices**
  Reduce heat stress with proper ventilation, cooling systems, and overcrowding. Avoid nephrotoxic medications (e.g., aminoglycosides) when possible. Monitor flock health regularly for early detection of renal dysfunction. Practice good litter management to reduce ammonia buildup, which can worsen dehydration and stress.
- **Disease Control**
  Vaccinating (when available) against nephropathogenic IBV where it is prevalent. Maintain biosecurity to prevent the introduction of viruses that damage kidneys (e.g., IBV, avian nephritis virus). Control other immunosuppressive diseases (e.g., infectious bursa disease [IBD], Marek's) that exacerbate susceptibility.

12.3.7 Nursing Considerations

Nursing care of gout in chickens emphasizes supportive care, dietary modification, and prevention of further uric acid accumulation. Birds should be provided with clean, fresh water to support kidney function and prevent dehydration. Diets should be balanced with appropriate protein, calcium, and vitamin levels, avoiding excessive dietary protein or imbalances that contribute to hyperuricemia. Affected birds should be housed on soft, dry bedding to reduce pressure on swollen joints and minimize discomfort. Cold laser therapy or cool packing of affected joints. Monitoring clinical signs such as lameness, joint swelling, or lethargy is essential, and birds showing severe pain or systemic illness may require humane euthanasia. Addressing underlying causes, such as kidney dysfunction or nutritional deficiencies, is critical to prevent recurrence. Maintaining optimal environmental conditions, minimizing stress, and ensuring easy access to feed and water support recovery and overall welfare. Humane euthanasia if treatment is unsuccessful.

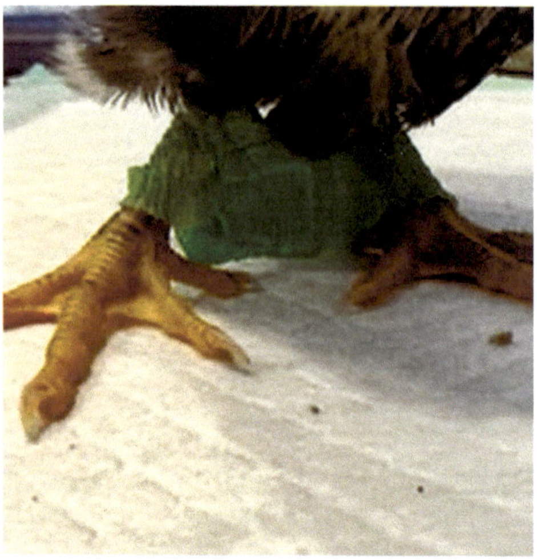

Figure 12.2 Splay leg with bandage hobbles. Courtesy of Funky Chicken Rescue.

12.4 Splay Leg

12.4.1 Overview and Pathogenesis

Splay leg, also called spraddle leg, is a musculoskeletal disorder observed primarily in newly hatched chicks, characterized by lateral abduction of one or both legs, resulting in an inability to stand or walk properly. The condition is typically associated with a combination of genetic, nutritional, and environmental factors.

Pathogenesis involves weakness or underdevelopment of the muscles and ligaments responsible for limb adduction, often exacerbated by slippery or uneven hatching surfaces that prevent proper limb positioning. Nutritional deficiencies, particularly in trace minerals such as manganese, copper, or biotin, as well as improper incubation conditions, may impair normal neuromuscular development. Clinically, affected chicks show lateral leg splaying, inability to bear weight, and impaired mobility, which can lead to starvation, dehydration, or secondary injuries. Histological examination reveals underdeveloped or poorly organized muscle fibers, and in some cases, laxity or malformation of ligaments and tendons controlling limb alignment (Figure 12.2).

12.4.2 Risk Factors

- **Incubation-Related Factors**
  Incorrect incubator temperature or humidity. Slippery hatching surfaces (e.g., plastic and smooth cardboard without grip). Malpositioning of the chick inside the egg.
- **Nutritional Deficiencies**
  B vitamin deficiencies, especially riboflavin (B2), impair tendon and muscle development. Deficiencies in manganese or other trace minerals affect cartilage and joint strength.
- **Genetic and Developmental Factors**
  Congenital musculoskeletal weakness. Rapid growth or weak leg confirmation in certain breeds (notably heavy meat-type birds).
- **Environmental and Management Factors**
  Slippery brooder flooring (newspaper, smooth plastic) prevents proper leg traction. Overcrowding or rough handling of chicks. Inadequate brooder temperature causes chilling and muscular weakness.
- **Injury and Secondary Causes**
  Trauma to legs during hatching, transport, or early brooding. Secondary to other leg deformities (twisted legs, slipped tendon).

12.4.3 Clinical Signs and Pathology

- **External Findings**
  One or both legs extend sideways (laterally) instead of being under the body. Birds may "swim" or paddle with wings for balance. Soiled down feathers, dehydration, malnutrition, or trampling by other chicks.

- **Necropsy Findings**
  Inability of the tendons and muscles of the hip and hock to hold the leg in normal alignment. Degeneration of peripheral nerves supplying the legs. Atrophy of leg muscles.

12.4.4 Diagnostic Imaging

- **Radiographs**
  May help differentiate tendon or joint malformations from fractures or slipped tendon.

12.4.5 Treatment and Therapeutic Interventions

- **Early Physical Correction**
  Use a soft band (e.g., vet wrap, tape, or rubber band with padding) to hold the legs in correct alignment under the body. Keep for 4–7 days, adjusting as the chick grows. Provide non-slip flooring (paper towel, rubber matting, or textured bedding) to help grip and strengthen legs. Avoid shavings as they will impede mobility.
- **Nutritional Support**
  Riboflavin (Vitamin B2) supplements oral or water-soluble formulations if deficiency is suspected. Ensure correct levels of manganese, biotin, choline, and protein to support musculoskeletal development.
- **Supportive Care**
  Hand-feed or use shallow feeders/drinkers if mobility is impaired. Gentle leg stretching and positioning exercises, passive range of motion, may improve tendon strength.

12.4.6 Prevention and Control

- **Incubation and Hatching Management**
  Maintain optimal incubator temperature and humidity to ensure proper embryonic development (discussed in Chapter 2). Use hatch trays with textured surfaces to provide traction at the hatch. Avoid prolonged delays in removing chicks from incubators, which can lead to fatigue and leg weakness.
- **Brooder Environmental**
  Provide non-slip flooring (paper towels, textured rubber mats, or non-slick bedding) for the first week of life. Avoid slippery materials such as newspaper or smooth plastic. Maintain appropriate brooder temperature to prevent chilling or overheating, both of which weaken chicks. Prevent overcrowding, which increases the risk of trampling and leg injuries.
- **Nutritional Prevention**
  Ensure balanced starter diets with adequate vitamins and minerals, especially riboflavin (B2), manganese, and biotin. Avoid feed formulation errors that result in deficiencies or imbalances. Reputable, high-quality chick feeds.
- **Handling and Management**
  Handle chicks carefully during transport and placement to reduce injuries. Monitor daily for early signs of splay leg and correct promptly. Separate weak or affected chicks to prevent bullying or trampling.

12.4.7 Nursing Considerations

Nursing care of splay leg focuses on supporting mobility, correcting limb alignment, and preventing secondary complications. Affected chicks should be housed on non-slippery, textured surfaces such as rubber mats or paper towels to provide traction and reduce further splaying. Early intervention with gentle splinting or hobbling of the legs can help align limbs and promote normal walking. Keep brooder clean, warm, and dry. Nutritional support, including adequate protein and trace minerals like manganese, copper, and biotin, is essential to support muscle and ligament development. Birds should be closely monitored for access to feed and water, as impaired mobility can lead to dehydration, starvation, or injury. Regular observation for improvement or worsening is important, and severely affected chicks with no potential for recovery may require humane euthanasia to prevent prolonged suffering.

12.5 Rickets (Osteomalacia)

12.5.1 Overview and Pathogenesis

Rickets is a metabolic bone disease in chickens, primarily caused by deficiencies of vitamin D3, calcium, or phosphorus, or by imbalances in their dietary ratios. The disease predominantly affects growing chicks, leading to impaired mineralization of the bone matrix and softening and deformation of skeletal structures.

Pathogenesis involves insufficient calcium and phosphorus deposition into the osteoid, which results in enlarged growth plates, bowed legs, thickened long bones, and weak skeletal support. Vitamin D3 deficiency impairs intestinal absorption of calcium and phosphorus, exacerbating the mineral imbalance, while chronic phosphorus deficiency further hinders proper bone mineralization. Clinically, affected birds exhibit lameness, reluctance to move, crooked or bowed limbs, poor growth, and reduced productivity, with severe cases leading to permanent skeletal deformities. Environmental and management factors, such as low-quality feed, inadequate lighting, or lack of sunlight exposure, may contribute to the development of rickets by reducing endogenous vitamin D3 synthesis. Overall, rickets is a nutritional-metabolic disorder resulting from deficiencies or imbalances of key minerals and vitamins, leading to impaired bone formation, skeletal deformities, and compromised growth in young chickens.

12.5.2 Risk Factors

- **Nutritional Factors**
  Common in poorly balanced starter feeds or diets low in limestone or oyster shell. Diets low in dicalcium phosphate or with high calcium-to-phosphorus ratios (>2.5:1) predispose birds to rickets. It can occur with insufficient supplementation, degraded feed, or lack of exposure to UVB light. The ideal ratio in growing chicks is ~2:1; any significant deviation leads to impaired bone mineralization.
- **Environmental Factors**
  Indoor housing without adequate sunlight exposure limits endogenous vitamin D3 synthesis. Cold stress increases energy demand, which can indirectly exacerbate nutrient deficiency.
- **Genetic/Management Factors**
  Rapid growth in meat bird breeds increases demand for calcium, phosphorus, and vitamin D3. Overcrowding or uneven feed access as some birds may not receive sufficient nutrients. Poor quality feed or storage issues leading to vitamin D3 degradation.

12.5.3 Clinical Signs and Pathology

- **External Findings**
  Bowed legs (valgus or varus deformities), enlarged hocks and carpi, beaded or swollen ribs at the costochondral junction ("rachitis rosary"), and curved or deformed sternum in severe cases. Waddling or splay-legged stance and reluctance to move due to bone pain and weakness. Reduced body weight, delayed feathering, muscle weakness, especially in legs and breast muscles. Occasionally, susceptibility to fractures increases.
- **Necropsy Findings**
  Soft, pliable long bones; easy to bend or fracture, thickened and irregular epiphyseal growth plates, and widened growth plates with poor mineralization. Usually, internal organs appear normal, unless secondary infections occur.

12.5.4 Diagnostic Testing

- **Bloodwork**
  Calcium levels are often decreased in rickets. Phosphorus can be low or imbalanced relative to calcium. ALP is usually elevated due to increased osteoblastic activity attempting to mineralize bone. Low 25-hydroxyvitamin D3 indicates deficiency. Low 1,23-dehydroxyvitamin D3 affects calcium absorption and bone mineralization.
- **Radiographs**
  Detects poor bone mineralization. Common findings are widened growth plate, bowed or deformed long bones, and thinner cortical bone. Useful for differentiating rickets from leg deformities caused by other factors (e.g., tibial dyschondroplasia and chondrodystrophy).
- **Bone Ash Analysis**
  Measures mineral content of bones (calcium and phosphorus). Reduced bone ash percentage confirms hypomineralization typical of osteomalacia.

12.5.5 Treatment and Therapeutic Interventions

- **Supportive Treatment**
  Provide soft, dry bedding to prevent sternal or leg sores. Reduce flock density to ease access to feeders and waterers. Ensure adequate UVB exposure if kept outdoors (natural conversion of vitamin D).
- **Nutrition Correction**
  Correct dietary calcium and phosphorus to a 2:1 ratio. Ensure vitamin D3 supplementation at 2000–5000 IU/kg of feed. Add phytase enzymes if birds are on cereal-based diets to improve phosphorus absorption.
- **Medications**
  Calcium Lactate
  5–10 mg/kg intramuscular every 7 days as needed.

12.5.6 Prevention and Control

- **Nutritional Management**
  Rickets are primarily caused by deficiencies or imbalances in calcium, phosphorus, and vitamin D3. Proper nutrition is the cornerstone of prevention. Avoid over-supplementation of calcium without balancing phosphorus, as this can impair absorption. Provide adequate vitamin D3 in

the feed or water. Use UVB light exposure for indoor-reared birds to stimulate endogenous vitamin D3 production. Avoid moldy or spoiled feeds that can reduce nutrient availability.

- **Environmental and Management Control**
  Allow natural sunlight or UVB lamps for indoor flocks. Maintain clean, dry litter to support healthy growth. Avoid overcrowding to ensure uniform access to feed and water. Maintain optimal temperatures for chick growth to prevent stress and reduced nutrient utilization. Ensure water is free from excessive minerals (e.g., high iron or magnesium) that may interfere with calcium absorption.
- **Monitoring and Early Intervention**
  Observe chicks for early signs of lameness, growth retardation, or leg deformities. Periodically analyze feed samples for calcium, phosphorus, and vitamin D3 content. Adjust supplementation based on analysis and growth performance.
- **Genetic Considerations**
  Select fast-growing breeds carefully, as extremely rapid growth increases the risk of rickets if nutrition is inadequate. Implement breeding strategies that emphasize skeletal robustness alongside growth.

12.5.7 Nursing Considerations

Nursing care for chickens affected by rickets (osteomalacia) focuses on supportive management, nutritional correction, and minimizing stress to promote skeletal development. Affected birds should be provided with a balanced, high-quality diet containing adequate levels of calcium, phosphorus, and vitamin D3, either through fortified feed or supplementation, to support proper bone mineralization. Housing should be clean, dry, well-lit, and spacious, allowing birds to move freely without risk of injury from weakened or deformed limbs. Caregivers should monitor growth, mobility, and limb development closely, providing gentle handling to prevent fractures or further skeletal damage. Access to sunlight or UVB lighting may be beneficial to facilitate endogenous vitamin D3 synthesis. Nursing also involves monitoring for secondary complications, such as reduced mobility, poor weight gain, or susceptibility to infections due to immobility or stress. Overall, nursing considerations emphasize correcting nutritional deficiencies, supporting skeletal health, careful monitoring, injury prevention, and environmental management to enhance recovery and prevent long-term deformities in growing chickens.

12.6 Tibial Dyschondroplasia (TD)

12.6.1 Overview and Pathogenesis

Tibial dyschondroplasia (TD) is a skeletal disorder in chickens characterized by abnormal development of the proximal growth plate of the tibia, leading to impaired endochondral ossification. The condition predominantly affects rapidly growing meat-type birds, resulting in bone weakness, lameness, and gait abnormalities.

Pathogenesis involves failure of normal cartilage maturation and mineralization within the growth plate, leading to accumulation of avascular, unmineralized cartilage, which weakens the structural integrity of the tibia. This defect is influenced by genetic predisposition, rapid growth rates, nutritional imbalances (particularly calcium, phosphorus, and vitamin D3), and management factors such as overcrowding or insufficient exercise. Clinically affected birds show reluctance to walk, standing on hocks, bowed legs, and reduced weight gain, while severe cases may lead to fractures or secondary infections. Overall, TD is a developmental bone disorder caused by disruption of normal cartilage maturation and mineralization, resulting in skeletal weakness and locomotor dysfunction in growing chickens.

12.6.2 Risk Factors

- **Genetic Factors**
  Fast-growing commercial meat breed lines are predisposed. Selective breeding for rapid weight gain and large breast muscle mass increases skeletal stress.
- **Nutritional Factors**
  Imbalances in calcium, phosphorus, or vitamin D3 can impair ossification. Copper deficiency has been linked to TD (copper is required for collagen cross-linking and angiogenesis). Excess energy or protein promotes rapid growth, outpacing skeletal development. Use of certain feed additives (e.g., ionophores at high levels) may exacerbate TD.
- **Growth Rate and Metabolic Stress**
  Rapid weight gain places mechanical load on immature bones. Growth plate cartilage may not mineralize fast enough to support body weight.

12.6.3 Clinical Signs and Pathology

- **External Findings**
  Mild to severe; birds may sit more, show reluctance to walk, or exhibit splayed legs. Waddling, limping, or inability to bear full weight on affected legs. Bowed or twisted tibiotarsus, sometimes asymmetric. Swelling at the hock or tibiotarsal region may be visible in advanced cases. Increased risk of pododermatitis or femoral head necrosis due to altered weight-bearing.
- **Necropsy Findings**
  There is a proximal tibia growth plate with a plug or mass of white, firm, avascular cartilage. Lesion appears chalky white and fails to mineralize. Absence of blood vessel penetration into the abnormal cartilage zone. Reduced or absent endochondral ossification. Factures can occur if the cartilage plate is weak and cannot support body weight.

12.6.4 Diagnostic Testing

- **Radiographs**
  Thickened, poorly mineralized proximal tibiotarsal growth plate. Clear demarcation between abnormal cartilage and normal ossified bone.
- **Bloodwork**
  May show mild imbalances in calcium, phosphorus, or vitamin D3 metabolites, though not as pronounced as rickets.

12.6.5 Treatment and Therapeutic Interventions

- **Nutritional Interventions**
  Correct calcium, phosphorus, and vitamin D3 levels. Ensure dietary Ca:P ratio is ~2:1. Supplement vitamin D3 at recommended levels to improve mineralization. Supplementing copper at 8–10 ppm in the diet will help collagen cross-link and angiogenesis in cartilage.

- **Management Interventions**
  Intermittent lighting or reduced day length may slow growth and give bones time to mineralize. Prevent slipping or abnormal leg positioning. Reduce early growth rate by restricting energy-dense diets or implementing phase-feeding strategies. Lowering body weight gain in the first weeks reduces skeletal stress.
- **Supportive Care**
  Provide easy access to feed and water for lame birds. Analgesics/anti-inflammatories are rarely used in commercial settings but may be considered backyard birds. Soft, non-slip flooring and bedding. Cold laser therapy.

12.6.6 Prevention and Control

- **Genetic Selection**
  Choose breeder lines with improved skeletal integrity without compromising growth rate excessively. Avoid using extremely fast-growing birds if TD incidence is high. Breeder may not know or divulge this information.
- **Nutritional Management**
  Maintain optimal calcium, phosphorus, and vitamin D3 levels. This includes trace minerals (copper, manganese, and zinc) for bone development. Avoid excessive energy or protein in early growth phases to prevent skeletal overload. Lower energy and protein diets during early growth to slow bone stress. Adjust feed density as birds approach market weight to balance growth and skeletal support.
- **Management Practices**
  Reduce overcrowding to minimize mechanical stress and trauma to immature legs. Provide dry, non-slippery, soft litter and firm footing to reduce leg injuries. Use natural lighting and measured feeding to avoid excessive feed intake and overly rapid growth. Regularly weighing a sample bird to ensure that growth matches skeletal development.

12.6.7 Nursing Considerations

Nursing care for chickens affected by TD focuses on supportive management, minimizing stress and injury, and optimizing growth conditions. Affected birds should be housed in clean, dry, and well-bedded environments to reduce pressure on weakened tibia and prevent fractures. Providing ample space and avoiding overcrowding allows birds to move without undue stress on compromised legs. Nutritional management is crucial: diets should be balanced in calcium, phosphorus, and vitamin D3, and growth rates may need moderation to reduce skeletal stress. Caregivers should monitor mobility, gait, and limb alignment closely, and aid severely lame birds, including soft bedding, reduced competition for feed and water, and gentle handling. Environmental enrichment, such as perches or low platforms, can encourage safe movement and strengthen bones when appropriate. Nursing care also includes monitoring for secondary injuries or infections associated with immobility or abnormal posture. Overall, nursing considerations emphasize supportive care, nutritional optimization, injury prevention, careful observation, and environmental management to improve mobility and reduce morbidity in birds with TD. Humane euthanasia is always a treatment option for severely affected or suffering birds.

12.7 Perosis (Slipped Tendon)

12.7.1 Overview and Pathogenesis

Perosis, also known as slipped tendon, is a skeletal and musculoskeletal disorder in chickens characterized by the displacement of the gastrocnemius tendon from the intercondylar groove of the tibiotarsus, resulting in deformity of the hock joint and impaired locomotion. The condition primarily affects rapidly growing meat-type birds, although it can occur in other breeds under certain nutritional or management conditions.

Pathogenesis involves a combination of nutritional deficiencies, particularly in manganese, zinc, biotin, or choline, and imbalances in calcium and phosphorus, which impair proper cartilage and tendon development. Genetic predisposition and rapid growth rates can exacerbate susceptibility. Clinically affected birds exhibit swelling around the hock, outward rotation of the foot, lameness, reluctance to walk, and abnormal gait, which can lead to reduced feed intake, poor weight gain, and secondary injuries. The lesion is caused by weakening of the tibiotarsal cartilage and structural abnormalities in the tendon insertion, resulting in tendon slippage under normal locomotor stress. Overall, perosis is a nutritionally and developmentally mediated musculoskeletal disorder that compromises mobility and growth in young chickens.

12.7.2 Risk Factors

- **Nutritional Factors**
  The primary cause of perosis; manganese is essential for chondroitin sulfate synthesis, important for cartilage, tendons, and bone matrix. Both deficiency and low bioavailability in feed contribute to the disease. Choline is needed for normal growth; deficiency can exacerbate tendon displacement. Zinc deficiency impairs cartilage and connective tissue formation, contributing to tendon weakness. Imbalanced Ca:P ratio can interfere with manganese utilization, indirectly increasing risk. Vitamin D3 deficiency indirectly affects bone growth and tendon alignment by reducing mineralization.
- **Genetic Factors**
  Fast-growing commercial birds and turkeys are predisposed. Breeds selected for heavy muscling are at higher risk.
- **Management Factors**
  Rapid weight gain can increase mechanical stress on immature legs. Chicks on smooth surfaces are more likely to experience tendon displacement. Accelerated growth can outpace tendon development, making them more prone to slipping. Continuous or excessive lighting leading to rapid feed intake can exacerbate growth-related disorders.

12.7.3 Clinical Signs and Pathology

- **External Findings**
  Lameness or reluctance to walk, often evident in 2–6-week-old chicks. Valgus or varus hock appearance. Birds may drag one or both legs, reducing access to feed and water. Reduced growth rate in affected chicks. Hock is enlarged or flattened; tendon slips to the side of the hock. Affected chicks often sit on hocks with legs splayed. Often, it is bilateral in presentation but can be unilateral.
- **Necropsy Findings**
  Displaced gastrocnemius tendon from the condyle of the tibiotarsus. Soft tissue around the hock may be thickened due to chronic strain. Epiphyseal cartilage may appear underdeveloped.

The gastrocnemius muscle may appear shortened or atrophied in chronic cases. Tendon fibers may be weak or poorly aligned.

12.7.4 Diagnostic Testing

- **Feed Analysis**
  Determine manganese content, as well as choline, zinc, calcium, phosphorus, and vitamin D3 levels.
- **Bloodwork**
  May show mild mineral imbalances; used mainly to rule out other nutritional disorders.

12.7.5 Treatment and Therapeutic Interventions

- **Nutritional Intervention**
  Correct manganese deficiency in feed (40–60 ppm depending on formulation). Ensure adequate zinc, copper, and biotin levels. Balance calcium and phosphorus to optimize absorption of trace minerals.
- **Mechanical Correction**
  Rarely practical in commercial settings, but in backyard birds with dedicated caregivers, careful repositioning of tendon, splinting. Use soft, non-slip bedding to support walking.
- **Supportive Care**
  Ensure easy access to feed and water for lame birds. Supplemental feeding if indicated.
  Clean, warm, dry environment with non-slip flooring. Passive range of motion exercises.

12.7.6 Prevention and Control

- **Nutritional Prevention**
  Supplement manganese recommended levels are 40–60 ppm in starter and grower diets. Ensure feed meets phase-specific nutritional requirements. Avoid overly energy-dense or protein-rich diets in early growth stages to prevent skeletal overload.
- **Genetic Selection**
  Select breeds or lines with good skeletal conformation and tendon stability. Avoid excessively fast-growing breeds if high perosis incidence is observed. Do not breed birds with this predisposition.

12.7.7 Nursing Considerations

Nursing care for chickens affected by perosis (slipped tendon) focuses on supportive management, nutritional correction, and prevention of secondary injury. Affected birds should be housed in clean, dry, and well-bedded environments to reduce stress on the hock joint and prevent trauma from slipping or falling. Providing ample space and minimizing overcrowding helps avoid additional pressure on weakened limbs. Nutritional support is critical: diets should be adequate in manganese, zinc, biotin, choline, calcium, and phosphorus to support cartilage and tendon development and prevent further cases. Supplemental feeding if indicated. Caregivers should monitor mobility, gait, and feeding behavior, assisting severely affected birds with access to feed and water as needed. Gentle handling is important to avoid exacerbating tendon displacement or causing fractures, and environmental enrichment, such as soft perches or low platforms, may be introduced carefully. Padded splinting of legs for support. Overall, nursing considerations emphasize supportive care, nutritional optimization, environmental management, careful observation, and injury prevention to improve mobility and overall growth performance in birds affected by perosis. If quality of life is compromised, consider humane euthanasia.

12.8 Spondylolisthesis ("Kinky Back")

12.8.1 Overview and Pathogenesis

Spondylolisthesis, commonly referred to as "kinky back", is a genetic and developmental spinal disorder in chickens characterized by malformation or displacement of the sixth thoracic vertebra, leading to dorsal spinal deviation and compression of the spinal cord. The condition primarily affects rapidly growing meat-type birds, with males often more susceptible, and results in neurological deficits and impaired mobility.

Pathogenesis involves a combination of genetic predisposition, rapid growth rates, and nutritional imbalances, particularly deficiencies in vitamin D3, manganese, and other trace minerals, which interfere with proper vertebral ossification and spinal stability. Clinically, affected birds present with twisted or elevated tails, abnormal posture, weakness or paralysis of the hind limbs, reluctance to move, and, in severe cases, sudden death due to spinal cord compression. Histopathology may reveal vertebral malformations, spinal cord compression, and associated nerve degeneration. Overall, spondylolisthesis is a developmental and genetic skeletal disorder that compromises spinal integrity, neurological function, and mobility in growing chickens.

12.8.2 Risk Factors

- **Genetic Predisposition**
  Strongly linked to fast-growing commercial meat breeds. Certain families show heritable vertebral deformities, predisposing chicks to vertebral slippage.
- **Rapid Growth**
  Excessive weight gain in the first 2–6 weeks of age increases mechanical stress on immature vertebrae. Fast growth can outpace skeletal and cartilage development, leading to instability.
- **Nutritional Factors**
  Calcium, phosphorus, and vitamin D3 imbalances may compromise vertebral ossification. Overly energy-dense diets can accelerate growth beyond skeletal support capacity.

12.8.3 Clinical Signs and Pathology

- **External Findings**
  Sudden or progressive kinking of the back near the tail base. The tail and rear body may appear elevated or twisted. Weakness or inability to use posterior legs. Chickens may drag their legs or sit with legs extended forward. Usually, it manifests around 4–6 weeks of age. Reduced feed intake and poor growth. Increased mortality in severe cases due to immobility and inability to access feed/water (dehydration, starvation).
- **Necropsy Findings**
  Subluxation or dislocation of the vertebra, often toward one side. Kinking deformity is visible along the spine. Compression at the site of vertebral displacement. May show hemorrhage or

softening due to pressure. Flaccid paralysis; sometimes mild muscle atrophy if chronic. Other organs are usually unaffected, though secondary trauma or pressure sores may occur due to immobility. Abnormal development or malformation of the sixth thoracic (T6) vertebra.

12.8.4 Diagnostic Testing

- **Palpation**
  "Kinky" vertebral displacement can sometimes be felt along the spine. The T6 vertebra may palpate misaligned or protruding.
- **Radiology**
  Confirms subluxation or displacement of the T6 vertebra. May show vertebral malformation, narrowing of intervertebral spaces, or spinal cord compression. Helps distinguish it from other spinal deformities or trauma.

12.8.5 Treatment and Therapeutic Interventions

- **Supportive Care**
  Provide easy access to feed and water for affected birds. Supplemental crop feeding. Isolate paralyzed birds to prevent trampling and secondary injury. Soft bedding reduces pressure on the body and prevents decubital ulcers (sores), while analgesia provides pain relief.
- **Nutritional Management**
  Maintain balanced calcium, phosphorus, and vitamin D3 to support skeletal development in the flock. Avoid overfeeding or excessive energy-dense diets in early growth stages.
- **Medical Therapy**
  No specific drugs can reverse vertebral displacement or spinal cord damage. Anti-inflammatory agents (e.g., NSAIDs) are sometimes considered to reduce discomfort in mildly affected birds, but use is mostly experimental.

12.8.6 Prevention and Control

- **Genetic Control**
  Select breeder lines with a lower incidence of vertebral deformities. Avoid breeding birds with a history of spinal deformities.
- **Nutritional Management**
  Ensure adequate calcium, phosphorus, and vitamin D3 for proper bone development. Avoid excessively energy-dense diets that accelerate early growth. Monitor trace minerals (manganese, zinc, and copper) that support cartilage and bone formation.
- **Growth Management**
  Control early growth rates through feed restriction or phase feeding. Moderate activity and natural lighting prevent skeletal overload.
- **Environmental Management**
  Provide dry, firm flooring to minimize stress on the spine. Maintain an appropriate bird: enclosure ratio to reduce mechanical trauma. Ensure proper ventilation, temperature, and lighting for optimal skeletal development.

12.8.7 Nursing Considerations

Nursing care for chickens affected by spondylolisthesis ("kinky back") focuses on supportive management, minimizing stress and injury, and optimizing environmental conditions. Affected birds should be housed in clean, dry, well-bedded areas with ample space to reduce pressure on the spine and prevent trauma from slipping or crowding. Rapid growth should be monitored and moderated through balanced nutrition, ensuring adequate levels of vitamin D3, manganese, calcium, phosphorus, and other trace minerals to support skeletal development. Caregivers should closely observe posture, mobility, and feeding behavior, assisting birds that are weak or paralyzed with access to food and water. Gentle handling is essential to prevent further spinal injury, and severely affected birds may require isolation from the flock to avoid pecking or competition. Nursing care also involves monitoring for secondary infections, providing soft bedding, and maintaining a stress-free environment. Overall, nursing considerations emphasize supportive care, nutritional optimization, careful observation, injury prevention, and environmental management to maintain welfare and quality of life in birds affected by spondylolisthesis. Quality of life in these birds is questionable, and euthanasia is a humane option to be considered upon presentation to the clinical facility.

12.9 Cage-Layer Fatigue/(Osteoporosis)

12.9.1 Overview and Pathogenesis

Cage layer fatigue, also known as osteoporosis, is a metabolic and skeletal disorder in laying hens characterized by progressive bone demineralization, reduced bone strength, and increased susceptibility to fractures. The condition primarily affects high-producing hens in battery cages, where restricted movement limits mechanical loading of the bones, contributing to skeletal weakening.

Pathogenesis involves an imbalance between bone resorption and formation, driven by calcium deficiency, inadequate dietary vitamin D3, phosphorus imbalance, or hormonal demands of continuous egg production. Calcium mobilization from the medullary bone to support eggshell formation results in thinning of cortical and trabecular bone, while limited exercise reduces bone deposition and structural integrity. Clinically, affected hens may present with spinal deformities, weak or fractured bones, reduced mobility, reluctance to perch, decreased egg production, and sudden deaths from spontaneous fractures. Predisposing factors include high egg production, inadequate dietary calcium or vitamin D3, poor lighting, and restricted housing systems, which together exacerbate bone loss. Overall, cage layer fatigue/osteoporosis is a nutritional-metabolic and biomechanical disorder resulting from the combined effects of high egg-laying demand, nutrient deficiencies, and lack of exercise, leading to compromised skeletal strength and increased fracture risk in laying hens.

12.9.2 Risk Factors

- **Nutritional Factors**
  Calcium deficiency or low Ca:P ratio in feed. Vitamin D3 deficiency reduces calcium absorption. Imbalances in phosphorus, manganese, zinc, and copper affect bone mineralization. Excess energy or protein without sufficient calcium may worsen skeletal depletion.
- **Genetic Factors**
  High-producing layer strains are predisposed. Selection for rapid onset of lay and high egg production increases calcium demand and risk of osteoporosis.

- **Management Factors**
  Battery cages restrict movement, reducing the mechanical stimulation necessary for bone strength. High stocking density increases stress and risk of injury. Lighting programs that push early and intense production may accelerate bone loss.
- **Physiological Factors**
  High daily egg production (>300 eggs/year) increases bone mobilization. Older hens have progressively weaker bones due to cumulative calcium depletion.

12.9.3 Clinical Signs and Pathology

- **External Findings**
  Hens may be unable to stand or walk properly. Frequently sit on the hocks or splay legs. Reduced activity due to bone fragility. Drooping wings, curved back, or sitting on the keelbone. Spontaneous fractures are common, especially in the sternum, keel, or long bones. Egg output may drop due to metabolic stress or pain. Pain elicited pain upon palpation, increased mortality from fractures or cage injuries.
- **Necropsy Findings**
  Long bones (femur, tibiotarsus) are thin-walled, fragile, and prone to fractures. Keelbones may show compression fractures or deformities. Vertebrae may be osteopenic or fragile, leading to spinal deformities in severe cases. Fractures are often spontaneous or minimal-trauma fractures of long bones, sternum, or keel. Bones fracture easily during handling or postmortem examination.

12.9.4 Diagnostic Testing

- **Radiology**
  It will reveal thinned cortical bones, reduced trabecular density, and spontaneous or healed fractures in keel, sternum, or long bones.
- **Bone Mineral Density (BMD) Assessment**
  Using DEXA scanning or bone ash analysis to measure calcium content and bone strength. Reduced BMD confirms osteoporosis.
- **Bloodwork**
  May show low serum calcium, reduced phosphorus, or altered vitamin D3 metabolites in severe cases.

12.9.5 Treatment and Therapeutic Interventions

- **Nutritional Support**
  Increase calcium supplementation in feed (3–4% for layers in peak production). Ensure adequate vitamin D3 for calcium absorption. Balance Ca:P ratio (2:1 recommended). Consider trace mineral supplementation (manganese, zinc, and copper) for bone metabolism.
- **Supportive Care**
  Provide soft bedding or perches to reduce fracture risk. Isolate birds with fractures to prevent trampling. Ensure easy access to feed and water for weak or immobile hens. Gentle supplemental feeding. Handle birds gently to prevent additional fractures. Preventing competition and minimizing injury.
- **Medical Therapy**
  No specific drugs reverse established osteoporosis or fractures in layers. Anti-inflammatories and opioids may reduce nociception in birds with fractures.

12.9.6 Prevention and Control

- **Nutritional Management**
  Provide adequate calcium and vitamin D3, especially during peak lay. Supplement with trace minerals (manganese, zinc, and copper) as needed. Avoid rapid early growth or diets lacking in bone-supporting nutrients.
- **Housing and Environmental Management**
  Encourage movement and exercise. Use soft litter and perches to minimize fractures. Provide perches or allow floor access where feasible to improve bone strength through mechanical stress. Avoid continuous lighting that accelerates egg production, reducing calcium depletion. Reduce overcrowding to allow movement and decrease fracture risk.
- **Production Planning**
  Avoid excessive egg production stress early in the laying cycle. Monitor older hens for signs of osteoporosis; adjust diet and care accordingly.

12.9.7 Nursing Considerations

Nursing care for chickens affected by cage layer fatigue/osteoporosis focuses on supportive management, fracture prevention, and nutritional optimization. Affected hens should be housed in clean, dry, and well-bedded environments that minimize the risk of falls or collisions, with ample space to reduce stress and avoid injury. Providing dietary support ample in calcium, phosphorus, and vitamin D3, along with trace minerals such as manganese and zinc, is essential to support bone health and prevent further demineralization. Encouraging gentle exercise and perching where feasible helps stimulate bone deposition and maintain skeletal integrity. Caregivers should closely monitor mobility, posture, and signs of pain or fractures, aiding with access to feeders and water for birds with limited movement. Assisted feeding if indicated. Analgesics in every case of fracture. Nursing care also involves reducing environmental stressors, preventing overcrowding, and managing flock dynamics to avoid pecking or pressure on weakened birds. Overall, nursing considerations emphasize nutritional management, environmental modification, careful observation, injury prevention, and supportive care to maintain welfare and reduce morbidity in hens affected by cage layer fatigue and osteoporosis. Humane euthanasia is advisable for these birds if intensive nursing management is not planned or performed.

12.10 Infectious Arthritis and Osteomyelitis

12.10.1 Overview and Pathogenesis

Infectious arthritis and osteomyelitis in chickens are bacterial infections of the joints and bones, most caused by *S. aureus*, *E. coli*, or *Mycoplasma* species. These infections can occur via the bloodstream (hematogenous spread), direct inoculation through injuries, or ascending infection from the reproductive or respiratory tracts. Pathogenesis involves colonization of joint synovium or bone tissue by pathogens, leading to inflammation, purulent exudate formation, cartilage and bone destruction, and fibrosis in chronic cases. Clinically, affected birds exhibit lameness, swelling, and heat in affected joints, reluctance to move, reduced feed and water intake, and decreased weight gain or productivity. Predisposing factors include trauma, poor litter quality, overcrowding, immunosuppression, and concurrent infections, which facilitate bacterial invasion. Chronic infections can result in permanent joint deformities, reduced mobility, and secondary infections due to compromised circulation and tissue damage. Overall, infectious arthritis and osteomyelitis are bacterial musculoskeletal disorders characterized by inflammation, tissue destruction, and impaired locomotion, significantly impacting growth, welfare, and productivity in affected chickens.

12.10.2 Risk Factors

- **Pathogen-Related Factors**
  Highly virulent strains of *S. aureus*, *M. synoviae*, or *E. coli* are more likely to cause severe infection. Co-infections (e.g., *M. synoviae* plus *S. aureus*) increase severity.
- **Host-Related Factors**
  Young chicks are particularly susceptible due to immature immune systems. Fast-growing meat breeds are more prone to joint infections due to skeletal stress. Birds with immunosuppression (e.g., Marek's disease, IBD, or poor vaccination) have an increased risk.
- **Nutritional Factors**
  Low vitamin D3, calcium, phosphorus, or manganese can weaken bones and joints, predisposing them to infection. High-energy diets leading to rapid growth can cause microtrauma to joints, creating entry points for bacteria.
- **Management and Environmental Factors**
  Overcrowding increases trauma, stress, and pathogen load, facilitating infection. Wet, dirty litter predisposes to skin lesions, pododermatitis, and joint infections. Poor ventilation, elevated ammonia, and temperature extremes weaken immunity and skin/mucosal barriers. Trauma during catching, transport, or vaccination can provide a portal of entry.
- **Infection Portals and Transmission**
  Footpad lesions, hock burns, or scratches allow bacterial invasion. In chicks, navel infection at hatch can seed systemic infection leading to osteomyelitis. Infected eggs or poor hatchery hygiene can introduce pathogens. Close contact in crowded conditions facilitates spread.

12.10.3 Clinical Signs and Pathology

- **External Findings**
  Lame, reluctance to move, and decreased activity. Sitting on hocks or "dog-sitting" posture. Edema and heat of hock, stifle, or intertarsal joints. Reduced feed intake, poor weight gain.
- **Necropsy Findings**
  Enlarged, distended with serous, fibrinous, or purulent exudate. Thickened synovial membranes. Caseous material in chronic cases. Necrosis of the growth plate and metaphyseal regions. Deformed, thickened bones. Sequestra (dead bone fragments) in chronic osteomyelitis. Surrounding tendons and tendon sheaths may also show inflammation (tenosynovitis).

12.10.4 Diagnostic Testing

- **Culture**
  Synovial fluid, bone marrow, or lesions (e.g., *S. aureus*, *E. coli*, and *M. synoviae*). Identify the causative pathogen (commonly *S. aureus*, *M. synoviae*, or *E. coli*). Aerobic/anaerobic culture, sensitivity testing for antimicrobial therapy.
- **ELISA**
  Detect exposure to *M. synoviae* or other pathogens. Useful for flock-level screening and monitoring vaccination programs.

- **PCR**
  Target pathogens are *M. synoviae, M. gallisepticum*, and other bacteria that are fastidious or slow-growing. Rapid and highly specific, it can detect subclinical infections.
- **Diagnostic Imaging**
  Radiography detects osteolysis, bone lysis, periosteal reaction, or joint space widening. It is useful for distinguishing arthritis from trauma or metabolic bone disease.

12.10.5 Treatment and Therapeutic Interventions

- **Antimicrobial Therapy**
  Systemic antibiotics may be administered via drinking water or feed when bacterial arthritis/osteomyelitis is confirmed. Common classes are tetracyclines, aminoglycosides, and macrolides (depending on culture/sensitivity results). *S. aureus* infections can be difficult to eliminate due to resistance and deep tissue involvement.
- **Supportive Care**
  Opioids and anti-inflammatories alleviate pain and improve mobility. Ensure adequate vitamins and minerals, especially calcium, phosphorus, and vitamin D3 for skeletal health. Clean, dry, soft bedding to limit further infection and trauma.
- **Surgical or Local Interventions**
  Surgical drainage and lavage (chlorhexidine 0.5–1%) of infected joints using general anesthesia. Debridement of necrotic bone in osteomyelitis cases.

12.10.6 Prevention and Control

- **Biosecurity and Management**
  Limit the introduction of pathogens through visitors, equipment, and new birds. Disinfect housing and equipment between flocks. Keep bedding dry and clean to prevent footpad dermatitis and skin abrasions that serve as bacterial entry points. Proper airflow reduces moisture and ammonia levels, lowering respiratory stress and bacterial load.
- **Nutritional and Genetic Factors**
  Adequate levels of protein, vitamins (especially D3), and minerals (Ca, P, Mn, and Zn) support skeletal strength and immune function. Probiotics, prebiotics, and organic acids may reduce gut bacterial translocation and systemic spread. Breeding programs increasingly emphasize leg health and skeletal soundness to reduce susceptibility to bacterial chondronecrosis and osteomyelitis (BCO).
- **Disease Control**
  Control of immunosuppressive viruses (Marek's disease, infectious bursal disease, chicken anemia virus) through vaccination and good flock health programs. *M. synoviae* vaccines can reduce the incidence of infectious synovitis, indirectly lowering the risk of arthritis. No routine vaccines exist for *S. aureus* or *E. coli* arthritis in poultry, though research is ongoing.

12.10.7 Nursing Considerations

Nursing care for chickens affected by infectious arthritis and osteomyelitis focuses on supportive management, pain relief, prevention of secondary infections, and environmental modification. Affected birds should be housed in clean, dry, well-bedded areas with ample space to reduce pressure on inflamed or damaged joints and to prevent further injury. Caregivers should monitor lameness, joint swelling, mobility, feed and water intake, and overall body condition, aiding as needed to ensure access to nutrition and hydration. Nutritional support with high-quality, easily digestible feed and adequate vitamins and minerals can promote recovery and maintain strength.

Nursing care also involves gentle handling to reduce pain, management of bedding to prevent contamination, and isolation from healthy flock mates to limit disease spread if the infection is caused by a contagious pathogen such as *Mycoplasma* or *E. coli*. Appropriate antimicrobial therapy, analgesics, and long-term care planning for birds with chronic joint or bone damage. Overall, nursing considerations emphasize supportive care, environmental management, pain mitigation, and careful observation to optimize recovery and welfare in affected chickens.

12.11 Fractures/Trauma

12.11.1 Overview and Pathogenesis

Fractures and trauma are common clinical presentations in backyard, commercial, and rescue poultry, resulting from accidents, predator attacks, rough handling, collisions, falls, entrapment, or underlying metabolic bone disorders. The most frequently affected sites in chickens are the long bones of the wings (radius/ulna), legs (tibiotarsus, femur), keelbone, and digits, though skull and spinal trauma may also occur. The severity and type of fracture (simple, comminuted, open, or closed) depend on the magnitude and direction of the force, the age of the bird, and bone quality. Young, rapidly growing birds with immature skeletons are particularly prone to greenstick fractures, whereas laying hens with osteoporosis or calcium deficiencies are susceptible to spontaneous or low-impact fractures (Figure 12.3).

Pathogenesis involves the application of a traumatic force exceeding the bone's strength, resulting in disruption of the periosteum and cortical bone, hemorrhage, and soft tissue injury. Open fractures are especially concerning due to bacterial contamination and the subsequent risk of osteomyelitis or septicemia. In addition to bone damage, trauma may cause shock, hemorrhage, or internal

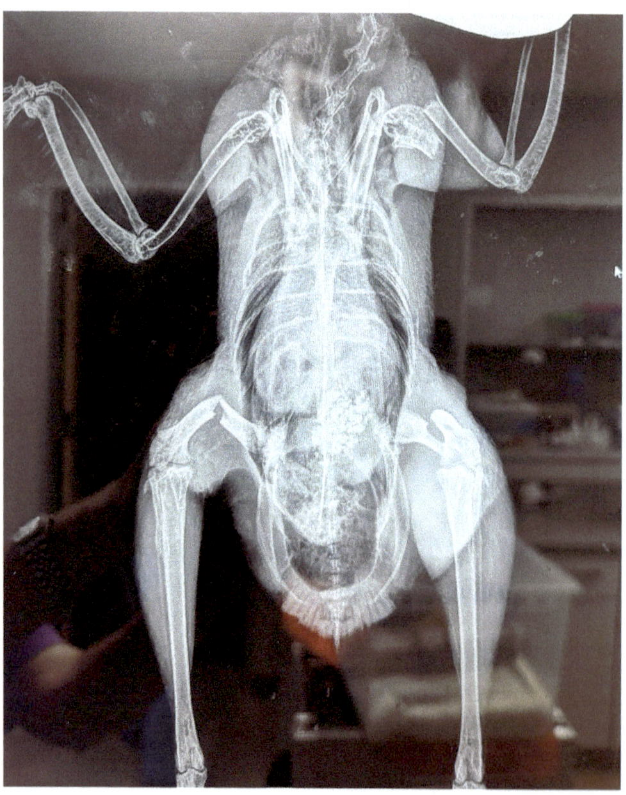

Figure 12.3 Radiographic image of chicken with bilateral femur fractures and left humerus fracture. Image courtesy of Funky Chicken Rescue.

organ injury, especially in high-impact events. Birds with fractures often present with lameness, are non-weight-bearing, wing droop, swelling, crepitus, abnormal limb angles, or reluctance to move. Skull or spinal trauma may result in neurological signs such as ataxia, head tilt, or paralysis. Prompt stabilization and appropriate management are crucial for successful, humane outcomes.

12.11.2 Risk Factors

- **Environmental and Housing Factors**
  Smooth or wet floors increase the risk of slips and falls, especially in young chicks with developing musculoskeletal systems. Abrupt footing changes or poorly maintained bedding in a pen can also contribute. High or unstable perches, steep ramps, or insufficient landing areas can result in wing or leg fractures during descent. Poor perch spacing increases collisions and missteps. Sharp edges, broken equipment, poorly secured feeders, or exposed nails can cause traumatic injuries. Sudden changes in light intensity can startle birds, leading to flight or panic reactions, which increase the risk of collision-related fractures. Rough handling during catching, crating, or transport often results in keel, wing, or leg fractures, especially in laying hens. Predator attacks or rough handling by caregivers or visitors.
- **Management Factors**
  Overcrowding leads to increased collisions, trampling, and aggression-related injuries. Pecking, fighting, or mounting can cause trauma, especially to the head, wings, and keel. Failure to address early signs of injuries or environmental hazards can allow minor traumas to progress to fractures.
- **Nutritional and Physiological Factors**
  Calcium, phosphorus, or vitamin D3 deficiencies, or imbalances, weaken bones and increase susceptibility to fractures even from mild impacts. Especially in broilers, bone development may lag body weight gain, predisposing to long bone fractures under normal activity. High egg production causes mobilization of calcium from bones, leading to fragile, brittle bones, particularly in the keel and long bones. Caged layers are at higher risk due to restricted exercise and lack of weight-bearing activity. Conditions like osteomalacia, TD, or osteomyelitis weaken skeletal integrity, increasing the probability of fractures.
- **Genetic and Age Factors**
  Certain breeds, especially fast-growing commercial meat birds, are more prone to skeletal weakness. Young chicks are more vulnerable to trauma due to immature skeletal structure and poor coordination. Older hens can develop osteoporosis and suffer from pathological fractures.
- **Stress and Behavioral Triggers**
  Startled birds may fly into walls, perches, or equipment, causing wings or keel fractures. Piling behavior (especially in overcrowded layers) can result in crushing injuries and fractures, particularly during sudden disturbances.

12.11.3 Clinical Signs and Pathology

- **External Findings**
  General Clinical Signs
  Lameness or non-weight-bearing on the affected limb is one of the most consistent signs. Reluctance or inability to stand, perch, or move, especially in fractures involving the pelvic limbs, keel, or wings. Visible deformity or abnormal angulation of a limb or wing. Swelling, bruising, or hematoma at the injury site. Pain elicited upon palpation, birds may vocalize, struggle, or flinch. Reduced feed and water intake due to pain and immobility. Depression and inactivity, often accompanied by ruffled feathers. In severe trauma (e.g., transport or panic-pile injuries), birds may be recumbent, in shock, or found dead.

Limb Fractures
Tibiotarsus, femur, humerus, radius/ulna, and metatarsals. Lame, inability to bear weight, drooping wing if the humerus is affected. Crepitus or instability on gentle palpation. Angular or spiral deformities depend on fracture type. Birds with femoral fractures may show acute, non-weight-bearing lameness, often sitting on their hocks.

Keelbone and Sternum Fractures
Common in laying hens, especially in cages or aviary systems, and during panic flights. Reluctance to perch or fly. Pain elicited upon palpation along the keel. Abnormal keel shape or palpable fractures. Decreased egg production or poor shell quality may be seen in chronic pain situations.

Wing Fractures
Drooping wings, inability to fly or flap normally. Asymmetrical wing carriage. Pain and swelling at the fracture site. Birds may hold the affected wing away from the body.

Head and Cervical Trauma
Neurological deficits (ataxia, head tilt, nystagmus, seizures) if brain or spinal cord is affected. Swelling around the head or comb, possible bleeding. Birds may be stuporous, disoriented, or blind if optical structures are involved.

- **Necropsy Findings**

Limb Fractures
Fracture edges may be sharp and clean in acute trauma or irregular if secondary to bone weakness (e.g., osteoporosis). Hemorrhage and soft tissue disruption are common. In chronic cases, malunion or callus formation may be observed.

Keelbone and Sternum Fractures
Fresh fractures show localized hemorrhage and periosteal disruption. Chronic injuries may show callus formation or fibrous healing, often palpable as bony lumps. In layers, fractures may be multiple and in different healing stages, indicating repetitive trauma.

Wing Fractures
Humeral fractures are often displaced and may damage nearby neurovascular structures. Radius/ulna fractures may be greenstick in younger birds or complete in older hens. Severe trauma can cause compound fractures with bone protrusion.

Head and Cervical Trauma
Subdural or intracerebral hemorrhage, skull fractures, or cervical vertebral luxation. Hematomas and bruises of soft tissues are frequent.

12.11.4 Diagnostic Imaging

- **Computed tomography** is the gold standard for diagnosing fractures. Radiographic images of at least two orthogonal views (lateral and dorsoventral/anteroposterior) are recommended. Confirm fracture location and type (transverse, oblique, comminuted, greenstick). Evaluate degrees of displacement and involvement of joints. Detect chronic lesions (e.g., old callus, malunion) in laying hens.

12.11.5 Treatment and Therapeutic Interventions

- **Initial Emergency Care**
Stabilization is the top priority, especially in trauma cases with potential internal injuries. Isolate the bird in a warm, quiet, dimly lit room and enclosure to minimize stress. Control hemorrhage with gentle pressure, hemostatic agents, or ligation under anesthesia if indicated. Provide

warmth and subcutaneous fluids at 30–50 mL/kg to replace hydration. Assess airway and breathing if thoracic trauma is suspected (rib fractures may impair ventilation). Analgesia should start early. Open wounds should be cleaned with dilute antiseptic (chlorhexidine 0.5–1%) and covered with sterile dressing. Birds in severe respiratory distress, with massive internal hemorrhage, or multiple open fractures have a guarded to poor prognosis and may require humane euthanasia.

- **Medication**
  Meloxicam 0.5 mg/kg by mouth or intramuscularly every 12–24 hours.
  Carprofen 5–10 mg/kg by mouth or intramuscularly once daily.
  Butorphanol 1–4 mg/kg intramuscular or intravenous every 3 hours.
- **Fracture Stabilization Techniques**
  External Coaptation (Splints and Bandages)
  Best for non-displaced fractures of long bones, particularly tibiotarsus, radius/ulna, or metatarsals. Common methods include padded tape splints, wooden spatulas, or custom foam splints. Applied with adequate padding to prevent pressure necrosis. Wing fractures, figure-of-eight bandage, or body wrap to immobilize humerus or radius/ulna. Leave splint intact for 2–4 weeks, depending on age and fracture type (Figure 12.4).

  Intramedullary Pinning/External Skeletal Fixation (ESF)
  Used for displaced, unstable, or comminuted fractures, especially in humerus or femur. Requires avian surgical expertise and general anesthesia. ESF frames with small pins or Kirschner wires can provide rigid stabilization while preserving blood supply.

  Keelbone Fractures
  Usually managed conservatively with analgesia, rest, and supportive care. Surgical intervention is rare and reserved for severe displacement or open fractures. Reduce perching height and provide soft bedding to minimize further trauma.
- **Wound Management and Infection Control**
  Open fractures should be lavaged thoroughly (chlorhexidine 0.5–1%) and debrided under aseptic conditions. Broad-spectrum antibiotics may be used if infection risk is high, ideally guided by culture and sensitivity. Regular bandage changes or in case of strike-through.

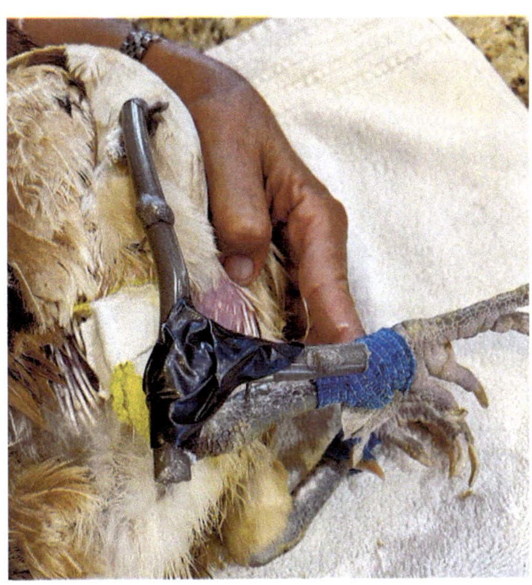

Figure 12.4 External Skeletal Fixation. Photo courtesy of Funky Chicken Rescue.

- **Nutritional and Supportive Therapy**
  Provide high-quality, balanced food with a correct Ca:P ratio and vitamin D3 to support bone healing. Supplemental calcium may be given short term, especially in laying hens or birds with metabolic bone disease. Vitamin supplementation (A, D, E, and trace minerals) can improve recovery. Assisted feedings if indicated.
- **Rehabilitation and Monitoring**
  Recheck splints weekly for tightness, soiling, or displacement. Remove bandages gradually after radiographic or clinical evidence of callus formation. Physical therapy (gentle range of motion) may be needed for wing injuries to prevent joint stiffness. Birds with severe or multiple fractures may be reassessed for quality of life and long-term prognosis.

12.11.6 Prevention and Control

- **Housing and Environmental Management**
  Provide non-slip flooring and dry, friable litter/bedding to reduce slipping and falls. Avoid abrupt changes in floor texture; maintain even surfaces. Ensure perches are stable, smooth, and appropriately spaced. Ramps should have gentle slopes and non-slip surfaces. Avoid high or unstable perches that may lead to wing or keel fractures. Gradual light changes prevent panicked flights. Avoid intense, flashing, or sudden bright lights that startle birds. Remove sharp edges, exposed nails, and broken equipment. Ensure adequate space for movement to minimize collisions and piling. Provide perches and enrichment to reduce stress and panic-induced injuries. Maintain appropriate temperatures to reduce stress-related collisions. Sudden chilling can cause birds to huddle or pile, leading to crushing trauma. Encourage normal movement and perching in young birds to strengthen bones and coordination. Prevent predator access and inexperienced handlers.
- **Flock Management**
  Avoid overcrowding to reduce trampling, collisions, and aggressive encounters. Monitor for aggression or pecking and manage environmental enrichment or flock separation if necessary.
- **Nutrition and Bone Health**
  Maintain BMD, particularly in laying hens and fast-growing broilers. Ensure manganese, zinc, and copper are adequate to support proper skeletal development. Avoid excessively rapid growth in broilers, which predisposes to long bone fractures. Adjust diet energy content to reduce metabolic bone stress. Short-term vitamin/mineral supplements may help during high-risk periods.
- **Stress Reduction**
  Avoid sudden loud noises, rapid movements, or startling light changes. Minimize disturbances during peak activity periods. Desensitize birds to noises and novel experiences.

12.11.7 Nursing Considerations

Nursing care for chickens with fractures or traumatic injuries focuses on pain management, stabilization, supportive care, and prevention of secondary complications. Veterinary technicians should assess the bird for shock, hemorrhage, or internal injuries. Provide warmth, fluid therapy, and analgesics as prescribed by a veterinarian. Handling should be gentle and minimal to prevent further injury or stress. Fractured limbs should be immobilized using splints, bandages, or external fixation, ensuring proper alignment to facilitate healing, while open wounds require thorough aseptic cleaning and monitoring for infection. Affected birds should be housed in a confined, padded area with non-slip surfaces and minimal obstacles to reduce movement and stress, preventing further trauma to the injured site. Nutrition is important for healing; diets should be high in protein, calcium, phosphorus, and vitamin D3 to support bone repair. Monitor for clinical signs of infection, delayed healing, or abnormal callus formation and report any changes promptly to the veterinarian. For severe trauma or spinal injuries, euthanasia may be considered for humane reasons if recovery and quality of life are unlikely. Additionally, technicians play a key role in educating caretakers on safe handling, preventing accidents, and proper housing to reduce the risk of fractures in the flock.

12.12 Chondrodystrophy/Dwarfism

12.12.1 Overview and Pathogenesis

Chondrodystrophy, commonly referred to as dwarfism in poultry, is a genetic skeletal disorder characterized by abnormal cartilage and bone development, leading to stunted growth, limb deformities, and reduced overall body size. This condition may arise from autosomal recessive genetic mutations affecting cartilage formation and endochondral ossification, often seen in certain inbred lines or strains. Environmental factors, such as nutritional deficiencies (particularly calcium, phosphorus, vitamin D3, or protein) during embryonic development, may exacerbate the severity of the disorder, but the primary etiology is hereditary.

Pathogenesis involves defective chondrocyte proliferation and differentiation within the growth plates of long bones, which impairs normal endochondral ossification. As a result, affected chicks exhibit shortened and thickened long bones, bowing of limbs, angular deformities, and disproportionate body conformation. The keel, sternum, and metatarsals may also be affected, leading to reduced mobility, difficulty perching, and impaired locomotion. Birds with severe chondrodystrophy may demonstrate slow growth, low body weight, and increased susceptibility to fractures, as the abnormal bone structure compromises mechanical strength. Although dwarf birds can survive and reproduce, they often have reduced productivity and performance, especially in commercial meat or layer operations.

12.12.2 Risk Factors

- **Genetic Factors**
  Autosomal recessive inheritance in many commercial and heritage breeds. Selection to rapid growth or extreme body conformation can increase prevalence. Certain meat or layer strains are more prone. Carrier parents increase the likelihood of affected offspring.
- **Incubation and Early Development**
  Improper incubation temperature or humidity due to abnormal cartilage growth may occur under hyper- or hypothermic conditions. Cracked or compromised eggs may produce weaker chicks with skeletal abnormalities.
- **Nutritional Factors (Exacerbating)**
  Deficiencies in vitamins or trace minerals (e.g., riboflavin, manganese, zinc) may exacerbate bone deformities, although they are primarily congenital. Imbalanced calcium-phosphorus ratios can contribute to secondary bone weakness, affecting growth plate development. Rapid growth diets in susceptible breeds may exacerbate skeletal abnormalities.

12.12.3 Clinical Signs and Pathology

- **External Findings**
  Legs appear disproportionately short relative to body size. Tibiotarsus and femur are most affected. Varus or valgus deviation of the legs may occur. Overall body size and weight are below

normal for age. Disproportion between head, trunk, and limbs may be noticeable. Difficulty ambulating or perching. Reluctance to move, which can affect feed and water intake. Birds may develop calluses on hocks or metatarsal pads due to abnormal posture.

- **Necropsy Findings**
  Disorganized growth plates at proximal and distal long bones. Chondrocytes fail to align properly, leading to defective endochondral ossification. Femur, tibiotarsus, humerus, and metatarsals are often affected. Bones appear thickened or widened at metaphysis in some cases. Secondary stress on ligaments and tendons can lead to tenosynovitis or chronic inflammation.

12.12.4 Diagnostic Testing

- **Radiographs**
  Lateral and dorsoventral (or craniocaudal for wings/limbs). Shortened long bones, disorganized growth plates and metaphyseal irregularities, and delayed ossification or irregular mineralization. Distinguish chondrodystrophy from osteomalacia, TD, fractures, or metabolic bone disease.

12.12.5 Treatment and Therapeutic Interventions

Chondrodystrophy is congenital and irreversible, so treatment is palliative rather than curative. Severely affected birds may require humane euthanasia to prevent prolonged suffering.

12.12.6 Prevention and Control

- **Genetic and Breeding Strategies**
  Segregate dwarves and those with significant skeletal deformities from breeding stock. Avoid inbreeding, which increases the risk of chondrodystrophy expression.
- **Nutrition and Growth Management**
  Adequate calcium, phosphorus, vitamin D3, and trace minerals (manganese, zinc, and copper) to support normal skeletal growth. Avoid excessively high-energy diets that accelerate growth in genetically predisposed birds. Vitamins and minerals during incubation and the first few weeks may support cartilage development.
- **Environmental and Management Measures**
  Provide soft, dry litter to reduce trauma from falls or abnormal gait. Lower and stabilize perches to reduce the risk of fractures in birds with short or deformed limbs. Observe the proper bird: enclosure ratio to allow safe movement and reduce collisions. Avoid sudden noises and abrupt lighting changes, which can cause panic and secondary injuries.

12.12.7 Nursing Considerations

Nursing care for chickens affected by chondrodystrophy or dwarfism focuses on supporting mobility, minimizing stress, and optimizing nutrition to enhance growth and overall welfare. Veterinary technicians should monitor birds for difficult ambulation, limb deformities, and poor body condition. Provide soft, level bedding and non-slip surfaces to reduce the risk of fractures or leg injuries. Perches, ramps, and feeders should be adjusted to bird height to allow easy access to food and water. Nutrition plays a key role in supporting skeletal health. Diets should be balanced and rich in protein, calcium, phosphorus, and vitamin D3 to maximize bone strength, even though genetic defects cannot be corrected. Technicians should also monitor growth rates and body condition, assisting weak or slow-growing birds with hand-feeding or supplemental nutrition if necessary. Regular handling should be gentle to prevent stress and injury, as abnormal bone structure makes these birds more prone to fractures. Breeding programs should consider removing affected individuals from the breeding population to prevent the perpetuation of genetic defects. Education of caretakers regarding housing modifications, safe handling, and monitoring for complications is essential to maintain welfare and reduce mortality in affected flocks.

12.13 Angular Leg Deformities (Varus/Valgus)

12.13.1 Overview and Pathogenesis

Angular leg deformities in chickens, commonly referred to as varus (inward angulation) or valgus (outward angulation) deformities, are developmental skeletal disorders affecting tibiotarsus and tarsometatarsus. These deformities are often seen in rapidly growing meat breeds, birds with nutritional deficiencies, or genetically predisposed lines, and can significantly impact locomotion, welfare, and productivity. Etiology is typically multifactorial, involving a combination of genetic predisposition, rapid growth rates, imbalanced nutrition (particularly deficiencies or imbalances of calcium, phosphorus, vitamin D3, and protein), and mechanical stress on the developing bones. Environmental factors, such as uneven flooring, inadequate perches, or overcrowding, can exacerbate the condition.

Pathogenesis involves disrupted endochondral ossification at the growth plates, leading to asymmetrical bone growth. In varus deformities, the distal portion of the tibiotarsus deviates medially, while in valgus deformities it deviates laterally. Abnormal mechanical loading on asymmetrically growing bones further stresses the joints and supporting ligaments, leading to angular angulation and compensatory postural changes. Clinically affected birds exhibit bowed legs, altered gait, decreased weight-bearing, lameness, and difficulty perching or walking, which increases susceptibility to secondary injuries such as fractures or pododermatitis. Birds with severe deformities may show reduced feed intake and growth, contributing to economic losses in production systems. Early detection and correction during growth stages are critical to prevent permanent skeletal malformations.

12.13.2 Risk Factors

- **Genetic Factors**
  Certain breeds or lines, particularly fast-growing meat birds, are more susceptible. Inbreeding increases the incidence of angular limb deformities. Poor limb alignment in breeding stock increases the risk in offspring.
- **Nutritional Factors**
  Low Ca:P ratio affects bone mineralization and growth plate development. Vitamin D3 deficiency leads to impaired calcium absorption, weaker bones, and abnormal limb alignment. Manganese is essential for cartilage and joint integrity; deficiency leads to abnormal epiphyseal cartilage. Zinc and copper contribute to connective tissue strength. Excess energy or protein intake accelerates skeletal growth, outpacing cartilage and tendon development.
- **Environmental and Management Factors**
  Hard, uneven, or slippery floors increase stress on developing limbs. Overcrowding limits movement, contributing to abnormal limb loading and angular deviations. Limited movement prevents proper musculoskeletal development and alignment. Sudden changes in lighting can cause panic, falls, and limb injuries in chicks with soft bones.

- **Early Life and Developmental Factors**
  Improper incubation temperatures or humidity can affect cartilage and bone development. Rough handling or transport of day-old chicks may predispose to growth plate injury. Rapidly growing chicks with soft bones are more susceptible to mechanical stress.

12.13.3 Clinical Signs and Pathology

- **External Findings**
  Usually evident within the first 2–6 weeks of life, coinciding with rapid skeletal growth. Visible limb deviation varus or valgus. Waddling, hopping, or limping. Reduced mobility or reluctance to move. One limb may be affected more than the other. Bilateral involvement may occur, especially in severe nutritional deficiencies. Pressure sores or calluses on hocks/metatarsal pads due to abnormal weight bearing. Moderate cases may show slowed weight gain compared to unaffected flock mates.
- **Necropsy Findings**
  Disorganized or uneven chondrocyte columns at the proximal and distal growth plates. Impaired endochondral ossification contributing to angular deviation. Shortened or twisted long bones (tibiotarsus, metatarsus, femur). Metaphyseal widening may be observed in valgus deformities. Malalignment leads to unequal weight distribution, stretching ligaments and tendons. Chronic cases may develop tendon contractures or joint subluxation. Muscle adaptation around deformed bones may occur, sometimes causing hypertrophy or atrophy depending on usage.

12.13.4 Diagnostic Testing

- **Diagnostic Imaging**
  Confirms the degree of angular deviation and identifies associated bone or growth plate abnormalities. Lateral, dorsoventral, and craniocaudal projection of the affected limb are needed. Differentiates angular deformities from fractures, perosis, rickets, or other metabolic bone disorders. Radiograph findings are bowing or tibiotarsus or metatarsus, asymmetric growth plates or metaphyseal widening, and secondary microfractures or subluxation of joints.
- **Bloodwork**
  Blood biochemistry may reveal low calcium, phosphorus, or vitamin D levels in nutritional deficiency cases.

12.13.5 Treatment and Therapeutic Interventions

- **Orthopedic and Mechanical Correction**
  Optimal results are achieved in young chicks, as growth plates are still open. Light splints or corrective bandages can gradually realign limbs. Use soft padding to prevent pressure sores. Splints need to be in place for 1–2 weeks, reassessing the limb alignment daily. In mild valgus or varus, toe alignment with gentle taping can redirect weight-bearing forces. Requires close monitoring for circulation and comfort. May include osteotomy and fixation in severe, nonresponsive deformities.
- **Medication**
  Birds with angular deformities may experience secondary joint stress or discomfort.
  Meloxicam 0.5 mg/kg by mouth or intramuscularly every 12–24 hours, no longer than 5 days.
  Carprofen 5–10 mg/kg by mouth or intramuscularly once daily, no longer than 5 days duration.

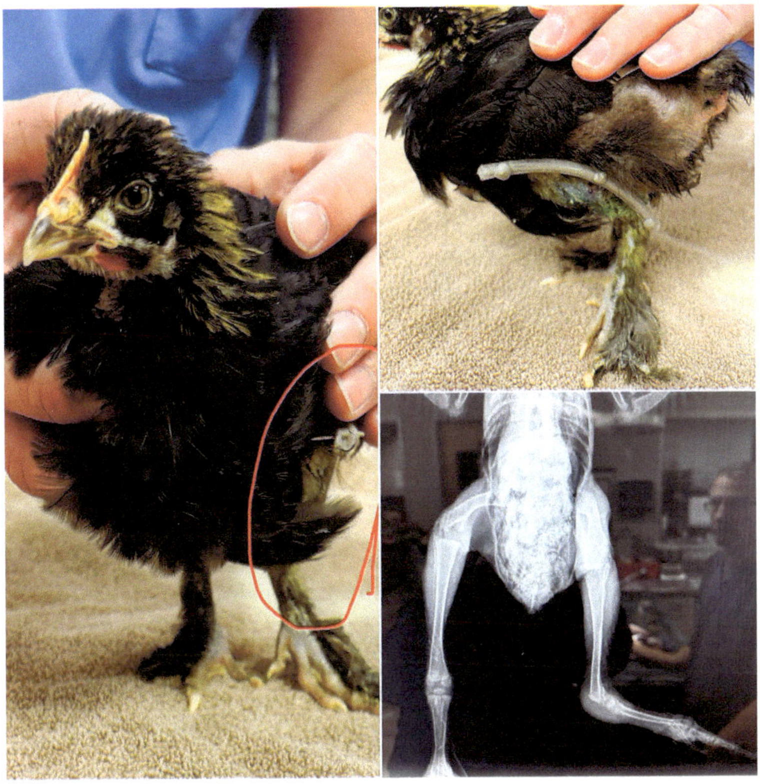

Figure 12.5 Angular limb deformity correction with external fixation. Courtesy of Funky Chicken Rescue.

- **Supportive Care**
  Soft, clean bedding to reduce pressure on deformed limbs. Low perches or ramps to prevent falls. Monitor gait and activity to prevent secondary injuries.
- **Follow-Up and Monitoring**
  Reassess limb alignment weekly. Monitor growth and weight gain. Remove or adjust splints as needed to prevent pressure sores. Severely affected birds with poor prognosis may require euthanasia to discontinue suffering (Figure 12.5).

12.13.6 Prevention and Control

- **Nutritional Management**
  Maintain a proper calcium-phosphorus ratio. Adequate vitamin D3 to support bone mineralization. Ensure sufficient manganese, zinc, and copper for cartilage and joint development. Avoid overfeeding high-energy diets that accelerate skeletal growth beyond cartilage support capacity. Vitamins and minerals during incubation and the first 2–3 weeks may support healthy limb development.
- **Environmental and Management Measures**
  Use soft, dry bedding and avoid slippery surfaces to reduce stress on developing limbs. Provide stable, low perches to reduce fall risk in growing chicks. Avoid overcrowding; sufficient space prevents collisions and reduces limb injuries. Encourage natural movement and weight-bearing

activities to strengthen bones and joints. Avoid sudden or intense light changes that can cause panic flights.

12.13.7 Nursing Considerations

Nursing care for chickens with angular leg deformities focuses on supporting mobility, preventing secondary injuries, and optimizing nutrition during critical growth periods. Veterinary technicians should monitor affected birds for lameness, altered gait, difficulty perching, and abnormal weight distribution, providing soft, non-slip bedding and spacious enclosures to reduce stress on joints and prevent pododermatitis or fractures. Early intervention with splints, braces, or corrective bandaging may be indicated under veterinary guidance to help realign developing bones in young chicks. Nutritional management is essential; diets should be balanced for protein, calcium, phosphorus, and vitamin D3, and growth rates monitored to avoid overloading developing bones. Technicians should assist weak birds with easy access to feed and water and remove them from overcrowded areas to reduce competition and stress. Long-term monitoring is necessary, as severe deformities may permanently impair locomotion, requiring lifetime adjustments to housing, perching, and feeding systems. Educating caretakers about genetic predisposition, early detection, proper husbandry, and environmental modifications is key to minimizing welfare issues.

12.14 Cross Beak

12.14.1 Overview and Pathogenesis

Cross beak, also known as *scissor beak*, is a developmental deformity of the skull/beak in which the upper and lower mandibles do not align properly, resulting in lateral deviation or twisting of one or both beak components. This condition is most observed in chickens but can occur in other avian species. It may manifest at hatch or develop gradually as the bird grows, leading to difficulty in grasping, manipulating, and ingesting feed, which can result in reduced body weight, poor growth, and failure to thrive. In severe cases, affected birds may require special feeding management or humane euthanasia if they cannot maintain adequate nutrition (Figure 12.6).

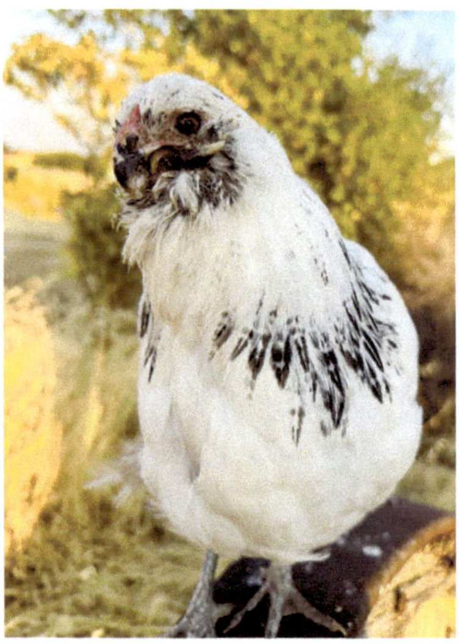

Figure 12.6 Severe crossbeak in Easter Egger hen. Photo courtesy of Funky Chicken Rescue.

The pathogenesis of cross beak is multifactorial, involving both genetic and environmental components. Genetic predisposition plays a significant role, with certain breeds, particularly those selectively bred for specific traits, such as high egg production or unique beak shapes being more susceptible. Embryonic malposition within the egg can also contribute, as uneven pressure during development may distort the growth plates of the beak. Nutritional deficiencies, especially in essential vitamins and minerals such as manganese, vitamin D3, and calcium, can interfere with normal skeletal and keratin formation during embryogenesis, predisposing chicks to craniofacial abnormalities. Additionally, trauma to the beak during the early post-hatch period or improper incubation temperatures and humidity levels may disrupt the normal ossification and alignment of the premaxilla and mandible. Morphologically, cross beak arises from asymmetric growth of the bones forming the upper and lower beak, often involving the premaxillary, nasal, and mandibular bones. This asymmetry leads to deviation of the beak tip away from the midline, producing the characteristic crossed or scissored appearance. Over time, the deformity may worsen as the bird grows, particularly if the upper and lower beak surfaces wear unevenly due to misalignment. The condition is not typically self-correcting and may progress if supportive care is not provided.

12.14.2 Risk Factors

- **Genetic and Hereditary Factors**
  Many cases have a genetic basis; hereditary transmission is observed particularly in certain breeds and lines. Breeding birds with even mild beak deformities increases the likelihood of offspring developing cross beak. Mutations affecting skull and beak formation (such as deviations in premaxilla or mandible development) contribute to congenital forms.
- **Nutritional Deficiencies**
  Deficiency of manganese, calcium, or vitamin D3 can interfere with normal skeletal and beak ossification. Inadequate protein and amino acids during embryonic development can affect keratin and bone growth. Hens lacking balanced nutrients can produce weak or malformed embryos prone to deformities.
- **Incubation and Hatching Conditions**
  Improper incubation temperature or humidity can cause craniofacial deformities during embryogenesis. Embryos developing in an abnormal orientation may experience uneven skull pressure, resulting in beak deviation. Physical strain during pipping can cause jaw displacement or asymmetric growth.
- **Trauma and Mechanical Injury**
  Physical trauma to the beak, especially in young chicks, can alter alignment as the bones harden. Damage to the developing maxilla or mandible can lead to permanent deformity if not corrected early. Rough handling during debeaking or trimming procedures can predispose to beak asymmetry.
- **Growth Abnormalities and Metabolic Disorders**
  Heavy-bodied breeds (e.g., broilers) may outgrow skeletal support systems, leading to deformities. Metabolic bone disease (rickets) disrupts mineralization and causes skeletal distortion, including the facial bones and beak.

12.14.3 Clinical Signs and Pathology

- **External Findings**
  The most obvious sign is lateral misalignment of the upper and lower beaks. The upper (maxillary) and lower (mandibular) portions of the beak may cross in either direction. Deviation often begins subtly and worsens progressively as the bird matures. In mild cases, birds can still eat and drink normally; in severe cases, feeding becomes difficult or impossible.
- **Necropsy Findings**
  The maxilla (upper beak) may curve to one side, while the mandible (lower beak) deviates in the opposite direction. In severe deformities, the nasal and frontal bones can also become

asymmetrical. The rami of the mandible may be unevenly developed, causing one side to elongate. The keratinized rhamphotheca (beak covering) becomes misshapen and can develop overgrowth or wear asymmetry due to uneven contact. Chronic rubbing or pressure at the beak tips can lead to ulceration, cracking, or necrosis.

12.14.4 Diagnostic Testing

Diagnosis of cross beak (also known as *scissor beak*) in chickens is primarily clinical, based on the visible deviation of the upper and lower mandibles.

12.14.5 Treatment and Therapeutic Interventions

- **Conservative Management**
  Mild beak deviations can be corrected or stabilized in chicks less than 2–3 weeks old due to the plasticity of growing bone and keratin structures. Frequent manual beak shaping and trimming can realign mild deviations before they become fixed. Soft diets (moistened crumble or mash) and deep feed dishes improve food access. Regular weight monitoring is critical; growth curves should be compared to normal flock averages.
- **Beak Trimming and Reshaping**
  The most common therapeutic intervention for functional improvement. Performed using emery boards or nail files (for minor reshaping), Dremel rotary tools with fine grit barrels (for moderate correction), or cautery unit and electric grinders in clinical settings under local anesthesia. The goal is to realign the beak tips to restore partial occlusion and feeding efficiency. Frequent maintenance trims (every 2–4 weeks) are often required, as the deformity continues to grow out of alignment. Avoid excessive trimming that may expose the vascular dermis or cause bleeding. Provide post-procedural antiseptic care and monitor for stress or pain behaviors.

12.14.6 Prevention and Control

- **Genetic Selection and Breeding Management**
  Genetic predisposition plays a key role in cross-beak development. The condition can occur sporadically or as a recessive inherited trait in some lines. Inbreeding increases the risk of expressing recessive deformity traits. Some breeds (e.g., Ameraucana, Araucana, Easter Egger, and Silkie) show higher incidence rates.
- **Incubation and Hatching Conditions**
  Embryonic skull development is highly sensitive to temperature, humidity, and positioning during incubation. Maintain incubator temperature at 99.5°F with minimal fluctuation. Overheating (>102°F) during early incubation is associated with craniofacial malformations. Keep relative humidity at 45–55% for the first 18 days; increase to 65–70% during hatching. Turn eggs at least 3–5 times daily until day 18 to prevent abnormal embryo orientation. Always hatch eggs large end up; mispositioning may lead to uneven cranial growth or malocclusion.
- **Nutritional and Metabolic Management**
  Nutrient deficiencies are among the most preventable risk factors for cross beak, especially during early growth. Maintain a 2:1 Ca:P ratio to support bone development. Ensure proper vitamin D3 levels to facilitate calcium absorption and skeletal ossification. Include adequate manganese, zinc, and copper, which are critical for cartilage and bone formation. Use a starter feed with 18–20% crude protein for chicks to support tissue growth.

12.14.7 Nursing Considerations

Nursing care for birds with cross beak focuses on maintaining adequate nutrition, monitoring body condition, and providing supportive husbandry to improve quality of life. Because affected birds often struggle to pick up or manipulate feed, early identification and intervention are essential. Caregivers should regularly observe feeding behavior and ensure the bird is maintaining appropriate weight and hydration. Birds with moderate to severe deformities may require specialized feeding techniques, such as offering deep dishes, raised feeders, or bowls with mash, moist crumble, or pelleted feed softened with warm water to make ingestion easier. Handfeeding or syringe-feeding may be necessary in advanced cases or for young chicks that cannot self-feed effectively. Regular trimming and reshaping of the beak by a trained avian veterinarian or technician can help improve alignment and function. Minor adjustments may reduce overgrowth and enhance the bird's ability to prehend feed. However, excessive trimming should be avoided, as it may expose sensitive tissues or lead to secondary trauma. If a bird's beak becomes excessively misaligned or causes significant feeding impairment, humane euthanasia may need to be considered to prevent prolonged suffering. Birds with cross beak should be housed separately or with gentle flock mates to prevent bullying and to ensure equal access to feed and water. Feeders and waterers should be adjusted to appropriate heights, and spillage minimized to prevent contamination. Because these birds expend extra energy eating, a high-quality, nutrient-dense diet is important. Vitamin and mineral supplementation, particularly of vitamin D3, calcium, and manganese, may help in mild or early cases where growth is ongoing.

12.15 Myopathies

12.15.1 Overview and Pathogenesis

Myopathies in chickens are a group of muscle disorders characterized by degeneration, necrosis, and fibrosis of skeletal muscle, most commonly affecting fast-growing broilers. These conditions include "wooden breast" (broiler breast myopathy), "white striping," and "spaghetti meat," and they primarily impact breast (pectoralis major) muscles, though other skeletal muscles may also be involved.

The pathogenesis is multifactorial, involving genetic predisposition for rapid growth, excessive muscle hypertrophy, and high metabolic demand, which can outpace the vascular supply to the enlarging muscle fibers. This results in ischemia, oxidative stress, muscle fiber degeneration, infiltration by inflammatory cells, and replacement of muscle tissue with connective tissue and fat. Clinically, affected birds may appear reluctant to move, exhibit reduced exercise tolerance, and have firm, pale, or fibrotic breast muscles, with potential economic impacts due to meat quality defects. Nutritional imbalances, environmental stress, and management factors such as high stocking density or inadequate exercise further exacerbate myopathy development. Overall, myopathies are degenerative muscle disorders in rapidly growing chickens caused by a combination of genetic, metabolic, nutritional, and management-related factors, leading to impaired muscle integrity, reduced mobility, and compromised meat quality.

12.15.2 Risk Factors

- **Nutritional Factors**
  Deficiency of vitamin E and selenium (nutritional myopathy). Imbalance in dietary antioxidants or high levels of unsaturated fats (increase oxidative stress).

- **Genetic and Growth Rate**
  Fast-growing broilers with large breast muscle yield are predisposed to growth-related myopathies. Selection of production traits may inadvertently reduce vascular development and muscle resilience.
- **Management and Environment**
  Excessive wing activity (escape flights, struggling, rough handling) predisposes to deep pectoral myopathy. Heat stress increases metabolic demands and muscle oxygen requirements. High stocking density and poor ventilation exacerbate oxidative stress and muscle hypoxia.
- **Health Status**
  Concurrent diseases causing systemic hypoxia or oxidative stress (e.g., respiratory disease and immunosuppression). Poor welfare or stress conditions increase activity and metabolic strain.

12.15.3 Clinical Signs and Pathology

- **External Findings**
  Often subclinical (especially wooden breast and spaghetti meat, detected at processing). In severe cases, weakness or reluctance to move, reduced feed intake and slower growth, swelling or hardness in breast muscles, and pain on palpation in exertional cases.
- **Necropsy Findings**
  - Nutritional Myopathy (White Muscle Disease)
    - Pale, streaky muscles (pectorals, thighs, gizzard), due to oxidative necrosis.
  - Deep Pectoral Myopathy (Green Muscle Disease)
    - Supracoracoideus appears swollen, hemorrhagic, then greenish necrotic.
  - Wooden Breast
    - Firm, pale, bulging breast fillet with fibrosis.
  - Spaghetti Meat
    - Separation of muscle fibers, giving a stringy texture.
  - Exertional Myopathy
    - Hemorrhage, edema, and necrosis of wing/pectoral muscles.

12.15.4 Diagnostic Testing

- **Histopathology**
  Myofiber necrosis, hyaline degeneration, and vacuolization.
- **Diagnostic Imaging**
  Ultrasound may detect abnormal echogenicity in pectoral muscles.
- **Bloodwork**
  Elevated creatine kinase (CK) and aspartate aminotransferase (AST) indicate muscle damage. Low vitamin E, selenium, or other antioxidants support a nutritional myopathy diagnosis.

12.15.5 Treatment and Therapeutic Interventions

- **Nutritional Myopathy**
  Vitamin E Supplementation
  - Add dl-α-tocopherol acetate to feed at 50–100 IU/kg feed. Water-soluble vitamin E preparations may be given in acute cases (25–50 IU/L of drinking water for 3–5 days).

Selenium Supplementation
- Sodium selenite or organic selenium (selenomethionine) at 0.1–0.3 ppm in feed.
- Care must be taken as selenium has a narrow margin of safety and can be toxic if overdosed.

Supportive Care
- Isolate severely weak birds to prevent trampling. Provide easily accessible feed and water.

- **Exertional Myopathy**

  Stress Reduction
  - Minimize rough handling and heat stress.
  - Avoid overcrowding and sudden fright.

  Electrolyte Therapy
  - Oral electrolyte solutions contain potassium, sodium, and magnesium to restore muscle function.

  Vitamin Supplementation
  - Vitamin E (50 IU/L water for 3–5 days) and selenium (0.2 ppm feed) to mitigate muscle degeneration.

  Environmental Adjustment
  - Reduce heat stress with adequate ventilation. Ensure proper lighting programs to reduce sudden activity bursts.

- **Degenerative Myopathies (Wooden Breast)**

  Nutritional Management
  - Adjust feed formulation to slow growth rate (reduce excess energy and protein). Balance amino acids (lysine, methionine) support proper muscle metabolism. Supplement with antioxidants (vitamin E, selenium, vitamin C, carnitine) to reduce oxidative stress.

No direct cure; this condition is a largely production-related syndrome, so treatment is supportive and preventive.

12.15.6 Prevention and Control

- **Nutritional**

  Supplementation with vitamin E and selenium to prevent oxidative muscle damage. Balanced rations to avoid excess polyunsaturated fatty acids without antioxidant support.
- **Genetics and Management**

  Selective breeding for balanced growth, with a focus on skeletal and muscle health. Reduce wing flapping (calm handling, low-stress environments) to prevent deep pectoral myopathy. Adjust growth rates via feed restriction or phased nutrition programs to reduce the incidence of growth-related myopathies.
- **Environmental Measures**

  Good ventilation and temperature control to reduce heat stress. Adequate bird: enclosure ratio to minimize competition and stress. Training caregivers in careful bird handling to reduce exertional muscle damage.

12.15.7 Nursing Considerations

Nursing care for chickens with myopathies focuses on reducing stress, supporting mobility, and optimizing nutrition to slow disease progression and minimize welfare concerns. Affected birds should be housed in low-stress environments with soft bedding and adequate space to reduce pressure on weakened muscles and joints. Encouraging moderate movement without overexertion helps maintain muscle tone, while preventing overcrowding reduces the risk of injury and further muscle strain. Nutritional support is vital, including diets balanced in protein, amino acids (particularly methionine and lysine), antioxidants such as vitamin E and selenium, and omega-3 fatty acids, which can reduce oxidative stress and support muscle health. Birds should be carefully observed for reluctance to move, reduced feed intake, or lameness, with prompt interventions to maintain hydration and body condition. For commercial flocks, nursing efforts also include monitoring carcass quality and working with veterinarians to adjust growth rates through feed restriction or genetic selection strategies. Overall, nursing management aims to enhance comfort, reduce metabolic strain, and support flock health while addressing the welfare impacts of myopathies. Veterinary professionals in clinical practice will likely never observe backyard birds with these conditions unless caregivers are raising poorly managed large flocks of meat birds.

Further Reading

Julian R. [cited 2025 Dec 8]. Available from: https://aaap.memberclicks.net/assets/musculoskeletal%20preview.pdf

Lameness Disorders in Poultry | Animal Health Laboratory [Internet]. Uoguelph.ca. 2015 [cited 2025 Dec 8]. Available from: https://www.uoguelph.ca/ahl/lameness-disorders-poultry

Leg Health in Chickens (FS-1179) | University of Maryland Extension [Internet]. Umd.edu. University of Maryland Extension; 2022. Available from: https://extension.umd.edu/resource/leg-health-chickens-fs-1179/

Wettere V. Noninfectious Skeletal Disorders in Poultry [Internet]. Merck Veterinary Manual. 2025. Available from: https://www.merckvetmanual.com/poultry/disorders-of-the-skeletal-system-in-poultry/noninfectious-skeletal-disorders-in-poultry

Wettere V. Overview of Skeletal System Disorders in Poultry [Internet]. Merck Veterinary Manual. 2025 [cited 2025 Dec 8]. Available from: https://www.merckvetmanual.com/poultry/disorders-of-the-skeletal-system-in-poultry/overview-of-skeletal-system-disorders-in-poultry

13

Neurologic, Ophthalmic, and Aural Diseases

Neurologic diseases in chickens often present with symptoms such as incoordination, paralysis, tremors, or abnormal head positions, reflecting damage to the brain, spinal cord, or peripheral nerves. Common causes include viral infections (refer to Chapter 11) such as Marek's disease and Newcastle disease, bacterial infections such as Listeriosis, and nutritional deficiencies, particularly vitamin E or thiamine deficiency. Environmental toxins, trauma, and metabolic disorders can also affect the nervous system, emphasizing the importance of proper husbandry, available vaccinations, and balanced nutrition to prevent neurologic disorders.

13.1 Algae Poisoning

13.1.1 Overview and Pathogenesis

Algae poisoning in chickens is an acute or chronic toxicosis caused by the ingestion of certain cyanobacteria (blue-green algae) or algal toxins present in contaminated water sources. This condition typically occurs when birds have access to stagnant or nutrient-rich ponds, water troughs, or puddles that support algal blooms. Clinical signs vary depending on the type and concentration of toxins but often include depression, weakness, diarrhea, incoordination, respiratory distress, and sudden death in severe cases.

Pathogenesis involves the ingestion of algal toxins—most commonly hepatotoxins (microcystins), neurotoxins (anatoxins), or cytotoxins—that interfere with normal cellular function. Hepatotoxins cause liver cell necrosis, leading to impaired metabolism, coagulopathy, and icterus. Neurotoxins disrupt neuromuscular transmission, resulting in tremors, paralysis, and respiratory failure. Chronic low-level exposure may cause weight loss, reduced egg production, and immunosuppression. Factors such as warm temperatures, nutrient-rich water, and stagnant conditions favor algal proliferation, increasing the risk of exposure. Overall, the toxic effects of algae ingestion compromise multiple organ systems, with the severity of disease depending on the type of algae, toxin concentration, duration of exposure, and the age and health of the chickens.

13.1.2 Risk Factors

- **Water Source and Quality**
  Standing or stagnant water in ponds, troughs, or puddles promotes cyanobacterial growth. Contaminated water with high nutrient levels (nitrogen, phosphorus) from fertilizers, manure,

or runoff increases risk. Shallow water bodies that warm quickly in sunlight are particularly susceptible to algal blooms.

- **Environmental and Seasonal Factors**
  Warm temperatures and sunlight favor cyanobacterial proliferation. Low water flow or stagnant ponds allow algae accumulation. High organic matter (decaying vegetation, manure) enhances nutrient availability. Seasonal patterns, late spring through early fall in temperate regions.
- **Husbandry and Management Practices**
  Allowing chickens with unrestricted access to ponds, ditches, or stagnant water increases exposure. Poor maintenance of water containers, including infrequent cleaning, promotes algae growth. Overcrowding near water sources increases the likelihood of ingestion of contaminated water.
- **Host Factors**
  Young or immunocompromised birds may be more susceptible to toxic effects. Previous hepatic or renal compromises may exacerbate clinical outcomes. Free-range birds are at higher risk due to environmental water exposure.

13.1.3 Clinical Signs and Pathology

- **External Findings**
  Sudden onset of weakness, ataxia, and tremors (neurotoxic cyanotoxins). Diarrhea or greenish droppings due to gastrointestinal irritation. Drooping wings, lethargy, and prostration. Rapid mortality in severe acute exposure; multiple deaths may occur within hours if the entire flock is exposed.
- **Necropsy Findings**
  Hepatomegaly, pale or mottled liver, sometimes with hemorrhages (hepatotoxic cyanotoxins). Congestive renomegaly (nephrotoxic cyanotoxins). Intestinal irritation, thin walls, watery contents, and possibly mild hemorrhage. Neurological tissues (brain, spinal cord) often show congestion in neurotoxic cases.

13.1.4 Diagnostic Testing

- **Water Testing**
  Identify cyanobacterial species in drinking water or ponds. Measure cyanotoxin concentrations using enzyme-linked immunosorbent assay (ELISA), high-performance liquid chromatography (HPLC), , or mass spectrometry.
- **Tissue Analysis**
  Liver, kidney, and blood samples can be tested for cyanotoxins. Helps confirm exposure and determine the toxin type (hepatotoxin, neurotoxin, or gastrointestinal).

13.1.5 Treatment and Therapeutic Interventions

No specific antidote exists for cyanobacterial toxins in birds. Treatment is primarily supportive. In cases of secondary bacterial infection, veterinarians may prescribe appropriate antibiotics, but only after confirming bacterial involvement.

- **Supportive Care**
  Offer fresh water with electrolytes to support dehydrated or weak birds. Monitor for signs of dehydration. Provide high-quality, easily digestible food to support recovery. Assisted feeding for severely affected birds. Ensure ventilation and maintain proper ambient temperature. Keep bedding dry and clean. Passive range of motion for joints.

13.1.6 Prevention and Control

- **Water Source Management**
  Remove or drain ponds, puddles, or poorly maintained water troughs. Prevent nutrient buildup that promotes algal growth. Use clean waterers, especially during warm months.
- **Environmental and Husbandry Measures**
  Remove decaying vegetation and fecal matter from water sources. Keep the environment and pen dry. Control free-range access to potentially contaminated ponds or ditches.
- **Monitoring and Early Detection**
  Inspect water daily for algal blooms (green, blue-green, or reddish scum).

13.1.7 Nursing Considerations

Nursing care for chickens exposed to algal toxins focuses on removing the source of exposure, maintaining hydration, and supporting organ function. Veterinary technicians should immediately ensure that birds have access to clean, uncontaminated water and prevent further ingestion of affected water sources. Severely compromised, dehydrated birds may need fluid therapy and assisted feeding. Affected birds should be isolated to reduce stress, allow close observation, and prevent bullying. Since algal toxins primarily target the liver and nervous system, technicians should monitor for icterus, lethargy, incoordination, and sudden deaths, and report findings promptly to the attending veterinarian. Education of caretakers on preventing access to contaminated water, regular pond maintenance, and prompt recognition of clinical signs is key to reducing morbidity and mortality. Overall, nursing care emphasizes prevention, early detection, and supportive management while minimizing additional stressors. Birds whose quality of life is deemed poor should be humanely euthanized.

13.2 Avian Borreliosis

13.2.1 Overview and Pathogenesis

Avian borreliosis, also known as avian spirochetosis, is a tick-borne bacterial disease of chickens caused primarily by *Borrelia anserina*. The disease is most observed in tropical and subtropical regions where Argasid ticks (*Ornithodoros* spp.) act as vectors. Incidence is low in the United States; however, *Borrelia* species in birds are detected in the Northeast, Mid-Atlantic, Southeast, and Western United States, mirroring the distribution of human Lyme disease and their tick vectors. Clinically, affected birds present with a sudden onset of depression, ruffled feathers, pale combs and wattles, anorexia, diarrhea, anemia, and reduced egg production; mortality can be significant, particularly in young or immunocompromised birds.

The pathogenesis begins when infected ticks transmit *B. anserina* spirochetes into the bloodstream during blood feeding. The spirochetes rapidly disseminate, invading erythrocytes and endothelial cells, leading to hemolytic anemia, vascular damage, and systemic inflammation. The destruction of red blood cells contributes to pallor and weakness, while vascular injury can exacerbate tissue hypoxia and organ dysfunction. Concurrent stressors such as poor nutrition, high stocking density, or concurrent infections can intensify disease severity. If untreated, bacteremia may persist, causing chronic infection, immunosuppression, and increased susceptibility to secondary bacterial or viral infections. Overall, avian borreliosis represents a systemic spirochetal infection in which vector transmission, rapid hematogenous spread, and host factors converge to produce acute clinical disease and potential flock-level outbreaks.

13.2.2 Risk Factors

- **Tick Exposure**
  Argas persicus (soft tick) is responsible for transmission. Free-range birds may acquire ticks from wild birds or infested environments. *A. persicus* has a limited incidence in the United States, mainly appearing in poultry operations along the Gulf Coast and Mexican border.
- **Environmental and Seasonal Factors**
  Warm and humid climates favor tick survival and proliferation. Poorly ventilated housing increases tick infestation risk. Tick populations tend to peak in late spring through early autumn, coinciding with higher infection rates.
- **Flock Management Practices**
  The introduction of new birds without quarantine can introduce infected ticks. Infrequent cleaning of coops allows tick overpopulation. Multi-species housing (ducks, pigeons) can maintain tick populations. Overcrowding increases stress and exposure, making birds more susceptible.
- **Host-Related Factors**
  Young chicks are more susceptible to severe infection. Immunocompromised or stressed birds (from molting, transport, or concurrent disease) are at higher risk. Unvaccinated flocks in endemic areas are more prone to outbreaks (where vaccines are available, usually in endemic regions).

13.2.3 Clinical Signs and Pathology

- **External Findings**
  Birds may appear suddenly ill. Decreased feed intake. Drop in egg production in layers. Pale comb, wattles, and mucous membranes from anemia. Weakness and collapse due to reduced oxygen-carrying capacity. Tachypnea (rapid breathing) in severe cases. Ataxia, tremors, or paralysis in advanced or severe infections. Presence of ticks attached to the bird's skin.
- **Necropsy Findings**
  Marked anemia, pale muscles, and tissues. Enlarged spleen, soft and congested. Hepatomegaly with greenish discoloration or petechial hemorrhages. Intestinal congestion; sometimes catarrhal enteritis. Renomegaly with congestion. Heart shows petechiae or mild pericarditis in severe cases. Hemodilution.

13.2.4 Diagnostic Testing

- **Blood Smear**
  B. anserina spirochetes can often be seen in fresh blood smears stained with Giemsa, Wright's, or Leishman stain. It is best detected during the febrile stage of infection.
- **PCR**
  It can detect *B. anserina* DNA. More sensitive than microscopy, especially in chronic or low-level infections.

13.2.5 Treatment and Therapeutic Interventions

- **Medication**
  Oxytetracycline 5 mg/kg subcutaneous or intramuscularly every 12–24 hours. 2500 mg/L drinking water and 2500 mg/kg feed.

- Filtered whole blood collected (1% of body weight) from a screened, healthy, heavy bird (under sedation) for homologous transfusion into an anemic bird. Blood product transfusions are also discussed in Chapter 15.
- Supplemental oxygen therapy via mask or induction chamber

13.2.6 Prevention and Control

- **Vector Control**
  Apply poultry-safe acaricides (sprays and dusts) to coops, cracks, crevices, and perches. Replace or sanitize old wooden structures where ticks hide. Remove and dispose of contaminated bedding and nesting material. Fipronil can be applied topically to birds.
- **Housing and Environmental Management**
  Maintain clean, dry, and well-ventilated housing to discourage tick survival. Seal cracks and crevices in wood or walls where ticks hide during the day. Rotate or rest housing units, when possible, to break parasite cycles. Avoid overcrowding, which increases stress and tick exposure.
- **Biosecurity Measures**
  Quarantine new birds for 30 days to prevent the introduction of ticks or infection. Restrict access of wild birds that may carry ticks or spirochetes.

13.2.7 Nursing Considerations

Nursing care for chickens affected by avian borreliosis focuses on reducing stress, maintaining hydration and nutritional needs, and monitoring for complications such as anemia and weakness. Veterinary technicians should ensure that affected birds are adequately hydrated and receiving proper nutrition, as illness often reduces appetite and energy levels. Client education plays an important role, particularly regarding the importance of tick control, housing hygiene, and early recognition of signs such as diarrhea, depression, or sudden pale combs. By combining preventive husbandry and vector reduction, technicians can help minimize the impact of avian borreliosis on flock health.

13.3 Avian Encephalomyelitis

13.3.1 Overview and Pathogenesis

Avian encephalomyelitis (AE) is a viral disease of chickens, turkeys, and other gallinaceous birds caused by an enterovirus in the Picornaviridae family. It primarily affects young chicks, usually under 6 weeks of age, and is characterized by neurologic signs including ataxia, tremors, paralysis, and weakness, while in adults it may cause decreased egg production and hatchability.

The pathogenesis begins with horizontal or vertical transmission of the virus, most commonly through ingestion of contaminated feces or via transovarian passage from infected hens to embryos. In young chicks, the virus invades the gastrointestinal tract, then spreads hematogenously to the central nervous system, where it causes neuronal degeneration, perivascular cuffing, and gliosis in the cerebellum and spinal cord. These lesions lead to impaired motor coordination and tremors. Vertical transmission results in infected chicks hatching already viremic and showing signs within the first few days of life. In adult laying hens, infection is often subclinical but can lead to reduced egg quality and embryo mortality. Environmental factors such as poor hygiene, overcrowding, and lack of vaccination increase the risk of outbreaks. The combination of neurotropism, early-age susceptibility, and vertical transmission makes AE a significant disease for welfare in backyard flocks.

13.3.2 Risk Factors

- **Host-Related Factors**
  Chicks under 2–4 weeks old are at the highest risk for clinical disease. Adult birds usually show subclinical infection, but infected hens can transmit the virus vertically through eggs.
- **Flock Husbandry**
  Shared equipment and vectors spreading contaminated feces. Overcrowding increases stress and facilitates fecal–oral spread. Virus persists in contaminated bedding and housing.

13.3.3 Clinical Signs and Pathology

- **External Findings**
  - In chicks, neurological signs appear between 1 and 3 weeks of age. Ataxia, fine tremors of the head and neck, paralysis of one or both legs, and sitting on hocks or prostration. Lethargy, failure to thrive, and stunted growth are also clinical signs.
- **Necropsy Findings**
  May appear normal externally despite severe neurological signs. Occasionally small, pale, or congested livers.

13.3.4 Diagnostic Testing

- **RT-PCR/PCR**
  Detect AE virus RNA in tissues or feces.
- **ELISA or Virus Neutralization (VN)**
  Detects antibodies from AE virus.

13.3.5 Treatment and Therapeutic Interventions

- **Supportive Care**
  In severely weak chicks, technicians must assist with oral fluids and crop feeding. Severely affected chicks with persistent tremors or paralysis often do not recover; humane euthanasia may be indicated.

13.3.6 Prevention and Control

Because AE is a viral disease without a cure, prevention is the most effective strategy.

- **Biosecurity Measures**
  Restrict visitors and contaminated equipment, clothing, and footwear. Regularly clean and disinfect housing, feeders, waterers, and equipment. Dispose of bedding and dead birds promptly and properly. Prevent mechanical spread of the virus.
- **Environmental and Husbandry Practices**
  Maintain clean, dry bedding and good ventilation. Avoid overcrowding, which increases stress and viral spread. Ensure chicks are brooded under optimal conditions (clean, warm, with easy access to feed/water).

13.3.7 Nursing Considerations

Nursing care for AE focuses on managing neurologic impairment, maintaining hydration and nutrition, and preventing injury in affected chicks. Birds with tremors, ataxia, or paralysis should be housed in a quiet, well-bedded environment to reduce stress and minimize the risk of trampling or self-injury. Providing easy access to feed and water at ground level helps weak or uncoordinated chicks maintain intake. Monitoring weight gain, hydration status, and mobility is essential to detect deterioration early. Intensive nursing care may be indicated to include fluid therapy and nutritional support. Since AE is highly contagious and may spread vertically and horizontally, veterinary technicians in clinical practice should implement strict biosecurity and sanitation protocols, including isolation of symptomatic birds and careful disinfection of housing and equipment. Client education is critical, especially regarding the importance of availability of vaccination, recognition of early neurologic signs in chicks, and supportive management to reduce suffering in affected birds. While no direct treatment exists, diligent nursing care helps preserve flock welfare.

13.4 Brain Tumor

13.4.1 Overview and Pathogenesis

Brain tumors in chickens are uncommon neoplastic conditions that may arise as primary central nervous system neoplasms or, less frequently, as metastatic lesions. These tumors can occur in birds of any age but are more often reported in older hens and roosters. Clinical signs depend on tumor location and size, and may include ataxia, circling, head tilt, torticollis, seizures, behavioral changes, and sudden death.

Pathogenesis involves uncontrolled proliferation of neural or glial cells within the brain, leading to compression of surrounding neural tissue, disruption of normal neuronal pathways, and increased intracranial pressure. Some tumors, such as gliomas or medulloblastomas, originate from glial or progenitor cells, whereas metastatic lesions arise from neoplasms elsewhere in the body. The resultant neuronal dysfunction impairs motor coordination, sensory perception, and normal behavior, and may predispose birds to secondary trauma or malnutrition due to an inability to feed effectively. Factors contributing to tumor development in poultry are poorly understood but may include genetic predisposition, environmental carcinogens, or viral oncogenesis (e.g., avian leukosis virus (ALV) in certain neoplasms). Overall, brain tumors in chickens compromise neurologic function and welfare, and clinical outcomes are typically poor due to progressive neurologic deterioration.

13.4.2 Risk Factors

- **Genetic Predisposition**
  Certain breeds may be more susceptible to specific tumor types. Hereditary or familial lines with a history of neoplasia are at increased risk.
- **Viral Infections**
  ALV and reticuloendotheliosis virus (REV).
- **Environmental Factors**
  Chronic exposure to carcinogens (e.g., aflatoxins in feed) may contribute to tumor development.

- **Immunosuppression and Stress**
  Immunocompromised birds due to concurrent infections (e.g., Marek's disease and infectious bursal disease) are more susceptible to tumor development. Stress from overcrowding, transport, or poor nutrition may exacerbate tumor growth.

13.4.3 Clinical Signs and Pathology

- **External Findings**
  Uncoordinated gait or stumbling. Torticollis, especially with cerebellar or brainstem tumors. Circling behavior is often toward the side of the lesion. Seizures or tremors in severe or rapidly growing tumors. Paralysis or paresis and blindness or head-pressing.
- **Necropsy Findings**
  Visible tumors ranging from small nodules to large masses, often in the cerebrum, cerebellum, or brainstem. Tumors may be multicentric with associated lymphoid involvement (ALV or REV-induced).

13.4.4 Diagnostic Testing

- **CT or MRI Scans**
  Visualization of intracranial masses in anesthetized birds.

13.4.5 Treatment and Therapeutic Interventions

Treatment is primarily supportive and palliative. No proven pharmacological treatment exists to shrink or eliminate tumors. Analgesics, corticosteroids, and antiemetic agents can be administered as comfort measures.

13.4.6 Prevention and Control

Most brain tumors are virally induced (ALV, REV) or linked to genetic predisposition.

- **Biosecurity and Environmental Control**
  Limit contact with new or unknown birds. Prevent spread via equipment, visitors, and wild birds. Maintain clean housing, feeders, and waterers to reduce viral persistence.
- **Genetic and Breed Considerations**
  Avoid breeding lines with known predisposition to neoplasia.

13.4.7 Nursing Considerations

Nursing care for chickens with brain tumors focuses on maintaining safety, hydration, nutrition, and minimizing stress, as affected birds often exhibit neurologic deficits such as ataxia, circling, tremors, or seizures. Veterinary technicians should provide soft bedding and a quiet enclosure. Ensure easy access to feed and water at ground level to maintain nutrition in birds with impaired mobility. Monitoring signs of progressive neurological deterioration, weight loss, dehydration, or secondary trauma is essential, and records should be kept informing prognosis and management decisions. Intensive nursing therapies for severely compromised birds. Since brain tumors are generally irreversible and progressive, humane considerations, including euthanasia in severely affected birds, may be necessary to prevent suffering. Technicians should also educate caretakers about the importance of observation for early neurologic changes, maintaining flock safety, and reducing environmental stressors to protect other birds. Overall, nursing care emphasizes comfort, welfare, and careful monitoring while providing supportive husbandry tailored to the bird's neurologic limitations.

13.5 Cerebellar Hypoplasia

13.5.1 Overview and Pathogenesis

Cerebellar hypoplasia (CH) in chickens is a congenital or early-onset neurologic condition characterized by incomplete development of the cerebellum, resulting in impaired coordination and motor control. The disorder is most observed in young chicks and manifests as ataxia, tremors, unsteady gait, head bobbing, and difficulty perching or feeding, though affected birds may remain alert and feed adequately in mild cases.

Pathogenesis involves arrest or defective development of cerebellar neurons, particularly Purkinje cells and granule neurons, leading to reduced cerebellar size and impaired integration of motor signals. CH can arise due to genetic defects, in-ovo exposure to teratogenic viruses (such as ALV or chicken embryonic encephalomyelitis virus), nutritional deficiencies, or environmental insults during embryogenesis. The structural deficit in the cerebellum prevents proper coordination of voluntary movements and postural control, while other parts of the nervous system may remain intact. Unlike progressive neurodegenerative diseases, cerebellar hypoplasia is nonprogressive, but the functional impairment persists throughout life, potentially affecting growth, feeding efficiency, and overall welfare.

13.5.2 Risk Factors

- **Viral Infections During Embryogenesis**
  Avian encephalomyelitis virus (AEV) or infectious bursal disease virus (IBDV) infections during embryonic development can disrupt cerebellar formation. Virus exposure between 3 and 14 days of incubation is most critical. Vertical transmission from infected breeder hens is the primary pathway.
- **Genetic Predisposition**
  Certain lines may have higher susceptibility to developmental neurological defects.
- **Incubation and Hatchery Factors**
  Improper incubation temperatures or humidity can exacerbate cerebellar developmental issues. Mechanical shaking or handling of eggs during critical stages may increase risk.
- **Nutritional Factors**
  Vitamin or mineral deficiencies (e.g., vitamin E, folic acid) in breeder hens may contribute to defective cerebellar development.

13.5.3 Clinical Signs and Pathology

- **External Findings**
  Uncoordinated gait is the hallmark sign. Fine tremors, especially of the head and neck. Over- or under-shooting movements when walking or reaching for food. Birds may topple when attempting

to stand or walk. Slower progression in walking, running, and feeding. Normal alertness and appetite are usually preserved. Weight gain may be slightly reduced due to inefficiency in feeding. Present from hatching, as CH is congenital.

- **Necropsy Findings**
  Cerebellum is visually smaller or malformed in severe cases.

13.5.4 Diagnostic Testing

- **Clinical Diagnosis (Primary Tool)**
  Observation of neurologic signs from hatching is the most important diagnostic tool.

13.5.5 Treatment and Therapeutic Interventions

There is no curative treatment; care focuses on supportive management, welfare, and optimizing survival.

- **Supportive Care**
  Maintain warm and draft-free housing. Minimize obstacles to allow safer movement. Ensure easy access to feed and water, using shallow feeders and drinkers. Assist with handfeeding if necessary for weak or inefficient birds. Consider separating severely affected chicks to prevent bullying and ensure access to nutritional resources. Mildly affected birds may survive and thrive with supportive care.

13.5.6 Prevention and Control

- **Hatchery and Incubation Management**
  Proper temperature, humidity, and egg handling reduce embryonic stress that may exacerbate cerebellar development issues. Avoid mechanical shaking or rough transport of hatching eggs.
- **Biosecurity Measures**
  Limit introduction of AEV, IBDV, or other immunosuppressive viruses. Prevent mixing of multi-age flocks, which increases viral circulation.

13.5.7 Nursing Considerations

Since cerebellar hypoplasia is a nonprogressive but lifelong condition, nursing care focuses on ensuring comfort, safety, and quality of life. Affected birds often struggle with coordination, tremors, or difficulty perching, so veterinary technicians should recommend housing modifications such as soft bedding, low or no perches, and easy access to feed and water at ground level. Monitoring is important to ensure that affected birds can eat and drink adequately, as motor deficits may limit their ability to compete in a flock. Technicians should watch for secondary injuries due to falls or abnormal movement patterns, and intervene promptly if welfare is compromised. Stress reduction is also critical and handling should be minimized, and affected birds may benefit from separation or smaller group housing to reduce competition. Client education is key: caretakers should understand that the condition does not worsen over time, but supportive husbandry is essential to maintain welfare. In severe cases where birds cannot feed, walk, or perch safely, veterinary technicians should counsel owners on humane euthanasia decisions to prevent prolonged suffering.

13.6 Dactylariosis

13.6.1 Overview and Pathogenesis

Dactylariosis in chickens is a sporadic but often fatal fungal encephalitis caused by the dematiaceous thermophilic fungus *Dactylaria gallopava* (synonym *Ochroconis gallopava*). Birds become infected by inhalation of fungal spores from contaminated bedding, decaying wood, sawdust, mulch, or egg incubators, especially when such materials are damp or poorly sanitized. The fungus is ubiquitous in the environment—present in soil, wood, and decaying vegetation—and grows especially well in warm, acidic, and moist conditions. In young chicks (commonly 1–5 weeks old), the immune system and central nervous system barriers are less mature, rendering birds more susceptible to invasion. After inhalation, spores may initiate infection in respiratory tissues, but the defining pathology is invasion of the central nervous system.

The organism travels (hematogenously or via local spread) to the brain (both cerebrum and cerebellum), where it causes multifocal to coalescing areas of necrosis. Inflammatory responses include massive infiltration by heterophils, macrophages, and multinucleated giant cells. Pigmented (melanized) septate hyphae are seen in lesions, often with hemorrhage, edema, and discoloration in brain tissue. Clinically, infected chickens exhibit neurologic signs such as tremors, incoordination, head tilt (torticollis), paralysis, and death, which follows a short course. Grossly, lesions may be circumscribed, firm, grayish, or cream-colored areas in the cerebrum or cerebellum; sometimes pulmonary granulomas are also present if respiratory involvement occurs. Outbreaks are often associated with contaminated litter or incubators, and attempts to reproduce disease experimentally confirm that exposure to heavily contaminated wood-bark litter can result in neurologic disease. The pathogenesis thus combines environmental exposure, fungal virulence, immature host defenses (especially in young birds), and central nervous system (CNS) dissemination, resulting in neurologic destruction and high mortality.

13.6.2 Risk Factors

- **Environmental Reservoirs**
  The fungus is a soil- and litter-dwelling opportunistic mold. Thrives in warm, moist, poorly ventilated poultry houses, organic matter buildup, and contaminated feed or bedding materials.
- **Host-Related Factors**
  Immunocompromised birds are more susceptible. Young and growing birds are most frequently affected due to immature immune systems.
- **Housing and Management Practices**
  Overcrowding, poor sanitation, and poor ventilation increase stress and environmental contamination.
- **Geographic and Seasonal Factors**
  Endemic in warm, humid climates. Risk increases during rainy seasons when bedding may remain damp.

13.6.3 Clinical Signs and Pathology

- **External Findings**
  Ataxia, circling, tremors, paralysis, or seizures. Dyspnea, open-mouth breathing, and reduced activity. Weight loss, anorexia, weakness, and lethargy. Sudden death without premonitory signs is common. Dactylariosis is most often presented as a systemic or disseminated fungal infection.

- **Necropsy Findings**
  Lesions are usually multifocal, granulomatous, and necrotizing. Brain (meningoencephalitis, granulomas in cerebrum/cerebellum), lungs and air sacs (necrotic, granulomatous lesions), and occasionally other organs such as the liver, kidney, and heart. Lesions may mimic aspergillosis or other systemic mycoses.

13.6.4 Diagnostic Testing

- **Histopathology**
  Definitive diagnosis often requires microscopic evaluation; periodic acid-Schiff (PAS) and Grocott's Methenamine Stain (GMS) stains reveal dematiaceous fungal hyphae with granulomas.
- **Microbiological Culture**
  Tissue samples (brain, lung, and liver) can be cultured to isolate *D. gallopava* (*O. gallopava*).

13.6.5 Treatment and Therapeutic Interventions

Dactylariosis is a rare but severe systemic fungal infection. By the time clinical signs appear, prognosis is often poor to grave.

- **Medication**
  Itraconazole 5–10 mg/kg by mouth every 12–24 hours.
- **Supportive Care**
  Focus on reducing stress, providing comfort measures.
- **Euthanasia Considerations**
  Birds with severe neurological disease or unresponsive to supportive care often require humane euthanasia.

13.6.6 Prevention and Control

- **Environmental Management**
  Since *Dactylaria* spp. are opportunistic soil-borne fungi, control efforts should focus on minimizing environmental exposure. Keep bedding dry and clean. Replace wet, caked bedding promptly. Avoid moldy straw, hay, or shavings. Maintain good airflow in coops to reduce humidity. Prevent condensation, especially in cold weather housing. Fix leaking waterers, roofs. Use raised waterers to prevent bedding saturation.

13.6.7 Nursing Considerations

Because dactylariosis is an aggressive fungal encephalitis with a poor prognosis, nursing care centers on supportive management, prevention of suffering, and environmental control. Affected birds often show severe neurologic signs such as tremors, paralysis, or circling, so veterinary technicians should ensure housing is safe, padded, and free of high perches or sharp edges to reduce the risk of injury. Birds with impaired mobility may struggle to access feed and water. Nutritional and hydration support is indicated, and caretakers will need to hand-feed or crop feed. Since treatment options are limited and systemic antifungals are rarely effective in poultry, technicians must emphasize flock-level prevention, including removing contaminated wood-based bedding, sanitizing incubators, and improving ventilation to reduce fungal spore exposure. Clear communication with guardians is vital as birds showing advanced neurologic dysfunction are unlikely to recover, and humane euthanasia should be considered to prevent unnecessary suffering.

13.7 Ear Infections

13.7.1 Overview and Pathogenesis

Ear infections (otitis) in chickens most often involve bacterial invasion of the middle or inner ear, leading to localized inflammation, swelling, and neurologic dysfunction. The condition typically arises as a secondary complication of respiratory disease, since pathogens can ascend the auditory (eustachian) tube from the upper respiratory tract. Common bacteria include *Escherichia coli*, *Staphylococcus aureus*, *Pseudomonas* spp., and *Pasteurella multocida*. In some cases, fungal organisms such as *Aspergillus* may also colonize the ear canal.

Pathogenesis begins with mucosal irritation or damage, often associated with concurrent respiratory infections, poor ventilation, or high ammonia levels, which facilitates pathogen entry. Inflammation leads to pus accumulation and caseous exudate within the ear canal or tympanic cavity, producing visible swelling around the ear, head tilting, and sometimes neurologic signs if infection extends into the inner ear (vestibular system) or cranial bones. Chronic infections may lead to granuloma formation or bone erosion. Because balance organs lie within the inner ear, advanced otitis can result in ataxia, circling, or head shaking, mimicking central nervous system disease. Left untreated, the infection can become systemic or lead to permanent neurologic impairment.

13.7.2 Risk Factors

- **Environmental and Husbandry Factors**
  Dirty, dusty, or wet litter can harbor bacteria, fungi, and mites that migrate into the ear canal. High dust levels from bedding, feed, or dander irritate the ear canal, facilitating secondary infection. High humidity or damp housing creates favorable conditions for fungal and bacterial growth.
- **Nutritional Factors**
  Vitamin A deficiency leads to squamous metaplasia of epithelial tissues, including the ear canal lining, increasing susceptibility to bacterial and fungal infection. Weakened immune defenses predispose birds to opportunistic pathogens.
- **Infectious Disease Factors**
  Mycoplasma gallisepticum, *P. multocida*, *E. coli* can spread from the upper respiratory tract to the middle ear. Diseases like Marek's disease or infectious bursal disease weaken immunity, allowing secondary infections. Mites (e.g., *Ornithonyssus sylviarum*) and lice may irritate skin and ear openings, increasing secondary bacterial invasion.

13.7.3 Clinical Signs and Pathology

- **External Findings**
  Head shaking, scratching at ear, lethargy, and inappetence.

  Otitis Externa
  Erythema, edema, or dried exudate at the ear opening. Brown, caseous, or waxy discharge with foul odor. Presence of mites or debris. Feather loss around ear from self-trauma.

Otitis Media

Swelling just caudal to the eye, often firm or fluctuant. Caseous pus may build up behind the tympanic membrane. Head tilting as infection interferes with the vestibular system.

Otitis Interna

Severe head tilt, circling, loss of balance, or falling over. Involuntary eye movements, less common but possible. Even after infection is resolved, birds may retain head tilt or balance deficits.

- **Necropsy Findings**
- Caseous exudate filling the ear canal and tympanic cavity. Thickening of ear canal lining. Extension of infection to surrounding tissues (sinuses, skull bones).

13.7.4 Diagnostic Testing

- **Ear Cytology**
  Smears stained with Gram, Diff-Quik, or Wright-Giemsa to identify bacteria, yeast, and parasites.
- **Aerobic and Anaerobic Culture**
  Confirms bacterial involvement (common pathogens: *E. coli*, *M. gallisepticum*, *P. multocida*).
- **Radiographs**
  May show soft tissue density or caseous material in tympanic cavity.

13.7.5 Treatment and Therapeutic Interventions

- **Medication**
  Trimethoprim-Sulfamethoxazole 100 mg/kg by mouth every 12 hours for 5–7 days.
  Meloxicam 0.5 mg/kg by mouth or intramuscularly every 12–24 hours.
  Carprofen 5–10 mg/kg by mouth or intramuscularly once daily.
- **Abscess Drainage**
  Caseous pus in the middle ear may need general anesthesia, surgical opening, and curettage.
- **Supportive Care**
  Isolation of affected birds in a quiet, clean environment. Ensure easy access to feed and water; handfeeding may be necessary for neurological cases. Maintain optimum ambient temperature and ventilation.

13.7.6 Prevention and Control

- **Environmental Management**
  Replace wet or soiled bedding regularly in the house and pen. Prevent buildup of manure and organic debris. Ensure adequate airflow to reduce humidity, ammonia, and dust. Avoid drafts that stress birds while maintaining good air exchange. Use low-dust bedding when possible. Moisten dusty floors lightly during cleaning to reduce airborne particles.
- **Nutritional Prevention**
  Ensure chickens receive complete feed with essential vitamins and minerals. Vitamin A prevents squamous metaplasia and strengthens mucosal defense. Especially important for birds on homemade or forage-heavy diets.
- **Infectious Disease Control**
  Control *M. gallisepticum*, *E. coli*, and other pathogens through biosecurity and vaccination (where applicable). Regular monitoring and treatment for mites and lice to prevent ear canal irritation. Environmental acaricides to break parasite life cycles.

- **Biosecurity Practices**
  Quarantine new birds for 30-days before introducing them to a flock. Limit visitors and equipment sharing between flocks. Routine disinfection of housing and equipment.
- **Flock Husbandry**
  Avoid overcrowding, which increases aggression, dust, and pathogen transmission. Provide adequate feeder and waterer space to minimize pecking injuries near the head and ears. Routine inspection of crested breeds (Polish, Silkies) that may hide early ear lesions. Address respiratory or systemic infections early before they spread to the ear canal.

13.7.7 Nursing Considerations

Nursing care of chickens with ear infections focuses on supportive treatment, safe handling, and preventing recurrence. Birds with otitis often have painful swelling, head tilts, or impaired balance, so they should be housed in a quiet, well-bedded, low-perch environment to reduce the risk of falls and injuries. Veterinary technicians may need to assist with gentle cleaning of the ear canal to remove exudate and ensure prescribed topical or systemic agents are administered correctly. Hydration and nutrition are essential, as affected birds may have reduced feed intake; offering soft, palatable foods at ground level helps maintain body condition. Caretakers should monitor for signs of progressive neurologic dysfunction, such as circling, rolling, or severe head tilt, which may indicate deeper inner ear or CNS involvement. Isolation may be required both to prevent flock bullying of uncoordinated birds and to allow close monitoring. Education of owners is crucial: improving ventilation, reducing dust and ammonia, and promptly addressing respiratory disease lowers the risk of recurrent otitis. In chronic or nonresponsive cases, technicians should also prepare caretakers for discussions about long-term quality of life and, if appropriate, euthanasia.

13.8 Head Trauma

13.8.1 Overview and Pathogenesis

Head trauma in chickens is a relatively common injury that can occur from pecking, predator attacks, collisions, or falls, and it may result in damage ranging from superficial wounds to severe brain injury.

Pathogenesis depends on the severity and mechanism of trauma: blunt force, sharp impact, or crushing injury. External trauma can lead to lacerations, fractures of the skull, and bleeding, while internal injury may involve cerebral contusions, intracranial hemorrhage, edema, and secondary inflammation. Even mild trauma may impair neural function due to swelling within the confined space of the skull, causing increased intracranial pressure and disruption of normal brain activity. Clinically, birds may present with ataxia, head tilt, circling, seizures, blindness, or depression, depending on the region of the brain affected. In some cases, ocular or ear damage may accompany cranial injuries, further complicating the presentation. Secondary bacterial infections of open wounds are also a concern, particularly in flock settings where pecking can exacerbate injuries. The overall outcome varies widely from full recovery in mild cases to sudden death or long-term neurological impairment in severe trauma.

13.8.2 Risk Factors

- **Environmental and Housing Factors**
  Exposed nails, wires, or splintered wood in coops can cause direct injury. Birds startled into flight may strike roosts, feeders, or ceilings. Predators cause penetrating injuries. Falls from unstable or overcrowding roosts. Rough handling or overcrowding in crates increases the risk of collisions.
- **Flock Dynamics Factors**
  Dominant birds may peck or strike subordinates on the head. Overcrowding or competition for resources intensifies aggression. Multiple roosters in confined spaces may fight, causing comb and head injuries. Cannibalism is common in stressed or overcrowded flocks, leading to severe cranial wounds.
- **Management and Husbandry Factors**
  Overcrowding increases stress, aggression, and accidents. Bored birds may redirect pecking behavior toward flock mates. Feeders, waterers, enrichment equipment, or perches placed at head height can cause repeated impact injuries.
- **Host-Related Factors**
  Feathers can obscure vision, making birds more prone to collisions and pecking injuries. Thinner cranial bones predispose to more severe trauma. Sick birds may be pecked or bullied, increasing trauma risk.

13.8.3 Clinical Signs and Pathology

- **External Findings**
  Reduced activity, reluctance to move, localized swelling around eyes, comb, wattles, or skull. External lacerations or wounds from pecking or sharp objects. Uncoordinated movements, head tilt, circling, loss of balance, seizures, tremors, blindness, coma, or sudden death. Periorbital swelling from blunt trauma, corneal injury, and facial paralysis.
- **Necropsy Findings**
  Hematomas beneath the skin or within the cranial cavity. Skull fractures with displacement of bone fragments. Cerebral hemorrhage or edema (common with blunt force). Evidence of secondary infection in open wounds (abscesses).

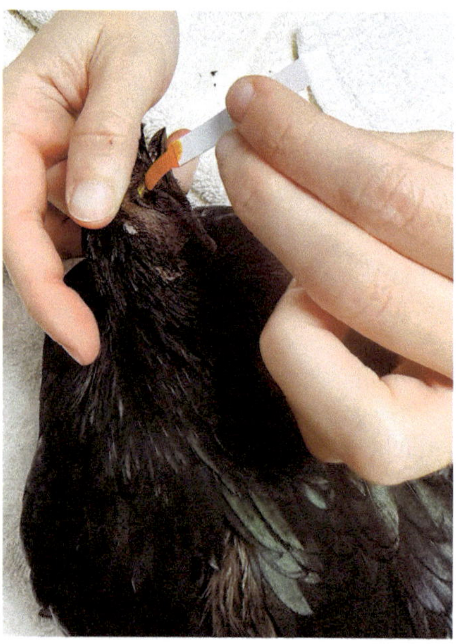

Figure 13.1 Fluorescein staining of cornea after head trauma. Courtesy of Funky Chicken Rescue.

13.8.4 Diagnostic Testing

- **Diagnostic Imaging**
  Skull radiographs help identify fractures, bone displacement, and metallic foreign bodies. Positioning may require analgesia and anesthesia to minimize stress.
- **Fluorescein Staining**
  Assess eyeballs for abrasions (Figure 13.1).

13.8.5 Treatment and Therapeutic Interventions

- **Wound Management**
  Appropriate level of anesthesia and analgesia. Gently flush lacerations with sterile saline or diluted antiseptic (povidone iodine; "weak tea"). Debride necrotic tissue where appropriate. Systemic antibiotics may be prescribed to prevent infection in open skull or skin wounds. Light bandaging if appropriate.

13.8.6 Prevention and Control

- **Housing and Environment**
  Avoid sharp edges, protruding nails, or low-hanging objects inside the coop. Ensure perches are sturdy, stable, and not placed at excessive heights that increase fall risk. Provide adequate bedding to cushion falls. Sudden changes in light intensity or predators can cause panic flights and collisions. Use gradual dimming or soft lighting to reduce startling behaviors. Provide sufficient space to minimize overcrowding, which can lead to trampling or aggressive pecking. Offer environmental enrichment (dust baths, perches, foraging areas) to reduce stress behaviors. Prevent predator access.

13.8.7 Nursing Considerations

Nursing care for chickens with head trauma focuses on minimizing stress, supporting recovery, and preventing complications. A quiet, dimly lit, and warm environment should be provided to reduce stimulation and allow the bird to rest, as stress can worsen neurological signs. Handling should be kept to a minimum, and the bird should be isolated from the flock to prevent pecking injuries and reduce competition for food and water. Careful observation is essential to monitor for progression of neurological signs, hemorrhage, edema, or changes in mentation. Soft, easily accessible feed and water should be provided, and in cases where the bird is unable to eat or drink independently, supportive feeding and hydration may be necessary. Prevention of aspiration during assisted feeding. Wound care should be performed gently if external injuries are present, while avoiding pressure to the head. Pain management and anti-inflammatory medications help reduce swelling and discomfort. Ongoing nursing care involves frequent reassessment of wound healing and clinical signs, gradual reintroduction to the flock if recovery occurs, and clear documentation of clinical progress to guide treatment decisions. If head wounds are severe, humane euthanasia is a considerate treatment option.

13.9 Ammonia Toxicity

13.9.1 Overview and Pathogenesis

Ammonia toxicity is a common environmental problem in poultry production, resulting from the breakdown of uric acid in manure by microbial activity, especially under conditions of poor ventilation, high moisture, and inadequate bedding/pen management. Ammonia is a colorless gas with a pungent odor, and concentrations above 25 ppm are considered harmful to chicken health. Chickens are particularly sensitive because of their constant exposure to the bedding environment and their relatively high respiratory rate. Chronic exposure contributes to reduced growth rates, poor feed conversion, and increased susceptibility to disease, making it a welfare concern.

The pathogenesis of ammonia toxicity primarily involves irritation and damage to the respiratory and ocular systems. Inhaled ammonia dissolves in the moisture of the respiratory tract, forming ammonium hydroxide, which is highly irritating to mucous membranes. This leads to ciliostasis, epithelial damage, and inflammation of the upper respiratory tract, compromising mucociliary clearance and predisposing birds to secondary infections such as colibacillosis, *Mycoplasma* infections, and Newcastle disease. Chronic exposure can result in tracheitis, keratoconjunctivitis, and corneal ulceration. Prolonged irritation also causes increased mucus production and thickening of respiratory tissues, which impair gas exchange and overall respiratory efficiency. Additionally, sustained exposure stresses the immune system, reducing vaccine effectiveness and lowering resistance to pathogens. Together, these effects explain the multifactorial role of ammonia toxicity with increased morbidity.

13.9.2 Risk Factors

- **Environmental and Housing Factors**
  Excessive fecal matter decomposition and inadequate air exchange increase ammonia concentration.
  Warm, humid conditions accelerate microbial breakdown of uric acid to ammonia.
- **Nutritional Factors**
  High-protein diets cause increased uric acid excretion in droppings. Imbalanced diets (excess nitrogen, low energy) cause higher nitrogen waste output.
- **Management Practices**
  Infrequent replacement or poor bedding quality. Leaking waterer moisture increases ammonia release.

13.9.3 Clinical Signs and Pathology

- **External Findings**
  Sneezing, coughing, tracheal rales, and open-mouth breathing. Watery eyes, conjunctivitis, keratoconjunctivitis, corneal ulceration, and blindness. Reluctance to move, reduced feed intake, and decreased egg production and shell quality.
- **Necropsy Findings**
  Hyperemia and inflammation of nasal passages and trachea. Thickened tracheal mucosa with excess mucus. Caseous exudate in severe cases or when secondary infections are present. Conjunctival swelling, clouded corneas, and corneal ulceration. Feather staining around eyes from excessive tearing and nasal discharge.

13.9.4 Diagnostic Testing

- **Environmental Testing**
  Use handheld ammonia meters or detector tubes. Clinical problems often begin when levels exceed 25 ppm; levels above 50 ppm are considered dangerous.

13.9.5 Treatment and Therapeutic Interventions

- **Supportive Care**
  Place birds with ocular ulceration or severe respiratory signs in a clean, dry environment. Rinse eyes with sterile saline to remove irritants. Saturated birds may benefit from a warm bath and

immediate forced warm-air drying. Apply prescribed ophthalmic ointments if corneal ulcers are present after fluorescein staining. Provide nebulization with sterile saline. If prescribed, administer antimicrobials/anti-inflammatory agents.

13.9.6 Prevention and Control

- **Housing and Ventilation**
  Ensure ventilation systems (fans, windows, and vents) provide a steady flow of fresh air. Avoid shutting down ventilation completely during cold weather. Balance heat conservation with air quality. Test ventilation where chickens live, not just at human height. Eliminate "dead zones" where air stagnates and ammonia accumulates.
- **Litter Management**
  Keep bedding dry with frequent cleaning, removing damp areas, and repairing leaky waterers. Use clean absorbent bedding materials (pine shavings and chopped straw).

13.9.7 Nursing Considerations

Nursing care for chickens suffering from ammonia toxicity requires supportive care and careful environmental correction to reduce further exposure and allow respiratory healing. Birds with ocular or respiratory irritation should be moved to a clean, well-ventilated area with fresh litter and appropriate bird: enclosure ratio, ensuring that ammonia levels are kept within safe limits (<25 ppm). Veterinary technicians should monitor affected birds for respiratory distress, ocular lesions, conjunctivitis, or corneal damage, providing supportive therapies such as ophthalmic rinses or lubricants under veterinary guidance. Ensuring adequate hydration and easy access to feed is important, since affected birds may eat or drink less due to eye pain or labored breathing. Administer prescribed medications and other therapeutics. Observation should also include assessing for secondary infections, particularly bacterial respiratory disease, which are common sequelae of ammonia-induced tissue damage. Client education plays a key role; caretakers should be instructed on proper husbandry, ventilation, humidity control, and bird: enclosure ratio adjustments to prevent recurrence. In severe cases where birds suffer permanent ocular or respiratory damage, technicians may need to assist caretakers with decisions regarding long-term welfare.

13.10 Anophthalmia

13.10.1 Overview and Pathogenesis

Anophthalmia in chickens is a rare congenital disorder characterized by the complete absence of one or both eyes due to failure of ocular development during embryogenesis. Unlike microphthalmia, where a small but malformed eye is present, anophthalmia involves a total lack of eye tissue, often accompanied by abnormalities of the optic nerve, orbit, or surrounding craniofacial structures.

Pathogenesis is linked to disruptions in early embryonic development of the optic vesicle and optic cup, which normally give rise to the retina and other ocular structures. Genetic mutations, hereditary defects, in ovo exposure to teratogenic agents (such as certain mycotoxins, vitamin A deficiency, or toxic chemicals), and viral infections during embryogenesis have all been implicated as potential causes. In some cases, anophthalmia is part of a broader craniofacial or neurologic malformation syndrome. Clinically, affected chicks hatch with one or both eyes absent, which may compromise vision, feeding ability, and navigation. While the condition is nonprogressive and not contagious, birds with bilateral anophthalmia are often severely handicapped and may struggle to thrive in normal flock environments.

13.10.2 Risk Factors

- **Genetic Factors**
  Certain lines or breeds may carry heritable mutations affecting ocular formation. Inbreeding increases the likelihood of expressing such defects. Errors in early embryogenesis may prevent normal optic vesicle formation.
- **Nutritional Deficiencies**
  Vitamin A is critical for ocular development; deficiency in breeder hens can cause malformations in embryos. Insufficient riboflavin or other essential vitamins may contribute to defective eye development.
- **Environmental and Incubation Factors**
  Excessive heat or humidity fluctuations during incubation may interfere with organogenesis. Contact with certain toxins, mycotoxins, or chemical contaminants during embryonic development may disrupt normal ocular growth. Some embryonic infections (e.g., avian encephalomyelitis, adenoviruses) have been linked to developmental anomalies.

13.10.3 Clinical Signs and Pathology

- **External Findings**
  A complete lack of an eye in the orbit(s) may be unilateral or bilateral. The orbital region may appear flattened, narrowed, or covered by skin. Skin folds may be fused or incomplete where the eye would normally be. Chicks may show poor coordination or abnormal head movements if brain or cranial nerve structures are affected during embryonic development.
- **Necropsy Findings**
  Primary lesion is a complete failure of optic vesicle or ocular tissue development. Orbit may contain only connective tissue, remnants of undeveloped ocular tissue, or be completely absent. In some cases, concurrent anomalies such as microphthalmia (abnormally small eye), cleft palate, or brain malformations may occur.

13.10.4 Diagnostic Testing

Because anophthalmia is a congenital defect, diagnosis is usually clinical and made by physical examination at hatch.

13.10.5 Treatment and Therapeutic Interventions

Anophthalmia is a congenital, irreversible defect. There are no surgical or medical interventions that can restore absent eyes.

13.10.6 Prevention and Control

- **Breeder Nutrition**
  Ensure breeder diets meet recommended vitamin A levels, which are critical for normal embryonic eye development. Adequate levels of riboflavin, folic acid, and other vitamins/minerals

support proper organogenesis. Avoid feed spoilage, mold, or toxin contamination that could affect embryo development.

- **Genetic Management**
  Inbreeding increases the risk of congenital defects, including anophthalmia.
- **Incubation and Hatching Practices**
  Maintain stable incubation conditions; avoid excessive heat, cold, or humidity fluctuations. Minimize mechanical shocks or improper turning that could disrupt embryonic development. Reduce exposure to infectious agents that may interfere with eye development (e.g., avian encephalomyelitis). Refer to Chapter 2, Incubation.

13.10.7 Nursing Considerations

Nursing care for chickens with anophthalmia focuses on ensuring safety, accessibility to feed and water, and minimizing stress, as affected birds have partial or complete loss of vision. Veterinary technicians should provide low perches or remove perches entirely, place feeders and waterers at ground level, and maintain a consistent and uncluttered environment to help visually impaired birds navigate safely. Observation is important to ensure the birds can feed, drink, and move without injury. Weak or underweight chicks may require hand-feeding or supplemental nutrition. In flocks with normal-sighted birds, social management is crucial, as visually impaired birds may be outcompeted for food or bullied; isolation or smaller groups may improve welfare. Since anophthalmia is nonprogressive and congenital, ongoing monitoring rather than treatment is appropriate, but humane considerations should guide decisions for birds that cannot thrive independently. Technicians should educate guardians on long-term husbandry adjustments, careful flock management, and welfare-focused interventions to maximize quality of life for affected birds.

13.11 Avian Philophthalmiasis

13.11.1 Overview and Pathogenesis

Avian philophthalmiasis, commonly referred to as "eye worm infection," is a parasitic condition caused by the trematode (fluke) *Thelazia* spp., which infects the conjunctival sac and lacrimal ducts of chickens and other birds. The disease is most prevalent in regions with abundant vector flies, such as *Musca* spp. or *Fannia* spp., which transmit infective larvae while feeding on ocular secretions. Incidents in North America are considered a rare zoonosis. Clinically affected birds present with conjunctivitis, excessive tearing, blepharospasm, corneal opacity, and ocular discharge, which can progress to corneal ulceration and impaired vision if untreated.

The pathogenesis involves the deposition of infective larvae into the conjunctival sac by flies, where the larvae mature into adult worms. These adult nematodes mechanically irritate the conjunctival epithelium and lacrimal ducts, causing inflammation, hyperemia, and increased tear production. Secondary bacterial infections frequently develop due to compromised ocular defenses, exacerbating inflammation and potentially leading to keratitis or corneal ulcers. Chronic infections may impair vision, reduce feeding efficiency, and predispose birds to trauma or predation. Environmental conditions such as warm, humid climates and high fly populations facilitate transmission, making control of both vectors and environmental contamination essential in managing the disease.

13.11.2 Risk Factors

- **Environmental Factors**
  Birds with access to outdoors have increased exposure to intermediate hosts, such as cockroaches, beetles, and other insects that carry infective larvae. Accumulation of feces and decaying matter supports insect populations, increasing transmission risk. Warm and humid climates are favorable for insect vectors and survival of infective larvae.

13.11.3 Clinical Signs and Pathology

- **External Findings**
  Epiphora, edema, conjunctivitis, and blepharospasm due to discomfort. Serous to mucopurulent ocular discharge. Crusting around eyelids, especially in chronic cases. Corneal opacity or ulceration in heavy infections. Head shaking or rubbing eyes and face on objects.
- **Necropsy Findings**
  Conjunctival hyperemia and edema. Lacrimal duct dilation due to parasite presence. Corneal opacity or ulceration in severe infections. Occasionally, secondary bacterial infections cause purulent exudate.

13.11.4 Diagnostic Testing

- **Direct Parasite Detection**
  Flush the conjunctival sac with sterile saline to collect larvae for microscopic examination. Adult *Oxyspirura mansoni* or larvae can be identified by morphology. Microscopic egg detection in conjunctival washings is also possible in chronic infections.

13.11.5 Treatment and Therapeutic Interventions

- **Mechanical Removal of Adult Worms**
  Adult nematodes can sometimes be carefully removed using fine forceps under anesthesia. Ensure proper restraint of the bird and gentle handling to avoid ocular injury. Conjunctival sac may be flushed with sterile saline to dislodge small worms or larvae.
- **Medication**
  Ivermectin 0.2–0.4 mg/kg once by mouth or topically, repeat in 10–14 days.

13.11.6 Prevention and Control

- **Vector Control**
  Prevent pests: cockroaches, beetles, grasshoppers, and other insects that act as intermediate hosts, with frequent cleaning. Use insecticides or traps safely around housing, following label instructions for poultry environments. Remove debris, decaying vegetation, and standing water that promote insect breeding.

13.11.7 Nursing Considerations

Nursing care for chickens with Avian Philophthalmus focuses on relieving ocular irritation, preventing secondary infections, and minimizing stress. Technicians should monitor affected birds for signs of conjunctivitis, corneal ulcers, excessive tearing, or visual impairment and provide clean, dust-free housing to reduce additional eye irritation. Manual removal of visible worms may be performed under anesthesia and veterinary guidance, and affected eyes should be kept clean and flushed with sterile saline or veterinary-recommended solutions. Because secondary bacterial infections are common, technicians should administer prescribed antimicrobial and analgesia therapy. Environmental management is crucial: reducing fly populations through hygiene, proper waste disposal, and fly control measures prevent further transmission. For severely affected or visually impaired birds, ensuring easy access to feed and water at ground level and minimizing competition within the flock is important. Client education on vector control, environmental sanitation, and early recognition of ocular signs is essential to reduce morbidity and prevent chronic infections.

13.12 Blindness

13.12.1 Overview and Pathogenesis

Blindness in chickens is a clinical condition characterized by partial or complete loss of vision, which can arise from congenital defects, trauma, infectious diseases, or environmental insults. Clinically, affected birds may display difficulty navigating their environment, decreased feeding efficiency, increased susceptibility to injury, and altered social behavior within the flock.

The pathogenesis depends on the underlying cause: congenital or hereditary defects (such as anophthalmia or microphthalmia) result from arrested ocular development during embryogenesis; infectious agents (including Newcastle disease virus, infectious laryngotracheitis (ILT) virus, or *M. gallisepticum*) cause ocular inflammation, corneal ulceration, or retinal damage; trauma or chemical exposure can lead to corneal perforation, lens rupture, or secondary uveitis; and environmental stressors such as high ammonia levels may damage the corneal epithelium and conjunctiva. Loss of visual input impairs coordination, feeding, and predator awareness, while secondary complications such as malnutrition, injuries, or social displacement may further compromise health. The severity and permanence of blindness vary depending on the type of insult, age at onset, and extent of ocular or neurologic damage.

13.12.2 Risk Factors

- **Genetic and Congenital Factors**
  Hereditary defects cause absent or underdeveloped eyes. Genetic malformations affect visual pathways. Inbreeding increases the likelihood of congenital ocular anomalies in certain breeds.
- **Nutritional Deficiencies**
  Vitamin A deficiency is the most significant nutritional cause; it leads to keratinization, corneal opacification, and eventual blindness. Riboflavin or other micronutrient deficiencies can impair ocular development in embryos or chicks.
- **Infectious Agents**
  Newcastle disease, ILT, Marek's disease (rare retinal lesions). *M. gallisepticum*, *E. coli*, *Staphylococcus* spp. causing conjunctivitis or keratitis. Eye worms (*O. mansoni*) and mites (e.g., *Knemidocoptes*) cause ocular damage.
- **Environmental and Management Factors**
  Chronic exposure to high ammonia levels causes conjunctival irritation and keratitis. Dusty or poorly ventilated housing leads to ocular irritation and secondary infection. Cleaning agents, pesticides, or smoke can damage corneal and conjunctival tissue.

13.12.3 Clinical Signs and Pathology

- **External Findings**
  Reduced responsiveness to visual stimuli (e.g., food, water, or movement in the environment). Hesitant or uncoordinated walking; frequent collisions with objects. Head shaking, eye rubbing, or flock mates pecking at the eyes if irritated. Cloudy or opaque corneas. Conjunctival swelling or redness (hyperemia). Excessive tearing (epiphora) or ocular discharge. Microphthalmia or anophthalmia in congenital cases. Corneal ulcers or scarring in chronic infections or trauma. Lens opacity (cataract formation) in some systemic infections or nutritional deficiencies
- **Necropsy Findings**
  Absence (anophthalmia) or underdevelopment (microphthalmia) of ocular structures. Retinal dysplasia or optic nerve hypoplasia leading to loss of visual function. Squamous metaplasia of conjunctival and corneal epithelium. Keratin deposition causing corneal opacification and xerophthalmia. Corneal ulceration, keratitis, conjunctivitis, or uveitis. Inflammatory infiltrates (heterophils, lymphocytes, plasma cells) in conjunctival tissue.

13.12.4 Diagnostic Testing

- **Menace Response**
  Move hand toward the eye to observe or use the cotton ball test.

13.12.5 Treatment and Therapeutic Interventions

- Unless vision loss is a result of glaucoma or cataracts, there is no treatment for this condition.

13.12.6 Prevention and Control

- Ensure nutritional requirements are met throughout the bird's lifespan. Strict biosecurity measures. Vaccination if available.

13.12.7 Nursing Considerations

Nursing care for blind or visually impaired chickens focuses on ensuring safety, accessibility to food and water, and minimizing stress. Veterinary technicians should provide low or no perches, soft bedding, and an uncluttered environment to reduce the risk of falls and injury. Feeders and waterers should be placed at ground level and in consistent locations to help blind birds locate them easily. Close observation is important to ensure that birds can feed, drink, and move without being bullied or outcompeted by sighted flock mates; in some cases, separation into smaller groups may be necessary. Blind birds should be monitored for weight loss, dehydration, or injuries, and supplemental feeding or hydration may be required for severely impaired individuals. Environmental consistency, gentle handling, and limiting sudden changes are crucial for stress reduction. Technicians should also educate caretakers on long-term management strategies, including safe housing, consistent flock routines, and monitoring for secondary complications, to maintain the welfare and quality of life for visually impaired birds.

13.13 Cataracts

13.13.1 Overview and Pathogenesis

Cataracts in chickens refer to an opacity of the lens of the eye that interferes with the passage of light and results in varying degrees of visual impairment. They can occur in birds of any age but are more common in older poultry or in association with certain nutritional, infectious, or management-related factors. Cataracts are significant because they may affect a bird's ability to find food and water, leading to reduced productivity, poor growth, or compromised welfare. In commercial settings, they are also associated with specific infectious diseases such as Marek's disease and AE, as well as with metabolic and nutritional imbalances.

The pathogenesis of cataracts in chickens generally involves disruption of normal lens metabolism and structure. The lens is normally avascular and relies on active transport mechanisms to maintain its transparency by regulating water, electrolytes, and protein stability. When these processes are disturbed, lens proteins (particularly crystallin) undergo denaturation and aggregation, leading to light scattering and lens opacity. Causes include oxidative stress, nutritional deficiencies (notably riboflavin and tryptophan), genetic predispositions, or damage secondary to viral infections that affect the nervous system and ocular tissues. Marek's disease, for example, induces lymphoid infiltration and metabolic disruption in the lens, while AE interferes with normal neural development, resulting in congenital cataracts in chicks. Over time, opacity may worsen, progressively impair vision, and increase susceptibility to trauma or starvation if the bird cannot navigate its environment effectively.

13.13.2 Risk Factors

- **Nutritional Factors**
  Deficiencies in niacin, riboflavin, vitamin E, and selenium. High oxidized fats or rancid feeds can lead to oxidative stress. Low antioxidant status leads to increased lens damage.
- **Infectious/Disease-Related Factors**
  AEV is the classic cause of cataracts in chicks. Marek's disease causes infiltration of lymphoid cells into the eye. Systemic infections cause high fever or metabolic stress.
- **Host-Related Factors**
  Older birds are more prone due to natural lens protein denaturation. Progressive oxidative damage with age. Certain strains and breeding lines show higher susceptibility. Inherited metabolic abnormalities affecting lens proteins.

13.13.3 Clinical Signs and Pathology

- **External Findings**
  Bumping into objects, difficulty finding feed/water. Startled or hesitant movements. Reduced activity, reluctance to move in bright light. Nervousness or abnormal pecking due to poor vision.
- **Necropsy Findings**
  Appears as cloudy, white, or pearly changes within the lens. May be unilateral or bilateral.

13.13.4 Diagnostic Testing

- **Ophthalmic Examination**
  Penlight or ophthalmoscope is used to detect lens opacity and determine its extent. Slit-lamp exam provides a detailed evaluation of lens structure.

13.13.5 Treatment and Therapeutic Interventions

There is no medical therapy for cataracts in chickens. Phacoemulsification performed by a veterinary ophthalmologist is a surgical corrective option. Minimal interventions focus on supportive care.

13.13.6 Prevention and Control

- **Nutritional Prevention**
  Provide balanced diets with adequate B vitamins (riboflavin, niacin), vitamin E, and selenium. Incorporate antioxidants (vitamin E, carotenoids, and selenium) to protect against oxidative damage to the lens. Avoid rancid or oxidized feed ingredients, which accelerate oxidative stress and lens protein damage.
- **Infectious Disease Control**
  Vaccinate against AEV and Marek's disease virus, both associated with cataract development (if available). Maintain strong biosecurity to reduce the introduction of viral pathogens.

13.13.7 Nursing Considerations

Nursing care for chickens with cataracts centers on maintaining quality of life, supporting vision impairment, and preventing secondary complications. Birds with cataracts should be housed in a safe, familiar, and low-stress environment to reduce the risk of injury from impaired navigation. Feeders and waterers must be kept in consistent, easily accessible locations, with wide, low-side containers to make access easier for birds with reduced eyesight. Monitoring feed and water intake is essential, since vision loss can lead to weight loss and dehydration; in severe cases, handfeeding or guiding the bird may be necessary. Isolation from aggressive flock members may be required to prevent pecking injuries, but social contact should be preserved, if possible, to reduce stress. Caregivers should also maintain good lighting and minimize sudden changes in the environment, as visually impaired birds rely on routine and spatial memory. Regular observation is important to detect signs of declining body condition, ocular irritation, or concurrent disease. Documentation on changes in vision and general health status ensures continuity of care and helps determine whether supportive management is adequate or if humane euthanasia may need to be considered in severe, welfare-compromising cases.

13.14 Conjunctivitis

13.14.1 Overview and Pathogenesis

Conjunctivitis in chickens refers to inflammation of the conjunctiva, the mucous membrane lining the eyelids and covering the sclera. It is a common clinical problem in poultry flocks and can occur as a primary condition or as part of a broader respiratory or systemic disease. Conjunctivitis is significant not only because it causes discomfort and reduced vision but also because it may signal underlying infectious, environmental, or management issues within the flock. Common causes include infectious agents such as *M. gallisepticum*, *Chlamydia psittaci*, *Avibacterium paragallinarum* (infectious coryza), Newcastle disease virus, and infectious bronchitis virus (IBV).

Noninfectious causes include high levels of dust, ammonia toxicity, trauma, or exposure to chemical irritants.

The pathogenesis of conjunctivitis depends on the underlying cause but generally follows a pattern of irritation or infection leading to inflammation of the conjunctival epithelium. Infectious organisms may adhere to or invade conjunctival tissues, triggering an inflammatory response characterized by hyperemia, edema, and exudate formation. In cases of *M. gallisepticum* infection, for example, the organism colonizes the respiratory mucosa, extends to the conjunctiva, and elicits a chronic inflammatory reaction that may lead to thickened conjunctiva and persistent ocular discharge. Ammonia or dust exposure causes direct chemical or mechanical irritation, damaging epithelial cells and compromising mucociliary defenses, which makes secondary infections more likely. In severe or chronic cases, conjunctival inflammation can extend to involve adjacent ocular structures, leading to keratoconjunctivitis, corneal ulcers, or impaired vision. The resulting discomfort, impaired feeding ability, and potential for systemic spread make conjunctivitis an important health and welfare concern in poultry production.

13.14.2 Risk Factors

- **Infectious Agents**
  Bacteria such as *M. gallisepticum*, *Mycoplasma synoviae*, *E. coli*, *C. psittaci*. Viruses like IBV, Newcastle disease virus, and avian influenza. *Aspergillus* spp. causes ocular mycoses. *O. mansoni* ("eyeworm") causing ocular irritation.
- **Environmental Factors**
  High ammonia levels from poor litter management irritate conjunctiva and respiratory mucosa. Dusty environments cause mechanical irritation and pathogen carriage.

13.14.3 Clinical Signs and Pathology

- **External Findings**
  Hyperemia and edema of the conjunctiva. Watery to mucoid or purulent discharge. Eyelid edema, sometimes the eye may be swollen shut. Rubbing eyes on wings or objects. Blepharospasm in bright light (photophobia). Reduced feed and water intake if vision is impaired.
- **Necropsy Findings**
  Conjunctiva is hyperemic, edematous, and thickened. Watery, mucopurulent, or caseous material in the conjunctival sac. Eyelids may be crusted, swollen, and adhered shut in advanced cases. The cornea may be cloudy, ulcerated, or perforated in severe infections. Infraorbital sinus swelling is common in *M. gallisepticum* or *E. coli* infections.

13.14.4 Diagnostic Testing

- **Conjunctival Swab**
  For bacterial culture (*Mycoplasma, E. coli, C. psittaci*) and sensitivity testing.
- **Fluorescein Staining** in case of present foreign body.
- **Exudate Cytology**
  Identifies inflammatory cells and infectious organisms.
- **Culture**
  Help guide antimicrobial therapy.

13.14.5 Treatment and Therapeutic Interventions

- **Supportive Care**
  Isolate affected birds to reduce spread in the flock. Clean eyes gently with sterile saline to remove crusts, discharge, foreign body, and keep cornea clean, moist. Reduce environmental irritants, lower ammonia, dust, and improve ventilation. Provide easy access to feed and water to prevent stress and weight loss.
- **Medication**
  Administer ophthalmic agents based on culture and sensitivity. Topical ophthalmic drops or ointments to reduce inflammation and discomfort. Systemic anti-inflammatories may be prescribed in severe cases.

13.14.6 Prevention and Control

- **Environmental Management**
  Maintaining proper ventilation prevents accumulation of ammonia and dust. Monitor litter moisture and replace wet or caked litter regularly. Reduce dust levels by using quality bedding materials and pelleted feed. Control light intensity to avoid ocular irritation.
- **Nutritional Strategies**
  Provide a balanced diet with sufficient vitamin A to support epithelial health and immune function. Supplement with antioxidants (vitamin E, selenium, carotenoids) to reduce oxidative stress. Ensure feed is fresh and uncontaminated (avoid mold and rancid fats).

13.14.7 Nursing Considerations

Nursing care for chickens with conjunctivitis focuses on reducing discomfort, preventing complications, and addressing underlying causes. Affected birds should be isolated from the main flock to prevent the spread of infectious agents and to protect them from pecking injuries, while still being housed within sight and sound of flock mates to minimize stress. The environment should be kept clean, well-ventilated, and low in dust and ammonia to reduce irritation of the eyes and respiratory tract. Gentle cleaning of the eyes with sterile saline or veterinarian-recommended solutions can help remove discharge and improve comfort, but care should be taken to avoid trauma to already inflamed tissues. Feed and water should be provided in easily accessible containers to support intake, as ocular pain and impaired vision may reduce feeding activity. Supportive care may include ensuring adequate hydration and providing soft, palatable foods. Strict biosecurity and sanitation practices are essential to prevent further spread, including dedicated equipment and hand hygiene when handling sick birds. Veterinary technicians should closely monitor for progressive ocular lesions, signs of systemic disease, or respiratory involvement and promptly implement veterinary-prescribed treatments such as antibiotics, anti-inflammatories, or ocular medications when indicated. Consistent documentation of progress helps guide ongoing management and determine when a bird can be safely reintroduced to the flock.

13.15 Glaucoma

13.15.1 Overview and Pathogenesis

Glaucoma in chickens is an ocular disorder characterized by increased intraocular pressure (IOP) resulting from impaired drainage of aqueous humor from the anterior chamber of the eye. Though relatively uncommon in poultry compared to mammals, it may occur as a spontaneous condition, secondary to trauma, intraocular inflammation (uveitis), or congenital malformations. It is clinically significant because the elevated IOP damages the retina and optic nerve, leading to progressive vision loss, ocular pain, and in severe cases, blindness. Vision impairment and pain can negatively impact feeding, social behavior, and quality of life.

The pathogenesis of glaucoma involves disruption of the normal balance between aqueous humor production and outflow. In chickens, aqueous humor is produced by the ciliary body and normally drains through the iridocorneal angle and associated outflow structures. When outflow is obstructed or reduced, whether by congenital anomalies, inflammatory debris, fibrosis, or space-occupying lesions, the continuous production of aqueous humor increases intraocular pressure. Sustained elevation of IOP causes mechanical stretching and compression of intraocular tissues, particularly the retina and optic nerve head, leading to degeneration and loss of visual function. Secondary glaucoma may develop from infectious processes (e.g., AE or ocular Marek's disease), neoplasia, or trauma that disrupts normal drainage pathways. Chronic disease results in irreversible ocular changes such as corneal edema, lens luxation, retinal degeneration, and buphthalmos (enlargement of the globe). Ultimately, progressive structural and functional damage explains the vision loss and quality of life concerns associated with this condition.

13.15.2 Risk Factors

- **Genetic and Developmental Factors**
  Congenital malformations of the anterior chamber or drainage angle cause impaired aqueous humor outflow. Hereditary predisposition in certain chicken lines is reported in research and experimental settings.
- **Ocular and Structural Factors**
  Lens luxation or cataracts may block aqueous humor flow. Ocular trauma can lead to scarring and damage to drainage pathways. Uveitis or intraocular inflammation obstructs aqueous humor outflow.
- **Infectious and Inflammatory Factors**
  Marek's disease virus can cause lymphoid infiltration and ocular tumors that disrupt intraocular fluid dynamics.
- **Environmental and Management Factors**
  Eye injuries from pecking or inadequate housing conditions. High dust or ammonia levels can predispose to ocular inflammation, increasing glaucoma risk secondarily.
- **Age-Related Factors**
  Older birds are more prone to degenerative changes in ocular tissues, increasing the risk of impaired aqueous drainage.

13.15.3 Clinical Signs and Pathology

- **External Findings**
  Enlarged, bulging eye (buphthalmia). Cloudy or bluish cornea due to edema. Dilated, fixed pupil with poor light response. Birds bump into objects and have a reduced ability to find feed and water. May show nervousness or hesitation in movement. Rubbing eyes on wings or objects due to intense pain. Blepharospasm or photophobia. Blindness is untreated or chronic.
- **Necropsy Findings**
  Enlarged globe with distended cornea and sclera. Corneal opacity or ulceration in advanced stages. The anterior chamber appears deepened, sometimes with aqueous flare. Optic nerve

head cupping (may be visible on dissection). Secondary lens displacement or cataract formation possible.

13.15.4 Diagnostic Testing

- **Tonometry**
  Measures intraocular pressure; elevated IOP confirms glaucoma. Parameter 9–22 mmHg.
- **Ophthalmoscopy**
  May show optic disc cupping or pallor. Retinal vascular attenuation and degeneration in chronic cases.

13.15.5 Treatment and Therapeutic Interventions

- **Supportive Care**
  Ensure easy access to feed and water, place in consistent, well-lit locations for visually impaired birds. Reduce obstacles in housing to prevent injury.
- **Medication**
  Topical intraocular pressure-lowering drugs:
  Dorzolamide, pilocarpine, or timolol to temporarily reduce intraocular pressure.
- **Surgical Interventions**
  Enucleation may be performed in birds if the eye is painful or severely enlarged. Lens removal or glaucoma filtration surgeries are not practical in avian-production settings.

13.15.6 Prevention and Control

- **Genetic and Developmental**
  Selective breeding, avoid using birds with congenital or hereditary ocular abnormalities.
- **Environmental Management**
  Avoid excessive brightness or continuous lighting systems that stress ocular tissues.
- **Nutritional Support**
  Provide balanced rations with adequate vitamin A, vitamin E, and selenium, supporting ocular tissue health. Ensure feed is fresh and uncontaminated to minimize oxidative stress on the eye.

13.15.7 Nursing Considerations

Nursing care for chickens with glaucoma emphasizes comfort, supportive management, and maintaining quality of life since the condition is often progressive and irreversible. Affected birds should be housed in a calm, well-lit, but not overly bright environment to minimize stress and avoid disorientation. If vision loss is present, feed and water should be kept in consistent, easily accessible locations, with wide containers to reduce difficulty in locating resources. Birds with impaired vision should be monitored closely for changes in body condition, dehydration, or inability to compete with flock mates; isolation or small-group housing may be necessary to prevent pecking injuries and ensure adequate intake. Handling should be minimized and performed gently, as IOP can make the eyes painful and fragile. If veterinary treatment is prescribed, such as topical medications to lower intraocular pressure or systemic anti-inflammatories, careful and consistent administration is required, with attention to proper technique to avoid additional ocular

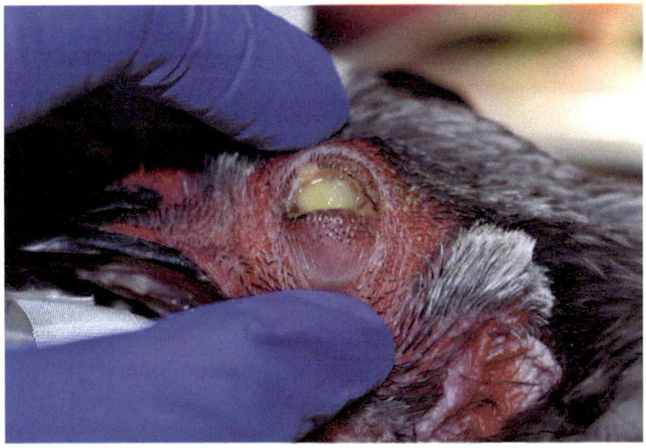

Figure 13.2 Hen with diseased eye requiring enucleation, before surgery. Courtesy of Unusual Pet Vets.

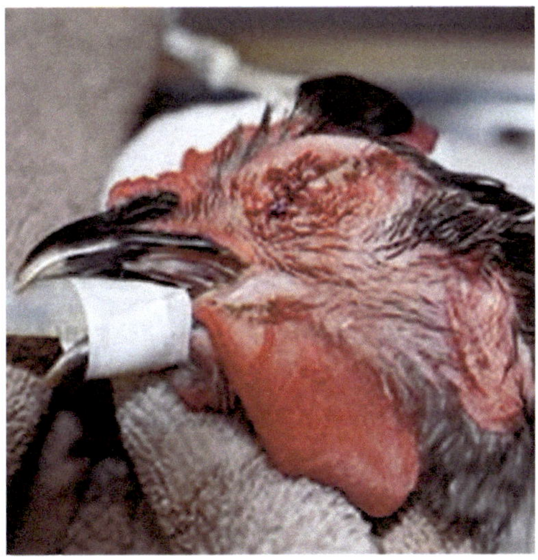

Figure 13.3 Postoperative enucleation. Courtesy of Unusual Pet Vets.

trauma. Caregivers should also regularly monitor for signs of discomfort, progressive eye enlargement, or blindness, documenting changes to guide treatment adjustments. In advanced cases in which pain and severe visual impairment compromise welfare, humane euthanasia may need to be considered (Figures 13.2 and 13.3).

Further Reading

Common Viral Diseases of Pet and Backyard Chickens | VCA Animal Hospitals [Internet]. Vca. Available from: https://vcahospitals.com/know-your-pet/common-viral-diseases-of-pet-and-backyard-chickens

Crispo M, Senties-Cué CG, Cooper GL, Mountainspring G, Corsiglia C, Bickford AA, et al. Otitis and meningoencephalitis associated with infectious coryza (*Avibacterium paragallinarum*) in commercial broiler chickens. *Journal of Veterinary Diagnostic Investigation.* 2018 Aug;30(5):784–788.

Diagnosing Neurologic Disease in Backyard Chickens | Animal Health Laboratory [Internet]. Uoguelph.ca. 2015. Available from: https://www.uoguelph.ca/ahl/diagnosing-neurologic-disease-backyard-chickens

PoultryDVM LLC. Ear Infections in Chickens: Signs, Treatment & Prevention [Internet]. PoultryDVM. Ear Infections in Chickens: Signs, Treatment & Prevention; 2017. Available from: https://poultrydvm.com/condition/ear-infection

PS47/PS044: Common Poultry Diseases [Internet]. http://edis.ifas.ufl.edu. Available from: https://ask.ifas.ufl.edu/publication/PS044

14

Anesthesia, Common Surgical Procedures, and Postoperative Care

Veterinarian surgical interventions are critical for the treatment of various conditions in chickens when medical therapies have been unsuccessful or in emergent cases. Credentialed veterinary technicians play an indispensable role in ensuring the success of these procedures through meticulous preparation and planning, anesthesia administration and patient monitoring, surgical assistance, and diligent postoperative care. This chapter aims to provide veterinary technicians with comprehensive knowledge and practical guidance on anesthesia, common surgical procedures, and postoperative care for chicken patients.

14.1 Preoperative Care: Patient Preparation

A preoperative assessment includes reviewing the chicken's signalment, previous medical history, obtaining vital signs, and ascertaining the current health status with a thorough physical examination. Performance of blood chemistry analysis, complete blood count including a manual blood smear, and diagnostic imaging (radiography, ultrasonography, advanced imaging) as indicated and ordered by the attending veterinarian provides additional patient data for planning.

Patient safety and outcome are directly affected by how well prepared the veterinary technician is for the planned procedure. Being well-prepared and having a robust minimum patient database empowers the veterinary team with information to make optimal treatment decisions, select tailored anesthetic drug protocol, assign an American Society of Anesthesiologists grade, and move forward with the procedure with confidence.

The anesthesia episode and recovery period must be documented for future ensuring patient safety, serving as a critical legal record, and improving future care through quality assurance. These records document the patient's response to anesthesia, which is vital for other veterinary healthcare providers, meet regulatory requirements, and facilitate reviews.

14.1.1 Anesthesia Preparation and Maintenance

The veterinary technician must be aware of the avian tendency to become apneic at the surgical plane of anesthesia; therefore, planning to administer assisted ventilation every 10–30 seconds. A non-cuffed endotracheal tube (preferably clear, PVC) is used to secure the airway. Anesthesia preparation involves patient fasting to avoid aspiration of crop contents. The larger the bird, the longer the fasting period (2–6 hours). Even if general anesthesia is not required or appropriate for the planned procedure, the veterinary technician must ensure all anesthesia equipment is properly maintained and operational, ready for use. Before any anesthetic agent is administered, flow-by or masked oxygenation is performed for a minimum of 5 minutes for hemoglobin saturation and hypoxemia prevention. The use of a nonrebreathing system for chickens weighing less than 7 kg is best practice once the uncuffed endotracheal tube is secured. Tidal volume is 15 mL/kg.

14.1.2 Premedication

As a part of a multimodal anesthetic plan, a premedication of an injectable opioid with sedative quality is administered intramuscularly for anxiolysis, facilitation of handling, analgesia, and the reduction of inhalant anesthetic required for surgical plane of anesthesia.

Opioids are administered preoperative, intraoperative, and/or postoperative to block pain receptors:

- Butorphanol 1–4 mg/kg (intramuscular [IM], intravenous [IV], per os [by mouth]) every 1–3 hours for kappa/weak mu receptor (mild) activity.
- Tramadol 15 mg/kg PO every 12 hours for mu agonist/weak kappa/delta activity.

Nonsteroidal anti-inflammatory agents are administered preoperatively or postoperatively to relieve acute and chronic musculoskeletal and visceral pain.

- **Carprofen:** 1–4 mg/kg PO, SQ, or IM q 12–24 hours for less than 7 days; weak inhibition of COX-1 and COX-2
- **Meloxicam:** 0.50–2.0 mg/kg PO or IM q12–24 hours; selective COX-2 inhibitor
- **Celecoxib:** 10–20 mg/kg PO q 24 hours; selective COX-2 inhibitor

Local anesthetics are administered for nerve blocks (injection or splash) by infusing into the intended tissues once the bird has reached surgical plane of anesthesias.

- Bupivicaine 5 mg/mL, 1–2 mg/kg
- Lidocaine 20 mg/mL, 2–3 mg/kg

Gabapentin 10–25 mg/kg PO q 8–12 hours pre- and postoperatively.

14.1.3 Induction and Maintenance Periods

Injectable agents, such as propofol, can be administered intravenously for induction prior to endotracheal intubation if desired at 20 mg/kg. Boluses of 3 mg/kg can be infused to maintain surgical anesthesia.

Volatile, inhalant agents are administered via induction mask and uncuffed endotracheal tube; in conjunction with analgesic premedication. Endotracheal intubation is recommended for all birds undergoing anesthesia to provide assisted ventilation and ensure adequate gas exchange. The oxygen flow rate is 0.5–2 L/min.

- Isoflurane at 3–4% induction, while the bird is gently restrained, until the veterinary technician performs endotracheal intubation for a secure airway. Maintain at the lowest surgical plane of

anesthesia (absence of reflexes, reduced vital signs) at 0.5–2.5%.
- Sevoflurane at 4–5% induction; 3–4% maintenance (Figure 14.1).

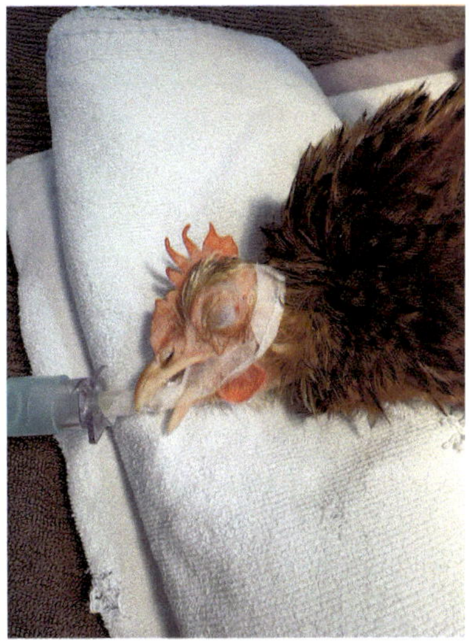

Figure 14.1 Endotracheal intubation of an anesthetized hen. Courtesy of Unusual Pet Vets.

14.1.4 Anesthetized Patient Monitoring

Patient vital sign monitoring devices include electrocardiogram (alcohol-soaked gauze on clips placed on the wings and at the base of the legs), Doppler blood flow for heart rate, and indirect blood pressure (using an oscillometric cuff). The Doppler crystal is placed over the medial metatarsal or brachial artery. SpO_2 (placement on the tongue, comb, wattle, or cloaca), end tidal carbon dioxide sampling attachment, and esophageal temperature probe (or manual thermometer in the cloaca) are also best practice to collect data and assess an anesthetized patient's condition.

Assisted ventilation regularly ensures proper gas exchange within the alveoli. If apnea occurs, lighten anesthesia and continue assisted ventilation. A Doppler blood pressure reading above 90 mmHg is considered acceptable in chickens. Ensure the chicken's body temperature is maintained as close to normal as possible to aid with anesthesia recovery. Body temperature can decrease significantly within 10–15 minutes. Forced warm air units and/or circulating water blankets are recommended. There is no piece of monitoring equipment that can replace the skill and diligence of a credentialed veterinary technician.

14.1.5 Surgical Site Preparation and Local Anesthetics

Pluck feathers at the intended surgical site and the surrounding area. Using warm antiseptic solutions and cotton (chlorhexidine scrub and chlorhexidine 0.5–1% or povidone iodine scrub and "paint" solution), prepare the site according to the anatomic location (target pattern, striping, etc.). Once the site has been prepared and dried, nerve blocks with lidocaine or bupivicaine (line or splash) may be performed, avoiding contamination of the freshly prepared site.

14.2 Intraoperative Care

Constant anesthetized patient monitoring: heart rate, respiratory rate, oxygen saturation, blood pressure, and temperature, along with assessing the bird's reflexes, determine its depth of anesthesia. Monitor the endotracheal tube for occlusions. Birds do not tolerate apnea; during assisted ventilation, do not exceed 15–20 cm H_2O. Administering intravenous crystalloid fluids (100 mL/kg) to maintain blood pressure, tissue perfusion, and hydration to increase the likelihood of a favorable patient outcome. Burette usage is recommended for accurate fluid delivery. If the patient is anesthetized for an hour or longer, additional opioids are administered parenterally until medications can be administered via the enteral route. Alert the surgeon of any abnormal occurrences during the procedure.

Parameter	Normal range	Notes
Body temperature	104–107.6°F	Esophageal probe or cloaca thermometer
Heart rate	250–325 bpm	Chicks: 300–400 bpm
Respiratory rate	15–30 bpm	Monitor for panting, wheezing, or increased effort
Capillary refill time	<2 seconds	Check by blanching comb or wattle; prolonged CRT indicates poor perfusion
SpO_2	95–100%	Comb or wattle; monitor color
End tidal carbon dioxide ($ETCO_2$)	30–45 mmHg	Side-stream or mainstream sample
Blood pressure (Systolic)	>90 mmHg	Doppler, oscillometric cuff

Table courtesy of Sarah Meyer.

14.3 Postoperative Care

Recovery from anesthesia begins the moment after the inhalant vaporizer is turned off. Chickens are allowed to breathe 100% oxygen until extubation and are safely recovered being lightly wrapped in a towel to prevent self-trauma. Unless otherwise indicated (crop surgery, etc.), chickens can begin eating regular foodstuffs and drinking once alert. Maintain postoperative patients in a warm (preferably humid), darkened, quiet, and clean enclosure and sternal recumbency. Avoid hyperthermia. Some sources recommend lightly wrapping the chicken in a towel to prevent self-trauma from flapping and struggling to recover from anesthesia. Once fully recovered and standing, the chicken can return to a normal enclosure. A painful chicken will exhibit avoidance behavior, withdrawal, vocalization, elevated heart rate, and blood pressure. Provide analgesia on a regular basis to prevent spinal wind-up.

Surgical wounds are monitored at least once daily for dehiscence, discharge, signs of infection, or hemorrhage. A dilute, warm antiseptic solution is used to cleanse wounds as necessary. Bandages are kept clean and changed when soiled or as directed by the veterinarian. Oral medications are prescribed and dispensed, and guardians should receive a discharge appointment to discuss home care and address any concerns. Follow-up appointments are scheduled to assess wound healing and document progress.

14.4 Surgical Procedures

14.4.1 Impacted Crop

14.4.1.1 Overview

The crop is a thin-walled diverticulum of the esophagus in chickens, serving as a temporary food storage organ. Surgical intervention is sometimes required when impaction cannot be resolved through medical management. Impacted crop surgery, or ingluviotomy, is a relatively common avian surgical procedure and, when performed correctly, results in rapid return to function.

14.4.1.2 Surgical Procedure

Per surgeons' preference, the patient may be in dorsal recumbency under general anesthesia or a local line nerve block performed, and the procedure may be performed under light sedation only. The feathers of the anterior area cranial to the breast are plucked, and the area is aseptically prepared. A longitudinal skin incision is made over the right lateral crop region. A second incision is made through the crop wall, avoiding alignment with the skin incision. Impacted material is carefully removed; the crop is lavaged using warm sterile saline. The crop is closed with fine absorbable sutures in a simple continuous pattern, and the skin is closed separately, ideally in a pattern offset from the crop incision to minimize fistula formation (Figures 14.2–14.4).

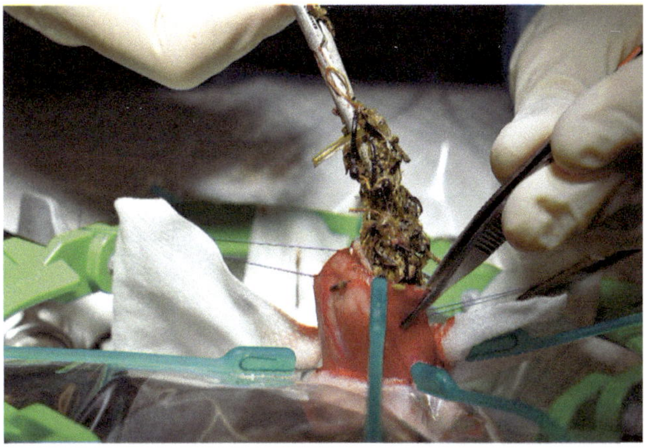

Figure 14.2 Impacted crop contents being removed with the hen under general anesthesia. Courtesy of Unusual Pet Vets.

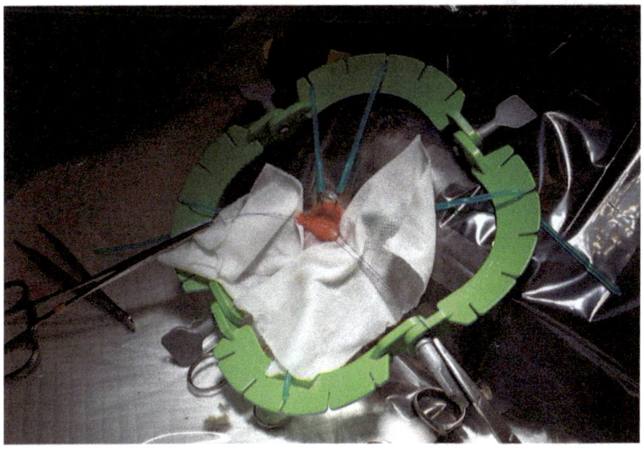

Figure 14.3 Crop completely emptied and flushed. Courtesy of Unusual Pet Vets.

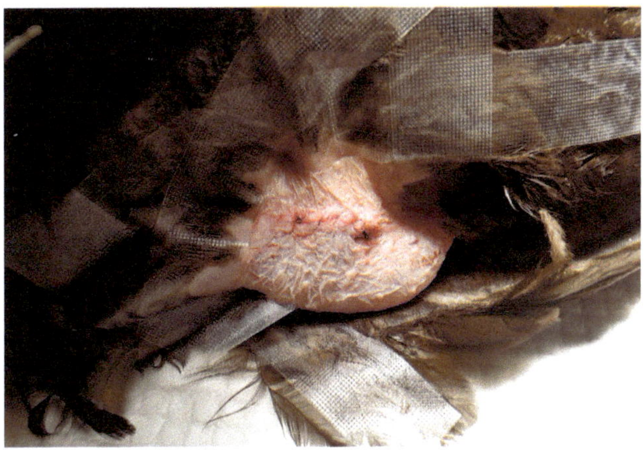

Figure 14.4 Small incision over crop sutured. Courtesy of Unusual Pet Vets.

14.4.1.3 Postoperative Care

An anti-inflammatory agent and an additional dose of opioids are administered as analgesia. The veterinarian will consider antibiotics based on contamination level and crop wall integrity. Provide a soft diet for the first 24–48 hours, gradually transitioning to normal food. Prebiotics and probiotics are recommended. Check for regurgitation, wound swelling or discharge, or dehiscence. Hospitalize the bird in a quiet, warm enclosure until discharge. A "crop bra" may be placed to protect the wound during healing, prevent self-trauma, or pecking from flock mates.

14.4.2 Oviduct Surgery

14.4.2.1 Overview

Reproductive tract disorders are among the most frequent reasons chickens require surgical intervention. Conditions such as egg binding (dystocia), salpingitis, oviduct impaction, and egg yolk peritonitis may necessitate surgical management when conservative therapy fails. Oviduct surgery, ranging from removal of obstructive material to partial salpingectomy, can be lifesaving.

14.4.2.2 Surgical Procedure

Place the anesthetized bird in dorsal recumbency, with legs secured. Pluck the feathers from the ventral abdomen; prepare the site aseptically. A midline or left lateral coelomic incision is made, depending on the access required. Gently retract the viscera to visualize the oviduct. For simple impaction or egg removal, carefully extract the obstructing material. For severe or recurrent disease, a partial salpingectomy may be performed, removing diseased sections of the oviduct. Ligate blood vessels carefully, as avian tissues bleed readily. Close the coelomic wall with absorbable suture; close the skin separately, avoiding alignment of suture lines to reduce fistula risk.

14.4.2.3 Postoperative Care

An anti-inflammatory agent and an additional dose of opioids are administered as analgesia. The veterinarian will consider antibiotics based on contamination level and crop wall integrity. Offer easily digestible feeds and fresh water once the bird is alert. Prebiotics and probiotics are recommended. Hospitalize the bird in a quiet, warm enclosure until discharge. A "bodysuit" may be placed to protect the wound during healing, prevent self-trauma, or pecking from flock mates. Antibiotics based on bacterial culture or empirical choice (commonly broad spectrum). Monitor for signs of tenesmus, anorexia, abnormal posturing, and coelomic swelling.

14.4.3 Abscess Debridement

14.4.3.1 Overview

Abscesses are common surgical presentations in chickens, most frequently associated with pododermatitis ("bumblefoot"), localized traumatic wounds, or chronic bacterial infections. Unlike mammalian abscesses, avian abscesses contain thick, caseous pus that does not drain easily. Therefore, surgical debridement is often required.

14.4.3.2 Surgical Procedure

Place the anesthetized bird in dorsal or lateral recumbency depending on the anatomic location of the lesion site. Feathers are plucked or trimmed around the abscess, and the skin is aseptically prepared. A careful incision is made over the lesion to expose the abscess capsule. Caseous pus is extracted using hemostatic forceps and curettes. The fibrous capsule and necrotic tissue are excised until healthy, viable tissue is reached. Irrigation with warm sterile saline or dilute chlorhexidine solution is performed. Depending on the site, wounds may be left partially open to heal by secondary intention or lightly closed with absorbable sutures if contamination risk is minimal (if the bird is hospitalized or kept in a stringently clean enclosure at home).

14.4.3.3 Postoperative Care

An anti-inflammatory agent and an additional dose of opioids are administered as analgesia. Offer easily digestible feeds and fresh water once the bird is alert. Prebiotics and probiotics are recommended. Hospitalize the bird in a quiet, warm enclosure until discharge. Antibiotics based on bacterial culture or empirical choice (commonly broad-spectrum). Monitor for signs of tenesmus, anorexia, abnormal posturing, and coelomic swelling.

A "bodysuit" may be placed to protect the wound during healing, prevent self-trauma, or pecking from flock mates. In pododermatitis cases, padded bandages are applied. A nonadherent pad, gauze pad, and cling bandage are used for a three-layer bandage that is changed regularly. Provide soft bedding, reduce abrasive surfaces, and ensure clean housing to prevent reinfection. Inspect for recurrence, wound dehiscence, or osteomyelitis. For chronic cases of pododermatitis, boots can be placed on chickens to provide protective padding for the plantar surface(s).

14.4.4 Vent/Cloacal Surgery

14.4.4.1 Overview

Cloacal (vent) surgery in chickens is most frequently performed to address conditions such as cloacal prolapse, papilloma, abscesses, or neoplastic growth. The cloaca is a critical anatomical structure, serving as the common exit point for gastrointestinal, urinary, and reproductive systems. Because of its complexity and constant exposure to contaminants, surgical procedures in this area are delicate and require meticulous techniques.

14.4.4.2 Surgical Procedure

Place the anesthetized bird in dorsal or lateral recumbency. Gently retract feathers around the vent and aseptically prepare the surgical field. Depending on the indication, stay sutures or gentle traction may be applied to improve visibility of cloacal tissues. Prolapse correction, necrotic or devitalized tissue is excised. Remaining mucosa is lubricated and replaced into the cloacal lumen. Temporary purse-string sutures may be placed at the vent margins, leaving sufficient space for fecal passage. For mass or abscess removal, lesions are carefully excised with attention to preserving cloacal function. Hemostasis is achieved using electrocautery or manual pressure. The site is flushed with warm sterile saline or diluted chlorhexidine. Absorbable monofilament sutures are used for deeper layers; skin or mucosal margins may be left open for drainage if infection risk is high.

14.4.4.3 Postoperative Care

An anti-inflammatory agent and an additional dose of opioids are administered as analgesia. Offer easily digestible feeds and fresh water once the bird is alert. Prebiotics and probiotics are recommended. Hospitalize the bird in a quiet, warm enclosure until discharge. Antibiotics based on bacterial culture or empirical choice (commonly broad-spectrum). Monitor for signs of tenesmus, anorexia, abnormal posturing, and coelomic swelling.

In prolapse cases, external protective dressings or a "body suit" with a disposable pad may be applied to prevent pecking by flock mates. Frequent monitoring for the ability to defecate, recurrence of prolapse, wound dehiscence, or stricture formation.

14.4.5 Tumor Excision

14.4.5.1 Overview

Neoplastic conditions in chickens are increasingly being diagnosed as companion birds and backyard flocks receive regular preventive and advanced veterinary care. Common tumors include squamous cell carcinoma, fibrosarcoma, lipoma, and lymphoid tumors associated with Marek's disease or avian leukosis virus. Tumor excision can provide therapeutic and palliative benefits, improving quality of life. Due to the small patient size, fragile tissues, and high anesthetic risk, surgery requires precise technique and diligent perioperative care.

14.4.5.2 Surgical Procedure

Position the bird for optimal surgical access; pluck and aseptically prepare the surgical field. A skin incision is made directly over the tumor, extending beyond the visible margins. Sharp and blunt dissection are performed to separate tumor tissue from the surrounding structures. Hemostasis is achieved with electrocautery or manual pressure. Care is taken to preserve vital vessels, nerves, and adjacent organs. The mass is excised with wide margins, when possible, to reduce recurrence. Wound edges are apposed using absorbable monofilament sutures. Tension-free closure is preferred; in some cases, secondary intention healing may be chosen if tissue loss is significant.

14.4.5.3 Postoperative Care

An anti-inflammatory agent and an additional dose of opioids are administered as analgesia. Offer easily digestible feeds and fresh water once the bird is alert. Prebiotics and probiotics are recommended. Hospitalize the bird in a quiet, warm enclosure until discharge. Antibiotics based on bacterial culture or empirical choice (commonly broad-spectrum). Monitor for signs of tenesmus, anorexia, abnormal posturing, and coelomic swelling.

External protective bandaging or a "body suit" may be applied to prevent pecking by flock mates. Frequent monitoring for the hemorrhage, wound dehiscence, and signs of incision infection.

14.4.6 Enucleation

14.4.6.1 Overview

Enucleation is indicated when the eye is painful, irreversibly damaged, blind, or harboring neoplasia or severe infection. Irreversible ocular disease, such as severe corneal ulcers or chronic infection. Birds typically adapt well to monocular vision.

14.4.6.2 Surgical Steps

Make a circular incision around the eyelids. Carefully dissect the orbital muscles and connective tissue from the globe. Identify and gently ligate the optic nerve and associated blood vessels. Excise the eye carefully, ensuring complete removal of the globe. Achieve hemostasis with gentle pressure, cautery, or absorbable suture as needed. Close the conjunctival sac and surrounding tissues with absorbable suture. Consider leaving eyelids partially open or using a temporary tarsorrhaphy if swelling is expected. In cases with significant inflammation or exudate, a small drain may be placed (Figures 14.5–14.7).

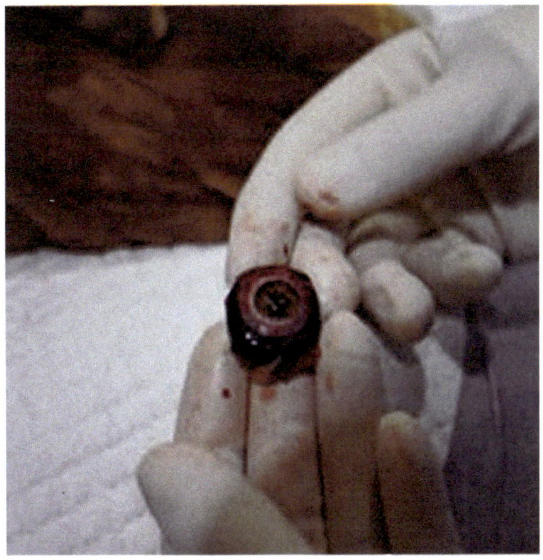

Figure 14.5 Enucleated eye from a hen. Courtesy of Unusual Pet Vets.

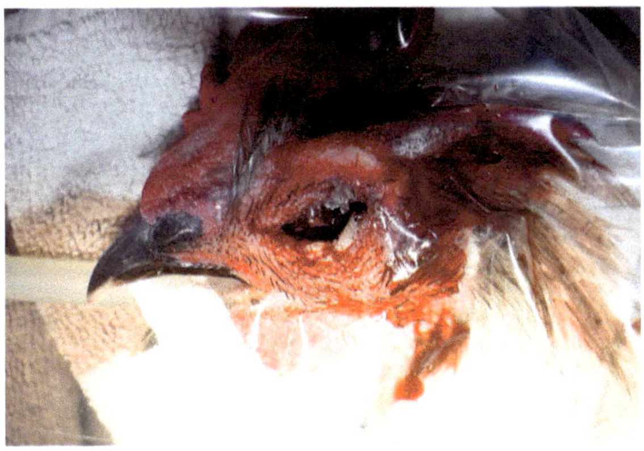

Figure 14.6 Hen under general anesthesia with the eye freshly enucleated. Courtesy of Unusual Pet Vets.

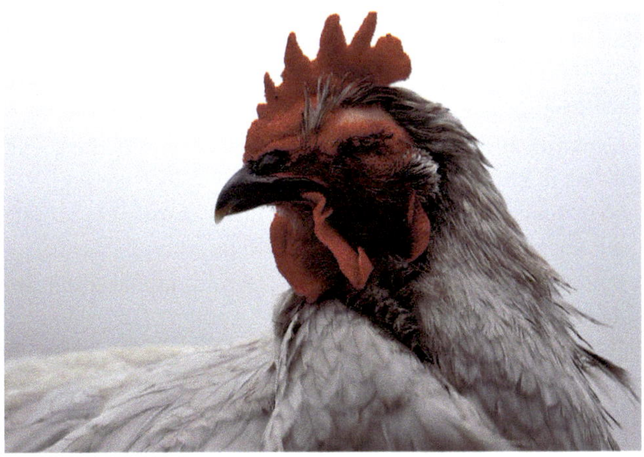

Figure 14.7 Hen recovered from the eyeball enucleation procedure. Courtesy of Unusual Pet Vets.

14.4.6.3 Postoperative Care

An anti-inflammatory agent and an additional dose of opioids are administered as analgesia. Offer easily digestible feeds and fresh water once the bird is alert. Prebiotics and probiotics are recommended. A cool/cold pack applied to the surgical site reduces swelling if the patient tolerates this treatment. Hospitalize the bird in a quiet, warm enclosure until discharge.

Topical or systemic antibiotics may be used to prevent secondary infection, particularly if preoperative infection was present. Keep the bird isolated from other birds initially to reduce stress and risk of trauma. Provide a quiet, low-light environment to minimize agitation. Ensure easy access to feed and water, as birds may be disoriented initially, and monitor intake to prevent dehydration or weight loss. Frequent monitoring for the hemorrhage, wound dehiscence, and signs of incision infection. Ensure sutures are intact, and no necrotic tissue develops. If placed, remove nonabsorbable sutures as directed (usually 7–10 days).

14.5 Conclusion

While the veterinarian performs the surgical procedures described in this chapter, the credentialed veterinary technician provides the care necessary as an anesthetist, surgical nurse, and postoperative caregiver. Patient outcomes depend on thorough preparation, planning, and communication within the veterinary healthcare team. Regular protocol reviews, case debriefing, and continuing education ensure robust, relevant patient care.

For in-depth surgical techniques, refer to *Backyard Poultry Medicine and Surgery: A Guide for Veterinary Practitioners*, Second Edition. For more information regarding chicken home care, see Client Education and Discharge Instructions in Chapter 17.

Further Reading

Çelik Y, Atalan G, Güneş V, Alpman U, Yönez MK. Use of medetomidine, midazolam, ketamine and sevoflurane as an anesthetic protocol for domestic chickens. *Veterinaria México OA*. 2020 Mar;7(1).

Gregory A. Pain Management in the Avian Patient [Internet]. Improveinternational.com. Improve International Limited; 2022 [cited 2025 Dec 8]. Available from: https://improveinternational.com/uk/clinical-library/pain-management-in-the-avian-patient

Hatt J-M, Kreyenbühl K, Kummrow M. Methods of analgesia and euthanasia in backyard poultry. *Schweizer Archiv Fur Tierheilkunde*. 2023 Jul;165(7):503–511.

Muir WW, Al E. Handbook of Veterinary Anesthesia. St. Louis, Elsevier Mosby; 2013.

Santos EA, Monteiro ER, Herrera JR, Mombach VS, Boos MZ, Gutierrez LG, et al. Total intravenous anesthesia in domestic chicken (*Gallus gallus domesticus*) with propofol alone or in combination with methadone, nalbuphine or fentanyl for ulna osteotomy. *Veterinary Anaesthesia and Analgesia [Internet]*. 2020 May;47(3):347–355. Available from: https://pubmed.ncbi.nlm.nih.gov/32222345

Sedation in Birds - ExoticsCon Virtual 2020 - VIN [Internet]. Vin.com. 2020. Available from: https://www.vin.com/apputil/content/defaultadv1.aspx?pId=25844&catId=150703&id=9768898

Sha J, Kongara K, Singh P, Jacob A, Ponnampalam J. Pharmacokinetics and pharmacodynamics of butorphanol and dexmedetomidine after intranasal administration in broiler chickens (*Gallus gallus domesticus*). *Veterinary Sciences*. 2022 Apr;9(5):212.

World Small Animal Veterinary Association Congress Proceedings, 2017. VINcom [Internet]. 2017 Sep 25; Available from: https://www.vin.com/apputil/content/defaultadv1.aspx?id=8506509&pid=20539&

Wing Lin G. Long-Term Prognosis and Treatment of Crop Impaction in Chickens via Ingluviotomy with Local Infiltration Anesthetic: Case Report [Internet]. [cited 2025 Nov 24]. Available from: https://bioone.org/journals/avian-diseases/volume-66/issue-3/aviandiseases-D-22-00024/Long-Term-Prognosis-and-Treatment-of-Crop-Impaction-in-Chickens/10.1637/aviandiseases-D-22-00024.short

15

Emergent Care and Wound Management

15.1 Emergency Stabilization

Wounded chickens often arrive in shock, which must be addressed before diagnostic testing and definitive therapy. The veterinary team must assess the risk of stress versus the benefit of treatment. The same principles of calm/quiet/dark are applied, just as during a well-bird physical examination, but with a sense of urgency as to not exacerbate the patient's stress.

15.1.1 Oxygen Supplementation

- Hyperbaric box with passive scavenge system
- Mask with nonrebreathing system and passive scavenge system
- Endotracheal intubation with non-cuffed clear, PVC tube

15.1.2 Fluid Therapy

- **Routes and locations**
  - IV (jugular, medial metatarsal vein)—preferred in unstable patients.
  - IO (dorsal distal ulna)—reliable for small or collapsed birds.
  - SQ (inguinal region, under the wing)—for mild dehydration only.
  - PO
  - Cloacal (Figure 15.1)
- **Crystalloid Fluids**: 5–10% dehydration estimate with trauma or severe illness.
  - **Lactated Ringer's for Shock**: 0.9% NaCl for metabolic acidosis. Warmed before administration.
  - **Initial Resuscitation (Shock)**: Bolus 30 mL/kg given as a single intravenous, intraosseous, or subcutaneous bolus, ideally warmed to 100–102°F.
    - **Further Boluses**: Additional crystalloid (10 mL/kg) and colloid (5 mL/kg) boluses can be given until systolic blood pressure exceeds 90 mmHg.
  - **Dosage**: 50–150 mL/kg/day maintenance, with boluses for shock (10–20 mL/kg, IV/IO).
- **Colloid Fluids:**
  - Oxyglobin single dose of 15 mL/kg IV or IO (avoid humerus, femur)
  - Whole blood (1% collected from donor) 0.5 mL/kg for 20 minutes; total volume within 4 hours; IV or IO.
  - Transfusion of blood is also discussed in Chapter 13.

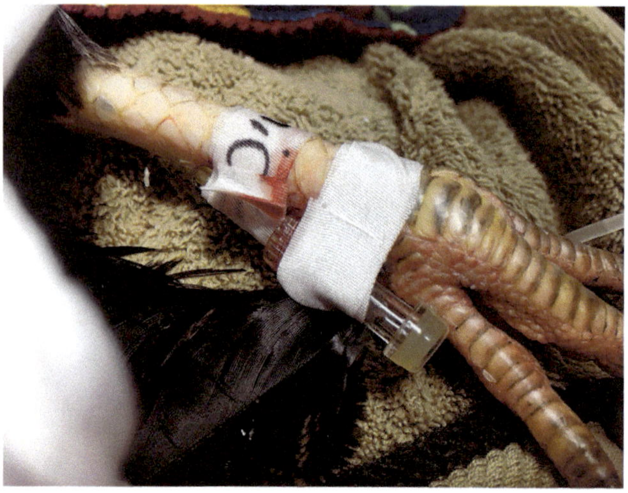

Figure 15.1 Medial metatarsal intravenous catheter in a hen's leg. Courtesy of Unusual Pet Vets.

15.1.3 Thermal Support

- Hypothermia is common due to shock and feather loss.
- Draft-free enclosure with soft, clean bedding (fleece blankets hold warmth).
- Provide external heat (warming pads, forced-air incubators).
- Avoid overheating (>103°F), which increases stress.

15.1.4 Hemorrhage Mitigation

- Apply direct pressure with gauze.
- Pluck the blood feather and apply pressure with gauze.
- Use hemostatic agents (styptic powder, silver nitrate) sparingly as they are caustic.
- Surgical ligation or cautery under anesthesia for arterial bleeds (Figures 15.2 and 15.3).

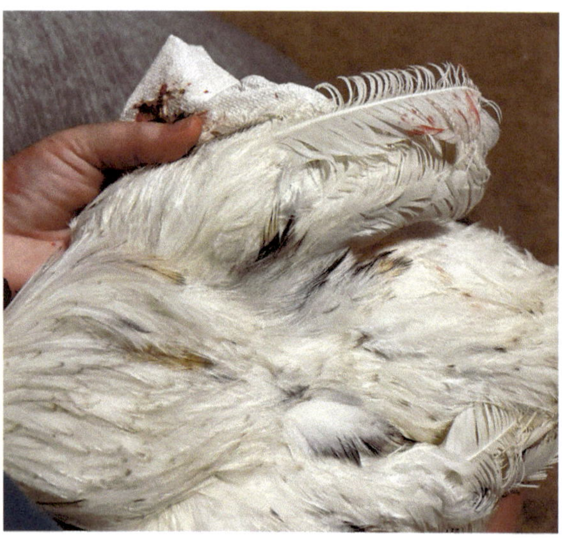

Figure 15.2 Broken blood feathers. Affected feathers were plucked, and direct pressure was applied until bleeding ceased. Courtesy of Stephanie Freeman.

15.1.5 Analgesia

There is a more extensive list of analgesics for use in chickens in Chapter 16; this is an abbreviated list for use in emergent cases.

- Butorphanol 1–4 mg/kg IM/IV/IN every 1–3 hours, up to every 12 hours
- Carprofen 1–4 mg/kg PO, SQ, or IM q 12–24 hours; no longer than 7 days
- Meloxicam 0.50–2.0 mg/kg PO or IM q12–24 hours; no longer than 7 days
- Bupivicaine 5 mg/mL, 1–2 mg/kg for perineural blockades
- Lidocaine 20 mg/mL, 2–3 mg/kg for perineural blockades

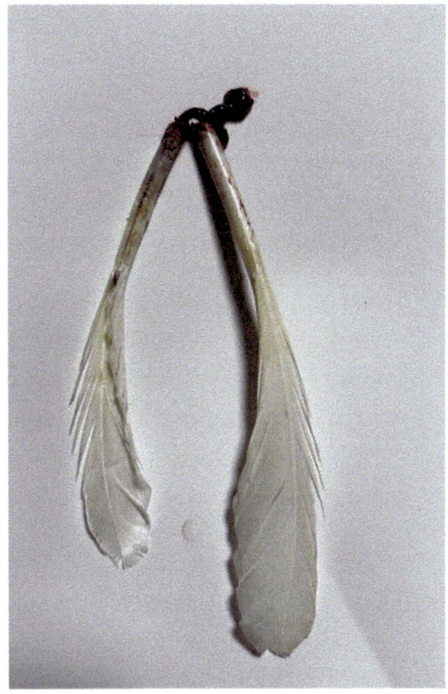

Figure 15.3 Removed feather; note the blood clot. Courtesy of Stephanie Freeman.

15.2 When to Seek Immediate Veterinary Attention

Provide guardians with "red flag" requiring urgent care or necropsy:

- Hemorrhage from wounds, broken blood feathers
- Sudden death or rapid deterioration
- Severe respiratory distress
- Neurological signs (seizures, head tremors, paralysis)
- Profuse diarrhea, bloody droppings, or persistent anorexia
- Swollen joints, severe lameness, or bone fractures
- Any signs of pain, distress, or unresponsive behavior

15.3 Wound Management

Wounds are a common clinical presentation in backyard poultry medicine and may occur due to predator attacks, conspecific aggression, environmental hazards, or iatrogenic causes. While many wounds appear superficial, chickens are highly susceptible to shock, rapid infection, and systemic decline, making prompt assessment and appropriate nursing care essential.

Unlike companion mammals, chickens present unique challenges in wound management due to their:

- Distinct integumentary system (thin skin, feather coverage, limited subcutaneous tissue).
- Rapid onset of shock following trauma.
- High risk of septicemia from Gram-negative bacteria such as *Escherichia coli* and *Pseudomonas*.
- Prey species behavior, which leads them to hide signs of pain or illness until late stages.

Credentialed veterinary technicians play a pivotal role in wound management, from triage and stabilization to bandage changes, monitoring, and client education. An understanding of avian anatomy, wound classification, and early clinical signs is crucial to developing an effective therapeutic plan.

15.4 Avian Integument and Wound Healing Physiology

15.4.1 Structure of Chicken Skin

The chicken's skin is the largest organ of the body, serving as the first line of defense against pathogens, trauma, and environmental injury. It is structurally thinner and more fragile than mammalian skin, with less subcutaneous fat (except in certain regions such as the keel and abdomen).

- **Epidermis**: thin, stratified squamous epithelium, keratinized in older birds.
- **Dermis**: relatively sparse connective tissue with limited elasticity.
- **Feather Follicles**: densely populate most of the body, complicating wound visualization.
- **Apteria (Featherless Tracts)**: common sites of injury due to less protective coverage.

15.4.2 Vascular Supply and Healing

Avian skin is well vascularized, allowing for rapid clot formation, but limited dermal thickness results in decreased tissue reserves for suturing. Chickens tend to rely more on secondary intention healing than mammals, especially for contaminated or extensive wounds. Integument diseases are discussed in Chapter 7.

Phases of Avian Wound Healing:

- **Hemostasis**: rapid clotting, often visible within minutes.
- **Inflammation**: infiltration of heterophils (avian equivalent of neutrophils), macrophages.
- **Proliferation**: fibroblast and keratinocyte migration, granulation tissue formation.
- **Maturation/Remodeling**: epithelialization and scar formation.

Feathers regrow in healed areas only if follicles remain intact. Severe tissue and follicular trauma can lead to permanent feather loss.

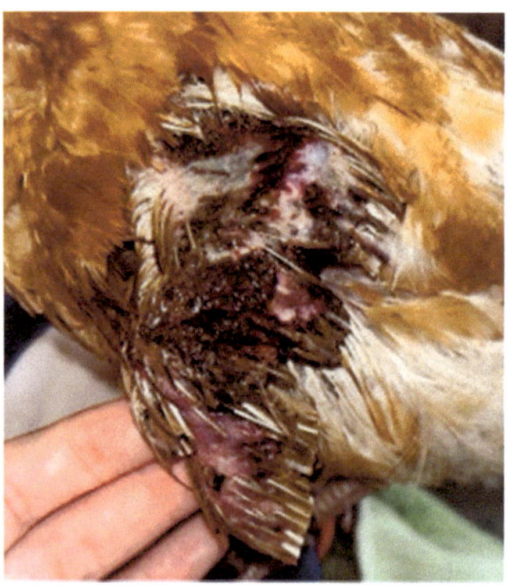

Figure 15.4 Young cockerel with wing wounds from predator attack. Day 1. Courtesy of Stephanie Freeman.

15.4.3 Comparative Anatomy with Mammals

- Less subcutaneous fat resulting in reduced insulation, higher risk of hypothermia during treatments or surgical procedures requiring anesthesia.
- Friable skin makes it more prone to tearing with aggressive handling or suturing.
- High metabolic rate making wounds progress more rapidly through inflammatory phases.

15.5 Classification of Wounds in Chickens

Veterinary professionals classify wounds by etiology, depth, contamination, and chronicity. Understanding wound type guides decisions regarding debridement, closure, and antimicrobial use (Figures 15.4–15.7).

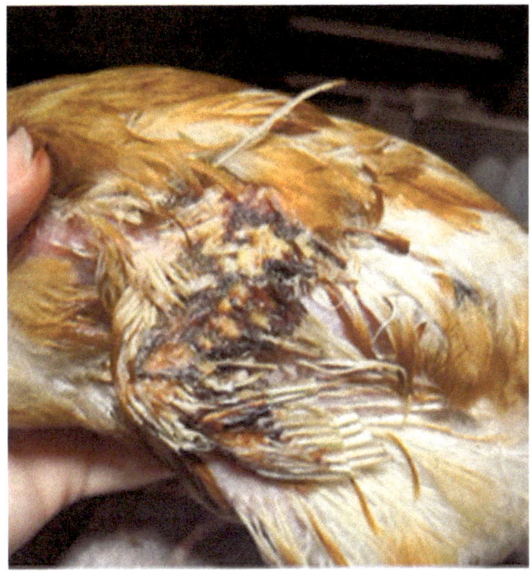

Figure 15.5 Day 7 of wound healing. Courtesy of Stephanie Freeman.

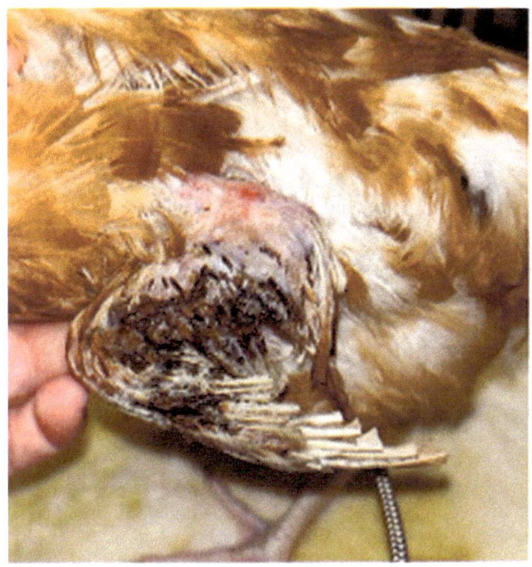

Figure 15.6 Day 14 of wound healing. Note the feathers regrowing from being clipped for treatment. Courtesy of Stephanie Freeman.

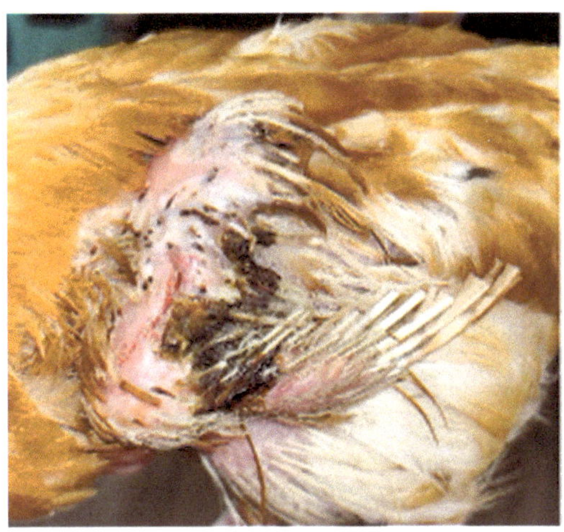

Figure 15.7 Day 18. Severe traumatic wound on the wing of a cockerel. Supportive care, antibiotics, and anti-inflammatory agents were administered. The wound was fully healed within a month's duration. Courtesy of Stephanie Freeman.

15.5.1 By Etiology

- **Incised Wounds**: sharp objects (wire, glass, metal); clean edges; amenable to surgical closure.
- **Lacerations**: tearing of skin/tissue; irregular edges; common from predator claws or sharp coop hardware.
- **Puncture Wounds**: caused by beaks, talons, nails, or teeth; high risk of anaerobic infection and abscess formation.
- **Degloving/Avulsion Injuries**: shearing trauma with tissue loss, often on legs, wings, dorsum.
- **Burns/Frostbite**: thermal damage from heat lamps, fires, or freezing temperatures; can cause necrosis and secondary infection.
- **Pressure Sores**: keel or hock lesions from poor bedding, prolonged recumbency, or obesity.

15.5.2 By Depth

- **Superficial Wounds**: epidermis and partial dermis; heal quickly with minimal intervention.
- **Partial-thickness Wounds**: extend through dermis; may require closure or bandaging.
- **Full-thickness Wounds**: involve subcutaneous tissue, muscle, or bone; require aggressive management.

15.5.3 By Contamination

- **Clean Wounds**: minimal contamination, fresh (<6 hours old).
- **Contaminated Wounds**: exposed to bacteria or debris, moderate risk of infection.
- **Infected Wounds**: established microbial colonization, purulent discharge, necrotic tissue.

15.5.4 By Chronicity

- **Acute Wounds**: recent trauma, active bleeding, better prognosis.
- **Chronic Wounds**: delayed healing due to infection, poor perfusion, or repeated trauma; examples include bumblefoot and pressure sores.

15.6 Clinical Signs Associated with Wounds in Chickens

Chickens are stoic and mask illness well, but careful observation and thorough physical examination can reveal significant injuries and systemic compromise. Analgesics should be administered prior to examination. Caregivers should wear either exam or sterile gloves during wound examination and treatment, including bandage changes.

15.6.1 Local Clinical Signs

- Visible lacerations, abrasions, swelling, or bruising.
- Missing feathers or blood-soaked plumage.
- Purulent discharge, foul odor (suggestive of anaerobic infection).
- Tissue necrosis (black or brown, cold tissues).
- Heat, erythema, or edema around wound margins.

15.6.2 Systemic Clinical Signs

- Depression, lethargy, and reluctance to move.
- Decreased appetite and water intake; anorexia.
- Shock: pale comb, tachypnea, cold extremities, collapse.
- Lameness or wing droop if musculoskeletal structures are involved.
- Decreased egg production in hens under stress.
- Posturing, tenesmus, tense coelom upon palpation

15.6.3 Pain Indicators in Chickens

Recognizing pain is critical for welfare and recovery, yet chickens rarely vocalize except in times of sudden, severe pain. Veterinary technicians should advocate for analgesia therapy. Subtle pain signs include:

- Guarding posture or reluctance to be handled.
- Decreased activity, standing with eyes closed.
- Shifting weight or holding a limb off the ground.
- Feather fluffing and reduced preening.

15.7 Principles of Wound Cleaning and Debridement

Effective wound care requires thorough cleaning, removal of devitalized tissue, and preparation for closure or healing by secondary intention. Heavy sedation or general anesthesia facilitates the procedure (Figure 15.8). Caregivers should wear either exam or sterile gloves during wound examination and treatment, including bandage changes.

15.7.1 Feather Removal

- Pluck or trim feathers around wound margins to improve visibility, provide clean surgical field.
- Avoid excessive feather loss, which impairs thermoregulation.

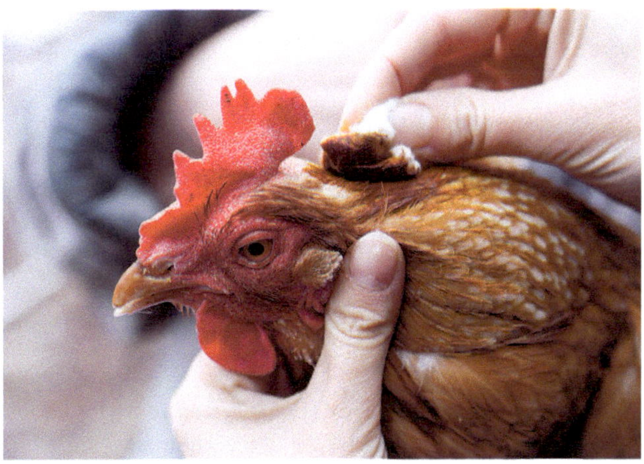

Figure 15.8 Use povidone iodine to cleanse wounds near the eyes and face. schankz / Adobe Stock Photos.

15.7.2 Wound Lavage

- Use copious irrigation/lavage with warm sterile saline or dilute chlorhexidine (0.5–1%).
- Avoid hydrogen peroxide or undiluted iodine tincture → cytotoxic to avian tissue.
- Pressure irrigation (35 mL syringe + 18-gauge needle) removes debris effectively.

15.7.3 Debridement

- Excision of necrotic skin, fascia, and nonviable muscle.
- Minimize removal of healthy tissue due to thin avian dermis.
- Repeated conservative debridement may be necessary in chronic cases.

15.7.4 Wound Closure Decisions

- **Primary Closure (Suturing)**: for clean, incised wounds <6–8 hours old.
- **Delayed Primary Closure**: after 2–3 days of infection control in contaminated wounds.
- **Secondary Intention Healing**: for large, infected, or heavily contaminated wounds; requires diligent bandage management.

15.8 Medications in Wound Management

15.8.1 Antimicrobials

15.8.1.1 Systemic Antibiotics

- **Amoxicillin/Clavulanic Acid**: 125–250 mg/kg PO q 8–12 hours for 5–7 days
  - Effective for Gram +/− bacteria.
- **Amoxicillin Sodium**: 50–250 mg/kg intramuscular every 8–12 hours for 5–7 days.
- **Amoxicillin Trihydrate**: 55–200 mg/kg by mouth, subcutaneous, or intramuscularly every 4–12 hours for 5–7 days.
- **Enrofloxacin**: 10 mg/kg PO/IM q24h
  - Broad-spectrum; extra-label in poultry in the U.S. (consider legal restrictions).
- Trimethoprim-sulfa (30 mg/kg PO q12h)
  - Effective for many soft tissue infections.
- **Cephalexin**: 50–125 mg/kg intramuscular or by mouth every 6–12 hours.

15.8.1.2 Topical Antimicrobials

Avoid contaminating the jar; use a tongue depressor to remove patient dose prior to application.

- **Silver Sulfadiazine Cream**:effective for burns and contaminated wounds.
- **Triple Antibiotic Ointments (Without Corticosteroids)**: effective for superficial wounds.

15.8.2 Analgesics

Opioids are administered preoperative, intraoperative, and postoperatively to block receptors:

- **Butorphanol**: 1–4 mg/kg IM/IV every 1–3 hours for kappa/weak mu receptor (mild) activity.
- **Nalbuphine**: 12.5 mg/kg IM/IV every 3 hours for kappa/partial mu receptor (mild) activity.
- **Tramadol**: 15 mg/kg PO every 12 hours for mu agonist/weak kappa/delta activity.

Nonsteroidal anti-inflammatory agents are administered preoperatively or postoperatively to relieve acute and chronic musculoskeletal and visceral pain.

- **Carprofen:** 1–4 mg/kg PO, SQ, or IM q 12–24 hours for less than 7 days; weak inhibition of COX-1 and COX-2
- **Meloxicam:** 0.50–2.0 mg/kg PO or IM q12–24 hours; selective COX-2 inhibitor
- **Celecoxib:** 10–20 mg/kg PO q 24 hours; selective COX-2 inhibitor

Local anesthetics are administered for nerve blocks (injection or splash) by infusing intended tissues.

- **Bupivicaine**: 5 mg/mL, 1–2 mg/kg
- **Lidocaine**: 20 mg/mL, 2–3 mg/kg
- **Gabapentin**: 10–25 mg/kg PO q 8–12 hours pre- and postoperatively.

15.8.3 Antifungals

Indicated wounds contaminated with organic material or after prolonged antibiotic use.

- Nystatin (100,000 U/kg PO q12h) for yeast infections in crop or GI wounds.
- Itraconazole (10 mg/kg PO q24h) systemic therapy for invasive fungal infections.

15.8.4 Additional Supportive Medications

- **Vitamin A and E Supplementation**: enhances epithelial healing.
- **Prebiotics and Probiotics**: support gut flora if antibiotics are used.
- **Calcium Gluconate**: if egg-laying hens present with concurrent hypocalcemia or cloacal tears.

15.9 Bandaging Techniques in Chickens

Bandaging is a cornerstone of wound management in chickens. Unlike dogs and cats, chickens present unique challenges due to their thin skin, feather coverage, small size, and active behavior. Proper bandaging protects wounds, prevents contamination, immobilizes injured tissues, prevents self-trauma, and promotes healing.

- Monitor for swelling of toes, bad odor, strike-through, skin irritation, toe color, skin temperature or slippage.
- Keep bandages dry and clean; soiled bandages act as infection reservoirs and compromise tissue integrity. If wet or strike-through occurs, change bandage expeditiously.
- Frequency of bandage changes depends on wound exudate and contamination risk.
- Never leave plastic over bandages; tissue requires oxygen for healing.

15.9.1 General Bandaging Principles

- Use nonadherent, semipermeable dressings as the primary layer to minimize wound trauma during changes. This can be wet-to-dry or dry depending on the contamination.
- Apply absorbent secondary layer (cotton, soft roll gauze) to manage exudate.
- Secure with outer tertiary cohesive wraps ensuring circulation is not compromised.
- Adhesive tape (i.e., Elastikon) is not recommended on chicken's friable skin.
- Adhesive removal spray.

15.9.2 Wing Bandages

- Figure-eight bandage immobilizes fractures or lacerations of the wing.
- Modified Robert Jones for more severe wing trauma requiring padding.
- Ensure crop is not compressed when immobilizing the wing to the body and the bird can still perch and balance.

15.9.3 Leg and Foot Bandages

- **Ball Bandage**: for plantar wounds such as bumblefoot; distributes weight and relieves pressure. "Donuts" can be made to add padding to the plantar surface for comfort and allow healing.
- **Spica or Spoon Splint**: for femoral or tibiotarsal stabilization; same as modified Robert Jones.
- Toe wraps for digit lacerations, taking care to avoid excessive tension. Similar technique as application of the ball bandage.

15.9.4 Body and Thoracic Bandages

- Used for large flank or keel wounds.
- Apply nonconstrictive wraps to allow normal respiration. A "onesie" bodysuit is often appropriate and less constrictive.
- Feather coverage often complicates adhesion, clip feathers judiciously.

15.9.5 Head and Neck Bandages

- Rarely used due to interference with vision, feeding, and thermoregulation.
- Collars (soft e-collars or improvised foam collars) may be necessary to prevent self-trauma.

15.10 Surgical Closure versus Secondary Intention Healing

15.10.1 Primary Closure (Suturing)

- Indicated for clean, sharp wounds <6–8 hours old.
- **Techniques**:
  - Simple interrupted sutures with absorbable monofilament.
  - Horizontal mattress for fragile skin.
- **Advantages**: faster healing, reduced infection risk.
- **Limitations**: fragile avian skin tears easily; infection risk if contaminated.

15.10.2 Delayed Primary Closure

- Wounds initially cleaned, debrided, and managed open for 48–72 hours.
- Once bacterial contamination is controlled, closure is performed.
- Useful for predator wounds or heavily soiled lacerations.

15.10.3 Secondary Intention Healing

- Common in avian practice due to delayed presentation and contamination.
- Relies on granulation tissue formation and epithelial migration.
- Requires diligent wound care, frequent bandage changes, and caregiver compliance.
- May lead to scarring and feather loss, but functional healing.

15.11 Types of Wounds

Certain wound presentations are especially common in backyard chickens, and each requires tailored management (Figures 15.9 and 15.10).

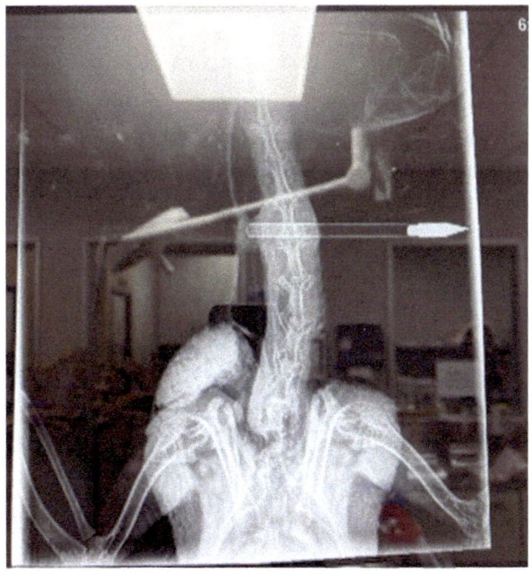

Figure 15.9 Radiographic image of a rooster that was shot with an arrow. With wound management, the rooster recovered. Courtesy of Funky Chicken Rescue.

15.12 Bumblefoot (Pododermatitis)

15.12.1 Overview and Pathogenesis

Bumblefoot, or pododermatitis, is a common condition in chickens and other poultry characterized by inflammation and infection of the footpad. It typically begins with minor abrasions, pressure sores, or skin damage caused by rough perches, hard flooring, obesity, poor litter quality, or prolonged standing

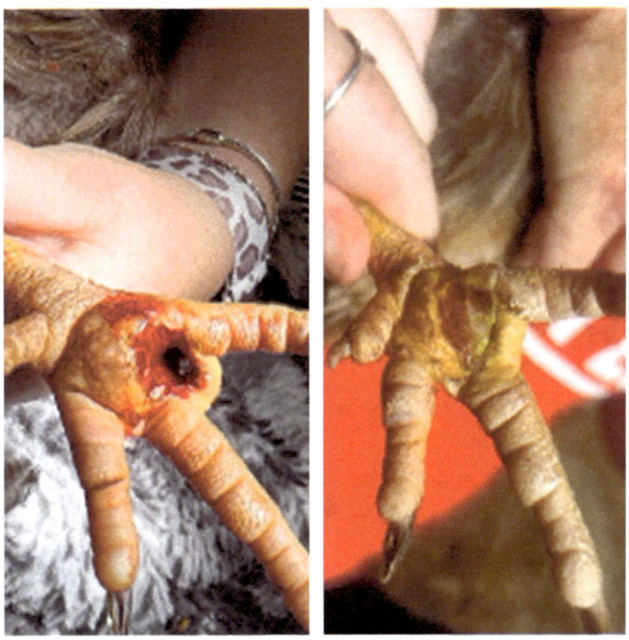

Figure 15.10 Pododermatitis wound, post-surgery, and 10 days later. Courtesy of Stephanie Freeman.

on wet or dirty surfaces. These minor injuries allow opportunistic bacteria, most commonly *Staphylococcus aureus*, to invade the underlying tissues. As the infection progresses, localized swelling, erythema, and pain develop, often leading to the formation of abscesses, caseous necrosis, and ulceration. Chronic cases can result in fibrosis, osteomyelitis, and septicemia if untreated.

Pathogenesis is strongly linked to mechanical trauma, poor husbandry, and compromised immunity, which together creates an environment for bacteria to colonize and persist. The condition not only affects welfare by causing pain and impaired mobility but also predisposes birds to reduced feed intake, poor growth, and decreased productivity.

15.12.2 Risk Factors

- **Mechanical & Environmental Factors**
  Rough or abrasive flooring (wire mesh, concrete). Wet or soiled litter that softens and damages skin. Unsanitary housing or flooring conditions. Unsuitable perches that are narrow, hard, or sharp-edged perches concentrate pressure on footpads.
- **Nutritional Factors**
  Vitamin A deficiency causes impaired skin integrity. Obesity causes excessive weight bearing on footpads, leading to trauma to the skin. Biotin deficiency weakens skin and keratin structures.
- **Management Factors**
  Overcrowding and poor perch designs such as too narrow and/or sharp. Soiled litter and infrequent changes cause ammonia buildup that then burns the footpad.

15.12.3 Clinical Signs and Pathology

- **External Findings**
  Edema, erythema, and heat of the footpad. Lameness or reluctance to walk. Firm, painful nodules on the plantar surface. In some cases, abscesses can form on the dorsal surface of the foot. In advanced cases, systemic illness, inappetence, and decreased egg production.
- **Necropsy Findings**
  Localized abscesses with central necrotic core (caseous plug). Chronic fibrosis and scarring of the footpad. Possible extension into tendons, joints, or bone (osteomyelitis).

15.12.4 Diagnostic Testing

- **Culture and Sensitivity Testing**
  Identifies causative bacteria and guides antibiotic selection for systemic therapy. Particularly important in recurrent or treatment-resistant cases.
- **Radiographs**
  Radiology can be used to detect osteomyelitis.
- **Bloodwork**
  May show leukocytosis if systemic infection is present and evaluates overall health before prolonged antibiotic use.

15.12.5 Treatment and Therapeutic Interventions

- **Mild Cases**
  Topical antiseptics such as dilute povidone-iodine ("weak tea") and chlorhexidine (0.5–1%) can be used in early and superficial wounds. Soaking feet in antiseptic solution to soften the ulcer.

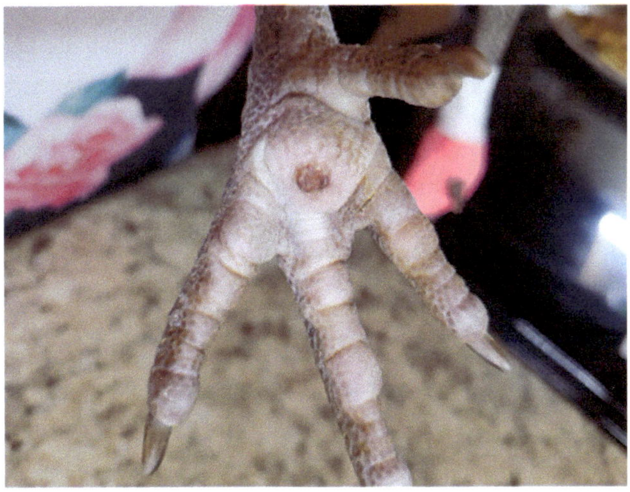

Figure 15.11 Mild case of pododermatitis treated daily with weak iodine soaks and bandaging. Courtesy of Sarah Meyer.

Repeat daily to flush deep wounds. Dry completely prior to bandage application. Bandaging to alleviate the pressure from the pressure point is also helpful (Figure 15.11).

- **Moderate to Severe Cases**
  Surgical debridement to remove abscess core (nidus, i.e., "kernel") and necrotic tissue is necessary at this point. Systemic antibiotics are also needed such as amoxicillin (20 mg/kg orally every 12 hours) or trimethoprim-sulfa (30 mg/kg orally every 12 hours).
- **Supportive Care**
  Analgesics such as meloxicam (0.5–1 mg/kg orally every 24 hours) will help with pain and inflammation. Warm water foot soaks in Epsom salt or diluted povidone iodine solution prior to debridement are also helpful in softening the surrounding tissue.

15.12.6 Prevention and Control

- **Environmental Management**
  Maintain clean, dry flooring; replace regularly to prevent soiling, moisture. Provide smooth, wide, rounded perches to distribute weight evenly. Avoid wire flooring or cover it with bedding. Cover perches with softer materials (rubber, padded wrapping) to reduce foot pressure. Provide ramps for access to perches/nests to limit jumping injuries.
- **Nutritional Strategies**
  Vitamin A supplementation supports epithelial and skin health, reducing susceptibility to cracks and infections. Biotin supplementation improves skin integrity and keratin formation in the footpads. Ensure adequate levels of protein, trace minerals (zinc, manganese, copper), and fatty acids for skin and tissue repair. A reputable, high-quality feed should be sufficient.

15.12.7 Nursing Considerations

Nursing care for chickens with bumblefoot focuses on both treatment of the lesion and improvement of management practices to prevent recurrence. Birds should be carefully examined for lameness, swelling, ulceration, or scab formation on the footpad, with affected individuals isolated to reduce stress and competition. Wound care involves cleaning and disinfecting the lesion, removing necrotic tissue if necessary, and applying topical antiseptics or antibiotics under veterinary guidance.

Bandaging may be used to protect the foot and promote healing, and perches or flooring should be padded to reduce pressure. Supportive care includes ensuring easy access to feed and water, monitoring body condition, and minimizing handling stress. Preventive measures are equally important, such as maintaining clean, dry flooring and substrate, providing smooth perches, and managing body weight to reduce pressure on the feet. Veterinary nurses should also monitor for systemic signs of infection, as chronic or severe cases may require systemic antibiotic therapy or even veterinarian surgical intervention. Regular bird and flock observation and early intervention are critical to safeguarding bird welfare.

15.13 Predator Bites and Claw Wounds

15.13.1 Overview and Pathogenesis

Predator bites and claw wounds in chickens are traumatic injuries most often caused by dogs, raccoons, foxes, hawks, or other predators. These wounds typically present as punctures, lacerations, crushing injuries, or tearing of skin, muscle, and sometimes bone, with varying degrees of hemorrhage and tissue damage.

Pathogenesis is primarily mechanical, where the predator's teeth or claws inflict penetrating trauma and tearing forces that compromise the skin barrier and deeper tissues. Secondary bacterial contamination is common, as predator mouths and claws harbor diverse pathogens such as *Pasteurella*, *Clostridium*, *E. coli*, and anaerobes, leading to localized cellulitis, abscesses, septicemia, or gangrene if untreated. The extent of injury depends on the size and strength of the predator, location of the wound, and the bird's ability to escape. Birds that survive initial trauma remain at high risk of shock, hemorrhage, and secondary infection, which can rapidly progress without prompt intervention (Figures 15.12).

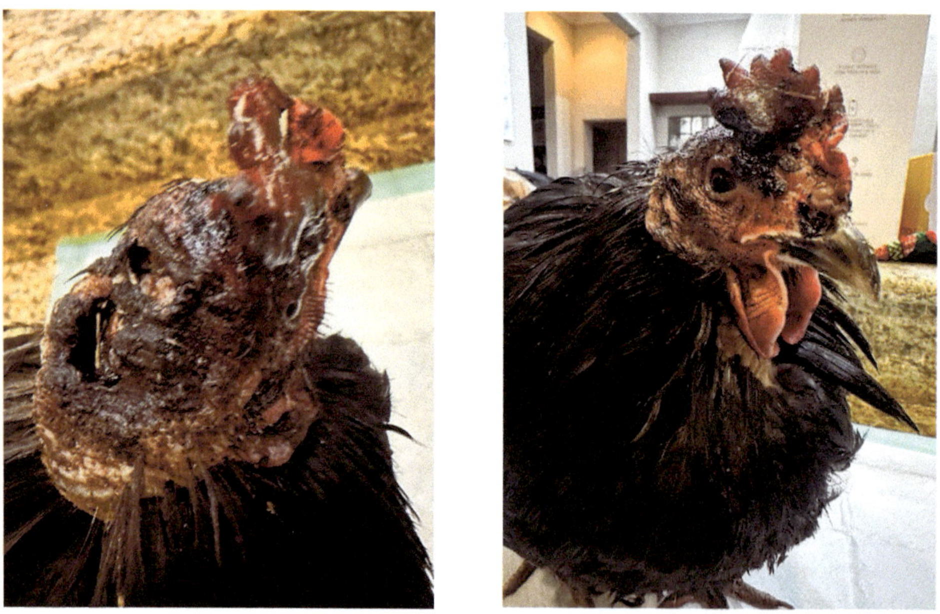

Figure 15.12 A hen after suspected predator attack. Head wounds exposed the bird's skull. Courtesy of Funky Chicken Rescue.

15.13.2 Risk Factors

- **Environmental Factors**
  Housing vulnerabilities such as poorly secured coops, open-top runs, and gaps in fencing. Free-range management also increases exposure to aerial and terrestrial predators. Proximity to predator habitats such as wooded areas and areas with stray dogs and cats.

15.13.3 Clinical Signs and Pathology

- **External Findings**
  Visible lacerations, puncture wounds, or feather loss. Hemorrhage, hematomas, suppuration. Signs of shock such as pale comb/wattles, lethargy, and collapse. Reluctance to move or difficulty moving if musculoskeletal injuries occur. Respiratory distress if thoracic trauma is present.
- **Necropsy Findings**
  Deep puncture wounds harboring necrotic tissue and purulent exudate. Septicemia with widespread infection. Fractures or dislocations from crushing trauma. Extensive subcutaneous emphysema (air under the skin) if the air sacs are damaged.

15.13.4 Diagnostic Testing

- **Diagnostic Imaging**
  Detect fractures, luxation, or crush injuries. Assess radiographs for foreign material. Evaluate coelomic cavity if puncture is suspected. Ultrasound can detect internal bleeding, air sac rupture, or fluid accumulation in the coelomic cavity.
- **Wound Culture & Sensitivity**
  Useful if infection is established or treatment fails. Recommended if infection is established or wounds are slow to heal. Identifies common pathogens and guides antibiotic choice.
- **Bloodwork**
  Assesses systemic infection, anemia, or dehydration. May reveal leukocytosis or anemia. Assess kidney and liver function, especially before prolonged antibiotic use.

15.13.5 Treatment & Therapeutic Interventions

- **Initial Stabilization**
  Administer analgesia including an opioid and anti-inflammatory agent prior to handling. Treat for shock with fluid therapy if indicated. K p the bird warm, quiet, and minimize handling.
- **Wound Management**
  Clip feathers surrounding the wound for improved visibility and aseptic preparation of the wound(s). Irrigate wound thoroughly with sterile saline, diluted chlorhexidine solution (0.05%), or diluted povidone iodine solution ("weak tea"). Avoid hydrogen peroxide as it is cytotoxic. Debride necrotic tissue, debris, and blood clots to reduce bacterial load. Fresh, clean wounds can be sutured. Older and contaminated wounds should be left open for drainage and cleaning.
- **Medications**
  Because predator saliva carries pathogenic bacteria (*Pasteurella*, *Streptococcus*, *Clostridium*), systemic antibiotics are indicated. Analgesics are indicated.

- **Supportive and Adjunctive Therapy**
  High-protein diet, vitamins A, C, and B-complex (reputable feed for complete nutrition) to aid healing. Keep injured bird separate from flock to prevent pecking and cannibalism. Apply light, semipermeable bandages if location permits and change as ordered by the attending veterinarian. Check wounds daily for progressive edema or discharge, or foul odor.
- **Advanced and Adjunctive Therapies**
  Laser therapy or photo biomodulation encourages wound healing. Honey or sugar dressings facilitate natural debridement and antimicrobial action.
- **Coaptation and Surgical Interventions**
  Splinting or surgical repair of fractures if feasible. Surgical exploration under general anesthesia for deep puncture wounds involving muscles or coelomic cavity. For air sac rupture or subcutaneous emphysema, use a small needle to puncture and decompress to release trapped air. Consider euthanasia if prognosis is poor.

15.13.6 Prevention and Control

- **Predator-Proof Housing**
  Use ½-inch hardware cloth instead of chicken wire (predators can bite or tear through chicken wire). Ensure all vents and windows are covered with hardware cloth. Raccoons can open simple latches; use padlocks, carabiners, or predator-proof locks. Always lock birds in the coop before dusk when most predators are active.
- **Outdoor Run Protection**
  Bury hardware cloth 12–18 inches into the ground or install an apron extending outward to stop digging predators (foxes, dogs, coyotes). Cover runs with netting or wire mesh to prevent hawks, owls, and climbing predator attacks. Electric fencing is an effective barrier against foxes, raccoons, dogs, and larger predators.
- **Environmental Management**
  Clear tall grass, shrubs, and woodpiles near coops that provide predator hiding spots. Secure feed storage prevents attracting rodents, which in turn attract larger predators. Motion-activated lighting or alarms deter nocturnal predators. Birds should be supervised during free range or any time outside of the pen or coop.

15.13.7 Nursing Considerations

Nursing care for chickens with bite and claw wounds centers on stabilization, wound management, and prevention of infection. Immediately after injury, affected birds should be placed in a quiet, stress-free environment to manage shock and allow close observation. Hemostasis through gentle pressure and careful cleaning of the wound with sterile saline or antiseptic solution is essential. Necrotic or contaminated tissue should be carefully debrided under veterinary guidance, and broad-spectrum antibiotics and analgesics may be required to manage infection and pain. Bandaging or protective coverings may be applied to severe wounds, though care must be taken to prevent restricting circulation. Supportive care includes ensuring proper nutrition and hydration, maintaining warmth, and reducing competition by housing the bird separately during recovery. Veterinary nursing staff should closely monitor signs of systemic infection, such as lethargy, anorexia, or edema, which may indicate septicemia requiring intensive treatment. Long-term considerations include reinforcing predator-proof housing, such as secure fencing and covered enclosures, to prevent recurrence and protect the flock.

15.14 Thermal Injuries (Burns and Frostbite)

See Figure 15.13

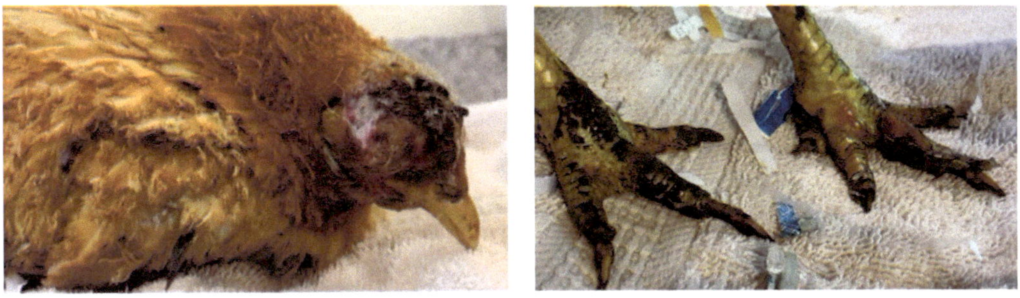

Figure 15.13 Hen with severe burns from coop/house fire. Courtesy of Funky Chicken Rescue.

15.14.1 Overview and Pathogenesis

Thermal injuries in chickens, including burns and frostbite, occur when birds are exposed to extreme heat, cold, or direct contact with caustic surfaces or substances. Burns most often result from exposure to heat lamps, faulty electrical equipment, overheated litter, or caustic chemicals such as disinfectants, leading to coagulation necrosis of tissues, blistering, and destruction of the skin barrier. Frostbite, on the other hand, is commonly seen in combs, wattles, and toes during prolonged exposure to freezing temperatures, particularly in high humidity, where ice crystal formation within tissues causes cellular rupture, impaired circulation, and ischemic necrosis.

The pathogenesis of both burns and frostbite involves direct tissue damage, disruption of skin integrity, and vascular injury, which predispose affected areas to secondary bacterial invasion. Severity ranges from superficial to deep tissue necrosis, with systemic effects such as dehydration, shock, and toxemia possible in severe cases. These injuries compromise welfare due to pain, stress, and impaired feeding or mobility.

15.14.2 Risk Factors

- **Environmental and Housing Factors**
  Exposed wires, faulty heating elements, heat lamps too close to birds. Heat lamps, brooders, or heated perches placed too near birds. Accumulation of heat in coops during hot weather. Straw or wood shavings near heaters; heat lamps increase fire risk. Birds are housed outdoors or in uninsulated coops during winter. Unprotected perches, windows, or gaps allowing cold air. Wet litter or damp conditions increase frostbite risk. Strong winds exacerbate cold injuries, especially on combs, wattles, and toes.

- **Host-Related Factors**
  Chicks and young birds are more susceptible to both heat stress and frostbite due to immature thermoregulation. Large-combed birds (e.g., Leghorns) are prone to frostbite; heavy-breasted meat birds may be more prone to burns under heat lamps. Poor feathering exposes skin to extreme temperatures. Sick or weak birds have impaired thermoregulation, increasing susceptibility.
- **Nutritional Factors**
  Poor nutrition (low vitamin A, E, or selenium) can impair tissue integrity and recovery from thermal injury. Birds with inadequate energy intake may tolerate cold poorly.

15.14.3 Clinical Signs and Pathology

- **External Findings**
  Burns
  - First-degree (superficial burns)
    - Erythema
    - Feathers singed or scorched.
    - Pain response (bird flinches when touched).
    - Often limited to exposed areas (legs, face, wings).
  - Second-degree (partial-thickness burns)
    - Blisters or vesicles filled with clear or serosanguinous fluid.
    - Moist, reddened, and swollen tissue after blisters rupture.
    - Feather loss over affected areas.
    - Severe pain, restlessness, and reduced activity.
  - Third-degree (full-thickness burns)
    - Blackened, leathery, or charred skin.
    - Necrosis extending through skin and into underlying muscle.
    - Loss of sensation in burned area (nerve endings destroyed).
    - Signs of systemic illness: weakness, dehydration, anorexia, or shock.
  - Systemic Complications
    Dehydration from fluid loss at burn sites. Septicemia due to open wounds colonized by bacteria (*Staphylococcus*, *Clostridium*). Respiratory distress if smoke inhalation or toxic fume exposure occurred.

  Frostbite
  - Early Stage (vasoconstriction)
    - Comb, wattles, or toes appear pale or white.
    - Cold to the touch, bird resists handling (pain).
    - Restlessness, reluctance to walk if feet are affected.
  - Intermediate Stage (ischemia and cellular injury)
    - Edema and erythema (reactive hyperemia).
    - Blisters filled with serous or serosanguinous fluid.
    - Comb and wattles turn dark bluish-purple (cyanotic).
    - Lameness, inappetence or anorexia, decreased egg production.
  - Severe Stage (necrosis and gangrene)
    - Tissue darkens to black, dry, and hard.
    - Auto-amputation of comb tips, wattles, or digits.

  - Loss of sensation in necrotic areas, but severe pain in surrounding tissues.
  - Secondary infection possible (cellulitis, septicemia).
- **Necropsy Findings**
  Burns
  - Coagulative necrosis of epidermis and dermis. Vascular thrombosis and edema in subcutaneous tissues. Secondary bacterial colonization of necrotic tissue.
- **Frostbite**
  - Ice crystal formation within cells causes mechanical rupture. Vascular congestion, thrombosis, and ischemia. Necrosis and tissue sloughing with bacterial infiltration in late stages.

15.14.4 Diagnostic Testing

- **Diagnostic Imaging**
  Indicated in severe frostbite to check for osteomyelitis or bone necrosis. Useful in burns if deep tissue involvement is suspected (especially over wings/legs). Ultrasonography can help identify fluid accumulation or assess deeper tissue damage.
- **Culture & Sensitivity**
  If infection is suspected (purulent discharge, foul odor, delayed healing). Common isolates: *Staphylococcus aureus*, *Escherichia coli*, *Clostridium spp*. Guides appropriate antibiotic therapy.
- **Bloodwork**
  Leukocytosis may indicate systemic infection. Anemia may result from chronic tissue damage or blood loss. Evaluates hydration status and organ function (important before systemic drug use).

15.14.5 Treatment and Therapeutic Interventions

- **Burns**
  Immediate Stabilization
  - Move bird away from heat source. Keep in a warm, quiet environment with minimal stress. Oral or subcutaneous fluids replace losses and prevent dehydration. Analgesia.

  Wound Care
  - Flush burns with tepid sterile saline or clean tap water. Gently remove necrotic feathers or tissue. Apply a thin layer of silver sulfadiazine cream to promote healing. Apply sterile nonadherent dressings to protect against contamination and reduce fluid loss.

  Supportive Care
  - High protein diet to support tissue repair. Ensure hydration. Assisted feeding if indicated. Vitamin A and E supplementation promote epithelial healing. Minimize stress and handling.
- **Frostbite**
  Immediate Stabilization
  - Move bird to a draft-free, warm environment. Apply warm (not hot) compresses or tepid water baths for 15–20 minutes. Never use direct heat (heating pads, heat lamps) as this can progress tissue necrosis.
- *Wound Care*
  - Do not massage or rub affected tissues; this can cause further cellular rupture. Leave blisters intact if possible; if ruptured, gently flush with sterile saline. Allow demarcation, surgical removal only if infection or severe gangrene. Apply protective ointments such as silver sulfadiazine.

- *Medications*
  - Antibiotics are indicated in cases of secondary infection.
  - Analgesics are indicated.
- *Supportive Care*
  - Provide easily accessible food and water (pain may limit mobility). Encourage intake of warm mash to support hydration. Assisted feeding if indicated. Vitamin and mineral supplements (especially vitamin E, selenium, zinc) to aid healing.
- In advanced cases of frostbite with necrotic toes or wattles, surgical removal may be required to prevent septicemia. Consider birds with extensive burns (>30% body surface) or severe frostbite with systemic compromise. Humane euthanasia is always a treatment option.

15.14.6 Prevention and Control

- **Prevention of Burns**
  1) *Safe Heating Practices*
     Use thermostat-controlled brooders or heaters instead of unprotected heat lamps. Heat lamps are the primary cause for coop/house fires and bird deaths. Position heating implements securely with protective covers and at safe distances from bedding. Secure dangling cords as chickens may peck or tangle them.
  2) *Coop and Equipment Safety*
     Insulate electrical wiring and check regularly for fraying or sparks. Use nonflammable bedding (avoid very fine dry shavings near heat lamps). Never place open flames, candles, or kerosene heaters in coops.
  3) *Chemical Safety*
     Store caustic disinfectants and cleaning agents securely away from birds. Dilute cleaning chemicals per manufacturer directions and rinse hard surfaces well to prevent skin burns.
- Prevention of Frostbite
  1) *Housing and Environment*
     Maintain dry, well-ventilated but draft-free housing. Provide deep, clean bedding to insulate feet. Elevate coops off damp ground.
  2) *Breed and Bird Factors*
     Large-combed breeds (e.g., Leghorns) are more prone to frostbite. Do not apply petroleum jelly as it masks the signs of frostbite. Roosting bars should be wide enough for chickens to cover their toes with feathers while resting.
  3) *Temperature Management*
     Insulate coops to buffer extreme temperature drops. Avoid excess humidity inside coops (from droppings, poor ventilation). Ensure water does not spill and freeze around the coop. Supplement heating if birds are shivering or signs of frostbite are present.

15.14.7 Nursing Considerations

Nursing care for chickens with thermal injuries focuses on pain management, wound care, prevention of secondary infections, and supportive care. Affected birds should be isolated in a clean, dry, and draft-free environment to reduce stress and facilitate monitoring. Burn wounds should be gently cleaned with sterile saline or antiseptic solutions, with necrotic tissue debrided under veterinary skill if indicated, and appropriate topical treatments and/or bandaging applied to protect the area. Frostbitten tissues should be gradually rewarmed without rubbing, and affected extremities may require protective padding to prevent further trauma. Birds should receive adequate hydration, high-quality feed, and supplemental vitamins or electrolytes to support healing and immune function.

Close observation for signs of infection, necrosis, or systemic illness is essential, with veterinary intervention sought promptly for antibiotic therapy and analgesia. Environmental management, including maintaining appropriate temperature and humidity, is critical to prevent recurrence. Overall, nursing considerations emphasize wound management, pain control, supportive care, environmental modification, and vigilant monitoring to optimize recovery and maintain welfare in birds with thermal injuries.

15.15 Degloving and Avulsion Injuries

15.15.1 Overview and Pathogenesis

Degloving and avulsion injuries in chickens are severe traumatic wounds in which skin and underlying tissues are forcibly separated from the underlying structures, often involving the feet, legs, comb, or wattles. These injuries typically result from predator attacks, mechanical trauma, or entanglement in equipment, and they can vary in severity from superficial skin loss to full-thickness tissue avulsion exposing muscle, tendons, or bone.

Pathogenesis involves mechanical disruption of skin, subcutaneous tissue, blood vessels, and nerves, which compromises tissue perfusion and creates a large, open wound susceptible to hemorrhage, ischemia, necrosis, and bacterial contamination. Secondary bacterial invasion, particularly by *Staphylococcus*, *E. coli*, and anaerobic organisms, can lead to cellulitis, abscess formation, or septicemia. Clinically, affected birds may show severe pain, lameness, bleeding, shock, or inability to use the injured limb, depending on the extent of tissue loss. Prompt recognition and intervention are critical to reduce morbidity and mortality associated with these traumatic injuries.

15.15.2 Risk Factors

- **Predatory Attacks**
  Carnivorous predators (dogs, cats, raccoons, foxes, and opossums) tend to grab the bird by the skin, wings, or legs and tear away tissue. Dogs often shake their prey, causing large areas of degloving. Avian predators (hawks and owls) use talons to grip, causing punctures and tearing of skin or muscle. Rodents may attack chicks or debilitated birds, often causing severe tissue damage on extremities (feet, comb, or cloaca).
- **Environmental Hazards**
  Wire flooring or mesh enclosures can cause limbs to become entrapped, and when birds struggle, skin may be stripped away. Rusted nails, broken wood, sharp metal edges, or damaged feeders/waterers can puncture or lacerate skin. Moving parts (doors, fans) can trap and avulse skin or appendages. Especially when panicked, chickens can be injured by claws and beaks of other birds.
- **Handling and Management Factors**
  Grabbing birds by the wings, legs, or feathers can inadvertently cause skin tears. Inadequate handling techniques may result in avulsion injuries. Birds confined in tight crates may injure one another or become caught in crate edges.

- **Anatomical Predispositions**
  A chicken's proximal leg and entire wing are covered by relatively thin, loose skin so it is easily torn. Their neck has fewer muscle layers, making them prone to tearing in predator attacks. Bare areas (vent, comb, wattles, feet) are more susceptible.
- **Nutritional and Health Factors**
  Poor protein, vitamin A, or zinc status may reduce skin strength and healing ability. Prior infection (mites, lice, dermatitis) can weaken skin, making avulsion more likely. Weak or immobile birds may fail to escape predators or entrapment situations.

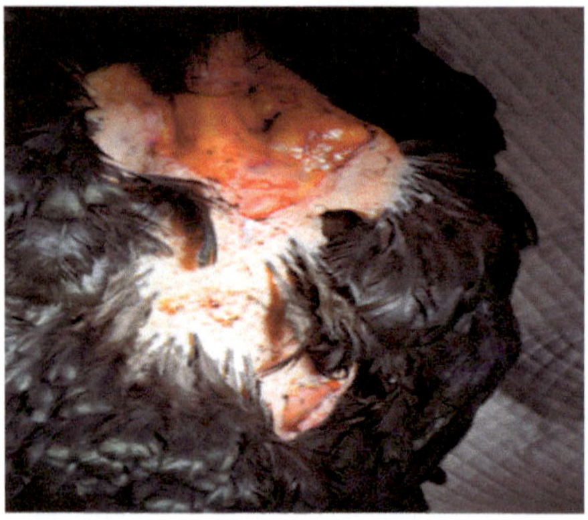

Figure 15.14 Avulsion injury to hen's dorsum. Courtesy of Unusual Pet Vets.

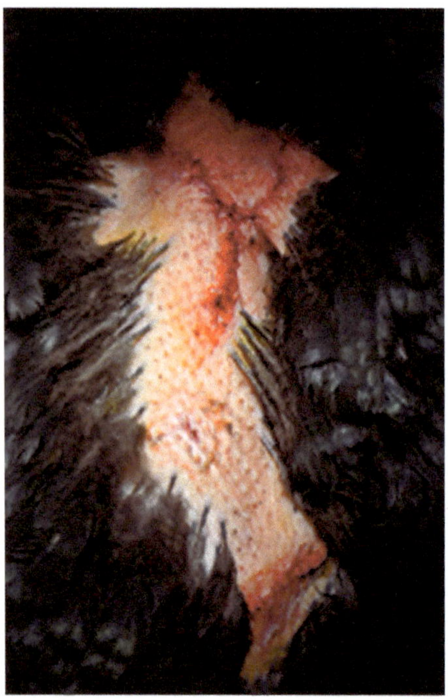

Figure 15.15 Avulsion wound closure. Courtesy of Unusual Pet Vets.

15.15.3 Clinical Signs and Pathology

- **External Findings**
  Profuse hemorrhage initially; clotted or dried blood present in older wounds. Birds may show signs of hypovolemic shock such as pale or cyanotic combs and wattles, cold extremities, weakness, collapse, reluctance to move, and increased respiratory rate. Restlessness, vocalization, wing flapping, or guarding injured limbs. Lameness, drooping wings, or inability to perch. Decreased activity, inappetence, or anorexia. Swelling, erythema, and warmth around wound margins. Malodorous discharge (serous to purulent) with necrotic tissue. Abscess formation in deeper tissues if untreated. Fever, if septicemia develops.
- **Necropsy Findings**
  Necrosis of skin and subcutaneous tissue. Vascular thrombosis causes ischemia and sloughing of devitalized skin. In chronic wounds, granulation tissue formation, fibrosis, and chronic abscessation (Figures 15.14 and 15.15).

15.15.4 Diagnostic Testing

- **Diagnostic Imaging**
  Detect fractures, joint involvement, or bone exposure. Useful in wing and leg avulsion cases. Ultrasonography to assess underlying soft tissue damage. Identify hematomas or seromas.
- **Bloodwork**
  PCV/hematocrit will assess blood loss severity. Leukocytosis indicated infection or inflammation. Biochemistry evaluates hydration, electrolytes, and organ function in shock cases.
- **Culture**
  Identify infecting organisms and guide antibiotic therapy (aerobic and anaerobic culture recommended).

15.15.5 Treatment and Therapeutic Interventions

- **Emergency Stabilization**
  Analgesia administration. Hemostasis with pressure and hemostatic agents (e.g., ferric subsulfate, silver nitrate) if indicated. Provide warmth and fluid therapy (Lactated Ringer's Solution 30–50 mL/kg).
- **Wound Cleaning and Debridement**
  Trim away feathers around the wound margins. Flush with warm sterile saline or dilute antiseptic (0.05% chlorhexidine or 1:40 povidone-iodine). Avoid hydrogen peroxide or strong iodine as it is cytotoxic to viable tissue. Debride necrotic or devitalized tissue using aseptic technique. Retain any viable skin flaps for possible suturing.
- **Surgical Intervention**
  If wound edges are clean and skin is viable, suturing can restore coverage. Use absorbable sutures for deeper tissue and nonabsorbable for skin. In contaminated wounds, allow 24–48 hours of cleaning and antibiotic therapy before closure. Wet-to-dry bandaging may aid contamination removal. If tissue loss is extensive, wounds may need to granulate naturally via second-intention healing. Amputation is considered for nonviable limbs. Carts and chairs are available for amputees.
- **Medication**
  Antibiotics and analgesics are indicated at presentation and throughout treatment.
- **Wound Dressings and Bandaging**
  Moist wound healing environment, hydrogel, or sterile nonadherent dressing. For protective bandaging, use soft padding, and cohesive bandage material. Replace bandages every 24–48 hours or sooner if soiled or strike-through presents.
- **Supportive Care**
  High protein feed and vitamin supplementation to promote healing. Isolate in a clean, quiet recovery pen with soft bedding. Minimize stress and handling. Encourage appetite and hydration. Assisted feeding if indicated.
- **Advanced and Adjunctive Therapies**
  Laser therapy or photo biomodulation speeds wound healing. Honey or sugar dressings facilitate natural debridement and antimicrobial action (Figure 15.16).

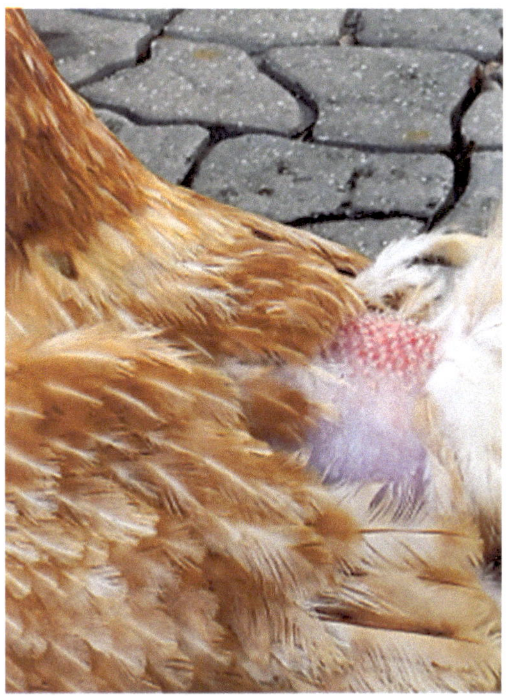

Figure 15.16 Avulsion wound in the healing process from a predator attack. Note the lack of follicles on the lighter colored skin that will not regrow feathers. Chart created by Stephanie Freeman.

15.15.6 Prevention and Control

- **Predator Management**
  Use hardware cloth (not chicken wire, which is easily breached). Cover outdoor runs with mesh or netting to prevent aerial predator

attacks. Lock coops at night with secure latches. Motion-activated lights, predator-proof fencing, and guard animals (e.g., dogs, geese). Remove food sources (leftover feed, spilled grain) that attract raccoons or rats. Regular monitoring and safe rodent-proofing to prevent attacks on chicks.

- **Environmental Modifications**
  Inspect and eliminate sharp edges, protruding nails, or broken wire. Repair damaged feeders, drinkers, and perches. Avoid wire-only flooring or provide pads to prevent limb entrapment. Ensure bedding is dry, soft, and deep enough to cushion falls. Protect birds from machinery, fans, and automatic doors where entrapment may occur.
- **Flock Management Practices**
  Overcrowding increases trampling, fighting, and traumatic injuries. Provide at least 4 sq. ft per bird in coops and 8–10 sq. ft in runs. Educate caregivers to pick up birds gently, supporting both wings and body. Avoid grabbing a bird by wings, legs, or feathers. Use smooth, secure crates free of gaps or sharp edges. Avoid overcrowding during transportation.
- **Nutritional and Health Support**
  Adequate protein, vitamins (A, E), and minerals (zinc, selenium) to support strong skin and tissue resilience. Treat mites, lice, and dermatitis promptly, as compromised skin is more vulnerable to avulsion. Monitoring weak or ill birds; these individuals are less mobile and more prone to attack or entrapment.

15.15.7 Nursing Considerations

Nursing care for chickens with degloving or avulsion injuries focuses on stabilization, pain management, infection prevention, and supportive care. Immediately after injury, affected birds should be placed in a quiet, clean, and dry environment to reduce stress and allow close monitoring. Hemorrhage should be controlled using gentle pressure or hemostatic agents, and the wound should be thoroughly cleaned with sterile saline or antiseptic solutions. Necrotic or contaminated tissue may require debridement under veterinary skill, and protective dressings or bandages can help prevent further trauma. Analgesics and systemic antibiotics should be administered to manage pain and reduce the risk of secondary infection. Supportive care includes ensuring easy access to feed and water, maintaining warmth, and minimizing stress.

Birds should be closely monitored for signs of shock, systemic infection, or progressive tissue necrosis, and severe cases may require surgical intervention. Preventive measures involve secure housing and predator-proofing to reduce the risk of such injuries. Overall, nursing considerations emphasize wound care, analgesia, infection treatment and prevention, environmental management, and close observation to optimize recovery and welfare in birds with degloving or avulsion injuries.

15.16 Optional Nutritional Support for Wound Healing

Nutritional status has a profound impact on recovery. Chicken with wounds require higher caloric intake, increased protein, and specific micronutrients to facilitate healing.

Nutrient/category	Role in wound healing	Sources for chickens
Protein and amino acids	Essential for tissue repair, collagen synthesis, immune function	Soybean meal, fish meal, peas, insects, mealworms
Methionine and cysteine	Keratin and collagen production, feather regrowth	Poultry feed supplements, sunflower meal, sesame
Arginine and glutamine	Supports immune response, nitric oxide production, cell proliferation	Protein-rich feeds, legumes, animal proteins
Vitamin A	Epithelial integrity, immune defense, collagen cross-linking	Carrots, pumpkin, sweet potato, dark leafy greens
Vitamin C	Collagen synthesis, antioxidant, reduces oxidative stress	Green leafy vegetables, citrus pulp (supplementation may be required)
Vitamin E	Antioxidant, reduces tissue damage, supports immune function	Wheat germ, vegetable oils, sunflower seeds
Vitamin K	Blood clotting, reduces risk of hemorrhage	Green leafy vegetables, alfalfa, commercial premixes
B-complex vitamins	Energy metabolism, cell division, RBC formation	Whole grains, brewer's yeast, legumes
Zinc	Collagen formation, DNA synthesis, epithelialization	Pumpkin seeds, fish meal, fortified premixes
Copper	Collagen cross-linking, RBC formation, angiogenesis	Legumes, seeds, mineral premixes
Iron	Oxygen transport, prevents anemia and delayed healing	Meat meal, leafy greens, mineral supplements
Selenium	Antioxidant defense, immune modulation	Grains (if soil adequate), yeast, premixes
Omega-3 fatty acids	Anti-inflammatory, supports membrane integrity	Flaxseed, fish oil, chia seed
Energy (carbohydrates and fats)	Provides calories for healing and immune activity	Corn, grains, vegetable oils

Chart created by Stephanie Freeman.

Wounds in chickens represent a frequent and serious clinical problem in backyard settings. Due to the fragility of avian skin, susceptibility to shock, and rapid onset of infection, successful management requires prompt veterinary attention, meticulous wound care, and strong nursing support. Veterinary technicians serve as the primary caregivers throughout this process, translating veterinary directives into consistent, compassionate, and practical care. Their role ensures that chickens receive not only medical treatment but also the supportive environment necessary for complete recovery.

Further Reading

Sabater González M, Calvo Carrasco D. Emergencies and critical care of commonly kept fowl. *Veterinary Clinics of North America: Exotic Animal Practice.* 2016 May;19(2):543–565.

Shaw S, Tully T. Avian Transfusion Medicine. Vetfolio. December, 2009. Accessed November 24, 2025. http://vetfolio-vetstreet.s3.amazonaws.com/mmah/d1/9cf789b8d5419bbc6ff868b5379979/filePV1209_Shaw.pdf

Wounds in Poultry [Internet]. Psu.edu. 2023. Available from: https://extension.psu.edu/wounds-in-poultry

16

Common Drug Therapies and Euthanasia

Therapeutic agents are essential tools in chicken health management, enabling the prevention, control, and treatment of bacterial, fungal, parasitic, and metabolic diseases. Proper use of these agents is crucial not only for animal welfare but also for flock safety and food chain safety. Even if the chicken or its eggs (ovary, follicles, and oviduct) will never be consumed by humans, veterinary professionals are obligated to inform guardians of drug withdrawal times in meat and eggs when administering any agent to a feathered friend.

The Federal Drug Administration (FDA) considers all chickens to be food-producing animals, and veterinarians can be held liable if meat or eggs (specifically the yolk) containing violative residues of prohibited drugs enter the human food chain. Agents are listed as approved, extra-label, and prohibited. Veterinarians and credentialed veterinary technicians can reference the Vet GRAM (Veterinarian's Guide to Residue Avoidance Management) website that is supported by FARAD (Food Animal Residue Avoidance Databank), for labeled use(s) of FDA-approved food animal drugs in the United States.

Veterinary technicians play a key role in calculating and administering drugs, monitoring responses, and educating chicken caregivers regarding the use of therapeutic agents. Unlike companion animals, production farm chickens are often treated at the flock level, which requires careful calculation of dosages per water or feed intake, observation of behavior and performance, and strict adherence to withdrawal times. Drug withdrawal begins when the last dose is administered. Guardians with small flocks are the focus of this text, so individual bird doses are listed. The same precautions and observations are required, but on a more "personalized" level.

The chapter covers major therapeutic classes, their uses, administration routes, and nursing considerations. Chicken caregivers should never attempt to diagnose conditions or prescribe any agent for their personal birds or others without veterinarian guidance. Strict adherence to drug stewardship prevents antibiotic resistance and misuse, resulting in animal, or human, injury. Responsible chicken-keeping goes beyond the backyard.

16.1 General Principles of Drug Use in Poultry

16.1.1 Routes of Administration

- **Oral**: drinking water, liquid dose, or solid dose
- **Injections**: intramuscular, subcutaneous, intraosseous, intravenous, intranasal
- **Topicals**: wounds of the skin, eye
- **Spray or Aerosol**: common for vaccines or respiratory medications

16.1.2 Withdrawal Times and Food Safety

Most therapeutic agents have specific withdrawal times to ensure residues do not enter eggs or meat. Those that do not are used in the extra-label manner at the veterinarian's discretion. Veterinary technicians must calculate available withdrawal time and communicate this information to caregivers. This information is not only recorded in the patient's medical record and given to the guardian at the time of discharge, but receipt of that information must also be documented, even with assurances from the guardian that the bird will never enter the food chain. With some drugs, FARAD cannot provide a blanket statement for withdrawal interval due to the lack of data, so the veterinarian can submit a withdrawal interval request to FARAD.

16.2 Antibacterial Agents

Antibacterial agents are widely used in chickens for the treatment of respiratory infections, enteric disease, septicemia, and wound infections. Classes commonly used include penicillins, tetracyclines, macrolides, sulfonamides, cephalosporins, and aminoglycosides. Choice of agent depends on the veterinarian's suspected or confirmed pathogenic microorganism, resistance patterns, and bird management practices.

Drug/class	Indication	Dosage	Route	Withdrawal time	Nursing notes
Amikacin	Septicemia, colibacillosis	10–20 mg/kg q8-12h	IM, SQ, IV	Meat: 30 days, eggs: not approved in laying hens	Ensure hydration; monitor for nephrotoxicity
Amoxicillin clavulanate	Respiratory infections, septicemia	125–250 mg/kg q8-12h or 500 mg/L drinking water	PO	Meat: 7 days, eggs: 1 day	Ensure full course; monitor for diarrhea
Amoxicillin sodium	Respiratory infections, septicemia	50–250 mg/kg q8-12h	IM, IV	Meat: 7 days, eggs: not approved in some regions	Ensure full course; monitor for diarrhea
Amoxicillin trihydrate	Respiratory infections, septicemia	55–200 mg/kg q4-12h or 200–1500 mg/L in drinking water	PO, SQ, IM, IV	Meat: 7 days, eggs: not approved in some regions	Ensure full course; monitor for diarrhea
Ampicillin sodium	Respiratory infections, septicemia, enteritis	100 mg/kg q4-12h or 528 mg/L in drinking water	PO	Meat: 5 days, eggs: not approved in laying hens producing eggs for human consumption	Ensure hydration; replace solution every 24 hours
Cefazolin	Septicemia, respiratory infections, osteomyelitis	25–75 mg/kg q12h	IM, IV (slowly)	No established withdrawal times	Not approved for poultry in food production

Drug/class	Indication	Dosage	Route	Withdrawal time	Nursing notes
Cephalexin	Skin infections, joint infections, septicemia	50–125 mg/kg q6-12h	PO, IM	Meat: no approved withdrawal times, Eggs: the United States, Ireland, the United Kingdom 0-day withdrawal	Watch for GI upset; ensure full course
Ciprofloxacin	Respiratory infection, enteric infection, septicemia	15–40 mg/kg q12h	PO, IM, IV, SQ	Meat: 14 days, eggs: no established withdrawal times	Should be reserved when no safer alternatives are available
Clindamycin	Anaerobic infections, joint infections, soft tissue infections	25–50 mg/kg q8-12h	PO, SQ, IM	No established withdrawal times	Monitor for GI upset; ensure hydration
Enrofloxacin	Respiratory infection, enteric infection, septicemia	10–15 mg/kg q12-24h or 50 mg/L in drinking water	PO, SQ, IM	Meat: 7–14 days, eggs: not approved in laying hens producing eggs for human consumption	Avoid in young, growing chicks; use is prohibited by FDA
Erythromycin	CRD, Mycoplasma	10–20 mg/kg × 5–7 days	PO	Meat: 7 days, eggs: the United States, Ireland, the United Kingdom, and Australia 0-day withdrawal	Ensure full course; ensure hydration
Gentamicin	Septicemia, joint infections	5–10 mg/kg q24h	IM	Meat: 21 days, eggs: not approved in laying hens producing eggs for human consumption	Use only under veterinary supervision; monitor for nephrotoxicity
Lincomycin	*C. perfringens*	25–50 mg/kg q 12hrs	PO	Meat: unknown, eggs: 1–10 days	Avoid with meloxicam, other antibiotics
Oxytetracycline	CRD, synovitis, enteritis	5 mg/kg q12-24h or 2500 mg/L of drinking water	SQ, IM, drinking water	Meat: 28 days, eggs: not approved in laying hens producing eggs for human consumption	Monitor water intake and flock response
Tiamulin	*Mycoplasma*	25–50 mg/kg q 24hrs x 3–5 days	PO	Mea: unknown, eggs: 72 hours	Ensure hydration

(*Continued*)

Drug/class	Indication	Dosage	Route	Withdrawal time	Nursing notes
Trimethoprim-sulfa	Coccidiosis, enteritis	100 mg/kg q12h or 360–400 mg/L of drinking water	PO	Meat: 10 days, eggs: not approved in laying hens producing eggs for human consumption	Ensure hydration; observe flock for adverse reactions
Tylosin	*Mycoplasmosis, synovitis*	15–30 mg/kg q6-12h (IM), 50 mg/kg q24h (PO), 50 mg/L drinking water	IM, PO, drinking water	Meat: 5 days, eggs: the United States, Ireland, the United Kingdom, and Australia 0-day withdrawal	Avoid abrupt withdrawal to prevent relapse

Chart by Stephanie Freeman.

16.3 Antifungal Agents

Fungal infections in chickens, such as candidiasis (crop or gastrointestinal yeast overgrowth) and aspergillosis (respiratory), can cause morbidity, reduced growth, and production losses. Candidiasis is most common in young chicks exposed to contaminated feed or water. Aspergillosis typically affects respiratory tissues, often after exposure to moldy litter or feed. Few antifungals are licensed for poultry; most therapy is supportive. Successful management depends on early detection, environmental control, and supportive care.

Drug	Indication	Dosage	Route	Withdrawal time	Nursing notes
Amphotericin B	*Aspergillosis*	7 mg/mL for 15 minutes (nebulized) q12h, 1.5 mg/kg (IV) q8h, 1 mg/kg intratracheal/nasal flush q8-12h diluted to 1 mL with sterile saline	Nebulized, IV, intratracheal/nasal	Unknown	If given rapidly or overdosing can result in heart arrhythmia and cardio-respiratory arrest
Fluconazole	*Cryptococcosis, Aspergillosis, Candidiasis,* Blastomycosis, and Histoplasmosis	2–5 mg/kg q24h x 7 days	PO	Unknown	With or without food; less effective than itraconazole
Itraconazole	Severe systemic candidiasis, *Aspergillosis*, Histoplasmosis, and *Cryptococcus*	5–10 mg/kg q12-24h	PO	Meat: 14 days	Limited poultry approval; use under veterinary guidance

Drug	Indication	Dosage	Route	Withdrawal time	Nursing notes
Nystatin	Candidiasis	100,000 U/L in drinking water or 300,000–600,000 U/kg q8-12h	Oral	None	Mix food thoroughly; safe for all ages; not absorbed systemically

Chart by Stephanie Freeman.

16.4 Antiparasitic Agents

Parasites are a major cause of reduced growth, poor feed conversion, anemia, and mortality in chickens. Correct dosing is critical to prevent resistance. Rotate anticoccidials to reduce drug resistance.

Drug	Indication	Dosage	Route	Withdrawal time	Nursing notes
Amprolium	Coccidiosis	13–30 mg/kg (PO), 1.25 mL/L in drinking water, 40–250 mg/kg in feed	PO, feed, drinking water	None	Ensure no concurrent thiamine deficiency; monitor water intake
Fenbendazole	Roundworms, *Capillaria, Heterakis*	1 mg/kg × 3–5 days, repeat in 10 days	PO	Meat: 6 days, Eggs: 17 days	Repeat treatment for lifecycle interruption if necessary
Ivermectin	Roundworms, Cecal worms, Gapeworms, Manson eyeworms	0.2–0.4 mg/kg once, repeat in 10–14 days	PO, SQ, IM, Topical	Meat: 21–28 days, Eggs: 7–14 days	Avoid using in very young chicks
Metronidazole	*Giardia*	10–50 mg/kg q12-24h	PO	Not approved for use in food-producing poultry.	Sometimes used for anaerobic bacterial infections
Piperazine	Ascarids	130–200 mg/kg	PO	Meat, eggs: 0 days	No longer available in the United States
Ponazuril	Toxoplasmosis, Coccidiosis, Sarcocystosis	10–20 mg/kg q24h	PO	No withdrawal periods are established	No known residues are approved for human food safety; hence, strict withdrawal precautions are necessary.
Praziquantel	Trematodes	10–20 mg/kg once and repeat in 10 days	SQ, PO, IM	No withdrawal periods are established	Acute toxicity is relatively low

(*Continued*)

Drug	Indication	Dosage	Route	Withdrawal time	Nursing notes
Pyrantel Pamoate	Roundworms, Capillaria, Heterakis	7 mg/kg once, repeat in 14 days	PO	No withdrawal periods are established	Use caution in severely debilitated animals
Selamectin	Scaly Leg Mites	23 mg/kg, repeat in 3–4 weeks	Topical	No withdrawal periods are established	Avoid use in very young chicks
Toltrazuril	Coccidiosis	6–25 mg/kg once; repeat in 5 days or 0.0125 g/L in drinking water x 2 days	PO, drinking water	Meat: 14 days, Eggs: Not approved in laying hens producing eggs for human consumption	Administer under veterinary guidance; potent drug

Chart by Stephanie Freeman.

16.5 Nutritional and Metabolic Therapeutics

Proper nutrition is critical in preventing myopathies, rickets, cage layer fatigue, and metabolic disorders. Therapeutic supplementation may be necessary when deficiencies occur or during stress periods.

Supplement	Indication	Dosage	Route	Nursing notes
Vitamin E	Nutritional myopathy, oxidative stress	50–100 IU/kg feed	Oral	Often combined with selenium; monitor for deficiency signs
Selenium	Nutritional myopathy, antioxidant support	0.1–0.3 ppm feed	Oral	Narrow safety margin; excess can be toxic
Vitamin D3	Rickets, cage layer fatigue	2000–5000 IU/kg feed	Oral	Ensure correct Ca:P ratio
Calcium (Oyster shell grit)	Eggshell quality, osteoporosis	Ad lib in feed	Oral	Provide constant access, especially in egg layers
Electrolytes	Heat stress, dehydration	ORS formulas as per label	Drinking water	Administer during heat waves or stress events
Probiotics	Gut flora health, immunity	As per manufacturer	Feed/ Water	Rotate strains to prevent resistance and maximize benefit

Chart by Stephanie Freeman.

16.6 Analgesics, Anti-Inflammatory Agents, and Local Anesthetic Agents

Pain management is an essential but often overlooked aspect of chicken care. Analgesics and anti-inflammatory drugs are used to alleviate discomfort from injuries, fractures, surgical procedures, or inflammatory conditions. Overuse or long-term use of anti-inflammatory agents can cause gastrointestinal irritation or renal toxicity.

Drug	Indication	Dosage	Route	Withdrawal time	Nursing notes
Aspirin	Pain, fever, inflammation	5 mg/kg q8h or 1.2 g/L in drinking water	PO, drinking water	Meat: 1–3 days, eggs: 24–48 hours	Usually flock-level; avoid overdose
Bupivacaine	Local anesthetic	1–2–5 mg/kg	SQ, splash, intra-articular, subarachnoid, brachial plexus	Unknown	Potential adverse cardiovascular effect if IV
Butorphanol	Mild pain, sedation	1–4 mg/kg q3-12h	IM, IV	Meat: 14 days, eggs: unknown	Can be used as a sole agent or in a multimodal protocol
Carprofen	Pain, inflammation	5–10 mg/kg q24h	PO, IM	Meat: 7–14 days, Eggs: 7 days	Can interact negatively with aspirin, cortisone-like drugs, and corticosteroids
Ibuprofen	Pain, inflammation, fever	5–10 mg/kg q8-12h	PO	No withdrawal periods are established.	Use for the shortest effective period to reduce the risk of side effects
Isoflurane	Induction, maintenance anesthesia	1–5%	Inhalation via nares, trachea	Unknown	Effectively metabolized, little residue
Ketamine	Pain, sedation	0.5 mg/kg	IM	Unknown	In conjunction with midazolam
Lidocaine	Local anesthetic	2–20 mg/kg	SQ, splash, brachial plexus, intra-articular, subarachnoid	Unknown	Potential adverse cardiovascular effect if IV
Medetomidine	Pain, sedation	50 ug/kg	IM	Unknown	In conjunction with midazolam, ketamine for induction
Meloxicam	Pain, inflammation	0.5–1 mg/kg q24h	PO	Meat: 7 days, Eggs: 14 days; some sources say unknown	Use for individual or small groups; monitor for GI upset; use 5 days or less
Methadone	Moderate to severe pain	6 mg/kg	IV, IM	Unknown	Used in conjunction with multimodal protocol

(*Continued*)

Drug	Indication	Dosage	Route	Withdrawal time	Nursing notes
Methylprednisolone acetate		200 mg/kg q24h	IM	No withdrawal periods are established.	Use caution in meat birds and layers due to potential effects on growth, egg production, and metabolism
Midazolam	Relaxation, anxiolytic	0.5 mg/kg	IM	Unknown	Used in conjunction with medetomidine, ketamine for induction
Sevoflurane	Induction, maintenance	1–5%	Inhalation via nares, trachea	Unknown	Lower blood:gas solubility quotient than isoflurane
Tramadol	Mild to moderate pain	15 mg/kg q12h	PO	Meat: 14 days, Eggs: Unknown	Can cause sedation

Chart by Stephanie Freeman.

16.7 Gastrointestinal Agents

Metoclopramide	Gastric motility	0.3–0.5 mg/kg	PO, IM	Meat: 14 days, eggs: 28 days (UK)	Crop emptying; avoid in chicks
Probiotics and prebiotics	Gut bacteria replenishment	Follow product directions In drinking water or powder on food.	PO	No known withdrawal time	Observe expiration dates and refrigeration recommendations
Sucralfate	GI protectant	25 mg/kg q 8h	PO	Unknown	Avoid use in certain antimicrobials and fat soluble vitamins

Chart by Stephanie Freeman.

16.8 Topical Agents and Antiseptics

Topical therapy is primarily used for wounds, pododermatitis, burns, and localized infections. Veterinary technicians play a critical role in proper cleaning, dressing, and monitoring for secondary infection. Clean and dry the affected area with warmed water, warm saline, or properly diluted antiseptic solution before applying medication. Bandaging or protective coverings may

Agent	Indication	Dosage/application	Route	Nursing notes
Povidone-iodine	Wound cleansing, antisepsis	Initial and subsequent cleansing; diluted 1:40	Topical	Avoid ingestion; protect surrounding feathers; safe around eyes, face
Chlorhexidine	Wound cleansing, pododermatitis	Initial and subsequent cleansing; diluted 0.5–1% solution	Topical	Mild antiseptic; less irritating than iodine; avoid eyes, face
Silver sulfadiazine	Burns, infected wounds	Thin layer daily or with bandage change	Topical	Monitor for contact dermatitis
Epsom salt in warm water	Foot soaks, abscess softening	1–2% solution × 10–15 min	Soak	Softens necrotic tissue prior to debridement

Chart by Stephanie Freeman.

be used to prevent trauma and contamination (refer to Chapter 15). Topical antimicrobial therapy is adjunctive, often combined with systemic therapy if infection is indicated and prescribed by the veterinarian.

16.9 Endocrine/Hormonal Intervention

Agent	Indication	Dosage/application	Route	Nursing notes
Deslorin acetate	Suppresses FSH and LH	4.7–9.4 mg implant every 4–8 months	SQ	Approved for ferrets only in the United States

Chart by Stephanie Freeman.

16.10 Euthanasia Protocol

To preserve the dignity of the bird and provide a "good" death, euthanasia must be discussed with guardians in cases of futile care. A pain-free death is the final gift the veterinary team can provide a patient. By explaining the procedure and its expectations to the guardian, it allows them to process the bird's loss in a rational manner. If available, gabapentin and tramadol are options for previsit sedation. Informed consent and handling of remains should be discussed and finalized prior to euthanasia.

While there are AVMA Guidelines for Euthanasia (manual and mechanical methods) for a chicken, the most humane is with premedication of injectable agents, inhalation of volatile anesthetic, and intravenous administration of pentobarbital. A common protocol is the administration of injectable agents, such as butorphanol and medetomidine (using the drug doses in this chapter), followed by inhalant anesthetic induction with isoflurane or sevoflurane which produces a desirable level of relaxation. An intravenous catheter (medial metatarsal, jugular, or ulnar vein) should be placed, or a winged infusion set can be used to avoid perivascular injection of sodium pentobarbital.

Agent	Indication	Dosage/ application	Route	Nursing notes
Sodium pentobarbital	Injectable chemical euthanasia	150–600 mg/kg	IV, intracoelomic, intrarenal, intrahepatic, intracardiac, intraosseous	IV catheter placement if procedure performed with guardian

Chart by Stephanie Freeman.

Once the patient is relaxed and calm, sodium pentobarbital is administered intravenously (150–600 mg/kg) for humane euthanasia. An alternative method can be performed by injecting into a kidney, liver, heart, or femur. Intra-organ, or intracoelomic, method will result in delayed death compared to the expedient intravenous or intraosseous methods. Two-person auscultation of heart cessation and lack of corneal reflex confirms patient death.

16.11 Handling of Remains

Many guardians will want to return home with their bird for burial. They must be advised of potential risks to scavengers (use of pentobarbital in the deceased bird) and the spread of contagious avian diseases (i.e., avian flu). Burial must follow local legal statutes for burial or disposal. Cremation is the preferable method of pentobarbital-euthanized remains handling, and private cremation is a service provided by most crematoriums.

16.12 Memorialization and Grief Support

A clay footprint or inked print can easily be made for the caregiver on the same day as euthanasia. A signed card or phone call a few days after the visit conveys sympathy, and the veterinary team can provide additional grief resources. Most veterinary colleges have social work departments that provide judgment-free, in-person or virtual grief support for animal guardians (Figure 16.1).

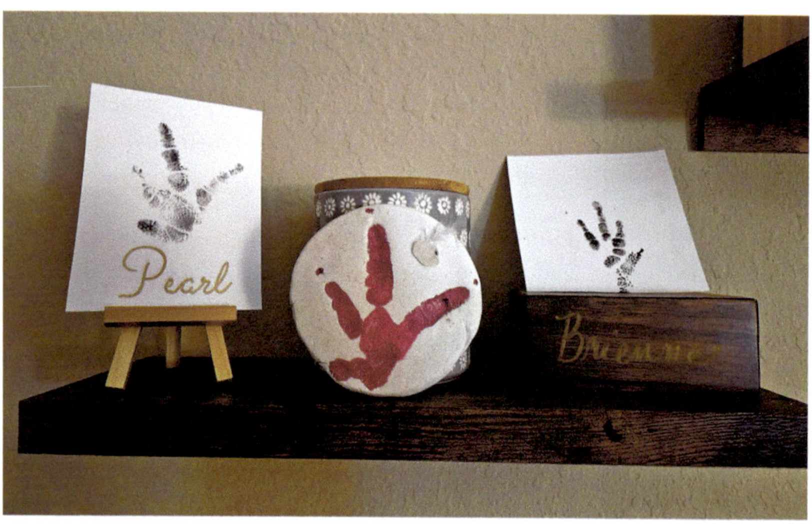

Figure 16.1 Footprints in clay and cardstock for the guardian's memories, displayed with boxed cremains. Courtesy of Sarah Meyer.

Further Reading

About: Vetgram: Farad [Internet]. [cited 2025 Nov 29]. Available from: chrome-extension://efaidnbmnnnibpcajpcglclefindmkaj/https://www.avma.org/sites/default/files/2020-02/Guidelines-on-Euthanasia-2020.pdf

Carpenter's Exotic Animal Formulary - 9780323833929 [Internet]. 2015 [cited 2025 Nov 29]. Available from: https://www.us.elsevierhealth.com/carpenters-exotic-animal-formulary-9780323833929.html?srsltid=AfmBOooP4t5p0HBmhJUlCNg3cgark4TOV4evPxYR3V8vB6aCTwxHzI84

Çelik Y, Atalan G, Güneş V, Alpman U, Yönez MK. Use of Medetomidine, Midazolam, Ketamine and Sevoflurane as an Anesthetic Protocol for Domestic Chickens [Internet]. [cited 2025 Nov 29]. Available from: https://www.redalyc.org/journal/423/42371733001/html/

Euthanasia for Broiler Chickens: Manual and Mechanical Cervical Dislocation Methods [Internet]. Vt.edu. 2019 [cited 2025 Dec 8]. Available from: https://www.pubs.ext.vt.edu/APSC/APSC-161/APSC-161.html

FARAD [Internet]. Farad.org. 2025. Available from: https://www.farad.org/

Help Prevent Euthanasia Drugs from Killing Bald Eagles and Other Wildlife | U.S. Fish & Wildlife Service [Internet]. www.fws.gov. 2022. Available from: https://www.fws.gov/story/help-prevent-euthanasia-drugs-killing-bald-eagles-and-other-wildlife

Leary S, Johnson C. AVMA Guidelines for the Euthanasia of Animals: 2020 Edition [Internet]. 2020. Available from: https://www.avma.org/sites/default/files/2020-02/Guidelines-on-Euthanasia-2020.pdf

Macdonald Campus Farm Poultry Unit Standard Operating Procedure # PU-520 POULTRY EUTHANASIA [Internet]. Available from: chrome-extension://efaidnbmnnnibpcajpcglclefindmkaj/https://www.mcgill.ca/research/files/research/pu-520_poultry_euthanasia.pdf

MSc M. Avian Euthanasia: Welfare Considerations & Clinical Techniques - LafeberVet [Internet]. LafeberVet. 2025 [cited 2025 Dec 12]. Available from: https://lafeber.com/vet/avian-euthanasia-welfare-and-techniques/?srsltid=AfmBOooOPCn-M68qLdwv_rXqAFn-ZicwpEaC22UVQIsmFbBBNoFmRoB

Pet Loss Support Information [Internet]. Vin.com. 2023 [cited 2025 Dec 8]. Available from: https://veterinarypartner.vin.com/default.aspx?pid=19239&id=6048074

17

Client Education and Patient Discharge Instructions

Guardian education is a cornerstone of patient outcomes. The clients' understanding of proper care, disease prevention, and post-treatment instructions directly impacts bird health and welfare. Veterinary technicians play a pivotal role in this education, bridging the gap between the veterinarian and clients' practical application. For the most effective retention of information, the veterinary technician should provide verbal instructions during the discharge appointment or phone conversation, written instructions (homecare information), and a scheduled follow-up appointment or phone call.

Key Points

- Chickens are highly sensitive to environmental, nutritional, and infectious challenges. Small errors in care can result in severe illness or death.
- Client education with credible information reduces recurrence of disease, improves compliance with treatment protocols, and enhances overall productivity and welfare.
- Veterinary technicians serve as primary educators, providing instructions on husbandry, nutrition, biosecurity, medication administration, monitoring, and follow-up care.

Why Education Matters

- Owners often underestimate the importance of proper housing, nutrition, and biosecurity, which are critical for disease prevention.
- Discharge instructions must translate complex medical advice into clear, actionable steps.
- Educated clients are more likely to recognize early signs of disease, reducing morbidity and mortality.

Challenges in Client Education

- Owners' prior experience and relationship with chickens vary widely.
- Availability to noncredible, anecdotal information can serve as a powerful barrier for scientific reasoning and evidence-based decision-making.
- Unintentional and willful ignorance can lead to abuse and neglect of chickens.
- Misconceptions about medications, supplements, or disease transmission can complicate care and have detrimental effects on birds and caregivers.
- Emotional attachment may influence willingness to implement certain interventions (e.g., euthanasia and isolation).

Effective Communication Ensures Clients Understand and Follow Instructions

1) Use clear, nontechnical language. Replace veterinary jargon with clear language.

2) Chunking Information: Provide instructions in manageable segments, then ask if they need clarification.
3) Repeat and reinforce: The client often retains only part of the information during a stressful visit. Repetition improves compliance.
4) Provide written discharge/home care instructions and review them verbally.
5) Visual aids such as diagrams, charts, and photos can help explain housing setups, bandage application, or medication administration.
6) Follow up with phone calls, emails, or text messages regularly (24 hours, 3 days, and/or 7 days post-discharge).

Provide discharge/home care instructions, summarizing key points. Use bold headings and bullet points for clarity. Never assume a caregiver knows how to perform home care. Examples of discharge instructions appear later in the chapter.

- Medication names, dosages, and frequency
- Feeding or water changes or nutritional guidance
- Daily monitoring checklist and signs that require immediate veterinary attention
- Contact information for emergencies

Demonstrations and Hands-On Training

- Show clients how to safely handle chickens.
- Demonstrate oral medication administration, crop tubing, or injections.
- Teach wound cleaning and dressing changes, highlighting hygiene to prevent secondary infections and zoonosis.
- Encourage clients to practice under supervision.

When to Seek Immediate Veterinary Attention

- Provide guardians with "red flag" signs requiring urgent care or necropsy
- Hemorrhage from wounds, broken blood feathers
- Sudden death or rapid deterioration
- Severe respiratory distress
- Neurological signs (seizures, head tremors, paralysis)
- Profuse diarrhea, bloody droppings, or persistent anorexia
- Swollen joints, severe lameness, or bone fractures
- Any signs of pain, distress, or unresponsive behavior

17.1 Basic Husbandry and Environmental Care

Proper husbandry and environmental management are fundamental to chicken health. Veterinary technicians must educate clients on optimal housing, bedding, nutrition, and water management to prevent disease and support recovery. Regular scooping of droppings, scrubbing and disinfection of hard surfaces, and cleaning of waterers and feeders are basic preventive measures caregivers can perform to ensure a sanitary environment. Chapter 3 details the importance of husbandry, housing, and biosecurity.

17.2 Housing Requirements and Hygiene

Show caregivers ideal coop designs or photos. Advise them to provide at least 2–3 sq. ft. per chicken in the coop and 8–10 sq. ft. per bird in the run. Overcrowding increases stress, aggression, and disease transmission. Ensure adequate airflow to reduce ammonia accumulation and respiratory disease risk. Avoid drafts directly on birds. Secure coops with hardware cloth, lockable doors, and buried fencing to prevent raccoons, foxes, or rodent access. Access to natural light and sunshine influences egg production and overall health. Demonstrate checking for drafts, leaks, or predator entry points. Explain the importance of seasonal adjustments (e.g., ventilation in summer, insulation in winter).

Recommend using dry, absorbent bedding such as pine shavings, hemp, or chopped hay. Maintain 2–4 inches of bedding and replace or add frequently to prevent moisture buildup. Daily removal of wet or soiled areas; full litter replacement every 4–6 weeks, depending on flock size and housing type. Wet litter promotes coccidiosis, respiratory infections, and footpad dermatitis. Accumulated droppings increase ammonia, causing eye irritation and respiratory issues. Specific cleaning protocols are described in Chapter 3, Husbandry, Housing, and Biosecurity.

17.3 Nutrition Education and Water Hygiene

Provide species-appropriate feed advisement based on age and production stage (starter, grower, layer). Supplement grit, which is necessary for digestion, especially with whole grains. Calcium is required by layer hens for strong eggshells. Ensure constant access to clean feed, adjust amounts based on age, breed, and production level. Show proper feeding techniques, measuring supplements, and mixing water-soluble vitamins. Educate on avoiding moldy feed and improper storage, which can lead to mycotoxicosis. Teach caregivers how to read feed bag labels to look for balanced nutrition and appropriate nutrients for life stages.

Monitor body condition and weight regularly. Avoid feeding excessive table scraps or high-fat treats. Teach clients how to recognize signs of nutritional deficiency, such as poor feathering, thin-shelled eggs, and lethargy.

Fresh water must be provided daily; ensure water is clean and free of debris. Use hanging drinkers or clean troughs to minimize contamination. Check water intake as a sudden reduction may indicate illness. Demonstrate or explain proper cleaning and sanitizing of waterers. Explain the importance of water for medication delivery and electrolyte supplementation during illness or heat stress. This is discussed further in Chapter 4, Nutrition.

17.4 Biosecurity Education

Biosecurity is critical to preventing infectious diseases in chicken flocks. Veterinary technicians must educate clients on practical strategies to limit exposure to pathogens and reduce disease transmission.

Wild birds can carry viruses, bacteria, and parasites. Minimize open access to feed, water, or housing areas. Restrict visitors' access to coops; instruct them to wear dedicated footwear and clothing.

Disease outbreaks are becoming an increasing concern for backyard flocks in different regions of the country, so caregivers cannot be too cautious. Footbaths with disinfectants at coop entrances reduce pathogen entry. Dedicated clothing and boots should be used in poultry areas; avoid using the same footwear outside. Handwashing before and after handling chickens is critical to prevent disease spread and zoonotic transmission. Biosecurity is discussed further in Chapter 3, Husbandry, Housing, and Biosecurity.

New birds should be quarantined for 4 weeks before introduction to the main flock. Monitor for clinical signs such as coughing, sneezing, diarrhea, lethargy, or abnormal behavior. Recommend screening for common infectious diseases (e.g., *Mycoplasma, Salmonella*, or Marek's disease) and internal and external parasites. Veterinary reference laboratories offer these diagnostic tests and offer specimen collection, preparation, and shipping information.

17.5 Disease Transmission Risks to Humans

Zoonotic pathogens such as *Salmonella* or *Campylobacter* can infect humans, especially children or immunocompromised individuals. Educate clients to wash hands thoroughly after handling birds, eggs, or feed. Wearing personal protective equipment while cleaning the chicken coop/house and pen can mitigate the risk of infection. Cook eggs and meat properly, according to the United States Department of Agriculture's Food Safety and Inspection Service guidelines, to avoid foodborne illness. It is recommended by human medical professionals to avoid kissing chickens to avoid pathogenic organisms.

17.6 Creating and Delivering Effective Discharge Instructions

Discharge instructions are vital for ensuring that guardians understand how to continue to care at home following veterinary treatment. Well-structured discharge plans improve recovery outcomes, reduce complications, and empower guardians to manage their birds confidently.

17.7 Components of Effective Discharge Instructions

1) Patient Identification
   - Bird's name or identification number
   - Breed, age, sex, and weight
   - Date of discharge and attending veterinarian
2) Diagnosis and Summary of Care
   - Clear, lay-language explanation of the condition diagnosed
   - Description of procedures performed, and treatments given during hospitalization
3) Medication Instructions
   - Drug name (generic or brand, if applicable)
   - Dosage (mg/kg or mL/bird), route, and frequency
   - Duration of treatment and refill instructions
   - Emphasize the importance of completing the full course of medication
   - Include withdrawal times for eggs and meat if applicable
4) Wound or Bandage Care (if applicable)
   - How to change bandages safely
   - Cleaning techniques and supplies to use/avoid
   - Signs of infection or complications to watch for

5) Feeding and Hydration Guidelines
   - Specific diet to offer, texture modifications (soft/moistened feed), and feeding frequency
   - Water supplementation (electrolytes, probiotics) if prescribed
   - How to monitor intake and what changes should prompt a call
6) Activity Restrictions and Housing Modifications
   - Confine the bird to a quiet area or hospital enclosure as needed
   - Avoid perches or ramps if mobility is impaired
   - Provide warmth, soft bedding, and minimal stress until recovery is complete
7) Monitoring and Follow-Up
   - Specific clinical signs to monitor (appetite, droppings, weight, respiratory effort, wound healing)
   - Exact date/time for recheck appointments
   - Contact information for emergencies

17.8 Examples of Discharge Instructions After Common Procedures and Treatments

Each example can be tailored to specific procedures, treatments:

Client Instructions for Home Care After Surgery

Common procedures such as wound repair, abscess drainage, enucleation, crop surgery, and reproductive surgeries.

Keep (*insert patient name*) in a clean, quiet, warm area with clean bedding. Provide enrichment and encourage drinking of water and eating. Weigh daily while recovering.

Restrict access to flock mates for 7–10 days, or until the sutures are removed. Slow reintroduction.

Limit activity and jumping to prevent injury to sutures or surgical sites. If the surgical site opens, contact us as soon as possible. Lower perches during recovery.

Monitor incision daily for redness, swelling, discharge, or odor. If a bandage is present, keep the bandage clean and dry; change or remove if it becomes soiled or wet. A onesie can be used and replaced as necessary.

Do not allow the bird to peck at sutures; use an avian collar if needed. A onesie can also be used.

Administer all prescribed medications as directed (*list each medication with its directions*). Complete the full course, even if (*insert patient name*) appears to be improved.

Observe appetite, droppings, and activity. Report any lethargy, anorexia, or active bleeding to the veterinarian as soon as possible.

Medications:

If the veterinarian has prescribed acupuncture/laser therapy/other therapy, make those appointments today.

A recheck appointment may be recommended and scheduled at the time of discharge.

Client Instructions: Fracture Repair or Orthopedic Care

Keep (*insert patient name*) in a clean, quiet, warm area with clean bedding. Provide enrichment and encourage drinking of water and eating. Provide a high-quality, balanced diet and supplemental calcium and vitamin D3 (*if prescribed*).

Restrict access to flock mates until the splint/bandage/external fixator is removed.

Strict confinement in a small, padded enclosure for 2–6 weeks depending on fracture type. No perches.

Keep splints and bandages dry and clean, monitor for swelling above or below the splint/bandage. Do not remove unless instructed. Limit activity and jumping to prevent injury to surgical sites. If the surgical site opens, splint slips, or bandage becomes soiled/wet, contact us as soon as possible.

Do not allow the bird to peck at the splint/bandage/external fixator; use an avian collar if needed.

Administer all prescribed medications as directed (*list each medication with its directions*). Complete the full course, even if (*insert patient name*) appears to be improved.

Observe appetite, droppings, and activity. Report any lethargy, anorexia, or active bleeding to the veterinarian as soon as possible. Weigh daily while recovering.

Physical rehabilitation directed by the veterinarian.

If the veterinarian has prescribed acupuncture/laser therapy/other therapy, make those appointments today.

Return for scheduled rechecks and radiographs as instructed.

Client Instructions: After Respiratory Illness Treatment

Common conditions are infectious bronchitis, Mycoplasmosis, and colibacillosis.

Keep (*insert patient name*) separate from the flock until fully symptom-free and cleared by the veterinarian. Reintroduce slowly.

Administer antibiotics or supportive medications as prescribed (*list all medications and directions for each*).

Gently clean nares and face of discharge as needed. Warm, wet cotton balls or baby wipes are ideal. Stop if the bird becomes stressed, begins open-beak breathing.

Improve ventilation and reduce dust and ammonia. Maintain warm, dry bedding.

Offer palatable food and water with added electrolytes if appetite is reduced. Encourage drinking and eating. Provide enrichment. Weigh daily while recovering.

Observe appetite, droppings, and activity. Report any lethargy, anorexia, or active bleeding to the veterinarian as soon as possible.

A recheck appointment may be recommended and scheduled at the time of discharge.

Client Instructions: Aftercare for Gastrointestinal Disease Treatment

Common conditions are coccidiosis, helminthiasis, crop impaction, sour crop, and enteritis.

Keep (*insert patient name*) in a clean, quiet, warm area with clean bedding. Provide enrichment and encourage drinking of water and eating. Weigh daily while recovering.

Restrict access to flock mates for 7–10 days, or until the sutures are removed. Reintroduce slowly.

Limit activity and jumping to prevent injury to sutures or surgical sites. If the surgical site opens, contact us as soon as possible.

Gradually return to regular feed. Provide easily digestible feed (crumbles, soaked pellets) during recovery. Offer clean water with prebiotics/probiotics or electrolytes if recommended.

Administer all prescribed medications as directed (*list each medication with its directions*). Complete the full course, even if (*insert patient name*) appears to be improved.

Observe appetite, droppings (monitor for change in character, blood), and activity. Report any lethargy, anorexia, or active bleeding to the veterinarian as soon as possible.

A recheck appointment may be recommended and scheduled at the time of discharge. Bring droppings for assessment or for submission to reference laboratory for parasite analysis if indicated.

Client Instructions: Aftercare for Wounds or Abscess Treatment

Keep (*insert patient name*) in a clean, quiet, warm area with clean bedding. Provide enrichment and encourage drinking of water and eating. Weigh daily while recovering.

Restrict access to flock mates for 7–10 days, or until the sutures are removed. Reintroduce slowly.

Limit activity and jumping to prevent injury to sutures or surgical sites. If the surgical site opens, contact us as soon as possible. Lower perches while recovering.

Monitor wound daily for signs of infection such as swelling, heat, discharge, odor, or lethargy.

If a bandage is present, keep the bandage clean and dry; change or remove if it becomes soiled or wet. A onesie can be used and replaced as necessary.

Flush wounds as instructed (often one to two times daily) with warm saline or dilute antiseptic solution (*dispense this diluted solution with the caregiver with directions for use*). Wear exam gloves during this procedure.

Do not allow (*insert patient name*) to peck at sutures; use an avian collar if needed. A onesie can also be used.

Encourage appetite, drinking during recovery. Offer clean water with prebiotics/probiotics or electrolytes if recommended. Weight daily during recovery.

Administer all prescribed medications as directed (*list each medication with its directions*). Complete the full course, even if (*insert patient name*) appears to be improved.

Observe appetite, droppings (monitor for change in character, blood), and activity. Report any lethargy, anorexia, or active bleeding to the veterinarian as soon as possible.

If the veterinarian has prescribed acupuncture/laser therapy/other therapy, make those appointments today.

A recheck appointment may be recommended and scheduled at the time of discharge.

Client Instructions: Aftercare for Reproductive Treatments

Keep (*insert patient name*) in a clean, quiet, warm area with clean bedding to minimize stress. Provide enrichment and encourage drinking of water and eating.

Restrict access to flock mates for 7–10 days or longer if necessary. Reintroduce slowly.

Limit activity and jumping for a couple of days, especially in the case of prolapse. Observe the bird to return to normal laying behavior and droppings; watch for straining, lethargy, or abdominal swelling.

Monitor the vent and cloaca daily for increased redness, swelling, discharge, or odor. Keep the cloacal area clean and dry.

If a bandage is present, keep the bandage clean and dry; change or remove if it becomes soiled or wet. A onesie can be used and replaced as necessary. Do not allow the bird to peck at sutures if present; use an avian collar if needed.

Transition to a balanced layer ration and monitor body condition to prevent recurrence. Gradually return to regular feed. Provide easily digestible feed (crumbles, soaked pellets) during recovery. Offer clean water with prebiotics/probiotics or electrolytes if recommended. Weigh daily while recovering.

Administer all prescribed medications as directed (*list each medication with its directions*). Complete the full course, even if (*insert patient name*) appears to be improved.

Observe appetite, droppings (monitor for change in character, blood), and activity. Report any lethargy, anorexia, or active bleeding to the veterinarian as soon as possible.

A recheck appointment may be recommended and scheduled at the time of discharge.

17.9 Vaccination, Parasite Prevention, and Preventative Health

This section guides veterinary technicians to educate chicken guardians on core preventive health measures, including vaccinations, parasite control, and health planning, which are crucial for disease prevention and flock productivity. Most major chick hatcheries offer chick vaccinations prior to shipment; guardians are encouraged to partake in this practice.

17.9.1 Core Vaccines

- Marek's Disease
  - Given at hatch (day-old chicks).
  - It prevents tumor formation and paralysis.
  - Lifelong protection, no boosters.
- Newcastle Disease/Infectious Bronchitis
  - Often given together as a combined vaccine.
  - Administered by eye/nose drops or drinking water.
  - Multiple boosters during the production period.
- Fowl Pox
  - Wing-web stab method in chicks 6–10 weeks old.
  - Provides long-lasting protection.
- Infectious bursal disease
  - Given at 2–3 weeks of age.
  - Protects immune system development.

- Optional/Region Specific Vaccines
  - Avian Encephalomyelitis (for breeding stock)
  - Infectious laryngotracheitis
  - Fowl cholera

17.9.2 Parasite Prevention Programs

- **External Parasites**
  - Common ectoparasites: poultry red mite, northern fowl mite, lice, and fleas.
  - Preventive Measures:
    - Inspect and clean birds and housing regularly.
    - Treat housing with approved permethrin or pyrethrin sprays/powders.
    - Provide dust baths with diatomaceous earth, sand, or natural soil.
    - Regular application of topical insecticide recommended by the veterinarian.
    - Isolate new birds and treat them with topical insecticide prior to integration.
- **Internal Parasites**
  - Common endoparasites: *Ascaridia galli, Heterakis gallinarum, Capillaria* spp., *Eimeria* spp.
  - Preventative Measures:
    - Rotate free-range areas to break parasite cycles.
    - Use fecal flotation exams for surveillance every 3–6 months. Veterinary reference laboratories have preparations for various parasites.
    - Administer dewormers when indicated and prescribed by the veterinarian.

17.9.3 Veterinary Recheck Appointments

Schedule follow-ups after the discharge appointment or as directed by the veterinarian.

Patient re-evaluation is important to:

- Confirm treatment success
- Perform repeat diagnostics (e.g., fecal test and blood work)
- Adjust medications or taper supportive care

Encourage clients to bring droppings, photos, or videos of behaviors to the recheck appointment. Digital data can also be emailed or texted to the veterinary hospital and entered into the patient's medical record.

17.10 Monitoring for Disease Spread

If the discharged bird was treated for an infectious disease, maintain isolation for at least 30 days, perform surveillance on flock mates (e.g., serologic or PCR testing), disinfect housing and equipment, and track new cases and report to the veterinarian immediately. Provide guardians with disease-specific literature and biosecurity information to be aware and vigilant.

Further Reading

Don't Be Chicken: Backyard Poultry Care and Medicine - WVMA [Internet]. WVMA. 2025 [cited 2025 Dec 8]. Available from: https://wvma.org/courses/dont-be-chicken-backyard-poultry-care-and-medicine/

Pollock C. Care of the Backyard Chicken - LafeberVet [Internet]. LafeberVet. 2021 [cited 2025 Dec 8]. Available from: https://lafeber.com/vet/care-of-the-backyard-chicken/?srsltid=AfmBOoqCeBcRqv7Zmo7JfBVDaP2bjyKqDVUCp4sdmqvk5xvnEKr1bdT8

Preventing Diseases in Pet Chickens With Client Education [Internet]. Dvm360.com. dvm360; 2018 [cited 2025 Dec 8]. Available from: https://www.dvm360.com/view/preventing-diseases-in-pet-chickens-with-client-education

Wallner-Pendleton E. Marek's Disease in Chickens [Internet]. Penn State Extension. 2023. Available from: https://extension.psu.edu/mareks-disease-in-chickens

Index

d

e